ALLE · ZEIT · WACH · 1842

H.G. Beger M. Büchler P. Malfertheiner (Eds.)

Standards in Pancreatic Surgery

With 242 Figures and 215 Tables

Springer-Verlag
Berlin Heidelberg New York
London Paris Tokyo
Hong Kong Barcelona
Budapest

Professor Dr. med. H.G. BEGER
Privatdozent Dr. med. M. BÜCHLER

Abteilung für Allgemeine Chirurgie
Universitätsklinik Ulm
Steinhövelstraße 9
W-7900 Ulm, FRG

Professor Dr. med. P. MALFERTHEINER

Abteilung Innere Medizin II
Universitätsklinik Ulm
Robert-Koch-Straße 8
W-7900 Ulm, FRG

ISBN 3-540-55360-6 Springer-Verlag Berlin Heidelberg New York
ISBN 0-387-55360-6 Springer-Verlag New York Berlin Heidelberg

Library of Congress Cataloging-in-Publication Data. Standards in pancreatic surgery / H.G. Beger, M. Büchler, P. Malfertheiner (eds.). p. cm. Includes bibliographical references and index. ISBN 3-540-55360-6 (alk. paper). — ISBN 0-387-55360-6 (alk. paper) 1. Pancreas—Surgery. 2. Pancreatitis. 3. Pancreas—Cancer. 4. Pancreas—Cysts. I. Beger, H. G. (Hans G.) II. Büchler, Markus, 1955- . III. Malfertheiner, P. (Peter), 1950- . [DNLM: 1. Pancreatic Neoplasms—surgery. 2. Pancreatic Pseudocyst—surgery. 3. Pancreatitis—surgery. WI 805 S785] RD546.S75 1993 617.5′57059—dc20 DNLM/DLC for Library of Congress 92-49286 CIP

Typesetting: Best-set Typesetter Ltd., Hong Kong
19/3130 – 5 4 3 2 1 0 – Printed on acid-free paper

Contents

List of Contributors

You will find the addresses at the beginning of the respective contribution

Surgical Anatomy of the Pancreas and Adjacent Structures

D.E. Bockman[1]

Introduction

The morphology of the pancreas and the basic relationships of the pancreas with other organs are well known to the pancreatic surgeon and others who have a particular interest in pancreatic function and pancreatic diseases. It does not seem worthwhile to restate these fundamental concepts. Rather, the approach of this presentation is to consider the ways the pancreas relates to other organs, and to concentrate on those anatomical and functional relationships that might have some relevance to the understanding and/or treatment of pancreatic disease. The goal is to give some anatomical correlates of inflammation, metastases, fibrosis, and pain, by considering selected observations that concern the pancreas proper as well as other structures.

The associations of the pancreas with other structures may be through direct contact, extension of cells and/or fluids, or through vascular (both blood and lymphatic vessels) or neural routes. Pertinent associations include those with gastrointestinal organs in the immediate vicinity, as well as with lungs, kidneys, and the brain. Because of the retroperitoneal location of the pancreas, distinct effects on adjacent muscle, connective tissue, and nerves during pancreatic disease is possible. The integral relationship of the pancreas with the liver, biliary tract, and duodenum is, of course, a key factor when considering either the etiologies or the consequences of pancreatic diseases.

Intimate Relationship with the Duodenum

The pancreas has a special relationship with the duodenum. The main and accessory pancreatic ducts empty into the duodenum. The epithelium of the ducts is continuous with that of the duodenum. The connective tissue surrounding the ducts is continuous with that of the duodenum. Furthermore, the intimate association of the pancreas with the duodenal wall

[1] Department of Cellular Biology and Anatomy, Medical College of Georgia, Augusta, GA 30912-2000 USA

Beger/Büchler/Malfertheiner (Eds.)
Standards in Pancreatic Surgery

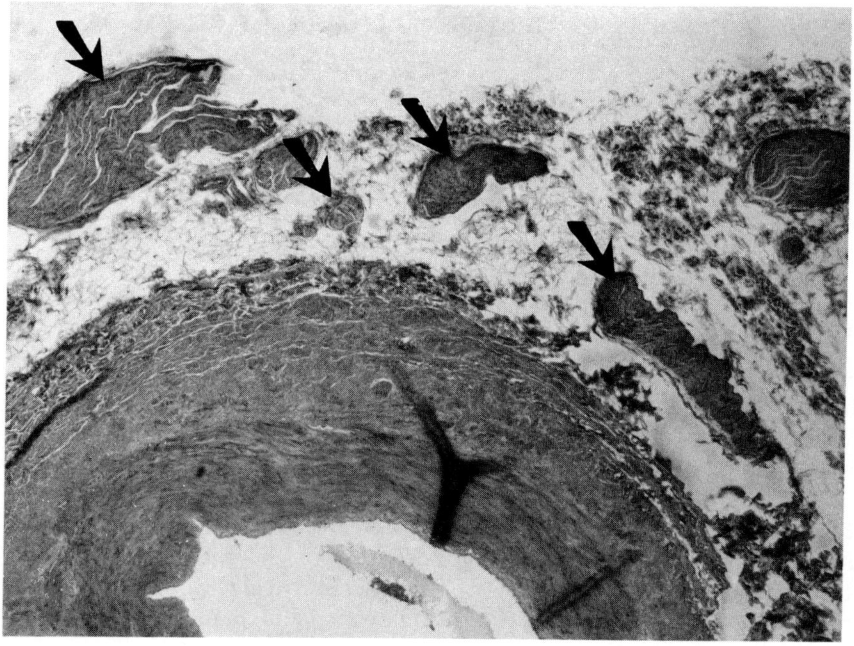

Fig. 1. Histological section of an artery supplying the human pancreas. Numerous nerve bundles (*arrows*) are present in the connective tissue immediately surrounding the artery. H&E, ×30

provides many areas where the connective tissue of one is continuous with the other [1]. Thus, a ready pathway exists, along which potentially damaging biologically active materials may be transmitted from pancreas to duodenum during inflammation.

Vessels pass freely back and forth between pancreas and duodenum. Arteries pass through the pancreas to ramify in the duodenal wall. Veins collecting blood from the duodenum pass through the pancreas as tributaries of the hepatic portal system.

Nerves transmitted through the pancreas ramify in the duodenum, making functional connections with the enteric nervous system. These include branches of the vagus nerve that have reached the duodenum without synapse, and nerve fibers of the sympathetic system that have synapsed in the celiac ganglion. Sensory fibers also are contained in the bundles of mainly unmyelinated nerves. Furthermore, axons originating from nerve cell bodies located in ganglia in the pancreas reach the duodenum, and axons from nerve cell bodies located in ganglia in the duodenum and lower stomach are transmitted to the pancreas [8]. Thus, the neural network provides for both centrally connected and locally directed responses.

Distribution of Nerves Along Arterial Walls

The nerve fibers from the pancreas that transmit impulses which are interpreted in the brain as pain travel mainly with the sympathetic nervous system. In the thoracic region, these fibers travel in the readily identifiable splanchnic nerves. Below the celiac plexus, however, the distribution of the fibers is highly irregular. Nerve fibers are distributed primarily along the arteries. Thus nerve fibers carrying pain from the pancreas may be expected along all of the arteries that make up the complex arterial system that serves the pancreas.

What may not be generally recognized is that the fibers do not simply occupy the same connective tissue intervals that are occupied by the blood vessels. Rather, the nerves are intimately associated with the arterial wall. Nerve bundles run in the connective tissue that is continuous with the adventitia of the arteries. The nerve bundles branch and recombine with each other. Smaller bundles accompany the arteries into the substance of the pancreas. Figure 1 illustrates both the quantity of nerve bundles that may be found around arteries serving the pancreas, and the close association of the bundles with the arterial wall. The knowledge of this relationship points out the likelihood of retaining nerve fibers, including pain fibers, when the arterial supply of a region is maintained and the arteries are not divided. Destroying the nerve bundles would require positive action aimed at removing the outer layers of connective tissue surrounding the artery or arteries in question.

Damage to Nerves in Pancreatitis and Pancreatic Cancer

Stimulation of the pain fibers of the pancreas may occur with increased pressure, such as that produced by edema or by distention of the ducts. Direct stimulation may take place when nerve endings are subjected to an inflammatory process. In addition, more permanent changes in nerves may be correlated with the chronic pain that usually accompanies chronic pancreatitis or pancreatic cancer.

The nerve bundles in and around the pancreas carry both motor and sensory fibers. The fibers are, for the most part, unmyelinated. The fibers are partially surrounded by Schwann cells and exist in a connective tissue environment, the endoneurium. This environment is separated from the general connective tissue of the pancreas by the perineurium, which is formed by multiple layers of epithelioid cells. Thus a specialized microenvironment is created inside the protective perineurium. The nerve fibers function normally within this microenvironment.

In chronic pancreatitis, foci of chronic inflammatory cells frequently locate around the nerve bundles. The perineurium may be damaged [4]. The perineurial cells may disappear. The basal lamina that normally separates the perineurial cells from the intervening layers of connective tissue may be damaged. It may be lost in some places. Thus, the specialized microenvironment surrounding the nerve fibers is lost. Biologically active products from the inflammatory cells, activated enzymes, and blood products may come into contact with the nerve fibers and cause them to discharge more or less continuously. The motor fibers may affect secretion, diameter of blood vessels, and sphincter function. Stimulation of the sensory fibers may cause pain.

The chronic pain associated with pancreatic cancer may share this mechanism. Pancreatic adenocarcinoma seems to have a particular affinity for nerve bundles. In a recent study, Pour et al. [12] reported that the incidence of nerve invasion reached 88% in experimentally induced pancreatic adenocarcinoma in hamsters. Drapiewski [6] reported that the pancreatic nerves had been invaded in 84% of 83 cases of carcinoma of the pancreas. Ngai et al. [11] reported nerve invasion in 75% of eight patients with pancreatic carcinoma, while Matsuda and Nimura [10] found neural invasion in all of the 14 cases of carcinoma of the head of the pancreas that they studied. Transmission of adenocarcinoma along nerves is not properly described as growth along perineural lymphatics [9], nor is it simply extension along the connective tissue space surrounding nerves. There is actual penetration of the carcinoma into the nerve bundle (Fig. 2). It is clear that this penetration breaches the barrier formed by the perineurium, destroying the specialized microenvironment inside. As was described for chronic pancreatitis, biologically active materials may enter the endoneurial space, triggering nerve impulses. In addition, direct contact of the cancer cells and their products with nerve fibers could induce nerve impulses.

It should be pointed out that the process of chronic nerve damage is not necessarily limited to the pancreas proper. With extension of inflammation into the retroperitoneum, and with extension of the adenocarcinoma, other nerves, including somatic sensory fibers, may be stimulated.

Involvement of the Lymphatic System

Pancreatic adenocarcinoma may spread by direct extension into adjacent organs and tissue, including along nerves. It may be transmitted through the blood, primarily through the hepatic portal system to the liver. It also may be transmitted through the lymphatic system.

The lymphatics of the pancreas begin as blind-ending capillaries in the connective tissue surrounding lobules. Lymphatic vessels drain first into lymph nodes that are within the substance of the pancreas or are located immediately outside the pancreas. The extrapancreatic lymphatic vessels and lymph nodes are generally distributed along the blood vessels which supply the pancreas. Lymphatics serving the pancreas are continuous with those serving the liver and biliary tract, as well as with those of the duodenum. Efferent lymphatic vessels from the primary lymph nodes

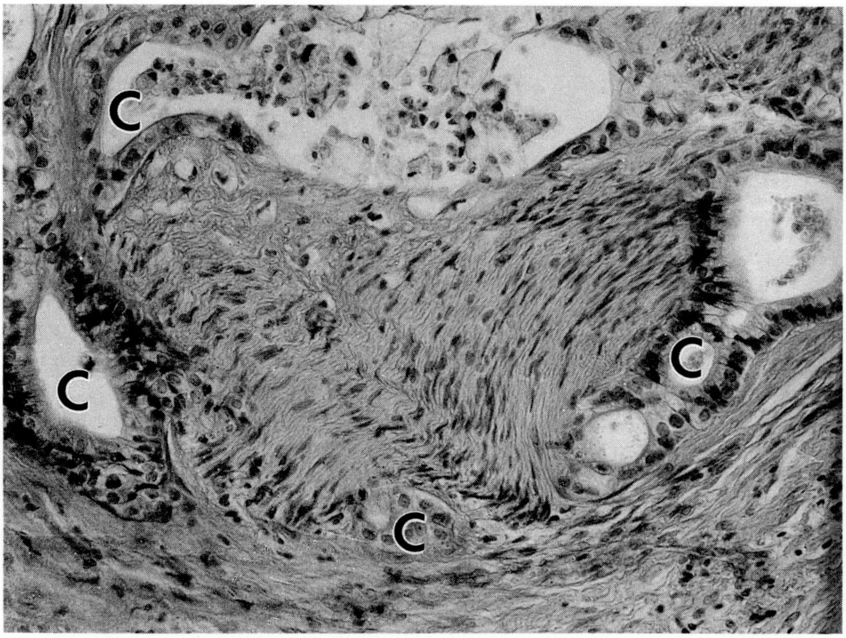

Fig. 2. Histological section of nerve in the pancreas from a patient with pancreatic adenocarcinoma. The carcinoma (*C*) has impinged upon and invaded a nerve, breaching the perineurium. H&E, ×240

accompanying such vessels as the splenic and pancreaticoduodenal drain into the regional lymph nodes. The celiac nodes and superior mesenteric nodes drain by way of their efferent vessels into the intestinal lymphatic trunk, and thence into the cisterna chyli. Subsequent drainage is by way of the thoracic duct into the great veins of the neck, through the heart, and eventually into the capillary bed of the lungs. A small portion of the lymph would be distributed so that the first capillary bed reached would be that of the heart itself.

Metastases from foci of pancreatic adenocarcinoma follow the pathway of lymphatic drainage and may be distributed while the tumor is still small. Cubilla et al. [5] conducted a study of the distribution of metastases from carcinomas of the head of the pancreas. They evaluated lymph nodes prospectively from 11 designated groups: superior head, superior body, gastric, inferior head, inferior body, anterior pancreaticoduodenal, pyloric, mesenteric, posterior pancreaticoduodenal, common bile duct, and splenic. The most common sites of matastasis were the superior head and posterior pancreaticoduodenal groups. Metastases were not found in the gastric or splenic groups. Since in 33% of the patients nodes not usually removed in the Whipple procedure were positive, Cubilla et al. suggested that the procedure was inadequate for removing adenocarcinoma of the head of the pancreas. Trapnell [14] has pointed out that the cystic node, located at the junction of the cystic duct with the common hepatic duct, frequently harbors metastases from pancreatic adenocarcinoma. He additionally indicated that small, normal-appearing lymph nodes often contain nests of tumor, while enlarged and hard nodes commonly show only reactive hyperplasia. It is interesting, with regard to tumor metastases in lymph nodes, that Pour et al. [12] reported transmission of tumor to lymph nodes via nerves when there was no evidence of transmission through the lymphatic vessels.

The lymphatics may be a route of transmission of other products of pancreatic disease. In an ultrastructural study of experimentally induced acute pancreatitis in dogs, it was demonstrated that breakdown products as large as segments of rough endoplasmic reticulum entered the pancreatic lymphatics [2]. This is a clear indication that in acute pancreatitis, many kinds of biologically active macromolecules may be carried away through the lymphatics, eventually entering the blood circulation and being carried to the lungs. It is perhaps significant in this regard that electron microscopic study of the lung after experimentally induced pancreatitis revealed granules from neutrophils free in the capillary lumen [3]. This would appear to indicate intravascular disintegration of neutrophils, a process that eventually could release potentially damaging proteolytic enzymes to affect endothelial cells.

Fibrosis in Transgenic Mice Overexpressing TGFα

There are changes in the pancreas proper that commonly are associated with pancreatic disease. Among these are fibrosis and the formation of tubular complexes. The mechanisms by which these are controlled have remained unknown. A recently constructed animal model promises to provide some understanding of these two processes. Transgenic mice have been produced [7, 13] which carry the human gene for transforming growth factor alpha (TGFα) along with a metallothionine promoter that makes it possible to induce increased expression of the gene by administering zinc. As these mice grow, with or without zinc in their drinking water, the pancreas becomes enlarged and hardened. Histological examination reveals that marked, progressive fibrosis, both intralobular and interlobular, is the cause of the alteration in consistency. Pancreatic acinar cells produce TGFα, and it has been suggested that receptors on fibroblasts are stimulated by TGFα to proliferate and to secrete collagen. It may be possible to determine whether the fibrosis that accompanies chronic pancreatitis and pancreatic carcinoma and, transiently, acute pancreatitis may be stimulated by this growth hormone or a similar one.

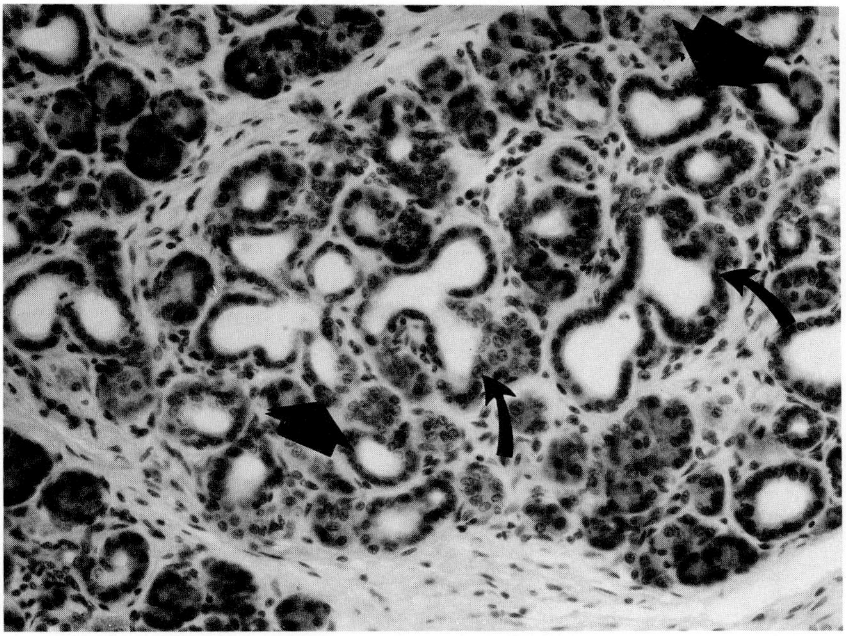

Fig. 3. Histological section of pancreas from a transgenic mouse overproducing transforming growth factor α. There is fibrosis within the lobule and around it. Tubular complexes with large lumina are evident. The larger tubules are composed mainly of duct-like cells. Some tubules are composed of acinar cells. In places, acinar cells may be seen forming part of a tubule (*arrows*). In other places, acini are being incorporated into an expanding tubular complex (*curved arrows*). H&E, ×240

Redifferentiation of Pancreatic Epithelial Cells

With pancreatic disease, the equilibrium normally maintained in the pancreas is disrupted. Whereas acinar cells normally are maintained in their fully differentiated state, they may be caused to redifferentiate into cells which have characteristics of other cells, such as ductal cells. This situation may be seen in pancreatitis, pancreatic adenocarcinoma, and cystic fibrosis, and with benign obstruction of the ductal system. The situation is evident in the TGFα transgenic mice as well. Histological examination of the pancreas in these mice (Fig. 3) reveals areas of tubular complexes that are composed mainly of cells with the morphology of ductular cells, but also of acinar cells. It is clear that the acinar cells are redifferentiating, presumably in response to the overproduction of TGFα, to a cell type that does not produce zymogens. In many areas further redifferentiation is evident, in that the tubular complexes are composed in part of cells that contain mucin (Fig. 4). Mucin-containing cells normally are confined to the larger ducts, and

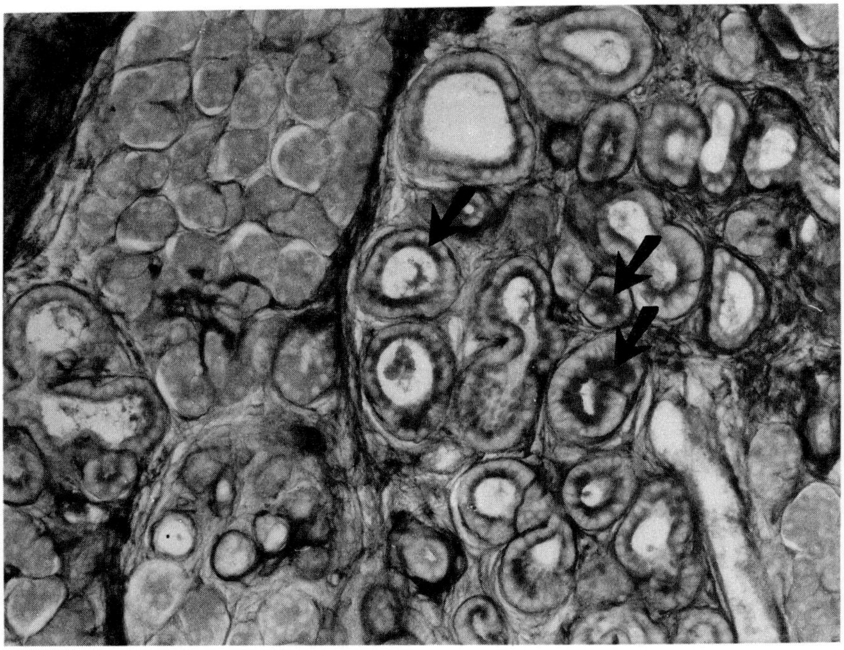

Fig. 4. Histological section of pancreas from a transgenic mouse overproducing transforming growth factor α. There are many areas in the tubular complexes where cells show PAS positivity (*arrows*), indicating the presence of mucins. The mucins are concentrated in the apical portions of cells. ×240

do not occur within pancreatic lobules. It is exciting to consider that the mechanisms controlling differentiation and maintenance of pancreatic parenchyma, a condition disrupted by pancreatic disease, may be revealed to suggest how the disruptions are caused.

Acknowledgements. The author would like to thank Dr. M. Büchler, Dr. H. Friess, and Prof. H. Beger for access to human tissue, Dr. G. Merlino for access to transgenic mice, and Mr. G. Oblak for technical assistance.

References

1. Bockman DE (1988) Systems underlying involvement of the duodenum in pancreatic disease. Pancreas 3:592
2. Bockman DE, Schiller WR, Suriyapa C, Mutchler JHW, Anderson MC (1973) Fine structure of early experimental acute pancreatitis in dogs. Lab Invest 28:584–592
3. Bockman DE, Schiller WR, Suriyapa C, Mutchler JHW, Anderson MC (1974) Intravascular degranulation of neutrophils in dog lungs secondary to experimental acute pancreatitis. In: Arceneaux CJ (ed) 32nd annual proceedings

of the Electron Microscopy Society of America. Claitor's, Baton Rouge, pp 22–23
4. Bockman DE, Büchler M, Malfertheiner P, Beger HG (1988) Analysis of nerves in chronic pancreatitis. Gastroenterology 94:1459–1469
5. Cubilla AL, Fortner J, Fitzgerald PJ (1978) Lymph node involvement in carcinoma of the head of the pancreas area. Cancer 41:880–887
6. Drapiewski JF (1944) Carcinoma of the pancreas: a study of neoplastic invasion of nerves and its possible clinical significance. Am J Clin Pathol 14:549–556
7. Jhappan C, Stahle C, Harkins RN, Fausto N, Smith GH, Merlino GT (1990) TGFα overexpression in transgenic mice induces liver neoplasia and abnormal development of the mammary gland and pancreas. Cell 61:1137–1146
8. Kirchgessner AL, Gershon MD (1990) Innervation of the pancreas by neurons in the gut. J Neurosci 10:1626–1642
9. Larson DL, Rodin AE, Roberts DK, Osteen WK, Rapperport AS, Lewis SR (1966) Perineural lymphatics: myth or fact. Am J Surg 112:488–492
10. Matsuda M, Nimura Y (1983) Perineural invasion of pancreas head carcinoma. J Jpn Surg Soc 84:719–728
11. Nagai H, Kuroda A, Morioka Y (1986) Lymphatic and local spread of T1 and T2 pancreatic cancer. Ann Surg 204:65–71
12. Pour PM, Egami H, Takiyama Y (1991) Patterns of growth and metastases of induced pancreatic cancer in relation to the prognosis and its clinical implications. Gastroenterology 100:529–536
13. Sandgren EP, Luetteke NC, Palmiter RD, Brinster RL, Lee DC (1990) Overexpression of TGFα in transgenic mice: induction of epithelial hyperplasia, pancreatic metaplasia, and carcinoma of the breast. Cell 61:1121–1135
14. Trapnell JE (1990) Staging of cancer of the pancreas. Int J Pancreatol 7:109–116

I. Acute Pancreatitis

Etiology and Pathogenesis of Acute Pancreatitis

M.L. STEER[1] and A.K. SALUJA[1]

Etiology of Acute Pancreatitis

Knowledge of the cellular events which lead to acute pancreatitis is severely limited and, as a result, concepts regarding the etiology of the disease are limited to epidemiologic data which identify disease states or conditions associated with acute pancreatitis [42].

Most patients with acute pancreatitis develop their disease in association with either alcohol abuse or biliary tract stone disease. Together, these two conditions account for 75%–80% of individuals in most series of patients with acute pancreatitis. The relative contribution of alcohol abuse and biliary tract stone disease in those series appears to depend upon the type of patient population being studied, i.e., alcohol abuse predominates when inner city urban groups are evaluated while biliary tract stone disease predominates when suburban groups are studied.

Alcohol Abuse

Most patients who develop an acute attack of pancreatitis as a result of alcohol abuse do so only after they have consumed large quantities of alcohol for many years [40]. It is likely that many, if not most, of these individuals have suffered silent alcohol-induced injury to the pancreas prior to their attack and that, had the gland been evaluated prior to the attack, evidence of chronic pancreatitis including fibrosis might have been detected. Thus, these individuals might more correctly have been diagnosed as having an acute attack of *chronic* pancreatitis. There remain, however, a substantial number of patients with alcohol-induced pancreatitis who develop acute symptoms after little or no prior abuse of alcohol. In such cases, the gland was most likely normal prior to the attack and the patient does, indeed, have acute pancreatitis. The mechanisms by which alcohol precipitates acute pancreatic injury in this setting are unknown.

[1] Beth Israel Hospital, Department of Surgery, 330 Brookline Avenue, Boston, MA 02215, USA

Beger/Büchler/Malfertheiner (Eds.)
Standards in Pancreatic Surgery

Biliary Tract Stones

The recent studies of Acosta and Ledesma [1, 2] as well as others [20] have indicated that patients with gallstone-induced acute pancreatitis develop their disease when a stone migrates into or through the distal biliary-pancreatic ductal system. The mechanisms by which such a stone might precipitate acute pancreatitis have been the subject of numerous studies over the past century. In a general sense, three theories have been proposed to explain the association between stone passage and acute pancreatitis.

The first or so-called "common channel" theory was proposed by Opie in 1901 [31] when he noted a patient who, at autopsy after death from acute pancreatitis, was found to have a stone impacted in the distal common bile duct at the ampulla. Opie suggested that such a stone might create, behind it, a common channel which would permit bile to reflux from the biliary duct into the pancreatic duct and he hypothesized that bile refluxing through this common channel might injure the gland and precipitate pancreatitis. Over the past 90 years, a substantial amount of evidence has accumulated which would suggest that the common channel theory is an unlikely explanation for clinical acute pancreatitis. Among the evidence against that theory is the observation that pancreatic secretory pressure usually exceeds biliary secretory pressure and, in the event that a distal obstruction were to create a common channel, pancreatic juice reflux into the biliary tree would be favored over bile reflux into the pancreatic duct [28]. Other arguments against the common channel theory include the observation that many patients develop gallstone pancreatitis without having a sufficiently long common channel to permit bile reflux [26] and the fact that bile, by itself, does not injure the pancreas when it is perfused, under normal pressure, through the pancreatic ductal system [34].

A second theory to explain the association between stone passage and acute pancreatitis is the so-called "duodenal reflux" theory [27]. According to this hypothesis, the stone passing through the sphincter of Oddi stretches that sphincter and renders it incompetent. Subsequent to stone passage, duodenal juice containing activated pancreatic enzymes can reflux through the incompetent sphincter into the pancreatic ductal system. Perhaps the strongest argument against this theory is the observation that surgical or endoscopic division of the sphincter does not invariably lead to acute pancreatitis although it would be expected to permit duodenal juice to freely reflux into the pancreatic ductal system. Furthermore, surgical procedures which allow intestinal contents to enter the pancreatic ductal system (e.g., pancreaticojejunostomy) also do not precipitate pancreatitis.

The third and final theory which has been proposed to explain the association between stone passage and acute pancreatitis is one which suggests that the offending stone or edema and inflammation resulting from stone passage cause pancreatic ductal obstruction and that, with continued secretion into the closed pancreatic ductal system, pancreatic ductal hypertension occurs. Early proponents of this theory suggested that the increased pressure within the pancreatic duct could lead to duct rupture and extravasation of pancreatic juice into the gland parenchyma. While this may be an important early event in the development of acute pancreatitis, it fails to provide a complete explanation for the basis of the disease since pancreatic juice in the pancreatic duct contains, for the most part, inactive proenzymes or zymogens. Thus, extravasation of inactive enzymes such as trypsinogen, chymotrypsinogen, and procarboxypeptidase into the gland parenchyma may not, by itself, be sufficient to cause injury to the gland. Rather, some other event must be superimposed upon these processes prior to gland injury in order to account for digestive enzyme activation. Recently, a number of studies have been reported which have attempted to explain events which might lead to intrapancreatic digestive enzyme activation during the early stages of acute pancreatitis. This issue is dealt with below.

Tumors

Acute pancreatitis may also be precipitated by tumors which obstruct pancreatic juice flow [6]. Thus, tumors originating in the duodenum, papilla, or pancreatic duct itself can precipitate acute pancreatitis. The severity of this form of pancreatitis is extremely variable. For the most part, only silent pancreatic inflammation is induced and the finding of acute pancreatitis is not made until the gland is examined microscopically. Occasionally, however, the patient may present with signs and symptoms of acute pancreatitis and the tumor may not be detected until subsequent studies are completed. Tumor induced pancreatitis should be suspected when a nonalcoholic patient presents without evidence of biliary tract stone disease.

Drugs

Administration of a number of drugs has been noted to be associated with the development of acute pancreatitis [14, 25, 45]. These drugs include the following: azathioprine, furosemide, methyldopa, nitrofurantoin, pentamidine, sulfonamides, procainamide, tetracycline, valproic acid, *l*-asparaginase, ethacrynic acid, isoniazide, thiazide diurectics, dideoxyinosine, estrogens, and 6-mercaptopurine.

For the most part, evidence implicating these drugs in the development of pancreatitis is rather meager and consists of the observation that a certain number of patients given that drug develop pancreatitis. In some cases, pancreatitis has been precipitated on a second occasion after rechallenge of the patient with the drug and, under those conditions, the evidence implicating the drug as the cause of pancreatitis would seem to be relatively strong. On the other hand, the mere observation that the incidence of pancreatitis is increased among the population of patients given a certain drug would seem to be relatively weak evidence incriminating that drug as a cause of pancreatitis. Examples of this latter situation include the observation that the incidence of acute pancreatitis is increased in patients receiving azathioprine for treatment of inflammatory bowel disease or dideoxyinosine [22] for treatment of the acquired immunodeficiency syndrome. It is certainly possible that it is the associated disease (e.g., inflammatory bowel disease, acquired immunodeficiency syndrome) which is the actual cause of the pancreatitis rather than the drug itself. Finally, there are a number of drugs which have been traditionally included in lists of agents capable of inducing pancreatitis but for which, in retrospect, there is little or no convincing evidence to support that association. This would appear to be the situation in the case of steroids which have been frequently referred to as a cause of acute pancreatitis but which, on close examination, have little or no evidence strongly incriminating them as a cause of the disease [44].

Infection

A number of infections have been associated with the development of acute pancreatitis. Those include mumps and coxsackie virus infection as well as infections with agents such as mycoplasma [11, 18]. In addition, certain parasitic infestations, such as *Ascaris lumbricoides* and *Clonorchis sinensis*, have also been associated with the development of pancreatitis [6]. The cellular basis for acute pancreatitis occurring in association with viral or mycoplasma infection is not known. Cases of pancreatitis occurring in association with parasitic infestation probably can be explained by obstruction of the pancreatic duct by the offending parasite.

Lipid Abnormalities

Acute pancreatitis has been noted to occur in patients with several types of lipid abnormalities. The most common of those lipid abnormalities is the hypertriglyceridemia which occurs with acute alcohol ingestion [5]. Some patients with acute pancreatitis may present with lactescent serum and the association of abdominal pain, lactescent serum, and a history of alcohol abuse has been considered to be pathognomonic of acute pancreatitis. Patients with types I, IV, and V familial hyperlipoproteinemia experience frequent attacks of abdominal pain associated with an elevated amylase level [10]. Such patients suffer repeated attacks of acute pancreatitis and correction of the hyperlipoproteinemia by dietary manipulation can sometimes reduce or eliminate the incidence of these attacks. The mechanism by which these various lipid abnormalities lead to pancreatitis is uncertain. It has been suggested that release of lipid breakdown products such as fatty acids into the microcirculation in or around the pancreas might result in pancreatic injury [15]. Convincing evidence for this conclusion, however, has not been presented.

Trauma

Acute pancreatitis has been noted after direct pancreatic trauma [16]. Acute traumatic pancreatitis usually is a transient phenomenon and may reflect a pancreatic contusion more than a real inflammatory process in the pancreas. On the other hand, some patients with blunt trauma to the pancreas suffer pancreatic ductal disruption which eventually leads to scarring and stricture formation. Those individuals may present months or years later with recurrent attacks of chronic pancreatitis. For the most part, the ductal injury occurs when the pancreas is pressed backwards against the spine and the area of chronic pancreatitis involves, primarily, the distal body and tail of the pancreas. Postoperative pancreatitis is, for the most part, a form of traumatic pancreatitis. Postoperative pancreatitis usually involves procedures in or around the area of the head of the pancreas. It has been presumed that, in most instances, interference with drainage of the ampulla is the basis for the pancreatitis which results [47]. On the other hand, postoperative pancreatitis has also been noted after procedures performed quite distant from the pancreas including groin hernia repairs and neck operations. The mechanism by which such procedures might lead to pancreatitis is certainly unknown.

Miscellaneous

A number of miscellaneous causes of acute pancreatitis have been identified. Acute pancreatitis in Trinidad is most commonly caused by the sting of a scorpion [4]. Acute pancreatitis has also been noted after translumbar aortography [18], after cardiac or renal transplantation [3, 19], and after cardiopulmonary bypass [33]. Some patients with afferent loop obstruction following Billroth II gastrectomy and gastrojejunostomy develop recurrent episodes of acute pancreatitis. They can be effectively treated by procedures which improve drainage from the afferent loop. Acute pancreatitis has also been noted in association with a number of autoimmune diseases including lupus [7]. The mechanisms by which these various miscellaneous causes of acute pancreatitis might trigger pancreatic injury is not clear.

Idiopathic

Idiopathic pancreatitis is felt to be present when acute pancreatitis is diagnosed but none of the above etiologies can be identified. The incidence of idiopathic pancreatitis among any group of patients being studied is, therefore, directly related to the vigor with which one of these underlying causes of acute pancreatitis is sought. In a general sense, the overall contribution of idiopathic pancreatitis to the total population of patients being studied is usually in the range of 10%–15%.

Pathogenesis of Acute Pancreatitis

Over the past decade, along with our colleagues, we have carried out a number of studies which have been aimed at elucidating the cellular events which might underlie the development of acute pancreatitis. In a general sense, these studies have attempted to provide an explanation for the association of stone passage through the distal biliopancreatic ductal system and the development of acute pancreatitis. As such, these studies are probably relevant only to the disease known as gallstone-induced pancreatitis. We have assumed that the offending stone causes pancreatic ductal obstruction and that, with continued secretion into the closed ductal space, pancreatic ductal hypertension occurs. Our studies have attempted to elucidate the mechanism by which pancreatic ductal hypertension might trigger pancreatic injury. Since pancreatic ductal contents include primarily inactive digestive enzymes such as trypsinogen, and chymotrypsinogen, our studies have been aimed at providing an explanation for the mechanism by which ductal obstruction could lead to intrapancreatic digestive enzyme activation.

We have employed a number of experimental models of acute pancreatitis. Features which might be common to each of the models studied have been sought with the expectation that such common features might also be of importance in the clinical disease. Four separate models of pancreatitis have been evaluated. The first is a form of acute hemorrhagic pancreatic necrosis which can be induced by administration of a choline deficient diet which is supplemented with eithionine [24]. When fed continuously and ad libitum to young female mice, all of the animals die by the fifth day of diet administration. We have modified that protocol by reducing the amount and duration of diet administration such that a mortality rate of approximately 50%–60% can be achieved [12]. Using this revised protocol, gross evidence of pancreatic injury does not occur prior to the third day of diet administration. As a result, studies performed during the 1st and 2nd days of diet administration directed at elucidating alterations in normal pancreatic cellular function can be performed and these studies can be completed prior to the appearance of evidence of cellular injury. The second model which we have evaluated is a form of acute edematous interstitial pancreatitis which occurs when rats are infused with a supramaximally stimulating dose of the secretagogue caerulein [23]. When given at a dose of $5\,\mu g\,kg^{-1}\,h^{-1}$, hyperamylasemia and pancreatic edema occur within 1 h, and these changes reach a maximum within 3–4 h of supramaximal stimulation. The third model which we have evaluated involves transient obstruction of the rabbit or rat pancreatic duct [38]. This manipulation causes mild pancreatic edema and hyperamylasemia but little or no evidence of acute pancreatic cellular injury. When maintained for a prolonged periods, pancreatic exocrine atrophy results. The final model which we have evaluated involves ligation of the opossum biliary-pancreatic duct at its point of entry into the duodenum. This procedure results in acute hemorrhagic pancreatitis which is usually lethal within 7 days of duct obstruction [41].

These models of pancreatitis have certain features in common. For example, in each there is a marked rise in the serum amylase level and the pancreatic wet to dry weight ratio increases indicating the presence of pancreatic edema. On the other hand, there are marked differences in the severity of the pancreatitis as well as the eventual outcome of these various models. For example, the diet model of pancreatitis is characterized by acute hemorrhagic pancreatic necrosis of the gland and death of the animal within 5 days if the ethionine-supplemented diet is administered continuously. Ligation of the opossum pancreatic duct results in acute hemorrhagic pancreatitis which is lethal within 7 days of duct ligation. In contrast, administration of a supramaximally stimulating dose of the secretagogue caerulein results in transient pancreatic edema and hyperamylasemia which begins to resolve within 12 h of supramaximal stimulation and which has completely resolved within several days. Finally, ligation of the rabbit pancreatic duct results in exocrine pancreatic atrophy with little or on evidence of acute pancreatic inflammation.

The pancreatic acinar cell is the most active protein synthesizing cell in the body. More that 90% of newly synthesized protein is destined for export out of the acinar cell as this protein is comprised of digestive enzyme zymogens. The acinar cell also synthesizes a number of other proteins some of which are destined for transport to specific locations within the cell itself. We were particularly interested in characterizing the process of lysosomal enzyme trafficking in the acinar cell because previous work by others had suggested that the lysosomal enzyme cathepsin B was capable of activating trypsinogen [9, 13]. Since trypsin can activate the remaining zymogens, activation of trypsinogen within the acinar cell by cathepsin B might be one mechanism by which premature digestive enzyme activation could occur during the early stages of pancreatitis.

We have found that in each of the models described above, protein synthesis remains normal but newly synthesized protein is not secreted from the acinar cell of the pancreas [12, 36, 38] (Fig. 1). The mechanisms by which digestive enzyme secretion is perturbed during the various models of pancreatitis appear to differ. For example, in the ethionine diet model, coupling between receptor and phospholipase C in the acinar cell membrane appears to be perturbed and, as a result, normal stimulus-secretion coupling cannot occur [32]. In the supramaximal stimulation model of pancreatitis, the secretagogue appears to interact with low-affinity cholecystokinin receptors that mediate the inhibition of digestive enzyme secretion [39].

We have studied the process of lysosomal enzyme trafficking within acinar cells during three of the models of pancreatitis. Those are the diet model, the secretagogue model, and the rabbit pancreatic duct-obstruction model. In each of those models, we have noted that the lysosomal enzyme cathepsin B is redistributed between the lysosome-enriched subcellular fraction and the zymogen granule-enriched subcellular fraction [30, 37, 38] (Fig. 2). In morphological studies using the techniques of immunolocalization at the light and electron microscope level, we have found that lysosomal

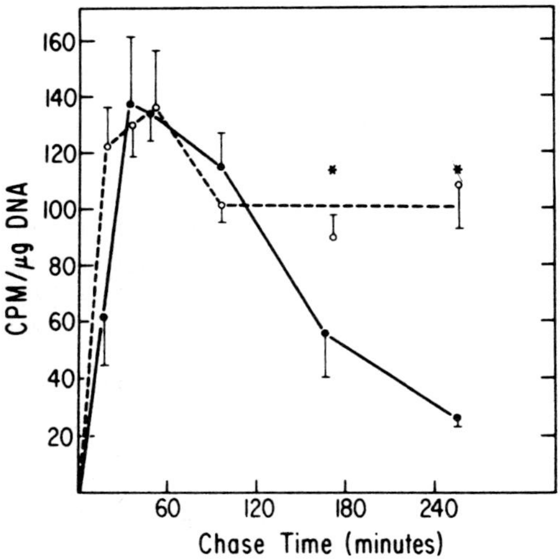

Fig. 1. Amino acid uptake, protein synthesis, and secretion during secretagogue-induced pancreatitis. Protein synthesis and discharge. Rats were preinfused with saline alone (●---●) or saline containing sufficient caerulein to deliver 5 μg kg^{-1} h^{-1} (○---○) for 1 h, given a pulse of [^{3}H]phenylalanine followed by a bolus of nonradioactive phenylalanine, and continued on infusion for varying times. At selected intervals, rats (n = 7) in each group were killed and trichloroacetic acid-precipitable radioactivity measured in pancreas homogenate. *Asterisks*, values in caerulein-infused animals that are significantly different from those found for saline-infused rats. (Reproduced from Saluja et al. [37] with permission of the publisher)

enzymes become colocalized along with digestive enzymes within large vacuoles in each of those three models of pancreatitis [21, 35, 38, 46] (Fig. 3). The mechanisms by which lysosomal enzymes become redistributed and colocalized with digestive enzymes during the early phases of these experimental forms of acute pancreatitis appear to differ. In some, lysosomes and zymogen granules appear to fuse by a process known as crinophagy [8]. In others, the normal events by which lysosomal enzymes are segregated from digestive zymogens as they traverse the trans Golgi network appear to be perturbed [46]. In any case, the net result is the colocalization of lysosomal enzymes with digestive zymogens. Others have noted that the structures containing these colocalized enzymes have an acidic pH [29]. We have suggested that this phenomenon, i.e., colocalization of digestive and lysosomal enzymes in acidic organelles, could lead to intra-acinar cell digestive enzyme activation. In other studies, we have noted that the lysosomal enzyme-containing structures become increasingly fragile during these models of pancreatitis and we have suggested that rupture of these organelles containing activated digestive enzymes could release those enzymes into the cell interior and, in this way, result in cell injury [43].

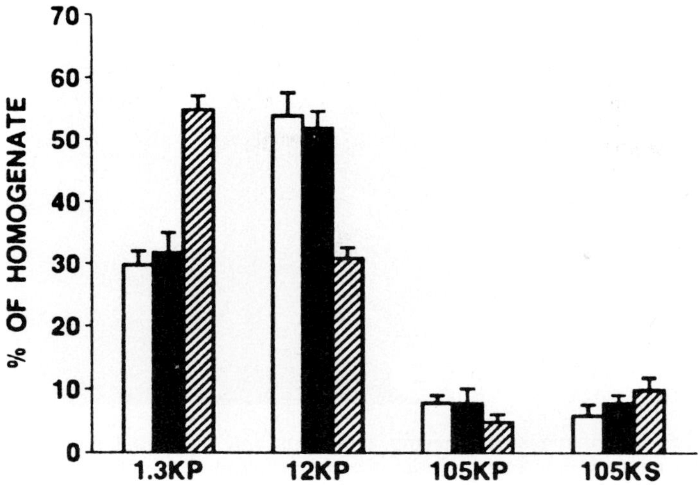

Fig. 2. Subcellular redistribution of cathepsin B during secretagogue-induced pancreatitis. Rats were infused with saline (*open bars*) or saline containing caerulein at a concentration designed to deliver either $0.25\,\mu g\,kg^{-1}\,h^{-1}$ (*solid bars*) or $5.0\,\mu g\,kg^{-1}\,h^{-1}$ (*hatched bars*) for 3.5 h prior to death, and pancreas was subcellularly fractioned. Cathepsin B activity, measured in each fraction, is expressed as percent of total found in postnuclear homogenate. *1.3 KP*, 1300 *g*/15-min pellet (primarily zymogen granules); *12 KP*, 12 000 *g*/12-min pellet (primarily lysosomes and mitochondria); *105 KP*, 105 000 *g*/60-min pellet (primarily microsomes); *105 KS*, 105 000 *g*/60-min supernatant (soluble fraction). Results represent mean values; *vertical bars*, SE obtained from four or more separate fractionations, each performed using samples from different animals. (Reproduced from Saluja et al. [36] with permission of the publisher)

There remain a number of important but as yet unanswered questions. These include the issue of where and how activated digestive enzymes might cause acinar cell injury. While it is known that activation of trypsinogen by cathepsin B can occur when that pH is in the range of 3.5–4.5, trypsin itself is not active at that pH. Thus, activation of trypsinogen by cathepsin B is, at best, an incomplete explanation for the mechanism by which acute pancreatitis is triggered. Some further insight into the events which enable active trypsin to activate the remaining zymogens and the mechanisms by which those enzymes are capable of injuring acinar cells must be defined. Another important but as of yet undefined issue is the question of what determines the ultimate severity of acute pancreatitis. The process of digestive enzyme and lysosomal enzyme colocalization appears to be common for each of the models we have studied yet the eventual outcome of these models varies considerably. Clearly, other events must be superimposed on the colocalization phenomenon and those events must be critical in determining the ultimate severity of the disease.

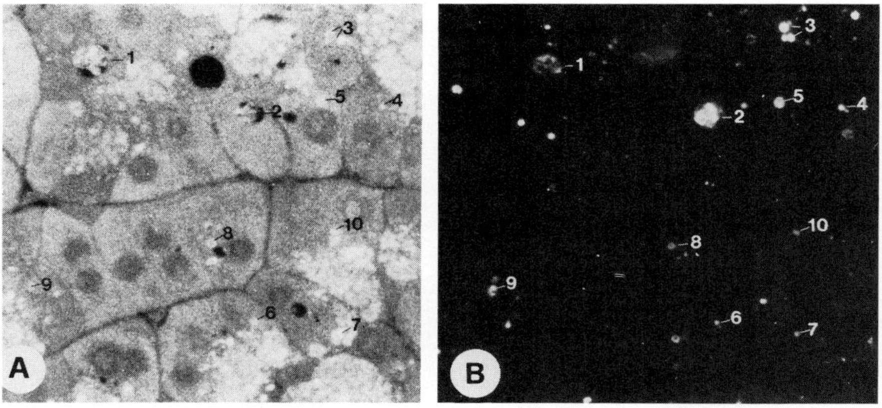

Fig. 3A,B. Colocalization of digestive enzyme zymogens and lysosomal hydrolase during secretagogue-induced pancreatitis. Indirect immunofluorescence of pancreatic acinar cells of rats infused with caerulein for 1 h. The two panels illustrate immunolabeling obtained with antizymogen (**A**) and anticathepsin D (**B**) sera in corresponding fields from two semithin (1-μm) sections cut next to each other from same block. Antizymogen immunolabeling appears diffuse in the whole cytoplasm with heavy reaction of zymogen granules (localized at cell apex) and, especially, on large, heterogeneous vacuoles localized preferentially in Golgi area. Anticathepsin labeling is restricted to vacuoles with latter localization. *Numbers* (*1–10*) point to vacuoles in two adjacent sections that were labeled by both sera used (×880). (Reproduced from Watanabe et al. [46] with permission of the publisher)

References

1. Acosta JL, Ledesma CL (1974) Gallstone migration as a cause for acute pancreatitis. N Engl J Med 290:484
2. Acosta JL, Ross R, Ledesma CL (1977) The usefulness of stool screening for diagnosing cholelithiasis in acute pancreatitis: a description of the technique. Am J Dig Dis 22:168
3. Adiseshia M (1983) Acute pancreatitis after cardiac transplantation. World J Surg 7:519
4. Bartholomew C (1970) Acute scorpion pancreatitis in Trinidad. Br Med J 1:666
5. Cameron JL, Capuzzi DM, Zuidema GD, Margolis S (1974) Acute pancreatitis with hyperlipemia. Evidence for a persistent defect in lipid metabolism. Am J Med 56:482–487
6. Durr GH (1979) Acute pancreatitis. In: Howatt HT, Sarles H (eds) The exocrine pancreas. Saunders, London, pp 352–401
7. Eaker EY, Toskes PP (1989) Systemic lupus erythematosus presenting initially with acute pancreatitis and a review of the literature. Am J Med Sci 197(1): 38–41
8. Farquhar MG (1977) Secretion and crinophagy in prolactin cells. In: Dellmann HD et al. (eds) Comparative endocrinology of prolactin. Plenum, New York, pp 37–94
9. Figarella C, Miszczuk-Jamska B, Barrett AJ (1988) Possible lysosomal activation of pancreatic zymogens. Activation of both human trypsinogens by cathepsin B and spontaneous acid activation of human trypsinogen 1. Biol Chem Hoppe Seyler 369:293–298

10. Fredrickson DS, Lees RS (1966) Familial hyperlipoproteinemia. In: Stanbury JB et al. (eds) The metabolic basis of inherited disease, 2nd edn. McGraw-Hill, New York, pp 429–485
11. Freeman R, McMahon MJ (1978) Acute pancreatitis and serological evidence of infection with *Mycoplasma pneumoniae*. Gut 19:367–370
12. Gilliland L, Steer ML (1980) Effects of ethionine on digestive enzyme synthesis and discharge by mouse pancreas. Am J Physiol 239 (Gastrointest Liver Physiol 2):G418–G426
13. Greenbaum LA, Hirshkowitz A (1961) Endogenous cathepsin activates trypsinogen in extracts of dog pancreas. Proc Soc Exp Biol Med 107:74–76
14. Greenberger NJ, Toskes P, Isselbacher KJ (1988) Diseases of the pancreas. In: Braunwald E et al. (eds) Harrison's principles of internal medicine. McGraw-Hill, New York, p 1372
15. Havel RJ (1969) Pathogenesis, differentiation and management of hypertriglyceridemia. Adv Intern Med 15:117–154
16. Heyse-Moore GH (1976) Blunt pancreatic and pancreaticoduodenal trauma. Br J Surg 63:226–238
17. Imrie CW, Ferguson JC, Sommerville RG (1977) Coxsackie and mumps virus infection in a prospective study of acute pancreatitis. Gut 18:53–56
18. Imrie CW, Goldring J, Pollock JG, Watt JK (1977) Acute pancreatitis after translumbar aortography. Br Med J 2:681
19. Johnson WC, Nasbeth DC (1969)Pancreatitis in renal transplantation. Ann Surg 171:309
20. Kelly TR (1976) Gallstone pancreatitis: pathophysiology. Surgery 80:488–492
21. Koike H, Steer ML, Meldolesi J (1982) Pancreatic effects of ethionine: blockade of exocytosis, crinophagy and autophagocytosis precede cellular necrosis. Am J Physiol 242:G297–G307
22. Lambert JS, Seidlin M, Reichman RC, Plank CS, Laverty M, Morse GD, Knupp C, McLaren C, Pettinelli C. Valentine FT (1990) 2′, 3′-Dideoxyinosine (ddI) in patients with the acquired immunodeficiency syndrome or AIDS-related complex. A phase I trial. N Engl J Med 322(19):1333–1340
23. Lampel M, Kern H (1977) Acute interstitial pancreatitis in the rat induced by excessive doses of a pancreatic secretagogue. Virchows Arch Pathol Anat Histol 373:97–117
24. Lombardi B, Rao NK (1975) Acute hemorrhagic pancreatic necrosis in mice. Influence of the age and sex of the animals and of dietary ethionine, choline, methionine and adenine sulfate. Am J Pathol 81:87–100
25. Mallory A, Kern F (1980) Drug-induced pancreatitis: a critical review. Gastroenterology 78:813
26. Mann FC, Giordano AS (1923) The bile factor in pancreatitis. Arch Surg 6:1
27. McCutcheon AD, Race D (1962) Experimental pancreatitis: a possible eitology of post-operative pancreatitis. Ann Surg 155:523–531
28. Menguy RB, Hallenbeck GA, Bollman JL, Grindlay JH (1958) Intraductal pressures and sphincteric resistance in canine pancreatic and biliary ducts after various stimuli. Surg Gynecol Obstet 106:306
29. Niederau C, Grendell JH (1988) Intracellular vacuoles in experimental acute pancreatitis in rats and mice are an acidified compartment. J Clin Invest 81(1):229–236
30. Ohshio G, Saluja A, Leli U, Sengupta A, Steer ML (1989) Esterase inhibitors prevent lysosomal enzyme redistribution in two non-invasive models of experimental pancreatitis. Gastroenterology 96:853–859
31. Opie EL (1901) The relationship of cholelithiasis to disease of the pancreas and fat necrosis. Am J Med Surg 12:27
32. Powers RE, Saluja AK, Houlihan MJ, Steer ML (1986) Diminished agonist-stimulated inositol trisphosphate generation blocks stimulus-secretion coupling in mouse pancreatic acini during diet-induced experimental pancreatitis. J Clin Invest 77:1668–1674

33. Rattner DW, Gu Zy, Vlahakes GJ, Warshaw AL (1989) Hyperamylasemia after cardiac surgery. Incidence, significance, and management. Ann Surg 209(3): 279–283
34. Robinson TM, Dunphy JE (1963) Continuous perfusion of bile protease activators through the pancreas. JAMA 183:530
35. Saito I, Hashimoto S, Saluja A, Steer ML, Meldolesi J (1987) Intracellular transport of pancreatic zymogens during caerulein supramaximal stimulation. Am J Physiol 251:G517–526
36. Saluja A, Saito I, Saluja M, Houlihan MJ, Powers RE, Meldolesi J, Steer M (1985) In vivo rat pancreatic acinar cell function during supramaximal stimulation with caerulein. Am J Physiol 249:G702–G710
37. Saluja AK, Hashimoto S, Saluja M, Powers RE, Meldolesi J, Steer ML (1987) Subcellular redistribution of lysosomal enzymes during caerulein-induced pancreatitis. Am J Physiol 251:G508–516
38. Saluja A, Saluja M, Villa A, Leli U, Rutledge P, Meldolesi J, Steer ML (1989a) Pancreatic duct obstruction in rabbits causes digestive zymogen and lysosomal enzyme colocalization. J Clin Invest 84:1260–1266
39. Saluja A, Saluja M, Printz H, Zavertnik A, Sengupta A, Steer ML (1989b) Experimental pancreatitis is mediated by low affinity CCK receptors which inhibit digestive enzyme secretion. Proc Natl Acad Sci USA 86:8969–8971
40. Sarles H (1986) Chronic pancreatitis: etiology and pathophysiology. In: Go VLW et al. (eds) The exocrine pancreas: biology, pathophysiology, and diseases. Raven, New York, p 37
41. Senninger N, Moody FG, Coelho JC, Van Buren DH (1986) The role of biliary obstruction in the pathogenesis of acute pancreatitis in the opossum. Surgery 99(6):688–693
42. Steer ML (1986) Etiology and pathophysiology of acute pancreatitis. In: Go VLW et al. (eds) The exocrine pancreas: biology, pathophysiology, and diseases. Raven, New York, p 465
43. Steer ML, Meldolesi J, Figarella C (1984) Pancreatitis: the role of lysosomes. Dig Dis Sci 29:934–938
44. Steinberg WM, Lewis JH (1981) Steroid-induced pancreatitis: does it really exist? Gastroenterology 81:799–808
45. Thomas FB (1982) Drug-induced pancreatitis: facts vs. fiction. Drug Ther Hosp 7(3):60
46. Watanabe O, Baccino FM, Steer ML, Meldolesi J (1984) Effects of supramaximal caerulein stimulation of the ultrastructure of rat pancreatic acinar cell: early morphological changes during the development of experimental pancreatitis. Am J Physiol 246:G457–467
47. White TT, Morgan A, Hopton D (1970) Postoperative pancreatitis: a study of seventy cases. Am J Surg 120:132

Epidemiology of Acute Pancreatitis

F. Carballo,[1] J.E. Dominguez-Muñoz,* C. Martinez-Pancorbo, and J. de la Morena

Introduction

Only few cases of acute pancreatitis are diagnosed by histology; therefore, the majority of patients are included in studies according to clinical, biological, and morphological criteria. Since there are no universal standard diagnostic criteria for acute pancreatitis, identical inclusion criteria are not used by different authors. This is a serious problem for epidemiological analysis and especially for the comparison of different studies.

Clinically, acute pancreatitis can be defined as a picture characterized by acute abdominal pain and increased pancreatic enzymes in blood and/or urine [1]. An international multicenter study published in 1979 indicates that 2.3% of acute abdominal pain is due to acute pancreatitis [2], and in our local experience this reaches 4.4% [3]. The number of undiagnosed cases of painful acute pancreatitis is proportionally inverse to the degree of clinical suspicion for disease, and this number also varies greatly among areas. More difficult is the approach to painless acute pancreatitis. Wilson and Imrie [4] report that about 42% of acute pancreatitis is diagnosed at necropsy without a previous clinical diagnosis. For only 13% of these misdiagnosed episodes was abdominal pain reported in the case record. In clinical practice, only typical painful acute pancreatitis is generally included in the epidemiological descriptive series.

In accordance with the clinical definition of disease, when a patient is evaluated in the emergency ward under clinical suspicion of acute pancreatitis, the first diagnostic step is the quantification of circulating pancreatic enzymes, usually total serum amylase activity. The definition of an optimal cut-off level is of great importance for the correct classification of disease. In our experience, as Fig. 1 shows, this cut-off is 250 U/l, approximately twice the upper normal limit for control population. Applying this cut-off, we obtain a sensitivity of 91% for total amylasemia with a specificity of 95% [5]. We obtain similar results with the determination of serum pancreatic

[1] Servicio de Medicina Interna, Hospital Universitario General, Universidad de Alcalá de Henares, c/Donante de Sangre s/n, 19002 – Guadalajara (Spain)
* Dr. Dominguez-Muñoz is actually the recipient of a grant from the Alexander von Humboldt Fundation in Ulm (Germany)

Beger/Büchler/Malfertheiner (Eds.)
Standards in Pancreatic Surgery

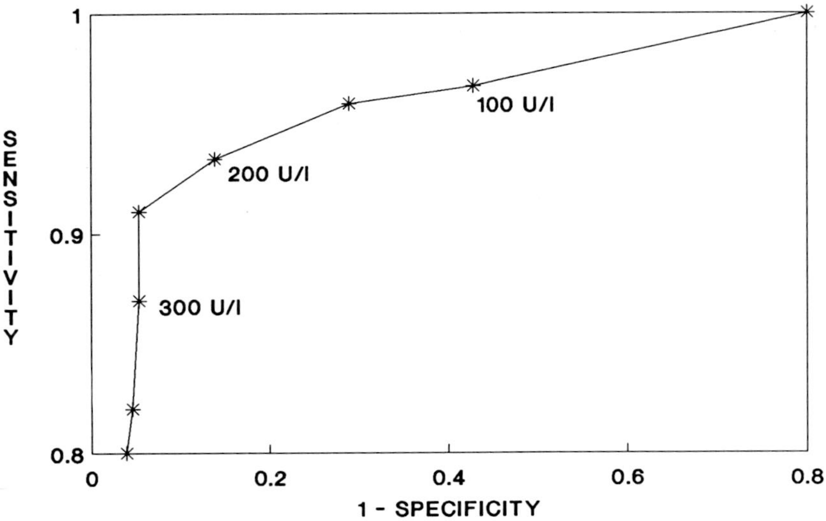

Fig. 1. Serum amylase ROC (receiver operator characteristics) curve in the diagnosis of acute pancreatitis

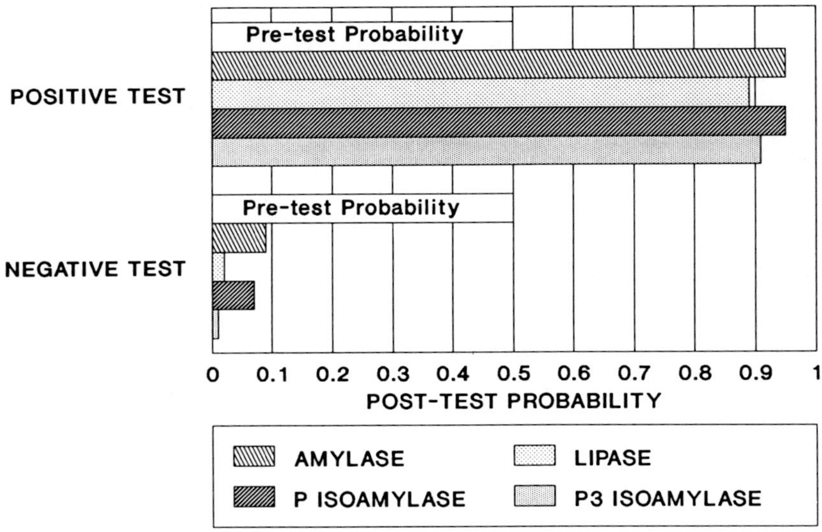

Fig. 2. Post-test probability of acute pancreatitis, starting with 50% pre-test probability of disease, using as tests the serum activities of amylase, lipase, and p-isoamylase, and applying the optimal cut-off levels

Table 1. Incidence of acute pancreatitis (cases/10^6 inhabitants and year) reported by various authors (modified from [7])

Author	Year/Period	Country	Study	Incidence
Thomson	1972–1979	UK	R	104
McMahon	1977	UK	R	110
Raga	1977–1987	Spain	R	163
Thomson	1981–1982	UK	P	195
CPSG	1978–1979	Denmark	P	281
Grilo	1983–1986	Spain	P	383

R, retrospective study; P, prospective study.

isoamylase also applying its optimal cut-off, with a sensitivity of 92% and identical specificity [6]. It is not correct to use the same values of diagnostic efficacy in different areas or different studies because the predictive value of tests changes with the prevalence of the disease. Therefore, each researcher should obtain his or her own values with the help of prospective studies. In spite of this problem, post-test probabilities of acute pancreatitis, starting from a pre-test probability of 50%, are similar, independent of the test applied: high for positive results and low for negative ones. At least, this is what occurs in our experience for an optimal cut-off level, as Fig. 2 shows. The raising of this cut-off leads to an infradiagnosis of the disease, and its decrease yields to an overdiagnosis.

Therefore, for a correct inclusion of patients into epidemiological studies it is necessary to keep in mind some standards: a good disease classification, inclusion of the whole clinical spectrum of the disease, knowledge of the prevalence of disease in the frame of the study, and a clinically correct sampling. Otherwise, the penalty for the infractor will be confusion. To summarize what has been said thus far, in acute pancreatitis the usual problems observed in the literature are: different inclusion criteria, variable suspicion for disease, different local prevalence, and infra- and overdiagnosis of disease.

Variability in Incidence and Proportion of Etiological Factors

It is difficult to determine the true worldwide incidence of acute pancreatitis. In addition to the problems mentioned above, there is an important difference in the reported incidences of acute pancreatitis between retrospective and prospective series [7], as shown in Table 1. Logically, the incidence is higher in prospective studies. Furthermore, the calculated incidence will be higher in prospective studies in which every episode of acute pancreatitis is correctly diagnosed, including very mild and rapidly self-limiting episodes.

Our local incidence rate is very high, around 460 cases per year and million inhabitants, and has apparently stablized in the past few years [8]. It

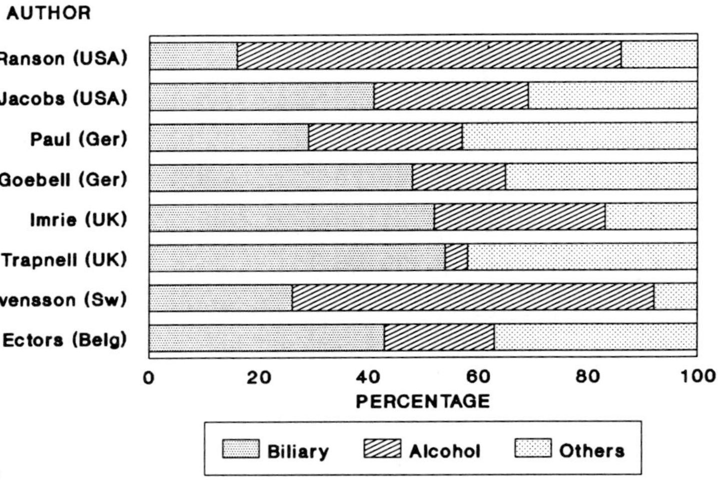

a

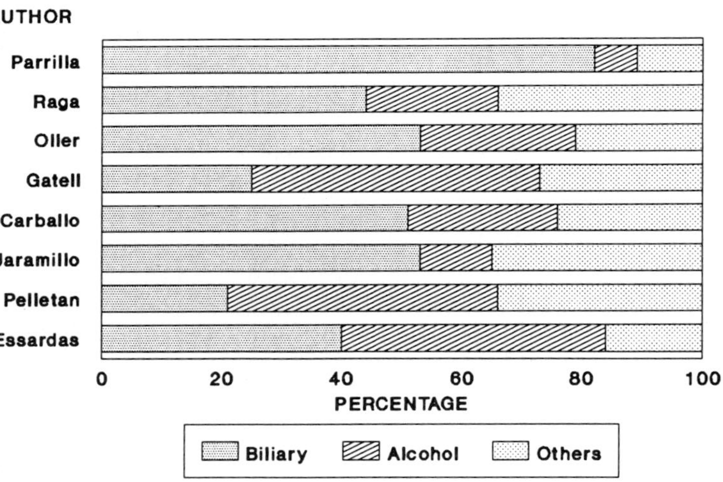

b

Fig. 3a,b. Variability in the proportion of etiological factors in acute pancreatitis: **a** Spanish reports, **b** worldwide series (modified from [7,9,10])

is important to note that this incidence was calculated taking into account only patients with a first episode of acute pancreatitis. This measure tends to correct the overdiagnosis secondary to the inclusion of recurrent attacks.

Another point of disagreement is the high variability in the proportion of different etiological factors in the reported series [7, 9, 10], as much among local – e.g., in Spain (Fig. 3a) – as among worldwide series (Fig. 3b). Probably, these studies are biased due to the various factors already mentioned.

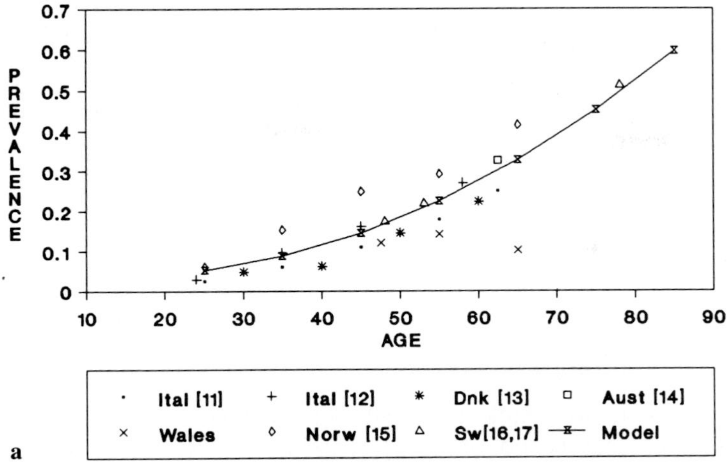

a

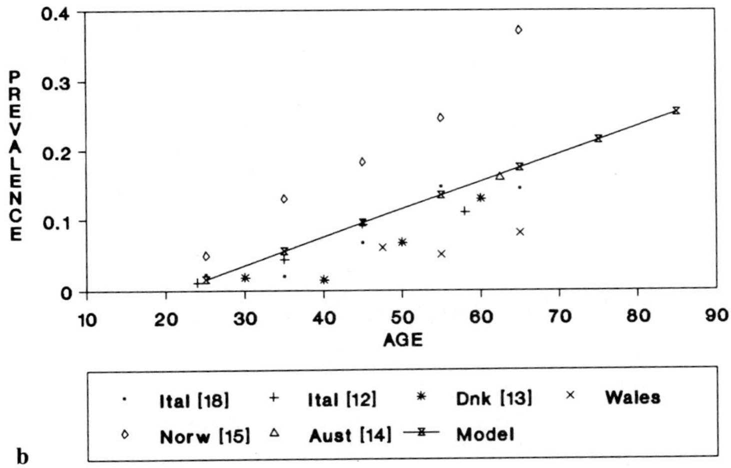

b

Fig. 4a,b. Prevalence of cholelithiasis in Europe according to published data [11–18] and two regression models: **a** polinomic regression model in women, **b** linear regression model in men (Wales data from [13])

This variability in the proportion of etiological factors is not easily understood, at least with respect to biliary lithiasis, if we observe the reported data on the prevalence of cholelithiasis. These data are clearly consistent among European series [11–18]. It is possible to obtain, by means of regression methods, a very good estimation of the average prevalence of cholelithiasis in Europe according to sex and age. The real data communicated in every country are the points defining the model. For women, as shown in Fig. 4a, the adjustment is almost perfect by means of a second-grade polynomic regression model, and we also obtain a very good adjustment by means of a simple linear regression model. For men (Fig. 4b) the best adjustment is obtained by means of simple linear regression. Using this simple linear model for both sexes, we have obtained good estimations for each interval, and the overall prevalence of cholelithiasis derived from this model is 12.2%. We have applied this design in constructing a stratified randomized sampling of the general population in a study performed in Guadalajara, the aim of which was to determine the local prevalence of cholelithiasis.

Standards in Epidemiological Studies

For the reasons given, we think that the performance of more local epidemiological studies based only on the description of series of cases is a useless exercise. The standard for new epidemiological studies designed to evaluate incidence should be: to perform prospective series, with a multicenter approach, useful for comparing incidence rates, always following the rules of identical inclusion criteria and consideration of the whole spectrum of the disease. To study etiological features, the standard should be: performing research in causality, obtaining measures of the intensity and direction of association by means of odds ratio or relative risk. With a multicenter approach the measures of association can be compared between different areas.

Estimation of the Risk to Develop Acute Pancreatitis

Since acute pancreatitis is a disease with low prevalence, in which the causal factors have a long induction time, and only a small percentage of those exposed develop the disease, cohort studies are very difficult and expensive to carry out. A case-control study is better and easier to perform.

In Guadalajara we carried out two retrospective case-control studies to estimate the association between cholelithiasis and acute pancreatitis. In the first one, our control group included patients undergoing abdominal sonography. In the second study, the controls were patients with acute abdominal pain.

In the first study estimating the risk of developing acute pancreatitis in the presence of cholelithiasis, all cases involved patients with acute pancreatitis diagnosed in our hospital during 1989 (n = 84); controls were a numerically identical randomized sample of all patients explored by sonography in the same year and hospital, excluding only acute pancreatitis. We performed crude and stratified analysis and nonconditional logistic regression analysis. The result of this study was an odds ratio adjusted by sex and age – which here play the role of confounders – of 6.0. A better

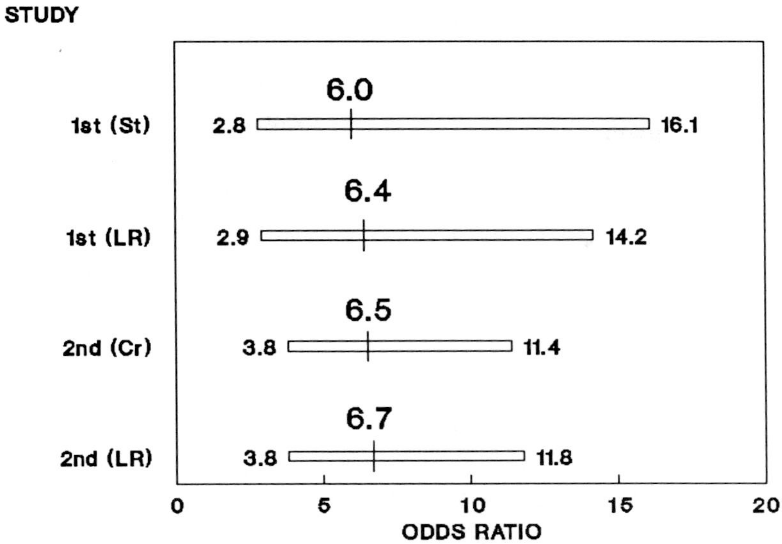

Fig. 5. Estimation of the risk to develop acute pancreatitis (odds ratio with its confidence interval at 95%) obtained by means of crude (*Cr*), stratified (*St*) or logistic regression (*LR*) analysis in two different studies carried out in Guadalajara (Spain). In the first study controls are patients undergoing sonography explorations; in the second controls are patients with acute abdominal pain

estimation was obtained by logistic regression, reaching an odds ratio of 6.4, with a confidence interval between 2.9 and 14.2.

In the second study, considering patients with acute abdominal pain as controls, it was possible to estimate also the risk of acute pancreatitis according to alcohol intake. Cases were patients with acute pancreatitis diagnosed over a period of 22 months (n = 133), and controls were 152 patients with acute abdominal pain not secondary to acute pancreatitis but in whom this diagnosis was suspected. An analysis similar to that in the first study was carried out. In this design, with respect to cholelithiasis as a risk factor, sex and age were not confounders and the crude odds ratio was 6.5. The measure of the risk of developing acute pancreatitis in the presence of cholelithiasis obtained by logistic regression in the best model, which includes alcohol intake and age, is 6.7, ranging between 3.8 and 11.8.

In Fig. 5 the results for cholelithiasis of both studies are summarized. It is remarkable that measures in both studies are almost identical, in spite of two different designs, in two different populations and over different time periods. The best final estimation of the risk to develop acute pancreatitis in presence of cholelithiasis is 6.7.

Concerning alcohol intake, it was possible to plot the logistic curve of the risk of acute pancreatitis according to the amount of alcohol consumption expressed as grams per day. As shown in Fig. 6, a risk for

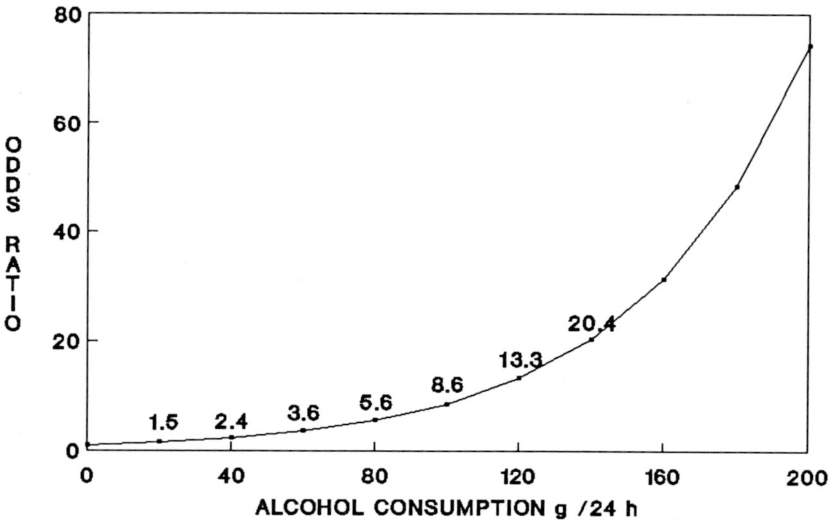

Fig. 6. Estimated risk (odds ratio) curve for acute pancreatitis in relation to daily alcohol consumption (logistic regression analysis controlled by sex and cholelithiasis)

developing acute pancreatitis similar to that in the presence of cholelithiasis is obtained with an intake of approximately 90 g of alcohol per day. Higher consumption yields a progressively higher risk.

References

1. Gyr KE, Singer MV, Sarles H (eds) Revised classification of pancreatitis – Marseille 1984: proceedings of the second international symposium on the classification of pancreatitis. Excerpta Med Int Congr Ser 624:xxiii
2. Dombal FT (1979) Acute abdominal pain. An OMGE survey. Scand J Gastroenterol 14:29–43
3. Carbonell MA, Carballo F, Martin A, Alonso MJ, Domínguez E, Fernández L, Beato I, de la Morena J (1989) Dolor abdominal agudo: características de los pacientes atendidos en un área de urgencia hospitalaria. Ann Med Interne 6:25
4. Wilson C, Imrie CW (1988) Deaths from acute pancreatitis. Why do we miss the diagnosis so frequently? Int J Pancreatol 3:273–282
5. Carballo F, Domínguez E, García A, García J, de la Morena J (1988) Diagnosis of acute pancreatitis: comparative study of enzymatic test. Gastroenterol Int 1:670
6. Carballo F, Domínguez E, de la Morena J (1990) Utilidad de las pruebas biológicas en el diagnóstico y pronóstico de la pancreatitis aguda. In: Diaz-Rubio M (ed) Avances en gastroenterología, vol 7. Aran, Madrid, pp 289–302
7. Aparisi L, Raga F (1990) Epidemiología de la pancreatitis aguda. Gastroenterol Hepatol 14:161–171
8. Carballo F (1990) ACAD multicentre hospital study of early prognostic evaluation in acute pancreatitis; case reports and epidemiological features. ACAD J 6:98–100

9. Cavallini G, Riela A, Brocco G, Bertelli G, Falconi M, Micciolo R, Pederzoli P, Scuro LA (1987) Epidemiology of acute pancreatitis. In: Beger HG, Büchler M (eds) Acute pancreatitis. Springer, Berlin Heidelberg New York, pp 25–31
10. Creutzfeldt W, Lankisch PG (1985) Acute pancreatitis: etiology and pathogenesis. In: Berk JE (ed) Bockus gastroenterology, 4th edn. Saunders, Philadelphia, pp 3971–3992
11. Rome group for the epidemiolopgy and prevention of cholelithiasis (GREPCO) (1984) Prevalence of gallstone disease in an Italian adult female population. Am J Epidemiol 119:796–805
12. Barbara L, Sama C, Morselli AM, Taroni F, Rusticalli AG, Festi D, Sapio C, Roda E, Banterle C, Puci A, Formentini F, Colasanti S, Nardin F (1987) A population study on the prevalence of gallstone disease: the Sirmione study. Hepatology 7:913–917
13. Jørgensen T (1987) Prevalence of gallstones in Danish population. Am J Epidemiol 126:912–921
14. Rhomberg HP, Judmair G, Lochs A (1984) How common are gallstones? Br Med J 289:1002
15. Glambek I, Kvaale G, Arnesjö B, Søreide O (1987) Prevalence of gallstones in a Norwegian population. Scand J Gastroenterol 22:1089–1094
16. Janzon L, Aspelin P, Eriksson S, Hildell J, Trell E, Östberg H (1985) Ultrasonographic screening for gallstone disease in middle-aged women. Scand J Gastroenterol 20:706–710
17. Mellströn D, Asztély M, Svanvik J (1988) Gallstones and previous cholecystectomy in 77- to 78-year-old women in an urban population in Sweden. Scand J Gastroenterol 23:1241–1244
18. The Rome group for the epidemiolopgy and prevention of cholelithiasis (GREPCO) (1988) The epidemiology of gallstone disease in Rome, Italy. I. Prevalence data in men. Hepatology 8:904–906

A Clinicopathological Classification of Acute Pancreatitis

W. Uhl, M. Büchler, and H.G. Beger[1]

Background

Inflammatory diseases of the pancreas can lead to a large variety of various different clinical pictures. In the past, many definitions have been used because of the lack of agreement for these clinical manifestations. Great progress was made in pancreatic research after the first international pancreatitis conference in Marseille, France, in 1963 with the etablishment of a worldwide accepted classification of pancreatic diseases [1]. In the following years, as knowledge increased, it became necessary to reclassify pancreatic diseases [2] because it was evident that in specific cases there were some problems with the old classification. For example, it was not possible to distinguish acute relapsing pancreatitis from an acute exacerbation of chronic pancreatitis or chronic relapsing pancreatitis on the basis of clinical or laboratory findings. This has made these categories difficult to use in clinical practice.

Up to now, two international workshops have been held, one in Marseille and one in Cambridge, UK, both in 1984, with the aim of bringing the classification and definitions of pancreatic inflammatory diseases up to date [3, 4]. In Cambridge, the definitions were entirely clinical, whereas in Marseille they were expanded to include descriptive histopathology. Mainly there was a reduction und simplification of chronic pancreatitis, and both conferences dropped the intermediately used terms of acute and chronic relapsing pancreatitis. Progress has, however, meanwhile been so dramatic that these new classification systems can only represent a minimum consensus level. For example, pancreatic abscess was not listed as a complication of acute pancreatitis by the second Marseille symposium on acute pancreatitis, while the Cambridge workshop failed to define the evolution from necrosis through infected necrosis to liquification and abscess formation.

In the last 10 years, considerable progress has been made in our understanding and knowledge of the natural history of acute pancreatitis based on findings from endoscopic retrograde cholangiopancreatography (ERCP),

[1] Department of General Surgery, University of Ulm, Steinhövelstr. 9, W-7900 Ulm, FRG

Beger/Büchler/Malfertheiner (Eds.)
Standards in Pancreatic Surgery

Table 1. Clinical and morphological terms used in the literature for necrotizing pancreatitis

Clinical	Morphological
Severe pancreatitis	Pancreatic necrosis
Fatal pancreatitis	Peripancreatic necrosis
Necrotizing pancreatitis	Fluid collection
Hemorrhagic pancreatitis	Phlegmon
Fulminant pancreatitis	Acute pseudocyst
	Infected pancreatic necrosis
	Pancreatic abscess
	Infected pseudocyst

contrast-enhanced computed tomography (CT) scanning, and fine needle aspiration and Gram staining of the aspirate. Today, none of the existing classification systems makes a stratification possible in clinical decision-making in patients with acute pancreatitis.

Pathophysiology and Clinical Course of Acute Pancreatitis

Acute pancreatitis can be classified histologically as interstitial–edematous or necrotizing inflammation of the pancreatic gland, and the clinical course in patients with acute pancreatitis varies from that of a mild, transitory illness to that of a rapidly fatal disease [5, 6]. Clinical and experimental observations have shown that in the early stage of severe acute pancreatitis biologically active compounds are released into ascitic fluids and circulation [7, 8]. Patients who die within the first weeks of necrotizing pancreatitis are those who suffer cardiovascular, pulmonary, and renal complications which determine the clinical course. Because of the improvements in intensive care measures, and particularly with early venous-pressure-adjusted fluid replacement, hardly any patients with acute pancreatitis die within this early phase of the disease. Septic complications prevail in the later stage of necrotizing pancreatitis, and, nowadays, local and systemic septic complications are the most frequent cause of death in severe acute pancreatitis [9–11].

Terminology of Acute Pancreatitis: Confusion

As shown in Table 1, various clinical and morphological terms in acute necrotizing pancreatitis have been used up to now in the literature, especially in infection of the necrotizing form of acute pancreatitis. Terms like "phlegmon" and "infected pancreatic necrosis" compound the confusion for clinicians and pancreatologists. Although the pathological–anatomical definition of a phlegmon is a purulent inflammation due to bacterial infection, the term is used to describe a solid mass of indurated

Table 2. Clinicopathological classification of acute pancreatitis

– Acute interstitial–edematous pancreatitis
– Necrotizing pancreatitis
Sterile
Infected
– Pancreatic abscess
– Postacute pseudocyst

pancreas and adjacent retroperitoneal tissue caused by edema, infiltration by inflammatory cells, and perhaps tissue necroses, which could be either sterile or infected [12, 13]. With regard to treatment modalities, infected necrosis reguires a different form of management than a pancreatic abscess or an infected pseudocyst. Furthermore, the development of a pseudocyst in the course of an acute attack of necrotizing pancreatitis is not a severe complication as was sometimes supposed in the most recent clinical studies [14, 15], if it is not infected, of course.

> "An ideal classification system should be simple, unequivocal, and must contain as much information as is needed to imply treatment and prognosis" [16].

Precise definitions of the most important conditions of acute pancreatitis are mandatory in order to be able to assess prognosis early and to treat the patients appropriately. In order to clarify this terminological variety and to improve the comparability of results of clinical studies, we would like to propose the following classification system on the basis of clinical and morphological criteria (Table 2).

Clinicopathological Classification of Acute Pancreatitis

On the basis of the clinicopathological classification we classified all 1099 patients hospitalized in the last 9 years at our hospital into 812 patients (74%) with acute interstitial-edematous and 201 patients (18%) with necrotizing pancreatitis (Table 3). Twenty-six patients (2.4%) and 60 patients (5.5%) were grouped into pancreatic abscess and postacute pseudocyst, respectively. The pancreatic necroses were sterile in 66% of cases and bacterially contaminated in 34%.

Acute Intersititial–Edematous Pancreatitis

Acute interstitial–edematous pancreatitis is morphologically characterized by a sterile periacinar and interstitial edema, an interstitial accumulation of inflammatory cells, and sometimes a fluid collection (previously referred to as "phlegmon", a term that should not be used); fatty tissue necroses may

Table 3. Classification of 1099 patients with acute pancreatitis ($n = 1099$)[a]

	No. of patients	Frequency (%)	Mortality (%)
Acute interstitial–edematous pancreatitis	812	74	0.5
Necrotizing pancreatitis	201	18	12.4
sterile	132	66	9.9
infected	69	34	17.3
Pancreatic abscess	26	2.4	19.2
Pancreatic pseudocyst	60	5.5	3.3

[a] All patients were hospitalized between May 1982 and May 1991 at the Departments of Surgery and Gastroenterology, University of Ulm, FRG.

Table 4. Morbidity and outcome in 812 patients with acute interstitial–edematous pancreatitis[a]

Morbidity (%)	
Pulmonary insufficiency[b]	10
Renal insufficiency[c]	4
Sepsis[d]	2
Metabolic disorders[e]	16
Shock[f]	2
Mean Ranson score (range)	1.2 (0–5)
Mean hospital stay in days (range)	18 (6–52)
Mortality (%)	0.5 (4/812)

[a] All patients were hospitalized between May 1982 and May 1991 at the Departments of Surgery and Gastroenterology, University of Ulm, FRG.
[b] pO_2 <60 mmHg.
[c] Serum creatinine >240 μmol/l.
[d] Leukocytes >12 g/l or <4 g/l; platelets <100 g/l; rectal temperature >38.5°C; positive blood culture; metabolic acidosis, base excess >−4 mmol/l.
[e] Hyperglycemia, blood glucose >8.4 mmol/l; hypocalcemia, calcium <2.0 mmol/l; coagulation disorders, prothrombin time <70% or partial thromboplastin time >45 s.
[f] Pulse rate >100 bpm; systolic blood pressure <80 mmHg for more than 10 min.

also be present if the inflammatory process involves the peripancreatic tissue. Clinically it is a mild and self-limiting disease with low morbidity and mortality below 1% [5, 6].

The morbidity and outcome in 812 patients suffering from interstitial–edematous pancreatitis are summarized in Table 4. The most frequent complications are pulmonary insufficiency and metabolic disorders such as hyperglycemia and hypocalcemia, in 10% and 16%, respectively. The mean Ranson score was 1.2 prognostic signs (range 0–5 points). The overall hospital stay was in mean 18 days (range 6–52 days), the mortality rate was 0.5% (4/812).

Acute Necrotizing Pancreatitis

Acute necrotizing pancreatitis regularly shows an interstitial edema with pancreatic parenchymal and peripancreatic fatty tissue necrosis. On contrast-enhanced CT scanning, there is evidence of local or diffuse areas of nonenhancement. In various studies it could be shown that these nonperfused areas correspond very well to the intraoperative necrotizing process [17–20]. Clinically, necrotizing pancreatitis ranges from a moderate to severe disease in which morbidity is still high and mortality is about 10%–25% [8, 10].

A subgroup of the patients develop signs of acute pancreatitis plus sepsis in the sense of bacterial contamination of the necroses. The condition of the infected necrosis can easily be identified using ultrasound or CT-guided fine needle aspiration [21, 22].

In prospective clinical studies, a bacterial contamination rate of about 40%–60% of patients treated surgically were found [9, 23–25].

Pancreatic Abscess

A pancreatic abscess is a collection of classically purulent material encapsulated by an inflammatory wall resulting from liquification of necrotic areas that have become secondarily infected. It must be stressed that pancreatic abscess and infected necrosis are two different local septic complications in acute pancreatitis [26, 27]. Clinically, pancreatic abscess shows signs of sepsis and is a late complication without the typical signs of acute pancreatitis that occurs in the third to sixth week after the onset of acute pancreatitis.

Table 5 summarizes the data from patients with infected pancreatic necrosis and pancreatic abscess. Although both entities show the clinical signs of sepsis (43% and 44%, respectively), there are considerable differences in laboratory parameters, particularly in preoperative morbidity. From these observations it could be concluded that patients with infected necrosis have a more severe type of the disease, which includes the risk of necrotizing pancreatitis plus sepsis. Among patients with infected necrosis, 75% exhibited increased serum enzyme levels and 52% metabolic disorders, the corresponding rates in patients with pancreatic abscess were 12% and 15%, respectively. Pulmonary and renal insufficiency and shock were observed in 74%, 45%, and 29%, respectively, of patients with infected necrosis, but only in 34%, 16% and 6% of patients with pancreatic abscess. The mean Ranson scores were 4.3 in infected necrosis and 2.5 in pancreatic

Table 5. Morbidity and outcome in patients with infected necrosis (n = 69) and pancreatic abscess (n = 26)[a]

	Infected necrosis	Abscess
Morbidity (%)[b]		
Pulmonary insufficiency	74	34
Renal insufficiency	45	16
Sepsis	43	44
Metabolic disorders	52	15
Shock	29	6
Enzyme elevation[c]	75	12
Ranson score	4.3	2.5
Mortality (%)	17.3	19.2
Time interval (days)[d]	14.2	35

[a] All patients hospitalized between May 1982 and May 1991 at the Departments of Surgery and Gastroenterology at the University of Ulm, FRG.
[b] For definitions of morbidity, see Table 4.
[c] Twofold specific pancreatic enzyme elevation.
[d] Time interval from onset of acute abdominal pain to surgical intervention.

abscess. In these patient populations the mortality rates were 17% in infected pancreatic necrosis and 19% in pancreatic abscess. The time interval between onset of acute pancreatitis and surgical intervention was a median of 2 weeks for infected and 5 weeks for pancreatic abscess.

Postacute Pseudocyst

Pancreatic postacute pseudocyst is characterized by pancreatic fluid collection in a cavity surrounded by a fibrous pseudoencapsulation around necrotic tissue. This fluid collection invariably exhibits a communication with the major duct system. Like pancreatic abscess, this entity is a late complication of acute pancreatitis that occurs 4–6 weeks after the initial symptoms. Patients with a postacute pseudocyst often develop upper abdominal pain and mostly moderate serum pancreatic enzyme elevations can seen in the laboratory examinations [28].

The data from 60 patients suffering from postacute pseudocyst are given in Table 6. The mortality rate was low (3.3%; 2/60). Almost all patients with this entity develop upper abdominal pain, and in 68% there was a secondary or persisting increase in pancreatic enzymes. The mean Ranson score was 1.5 points (range 1–3).

Differential Therapeutical Interventions

Using this clinicopathological classification, the following differential therapeutic interventions could be given (Table 7).

Table 6. Morbidity and outcome in 60 patients with postacute pseudocyst[a]

Morbidity (%)[b]	
Pulmonary insufficiency	10
Renal insufficiency	0
Sepsis	0
Metabolic disorders	18
Shock	0
Enzyme elevation[c]	68
Mean Ranson score (range)	1.5 (1–3)
Mean hospital stay in days (range)[d]	27 (16–76)
Mortality (%)	3.3 (2/60)

[a] All patients hospitalized between May 1982 and May 1991 at the Departments of Surgery and Gastroenterology, University of Ulm, FRG.
[b] For definitions of morbidity, see Table 4.
[c] Twofold specific pancreatic enzyme elevation.
[d] Hospital stay after conservative and surgical treatment.

Table 7. Therapeutic interventions based on the clinicopathologic classification

Condition	Intervention
Acute interstitial–edematous pancreatitis	Self-limiting disease
Necrotizing pancreatitis	
Sterile	Conservative treatment; surgery if nonresponsive to intensive care measures
Infected	Surgery
Pancreatic abscess	Percutaneous drainage; surgery
Pancreatic pseudocyst	Percutaneous drainage; surgery

Acute interstitial–edematous pancreatitis is a mild and self-limiting disease, which improves quickly and persistently on a zero-calorie diet, with electrolyte and albumin substitution, and with venous-pressure-adjusted correction of hypovolemia. Patients with necrotizing pancreatitis should be divided into two groups according to whether they have sterile or infected necrosis. Patients with proven necrotizing pancreatitis should be treated in the intensive care unit. Intensive care therapy comprises specific treatment of pulmonary, renal, and cardiocirculatory dysfunctions. A certain percentage (about 20%–25%) of patients with necrotizing pancreatitis and organ complications can be successfully treated by intensive care measures, thereby avoiding the necessity for an operation [29]. Patients who failed to respond to a 3–5 days of intensive care treatment are candidates for surgical management, as are patients with proven infected necrosis [28]. A pancreatic abscess could be treated by percutaneous catheter drainage with ultrasound or CT guidance [30], or by various surgical modalities [31–33]. The interventions for postacute pseudocysts are percutaneous or endoscopic drainage procedures or pseudocystojejunostomy [34, 35].

Summary

Since the last international conferences in 1984 there has been an enormous increase in our knowledge in pancreatic inflammatory diseases. In order to make further progress in the future in this field of clinical pancreatic research, it is extremely important to reclassify inflammatory diseases of the pancreatic gland to be able to objectively compare interinstitutional results and ultimately improve our patient care.

For clinical use, we propose a classification system of acute pancreatitis that is based on morphological and clinical criteria grouped into four different entities: interstitial–edematous pancreatitis, necrotizing pancreatitis (sterile/infected), pancreatic abscess, and postacute pseudocyst. For local infection, the terms infected necrosis and pancreatic abscess should be used. Although there is no absolute certainty in the differentiation between edematous and necrotizing pancreatitis, infected necrosis and pancreatic abscess, and postacute pseudocyst and pseudocyst in chronic pancreatitis, this classification has proved to be very efficient in our clinical practice. And since this clinicopathological classification system does not claim to be complete, an international consensus conference is urgently needed for worldwide acceptance.

References

1. Sarles H (ed) (1965) Pancreatitis: symposium of Marseille, 1963. Karger, Basel
2. Harrison RC (1982) Let's reclassify pancreatitis. Am J Surg 143:534–535
3. Sarner M, Cotton PB (1984) Classification of pancreatitis. Gut 25:756–759
4. Singer M, Gyr K, Sarles H (1985) Revised classification of pancreatitis. Report of the second international symposium on the classification of pancreatitis in Marseille, 1984. Gastroenterology 89:683–690
5. Warshaw AL (1980) A guide to pancreatitis. Compr Ther 6:49–55
6. Beger HG, Büchler M (1986) Decision-making in surgical treatment of acute pancreatitis: operative or conservative management of necrotizing pancreatitis? Theor Surg 1:61–68
7. Beger HG, Bittner R, Büchler M, Hess M, Schmitz JE (1986) Hemodynamic data pattern in patients with acute pancreatitis. Gastroenterology 90:74–79
8. Beger HG, Krautzberger W, Bittner R, Block S, Büchler M (1984) Results of surgical treatment of necrotizing pancreatitis. World J Surg 9:972–979
9. Beger HG, Krautzberger W, Bittner R, Büchler M, Block S (1986) Bacterial contamination of pancreatic necrosis. A prospective clinical study. Gastroenterology 91:433–438
10. Allardyce DB (1987) Incidence of necrotizing pancreatitis and factors related to mortality. Am J Surg 154:295–299
11. Buggy BP, Nostrant TT (1983) Lethal pancreatitis. Am J Gastroenterol 78: 810–814

12. Kune GA, King R (1973) The late complications of acute pancreatitis. Med J Aust 1:1241–1246
13. Warshaw AL (1974) Inflammatory masses following acute pancreatitis. Surg Clin North Am 54:621–632
14. Fan ST, Choi TK, Lai ECS, Wong J (1990) Prediction of severity of acute pancreatitis: an alternative approach. Gut 30:1591–1595
15. Leser H-G, Gross V, Scheibenbogen C, Heinisch A, Sal R, Lausen M, Rückauer K, Andreesen R, Farthmann EH, Schölmerich J (1991) Elevation of serum interleukin-6 concentration precedes acute-phase response and reflects severity in acute pancreatitis. Gastroenterology 101:782–785
16. Sarner M (1986) Pancreatitis: definitions and classification. In: The exocrine pancreas: biology, pathobiology, and diseases. Raven, New York, pp 459–464
17. Kivisaari L, Somer K, Standertskjöld-Nordenstam CG, Schröder T, Kivilaakso E, Lempinen M (1984) A new method for the diagnosis of acute hemorrhagic necrotising pancreatitis using contrast-enhanced CT. Gastrointest Radiol 9: 27–30
18. Block S, Maier W, Clausen C, Bittner R, Büchler M, Malfertheiner P, Beger HG (1986) Identification of pancreas necrosis in severe acute pancreatitis. Gut 27:1035–1042
19. Balhazar EJ (1989) CT diagnosis and staging of acute pancreatitis. Rad Clin North Am 27:19–37
20. Bradley EL, Murphy F, Ferguson C (1989) Prediction of pancreatic necrosis by dynamic pancreatography. Ann Surg 210:495–504
21. van Sonnenberg E, Wing VW, Casola G, Coons HG, Nakamoto SK, Müller PR, Ferrucci JT, Halasz NA, Simeone JF (1984) Temporizing effect of percutaneous drainage of complicated abscesses in critically ill patients. AJR 142:821–826
22. Gerzof SG, Banks PA, Robbins AH (1984) Role of guided percutaneous aspiration in early diagnosis of pancreatic sepsis. Dig Dis Sci 29:950 (abstract)
23. Gerzof SG, Banks PA, Robbins AH, Johnson WC, Spechler SJ, Watzner SM, Snider JM, Langevin RE, Jay ME (1987) Early diagnosis of pancreatic infection by computed tomography-guided aspiration. Gastroenterology 93:1315–1320
24. Büchler M, Malfertheiner P, Frieß H, Bittner R, Vanek E, Schlegel P, Beger HG (1989) The penetration of antibiotics into human pancreas. Infection 17: 20–25
25. Bassi C, Falconi M, Girelli R, Nifosi F, Elio A, Martini N, Pederzoli P (1989) Microbiological findings in severe pancreatitis. Surg Res Comm 5:1–4
26. Bittner R, Block S, Büchler S, Beger HG (1987) Pancreatic abscess and infected pancreatic necrosis: different local septic complications in acute pancreatitis. Dig Dis Sci 32:1082–1087
27. Frey CF, Bradley EL III, Beger HG (1988) Progress in acute pancreatitis. Surg Gynecol Obstet 176:282–286
28. Beger HG, Uhl W (1990) Severe acute pancreatitis. II: The surgical approach. Clin Int Care 1:223–227
29. Büchler M, Malfertheiner P, Uhl W, Beger HG (1988) Conservative treatment of necrotizing pancreatitis in patients with minor pancreatic necrosis. Pancreas 3:592 (abstract)
30. Warshaw AL, Jin G (1985) Improved survival in 45 patients with pancreatic abscess. Ann Surg 202, 408–417
31. Sarr MG, Nagorney DM, Mucha P, Farnell MB, Johnson CD (1991) Acute necrotizing pancreatitis: management by planned, staged pancreatic necrosectomy/debridement and delayed primary wound closure over drains. Br J Surg 78:576–581
32. Steiner E, Müller PR, Hahn PF, Saini S, Simeone JF, Wittenberg J, Warshaw AL, Ferrucci JT (1988) Complicated pancreatic abscesses: problems in interventional management. Radiology 167:443–446

33. Bradley EL III (1991) Operative management of acute pancreatitis: ventral open packing. Hepto-gastroenterol 38:134–138
34. Bastid C, Schönenberg P, Sahel J (1990) Treatment of pancreatic abscess using percutaneous catheters inserted under sonographic guidance: report of 13 cases in 7 patients. Digestion 46:129 (abstract)
35. Hancke S, Henrikson FW (1985) Percutaneous pancreatic cystogastrostomy guided by ultrasound scanning and gastroscopy Br J Surg 72:916–917

Morphology of Acute Pancreatitis

A.K. Foulis[1]

Introduction

Acute pancreatitis occurs in many different clinical settings, with varying causes. It is therefore very likely that factors as diverse as an impacted gall stone at the ampulla of Vater, hypothermia, or chronic alcoholism all initiate the disease process in different ways. Once an autodigestive process is started within the pancreas, however, a more uniform picture emerges.

The postmortem appearance of massive necrosis within the pancreas has been likened to the effects of a forest fire. There has been total destruction of all structures within the path of the process. Not surprisingly, in situations such as this, the site at which the process started cannot be readily identified. If, however, minor fires are consistently seen to be centred on picnic areas, it is a reasonable assumption that severe fires probably also start there.

The problem in studying the histopathology of very mild acute pancreatitis is that patients do not require surgical resection and do not die of it; access to histological material is therefore difficult. However, any pathological series which includes patients diagnosed as having acute pancreatitis solely at autopsy includes patients in whom pancreatitis was relatively mild and perhaps incidental to the patient's death. Lest it be assumed that these patients have quite a different disease from clinically recognised acute pancreatitis, it should perhaps be emphasised that the classical clinical associations of acute pancreatitis – such as cholelithiasis, alcohol abuse and shock – are also very common in these patients [8].

Is the Pancreatic Acinus or the Ductal System the Initial Site of Damage?

Ductal Inflammation and Periductal Necrosis

As can be seen from Table 1, which represents a personal autopsy series of 68 patients with acute pancreatitis of a full range of severity, duct

[1] Division of Pathology, University of Glasgow, Royal Infirmary, Glasgow G4 0SF, Scotland

Beger/Büchler/Malfertheiner (Eds.)
Standards in Pancreatic Surgery

Table 1. Incidence of duct inflammation and periductal necrosis in relation to aetiology in acute pancreatitis

Aetiology of acute pancreatitis	Number of patients (n = 44)	Number in whom duct inflammation and periductal necrosis were found
Gall stones	19	14
Alcohol abuse	11	9
Secondary to shock	8	0
Secondary to hypothermia	6	0

inflammation was present commonly in both alcohol-related and gall stone pancreatitis, but it was absent in patients with pancreatitis secondary to shock or primary hypotension. Involved ducts often had proteinaceous plugs within their lumens (Fig. 1). These plugs are probably derived from desquamated epithelial cells [13]. Within the duct lumen there was also a prominent polymorphonuclear infiltrate, and the epithelium of the duct lining was usually ulcerated. Evidence of acinar cell necrosis and associated inflammation was present around such ducts.

It was thus suggested that pancreatic excretory ducts are the site of initial damage in gall stone pancreatitis and pancreatitis secondary to alcohol abuse [8]. The initial pathological event in gall stone pancreatitis appears to be migration of a gall stone down the common bile duct with temporary impaction at the ampulla of Vater [1, 16]. Experiments in animals have shown that while sterile bile and primary bile acids do not damage the pancreatic mucosal barrier, when infused at low pressure, infected bile or bile preincubated with trypsin does result in a measurable loss of function of the barrier, allowing leakage of ions across the epithelium. This loss of function is first accompanied by mucin granule depletion of the duct epithelium and later by duct inflammation and periductal necrosis [17, 21]. Thus in the presence of an obstructing stone and common channel, bile may reflux into the pancreas where its composition may be altered, either because of infection [12], or by incubation with pancreatic proteolytic enzymes. Such altered bile may initiate gall stone pancreatitis in an analogous way to that described above in experimental animals.

Less is understood of how chronic alcohol exposure leads to pancreatic ductal damage. Reber et al. [21] showed that infusion of 5%–10% ethanol through the pancreatic duct caused moderate damage to the pancreatic mucosal barrier in cats, but alcohol levels in the pancreatic duct in man seldom exceed 0.5%. Possibly chronic alcohol exposure is more damaging. A point of interest is that in chronic calcifying pancreatitis there is little doubt that ductal epithelial damage is of major importance since ducts are usually focally ulcerated with underlying fibrosis. This eventually results in

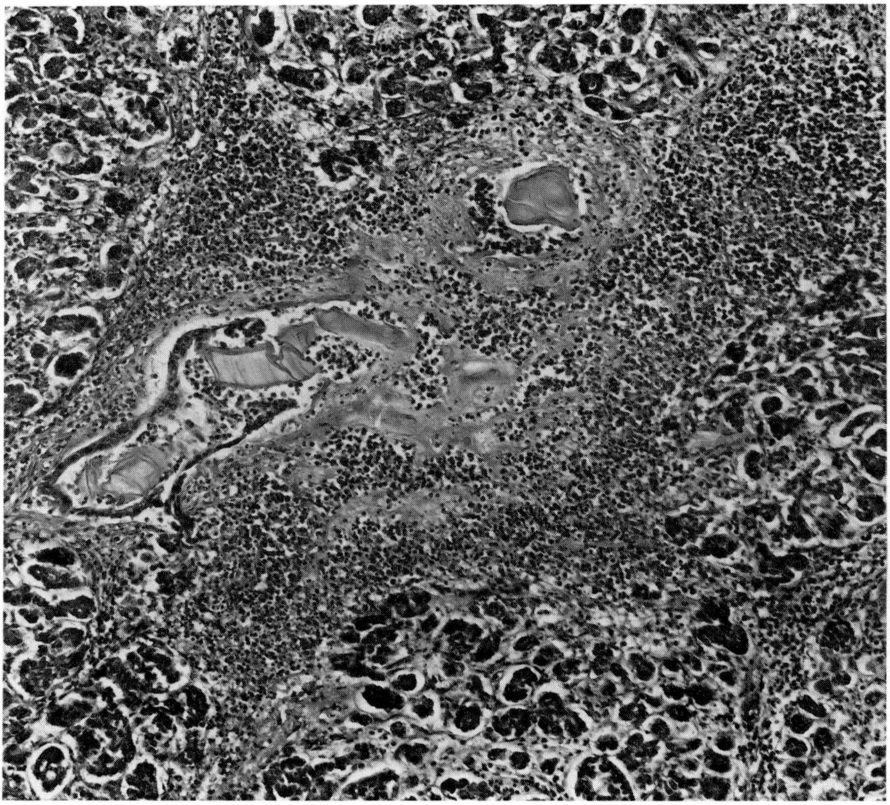

Fig. 1. Duct inflammation and periductal necrosis. There is an acute inflammatory infiltrate within the duct, and this extends out into surrounding pancreatic parenchyma where it is associated with acinar cell necrosis. Duct concretions are present within the duct lumen, and there is disruption of the lining epithelium. (H&E ×100)

duct stricture formation. Thus acute and chronic alcohol-related pancreatitis may be different manifestations of a similar toxic effect on duct epithelium.

Perilobular Necrosis

The pathogenesis of perilobular necrosis is best understood after a brief description of the pancreatic microvasculature (Fig. 2). Connective tissue septa divide the exocrine pancreas into secretory lobules which vary in size from about 2 to 10 mm in diameter. In rabbits, dogs and man it seems that lobules are supplied by one, or at most two lobular arteries [4, 25, 26]. Thus in most lobules the lobular artery can be regarded as an end artery and the

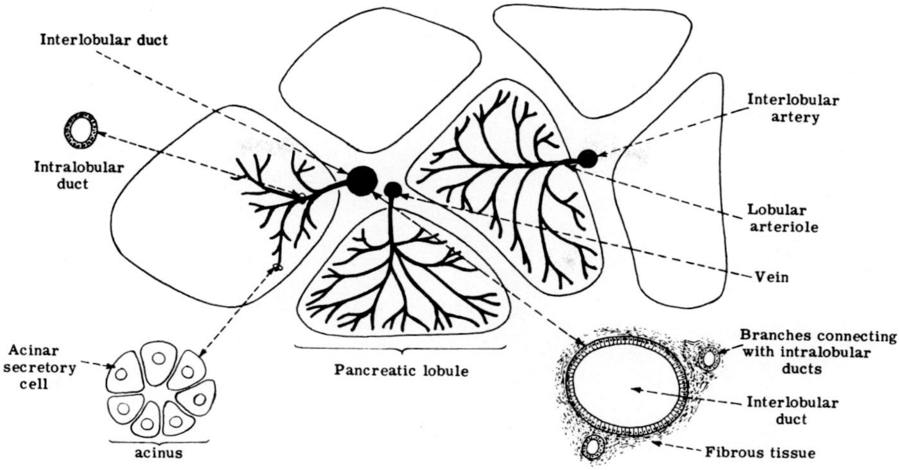

Fig. 2. Pancreatic microanatomy

branching of the artery is such that the periphery of the lobule is also the periphery of the lobular microcirculation. The venous drainage closely follows the arterial supply.

In states of profound hypotension or circulatory failure, therefore, ischaemic necrosis of acini at the periphery of lobules might be expected to occur (Fig. 3). Such perilobular necrosis is indeed the pattern observed in pancreatitis following cardiac surgery [7], shock or cardiac failure [8] and hypothermia accompanied by hypotension [9]. In these clinical states duct inflammation is absent, but acini at the periphery of lobules are necrotic, and here there is an associated acute inflammatory response. The situation is analogous to perivenular (centrilobular) necrosis in the liver in states of shock. The anatomical pattern of necrosis in each site is determined by the microanatomy of the blood supply.

Thus it can be seen that acute pancreatitis may be initiated primarily by a ductal lesion, in gall stone associated disease or pancreatitis secondary to alcohol abuse. By contrast, a completely different initial event – perilobular acinar cell necrosis – probably accounts for the pathogenesis of ischaemic pancreatitis. It seems likely, however, that either of these forms of disease can progress along a final common pathway leading to massive pancreatic necrosis [24].

Progression to Panlobular Necrosis

Wherever the initial autodigestive event takes place – whether around ducts or at the periphery of lobules – released enzymes may damage virtually any structure contained within or around the gland. Pancreatic ducts are

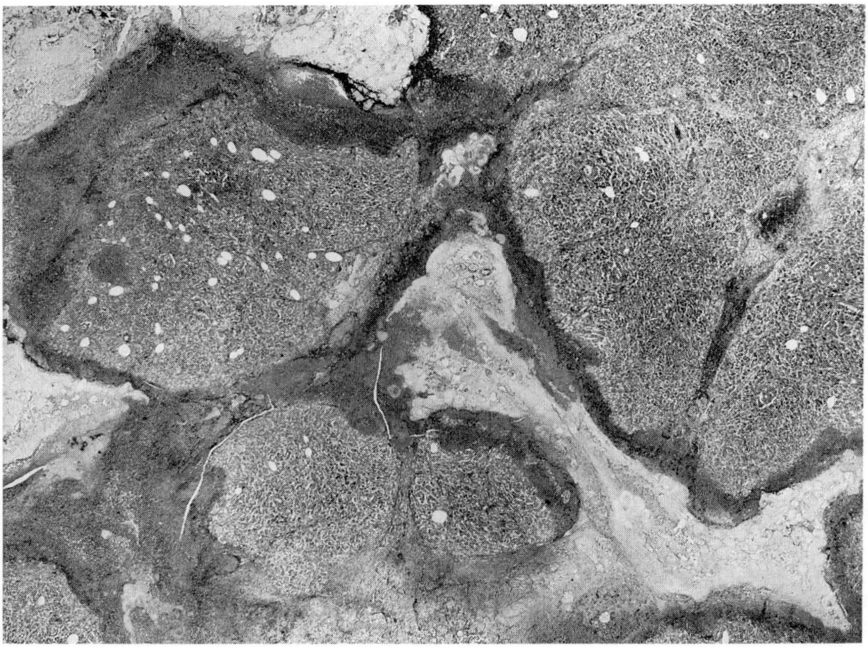

Fig. 3. Perilobular necrosis. There is necrosis of acini at the periphery of pancreatic lobules. Interlobular fat is also necrotic. (H&E ×16)

surrounded by a rich plexus of veins and arteries [14]. Release of enzymes in their vicinity results in a vasculitic process, first described by Rich and Duff [22]. The vessel wall becomes necrotic and damage to the endothelium results in thrombosis. If this process takes some days, there may be evidence of acute endarteritis as well. The veins, being thin walled, are generally affected earlier and more frequently than associated arteries. Since lobules are probably usually drained by single veins, thrombosis of such an efferent vessel results in ischaemic necrosis of the lobule with maximal early damage occurring at the periphery of the lobule. Thus perilobular necrosis can result not only from systemic hypotension but also from intrapancreatic vascular thrombosis secondary to autodigestive vasculitis. There is probably a third way in which this histological pattern may be produced in the evolving disease process. The pancreatic lobules are surrounded by loose connective tissue which often contains fat. Enzymes can probably track along this relatively minor barrier easily, producing perilobular fat necrosis. Necrosis of this adipose tissue is very common in acute pancreatitis and is always present in severe disease.

From this it can be seen that in gall stone or alcohol-related pancreatitis of any severity perilobular necrosis is almost invariable. However it is dif-

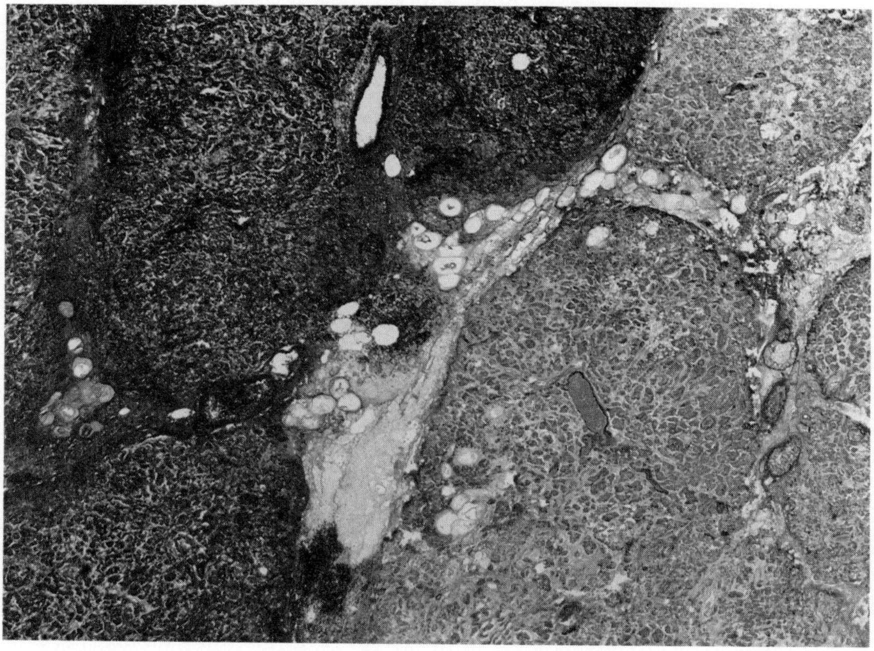

Fig. 4. Panlobular necrosis. *Top left*, viable tissue; *lower right*, coagulative necrosis. (H&E ×40)

ficult to conceive of a mechanism whereby ischaemic necrosis of perilobular acini leads to widespread duct inflammation, and this lesion is not seen in ischaemic pancreatitis (Table 1). Thus it is the presence of duct inflammation which distinguishes the two principal initial disease mechanisms.

Panlobular necrosis is the term which has been used to describe the histological appearances of the most advanced stage of pancreatic destruction [8]. Here entire lobules and intervening ducts, blood vessels, nerves and adipose tissue show the histological appearances of coagulative necrosis (Fig. 4) [23]. When the section is stained by haematoxylin and eosin, light pink ghost outlines of the pancreatic structures can be seen.

Several lines of evidence suggest that panlobular necrosis is the result of pancreatic infarction. Firstly, widespread venous thrombosis is readily seen in most cases [8, 18, 23]. Secondly, intravenous contrast-enhanced computed tomography shows that in widespread pancreatic necrosis the affected areas do not have a blood supply [2]. Thirdly, coagulative necrosis is a characteristic histological appearance of infarction in many organs, for example, heart, kidney and spleen. In the evolution towards panlobular necrosis lobules appear to become progressively necrotic. This starts at the periphery of the lobule, and the wave of necrosis extends towards the vascular pole of the lobule. This too is consistent with progressive ischaemic damage. Finally, in experimental pancreatitis reduced pancreatic blood flow is a characteristic terminal event of severe disease [6, 11].

Panlobular necrosis is recognised macroscopically by the pathologist, on sectioning the pancreas, as confluent dark red/black areas of pancreatic parenchyma. However the surgeon has difficulty in assessing the extent of this process when inspecting the gland surface at laparotomy. Peripancreatic fat necrosis is often accompanied by haemorrhage, presumably as a result of leakage from vessels damaged by autodigestion. In this circumstance the gland surface appears dark red or black, but it is difficult to predict the changes within the gland itself. In one series of pancreatic resections in which external assessment of the gland had suggested that the gland was subtotally/totally necrotic, 48% of the resections showed that less than a quarter of the pancreas was necrotic, and 11% of the resections showed no macroscopic pancreatic parenchymal necrosis at all [18, 19].

There is liable to be some confusion over the use of the term "pancreatic necrosis". From a histological point of view virtually all cases of human acute pancreatitis have evidence of pancreatic parenchymal necrosis. Purely "oedematous pancreatitis", with no necrosis, is seen in some animal models of pancreatitis and presumably occurs early in the course of any form of pancreatitis, but it is unlikely ever to be encountered surgically. However, the term "pancreatic necrosis" is also used in the surgical literature to describe widespread confluent macroscopic parenchymal necrosis [3]. This use of the term is clearly synonymous with "panlobular necrosis", as used here.

Local Complications of Acute Pancreatitis

Pancreatic Pseudocyst

Pancreatic pseudocysts occur in 5%–8% of cases [5, 15]. A pancreatic pseudocyst is a localised encapsulated effusion containing enzyme-rich fluid which may or may not communicate with the pancreatic ductal system. The mechanism involved in its production is probably leakage of pancreatic juice from a ductal system ruptured as a result of pancreatic parenchymal necrosis. The site of fluid accumulation depends on the site of leakage. The escaped juice causes acute inflammation in the structures into which it tracks. The consequence of this is the laying down of fibrous tissue at these sites in an attempt to wall off or localise the irritating fluid. The walls of the pseudocyst can include structures such as posterior wall of stomach, transverse mesocolon and posterior abdominal wall. Small pseudocysts may resolve spontaneously. In larger ones the fibrous wall tends to mature and strengthen so that at about 6 weeks of age it can be incorporated safely into a surgically created stoma, for example, a cystogastrostomy. At operation, pseudocysts often contain haemorrhagic fluid and necrotic debris. Histologically the pseudocyst is lined by granulation tissue. True pancreatic cysts, which are usually neoplastic, but which can be confused clinically with pseudocysts [3], are lined by an epithelium. If, in the absence of frank pus, culture of the pseudocyst fluid yields a positive bacterial growth, the preferred term is "infected pseudocyst" [10].

Infection Complicating Pancreatic Necrosis

In approximately 4%–8% of cases of acute pancreatitis infection complicates pancreatic necrosis [5, 20]. There is more confusion in the terminology of this subject than in the pathogenesis involved. It is generally agreed that infection of necrotic tissue is a secondary phenomenon, i.e., infection is not the primary cause of the pancreatic necrosis [3]. The avascular haemorrhagic necrotic mass is an ideal culture medium for many anaerobic bacteria. The necrosis, and hence the infection, may be very extensive, spreading in surgical planes. The necrotic tissue is relatively avascular and hence a good acute inflammatory response does not necessarily occur. This inhibits the ability of the body to localise the infection. Not surprisingly "infected pancreatic necrosis" normally carries a grave prognosis.

An "abscess" is normally defined as a localised collection of pus in a cavity formed by the disintegration of tissues. However the term "pancreatic abscess" is often used to describe infected pancreatic necrosis even although no pus may be present [3]. True abscesses do occur secondary to acute pancreatitis, but since the implication here is that the infection has been localised, the prognosis should be better than for infected pancreatic necrosis. Similarly, an infected pseudocyst or a pseudocyst abscess (pus in a pseudocyst) are localised infections, and the prognosis following drainage should be relatively good. The use of the term "pancreatic abscess" to cover all peripancreatic infections following acute pancreatitis is therefore to be avoided.

In conclusion, when a pathologist is faced with a pancreatic resection performed on a patient with acute pancreatitis, the two most important factors to assess are (a) the extent of pancreatic parenchymal necrosis and (b) the presence or absence of infection. It seems likely that these two factors most accurately determine the patient's prognosis [3, 18].

References

1. Acosta JM, Ledesma CL (1974) Gall stone migration as a cause of acute pancreatitis. New Eng J Med 290:484–487
2. Block S, Maier W, Bittner R, Büchler M, Malfertheiner P, Beger HG (1986) Identification of pancreas necrosis in severe acute pancreatitis: imaging procedures versus clinical staging. Gut 27:1035–1042
3. Bradley EL III (1988) Later complications of acute pancreatitis. In: Glazer G, Ranson JHC (eds) Acute pancreatitis. Baillière Tindall, London, pp 390–431

4. Cadete-Leite A (1973) The arteries of the pancreas of the dog. An injection-corrosion and microangiographic study. Am J Anat 137:151–158
5. Corfield AP, Cooper MJ, Williamson RCN et al. (1985) Prediction of severity in acute pancreatitis: prospective comparison of three prognostic indices. Lancet i:403–407
6. Donaldson LA, Williams RW, Schenk WG (1978) Experimental pancreatitis: effect of plasma and dextran on pancreatic blood flow. Surgery 84:313–321
7. Feiner H (1976) Pancreatitis after cardiac surgery: a morphologic study. Am J Surg 131:684–688
8. Foulis AK (1980) Histological evidence of initiating factors in acute pancreatitis in man. J Clin Pathol 33:1125–1131
9. Foulis AK (1982) Morphological study of the relation between accidental hypothermia and acute pancreatitis. J Clin Path 35:1244–1248
10. Glazer G (1988) Classification and definitions in acute and chronic pancreatitis. In: Glazer G, Ranson JHC (eds) Acute pancreatitis. Baillière Tindall, London, pp 37–50
11. Goodhead B (1969) Vascular factors in the pathogenesis of acute haemorrhagic pancreatitis. Ann R Coll Surg Engl 45:80–97
12. Graham DF, Wyllie FJ (1979) Prediction of gall-stone pancreatitis by computer. Br Med J i:515–517
13. Harada H, Ueda O, Yasuoka M et al. (1981) Histochemical studies on protein plugs obtained by endoscopic retrograde catheterization of the papilla. Gastroenterol Jpn 16:563–567
14. Harris PF (1979) In: Howat HT, Sarles H (eds) The exocrine pancreas. Saunders, London, p 21
15. Imrie CW, Benjamin IS, Ferguson JC et al. (1978) A single-centre double-blind trial of trasylol therapy in primary acute pancreatitis. Br J Surg 65:337–341
16. Kelly TR (1976) Gall stone pancreatitis – pathophysiology. Surgery 80:488–492
17. Konok GP, Thompson AG (1969) Pancreatic ductal mucosa as a protective barrier in the pathogenesis of pancreatitis. Am J Surg 117:18–23
18. Nordback I, Lauslahti K (1986) Clinical pathology of acute necrotising pancreatitis. J Clin Path 39:68–74
19. Nordback I, Pessi T, Auvinen O, Autio V (1985) Determination of necrosis in necrotizing pancreatitis. Br J Surg 225–227
20. Ranson JHC, Spencer FC (1977) Prevention, diagnosis and treatment of pancreatic abscess. Surgery 82:99–106
21. Reber HA, Roberts C, Way LW (1979) The pancreatic duct mucosal barrier. Am J Surg 137:128–134
22. Rich AR, Duff GL (1936) Experimental and pathological studies on the pathogenesis of acute haemorrhagic pancreatitis. Bull Johns Hopkins Hosp 58:212–258
23. Thal AP, Perry VF, Egner W (1957) A clinical and morphological study of 42 cases of fatal acute pancreatitis. Surg Gynecol Obstet 105:191–201
24. Warshaw AL, O'Hara PJ (1978) Susceptibility of the pancreas to ischemic injury in shock. Ann Surg 188:197–201
25. Wharton GK (1932) The blood supply of the pancreas with special reference to the islands of Langerhans. Anat Rec 53:55–81
26. Yaginuma N, Takahashi T, Saito K, Kyoguku M (1986) The microvasculature of the human pancreas and its relation to Langerhans islets and lobules. Pathol Res Pract 181:77–84

Diagnosis of Acute Pancreatitis

T.P. KEMMER and G. ADLER[1]

Introduction

Diagnosis of acute pancreatitis is based on clinical, morphological, and functional criteria with the currently employed definition based on the Second International Symposium on Classification of Pancreatitis [22]. This paper deals with the clinical symptoms and diagnostic procedures in establishing the diagnosis of acute pancreatitis.

Clinical Symptoms

The leading symptom in acute pancreatitis is severe abdominal pain localized in the epigastrium with a tendency to spread to the left or right upper abdomen and to irradiate to the back. The pain of acute pancreatitis, however, is not specific enough to be distinguished from that of other abdominal diseases. Other symptoms and signs are abdominal muscular rigidity, fever, nausea, vomiting, meteorism, ileus/subileus, jaundice, shock, and neurological symptoms [31, 33]. The most common diseases that should be considered for the differential diagnosis of acute pancreatitis are complications of peptic ulcer disease, acute cholecystitis, biliary colic, intestinal occlusion, mesenteric vessel thrombosis, peritonitis, colonic diverticulitis or perforation, basal pleuro-pulmonary inflammation, and myocardial infarction [31, 33]. Most patients with acute pancreatitis have a mild course of the disease, but up to 20% develop severe organ failure [6] and systemic complications (Table 1). Clinical signs such as abdominal wall ecchymosis around the umbilicus (Cullen's sign), below the inguinal ligament (Fox's sign), or on the flanks (Grey Turner's sign) are extremely rare and do not indicate a poor prognosis of the disease [16].

Etiological Factors

The definition of etiological factors involved in the pathogenesis of acute pancreatitis is important, since it may permit specific therapy. Alcohol and

[1] Universität Ulm, Abteilung Innere Medizin I, Robert-Koch-Straße 8, W-7900 Ulm, FRG

Beger/Büchler/Malfertheiner (Eds.)
Standards in Pancreatic Surgery

Table 1. Complications of acute pancreatitis [3, 26]

Local	Systemic
Necrosis	Pulmonary failure
Hemorrhagic collections	Renal failure
Abscess	Shock
Ileus	Sepsis
Pseudocyst	Encephalopathy
Ascites	Hyperglycemia
Pleural fluid	Hypocalcemia
Jaundice	Metabolic acidosis

gallstones are the most frequent pathogenic factors in acute pancreatitis. While alcohol has a higher prevalence among cases with acute pancreatitis in a series reported from North America [43], gallstones are the commonest etiological factor of acute pancreatitis in the United Kingdom, where they account for more than 50% of cases [15]. Several studies provide evidence that alcohol can cause acute pancreatic damage [11, 46]. In the study by Renner et al. [44], alcohol was the most common cause of fatal acute pancreatitis in chronic alcoholics lacking histologic evidence of chronic pancreatitis. Ultrasound (US) is indicated as first diagnostic step in all cases in the search for cholelithiasis [30], but the nonvisualization of the gallbladder in over 30% of patients should be taken into account [12]. Aspartate aminotransferase (AST >60 IU/liter) has recently been proposed as valid screening for the presence of biliary stones [35]. The gold standard for the detection of gallstones during an attack of acute pancreatitis is endoscopic retrograde cholangiopancreatography (ERCP). When stones are found to be impacted in the ampullary region or in the common bile duct, immediate treatment by endoscopic sphincterotomy is the method of choice [14].

In drug-related episodes of acute pancreatitis, the causal relationship is often difficult to establish. One study analyzed the occurrence rate of severe acute pancreatitis in a large group of metronidazole recipients [19]. New cases were reported during oral 5-aminosalicyclic acid therapy for inflammatory bowel disease [18] and high-dose interleukin-2 immunotherapy for malignant melanoma [10]. Severe pancreatitis was reported in two of nine patients after anticholinesterase insecticide (parathion) intoxication [28].

Diagnosis and Course of Acute Pancreatitis

Severe acute pancreatitis is often first diagnosed at autopsy. Lankisch et al. [29] analyzed whether recent improvements in diagnostic abilities had reduced the rate of undiagnosed cases. Between 1980 and 1985 acute pancreatitis was diagnosed at autopsy in 43 cases. In 13 cases (30.2%) diagnosis was first established at autopsy. Only one patient complained of abdominal pain. Twelve other patients received analgetics immediately on admission, which may have masked the most common symptom of acute pancreatitis. That serum amylase levels were often normal, not obtained, or obtained too late is a reminder that amylase levels do not correlate with the severity of pancreatitis. The absence of abdominal pain and serum markers in this study group resulted in few imaging procedures. Further, ultrasound examination in acute pancreatitis often gives inconclusive results because of intestinal gas. Finally, a normal or slightly elevated serum amylase level should not dissuade one from the diagnosis of acute pancreatitis in the appropriate clinical setting [1].

An increase in pancreatic serum enzymes, such as amylase, lipase, pancreatic isoamylase, immunoreactive trypsin, elastase, chymotrypsin, carboxyl ester hydrolase, and phospholipase A_2, is considered the gold standard for the diagnosis of acute pancreatitis. Nevertheless, several patients with acute pancreatitis have been reported to have normal pancreatic serum enzymes [8, 17, 23, 38]. Episodes of acute pancreatitis detected by imaging procedures with no elevation of pancreatic serum enzymes may sometimes be found during the course of chronic alcoholic pancreatitis with pancreatic parenchyma gradually replaced by fibrosis [47]. Another cause is a delay between the onset of symptoms and pancreatic enzyme – especially amylase – determination, since amylase is cleared from the circulation most rapidly.

Various methods based on the determination of enzyme activity, enzyme immunoassay, and radioimmunoassay determine several different pancreatic enzymes in the clinical setting. Since the traditional parameter of total amylase cannot represent the gold standard, several specific pancreatic enzymes (pancreatic amylase, lipase, immunoreactive trypsin or elastase) were routinely analyzed [31, 32]. The greatest accuracy for the detection of acute pancreatitis is achieved in clinical practice by the simultaneous determination of pancreatic amylase and lipase. The measurement of urinary enzymes is no longer of importance [39]. The determination of serum elastase is of particular interest, since elastase is the pancreatic enzyme least influenced by renal insufficiency [32]. In that respect, a comprehensive and critical overview on diagnostic tests for acute pancreatitis [4] suggested that lipase assays should be used more often due to their higher overall specificity when compared with amylase assays. There appears to be no additional diagnostic benefit in measuring other pancreatic enzymes in serum.

Besides the complex clinical and laboratory Ranson criteria [42] and contrast-enhanced CT, several biochemical parameters have been found to be valid for the detection of pancreatic necrosis: methemalbumin [36], ribonuclease [50], complement proteins [27], pO_2 [9], hemorrhagic peritoneal fluid [41], phospholipase A_2 [40], alpha$_2$ macroglobulin [37], C-reactive protein [34], PMN elastase [20, 48], and trypsinogen activation peptides [21]. Analysis of PMN elastase seems to be of similar value to lactate

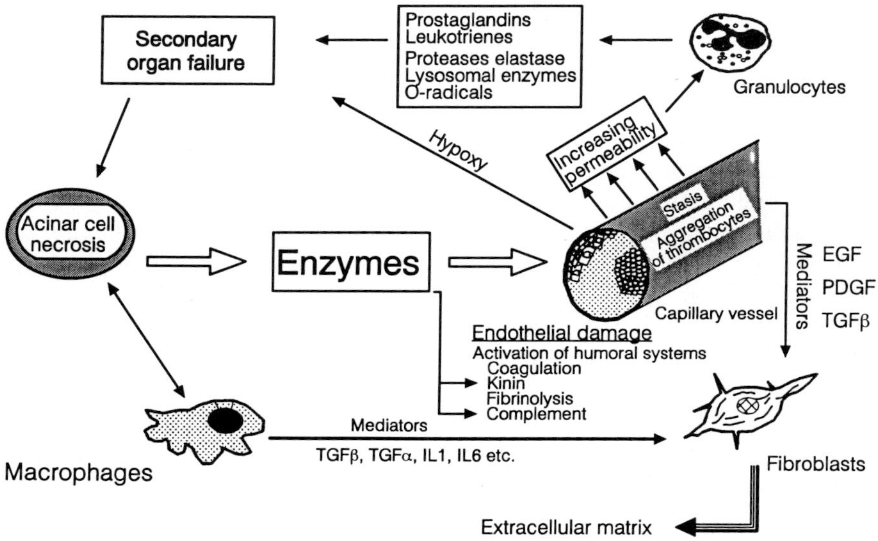

Fig. 1. Factors of inflammation and regeneration in acute pancreatitis

dehydrogenase and C-reactive protein in detecting necrotizing pancreatitis [49], whereas the value of serum ribonuclease is limited due to its low sensitivity [25]. The association of increased C-reactive protein and parenchymal necrosis is significant and is of definite prognostic value. The prognosis is poorer if the necrosis is infected [7, 13]. Recently, serum levels of extracellular biomatrix components such as procollagen peptide, laminin, fibronectin, and hyaluronate have been shown to correlate with the severity of acute pancreatitis [1, 2], reflecting inflammatory and reparative processes (Fig. 1). Complex pathological processes responsible for the high mortality in severe acute pancreatitis were explained as resulting from excessive stimulation of leukocytes (neutrophils, macrophages, basophils, etc.), whereas the role of pancreatic digestive enzymes in the complications is uncertain [45].

The major role of the imaging procedures US and CT is to reveal changes evolving within the pancreas and peripancreatic regions during and after an episode of acute pancreatitis, to aid in identifying etiological factors, and to aid in grading the severity of the disease and deciding therapeutic strategies [5, 24].

In summary, the diagnostic approach to acute pancreatitis is as complex as the etiological and pathogenetic factors (Fig. 1) of this disease. On the basis of the clinical picture, determination of specific pancreatic enzymes in the serum, and the imaging procedures US and CT, high diagnostic accuracy can be guaranteed and therapeutic strategies can be established.

References

1. Adler G (1991) Acute pancreatitis. Curr Opin Gastroenterol 7:714–719
2. Adler G, Kropf J, Grobe E, Gressner AM (1990) Follow-up of the serum levels of extracellular matrix components in acute and chronic pancreatitis. Eur J Clin Invest 20:494–501
3. Adler G, Reinshagen M, Bauerfeind U (1988) Die Akutdiagnostik der Pankreatitis. Diagn Lab 38:155–163
4. Agarwal N, Pitchumoni CS, Sivafrasad AV (1990) Evaluating tests for acute pancreatitis. Am J Gastroenterol 85:356–366
5. Balthazar EJ (1989) CT diagnosis and staging of acute pancreatitis. In: Freeny PC (ed) Radiology of the pancreas. The radiologic clinics of North America, vol 27. Saunders, Philadelphia, pp 19–37
6. Bank S, Wise L, Gersten M (1983) Risk factors in acute pancreatitis. Am J Gastroenterol 78:637–690
7. Beger HG, Block S, Bittner R (1987) The significance of bacterial infection in acute pancreatitis. In: Beger HG, Büchler M (eds) Acute pancreatitis. Springer, Berlin Heidelberg New York, pp 79–86
8. Berk JE (1978) New dimension in the laboratory diagnosis of pancreatic disease. Am J Gastroenterol 69:417–427
9. Berry AR, Taylor TV, Davies GC (1981) Pulmonary function and fibrinogen metabolism in acute pancreatitis. Br J Surg 68:870–873
10. Birchheld GR, Ward JH, Redman BG, Flaherty L, Samlowski WE (1990) Acute pancreatitis associated with high-dose interleukin-2 immunotherapy for malignant melanoma. West J Med 152:714–716
11. Blackstone MO (1990) Can alcohol cause true acute pancreatitis? Gastroenterology 99:1544–1546
12. Blamey SL, Osbourne DH, Gilmore WH (1983) The early identification of patients with gallstone-associated pancreatitis using clinical and biochemical factors only. Ann Surg 198:574–578
13. Büchler M, Uhl W, Malfertheiner P (1987) Biochemical staging of acute pancreatitis. In: Beger HG, Büchler M (eds) Acute pancreatitis. Springer, Berlin Heidelberg New York, pp 143–153
14. Carr-Locke DL (1990) Acute gallstone pancreatitis and endoscopic therapy. Endoscopy 22:180–183
15. Corfield AP, Cooper MJ, Williamson RCN (1985) Acute pancreatitis: a letal disease of increasing incidence. Gut 26:724–729
16. Dickson AP, Imrie CW (1984) The incidence and prognosis of body wall ecchymosis in acute pancreatitis. Surg Gynecol Obstet 159:343–347
17. Dürr GHK (1986) Value of pancreatic serum determination for diagnosis of acute pancreatitis. In: Malfertheiner P, Ditschuneit H (eds) Diagnostic procedures in pancreatic disease. Springer, Berlin Heidelberg New York, pp 84–91
18. Fiorentini MT, Fracchia M, Galatola G, Barlotta A, de la Pierre M (1990) Acute pancreatitis during oral 5-aminosalicyclic acid therapy. Dig Dis Sci 35: 1180–1182
19. Friedman GD, Selby JV (1990) How often does metronidazole induce pancreatitis? Gastroenterology 98:1702–1703
20. Gross V, Schölmerich J, Leser HG, Salma R, Lausen M, Ruckauer K, Schöffel U, Lay L, Heinisch A, Farthmann EH, Gerok W (1990) Granuolocyte elastase in assessment of severity of acute pancreatitis – comparison with acutephase proteins C-reactive protein, alpha-1-antitrypsin, and protease inhibitor alpha-2-macroglobulin. Dig Dis Sci 97–105
21. Gudgeon AM, Heath DI, Hurley P, Jehanli A, Patel G, Wilson C, Shenkin A, Austen BM, Imrie CW, Hermon-Taylor J (1990) Trypsinogen activation peptides assay in the early prediction of severity of acute pancreatitis. Lancet 335:4–8

22. Gyr K, Singer M, Sarles H (1984) Pancreatitis, concepts and classification. Elsevier, Amsterdam
23. Ihse I (1986) Is there a most useful parameter for the diagnosis of acute pancreatitis? In: Malfertheiner P, Ditschuneit H (eds) Diagnostic procedures in pancreatic disease. Springer, Berlin Heidelberg New York, pp 92–94
24. Jeffrey RB (1989) Sonography in acute pancreatitis. In: Freeny PC (ed) Radiology of the pancreas. The radiologic clinics of North America, vol 27. Saunders, Philadelphia, pp 5–17
25. Kemmer TP, Malfertheiner P, Büchler M, Kemmer ML, Ditschuneit H (1991) Serum ribonuclease activity in the diagnosis of pancreatic disease. Int J Pancreatol 8:23–33
26. Kemmer TP, Malfertheiner P (1991) Akute Pankreatitis. Klinikarzt 20:458–466
27. Lankisch PG, Koop H, Kaboth V (1981) Serum complement factors in human acute pancreatitis. Hepatogastroenterology 28:261–263
28. Lankisch PG, Müller CH, Niederstadt H, Brand A (1990) Painless acute pancreatitis subsequent to anticholinesterase insecticide (parathion) intoxication. Am J Gastroenterol 85:872–875
29. Lankisch PG, Schirren CA, Kunze E (1991) Undetected fatal acute pancreatitis: why is the disease so frequently overlooked? Am J Gastroenterol 86:322–326
30. Lees WR (1984) Pancreatic ultrasonography. Clin Gastroenterol 13:763–789
31. Malfertheiner P, Büchler M (1987) Clinical symptoms and signs and diagnostic requirements in acute pancreatitis. In: Beger HG, Büchler M (eds) Acute pancreatitis. Springer, Berlin Heidelberg New York, pp 103–109
32. Malfertheiner P, Büchler M, Stanescu A, Uhl W, Ditschuneit H (1987) Serum elastase 1 in inflammatory pancreatic and gastrointestinal diseases and in renal insufficiency. A comparison with other serum pancreatic enzymes. Int J Pancreatol 2:159–170
33. Malfertheiner P, Kemmer TP (1991) Clinical picture and diagnosis of acute pancreatitis. Hepatogastroenterology 38:97–100
34. Mayer AD, McMahon MJ, Bowen M, Cooper EH (1984) C-reactive protein: an aid to assessment and monitoring of acute pancreatitis. J Clin Pathol 37:207–211
35. Mayer AD, McMahon MJ (1985) Biochemical identification of patients with gallstones associated acute pancreatitis on the day of admission to hospital. Ann Surg 201:68–75
36. McKay AJ, Imrie CW, O'Neill J, Duncan JG (1982) Is an early ultrasound scan of value in acute pancreatitis? Br J Surg 69:369–372
37. McMahon MJ, Bowen M, Mayer AD, Cooper EH (1984) Relation of alpha-2-macroglobulin and other antiproteases to the clinical features of acute pancreatitis. Am J Surg 147:164–170
38. McMahon LF (1985) Pancreatitis: is total serum amylase misleading? J Clin Gastroenterol 7:17–19
39. Möller-Peterson J, Laustsen J, Klaerke M (1986) Serum and urinary pancreatic enzymes in diagnosis of acute pancreatitis. In: Malfertheiner P, Ditschuneit H (eds) Diagnostic procedures in pancreatic disease. Springer, Berlin Heidelberg New York, pp 95–106
40. Nevalainen TJ (1980) The role of phospholipase A in acute pancreatitis. Scand J Gastroenterol 15:641–650
41. Pickford IR, Blacklett RJ, McMahon MJ (1977) Early assessment of severity of acute pancreatitis using peritoneal lavage. Br Med J 2:1377–1379
42. Ranson JHC, Rifkind KM, Roses DF, Fink SD, Eng K, Spencer FC (1974) Prognostic signs and the role of operative management in acute pancreatitis. Surg Gynecol Obstet 139:69–81
43. Ranson JHC (1982) Etiological and prognostic factors in human acute pancreatitis: a review. Am J Gastroenterol 77:633–638
44. Renner JG, Savage WT, Pantoia JL, Renner VJ (1985) Death due to acute pancreatitis: a retrospective analysis of 405 autopsy cases. Dig Dis Sci 30: 1005–1018

45. Rinderknecht H (1988) Fatal pancreatitis, a consequence of excessive leukocyte stimulation? Int J Pancreatol 3:105–112
46. Singh M, Simsek H (1990) Ethanol and the pancreas. Gastroenterology 98: 1052–1062
47. Spechler SJ, Dalton JW, Robbins AH, Gerzof SG, Stern JS, Johnson WC, Nabseth DC, Schimmel EM (1983) Prevalence of normal serum amylase levels in patients with acute alcoholic pancreatitis. Dig Dis Sci 28:865–869
48. Uhl W, Büchler M, Malfertheiner P, Martini M, Beger HG (1989) PMN-elastase: a new serum marker for the staging of acute pancreatitis. Digestion 43:176–177
49. Uhl W, Büchler M, Malfertheiner P, Martini M, Beger HG (1991) PMN-elastase in comparison with CRP, antiproteases, and LDH as indicators of necrosis in human acute pancreatitis. Pancreas 6:253–259
50. Warshaw AL, Lee KH (1979) Serum ribonuclease elevations and pancreatic necrosis in acute pancreatitis. Surgery 86:227–234

Pancreatic Secretory Enzymes in the Diagnosis of Acute Pancreatitis

P.J. BLIND[1]

Introduction

During the past century great progress has been made in developing non-invasive methods, both imaging and biochemical, for the diagnosis of acute pancreatitis (AP). Computed tomography (CT) with contrast enhancement (CECT) [1] and ultrasonography (US) [2] are examples of recent diagnostic techniques which, along with clinical assement of the patient, provide the basis for a decision on therapy. CECT and US are usually not available in the emergency room. The diagnostic work-up of a patient with suspected AP always starts with laboratory tests. Laboratory tests for the diagnosis of AP are based on the assay of pancreatic secretory products and various other components in small samples of body fluids and tissues, which supposedly reflect the presence and extent of inflammatory changes in the pancreas and the consequences of these on the body. It should be noted that these biochemical tests yield only indirect evidence of the pathological process. New tests are continuously being explored, implying that the ideal test for diagnosing AP and monitoring its course has not yet been established. As early as in 1952, Thistlethwaite and Hill emphasized that in order to assess the value of any method for diagnosing AP, the presence of the disease must be objectively verified. At that time, pancreatic biopsy via laparotomy was the only feasible way to do this, while in fatal disease post-mortem examination was done [3]. The principle of objective verification of the diagnosis of AP was rarely adhered to in clinical studies until the introduction of CT and US. Since 80% of patients with AP present an uncomplicated course, operation to verify diagnosis is usually not justified. The lack of a reliable reference method for the diagnosis of AP has created substantial difficulties in the interpretation of published reports [4].

Aim and Method

The present review focuses on the value of determining pancreatic secretory enzymes in serum in making the diagnosis of AP. Among patients present-

[1] Department of Surgery, University of Umeå, Umeå, Sweden

Beger/Büchler/Malfertheiner (Eds.)
Standards in Pancreatic Surgery

ing with signs and symptoms of AP and hyperamylasemia, the diagnosis may be erroneous in as many as one third as judged by isoamylase determinations [5, 6]. Therefore, only publications stating verification of diagnosis using US, CT, CECT, laparotomy, or autopsy alone or combinations of these modalities are included.

Results and Discussion

The outcomes of diagnostic indices of assays designed to estimate pancreatic secretory enzymes are illustrated in Table 1 [7–18]. Sensitivities and specificities vary considerably for the same enzyme in different studies, a noteworthy observation with clinical consequences. In the case of amylase of supposedly pancreatic origin, for example, it makes a considerable difference if the suspicion of AP in a patient presenting with abdominal pain is further supported by the test in 67% or in 97.1% of patients (Table 1). The difference could be explained by differences in assay techniques used or by variations in performance of the assay between laboratories. Furthermore, the definition of cut-off levels between normal and elevated levels for the same assay in different laboratories may vary. The proportions of patients with AP associated with alcohol abuse or biliary disease may differ between studies. Patients with AP of alcoholic etiology present with normoamylasemia in a higher frequency than patients with AP associated with gallstone disease [17]. Inclusion criteria may differ. For example, when radiological methods are relied on for the diagnosis of AP, an unquantified interobserver variability is present, especially in borderline cases. A tissue sample taken for histopathological diagnosis may not be representative. Furthermore, histopathological diagnosis is dependent on the pathologist's opinion [19]. When assessing the diagnostic value of assays estimating lipolytic activity, it is important to scrutinize the method used, since many divergent results might be due to the use of different techniques for measuring lipase activity. The results depend on the assay technique, the substrate and its concentration, the emulsifier and its concentration, the stability of emulsion, the buffer, the temperature, the inhibitors and activators, the presence of colipase, the kinetics of hydrolasation, and the pH [20, 21]. Methods for determining the enzymatic activity of pancreatic lipases usually are not designed to discriminate between activities derived from carboxylic ester hydrolase (CEH) and colipase-dependent lipase (CLDL), although the existence of two different pancreatic lipases was proposed about 40 years ago [22]. Furthermore, methods estimating lipolytic activity are susceptible to contamination through lipolytic activities of extrapancreatic origin [23]. For example, in the presence of bile salts the predominant lipolytic activity derives from CEH, since bile salts inhibit CLDL activity in the absence of an excess of colipase. Colipase, a prerequisite for reliable determination of CLDL activity, overcomes inhibition by the high bile acid concentration

Table 1. Outcomes of diagnostic indices of assays designed to estimate pancreatic secretory enzymes

Pancreatic secretory enzyme	Sensitivity (%)	Specificity (%)	Predictive value		Efficiency (%)	Reference
			Positive (%)	Negative (%)		
Total amylase	67–100	84.8–98	94	88	86.7–90.4	[7–12]
Pancreatic isoamylase	67–97.1	82.6–97.6	95	95	88	[7, 10, 11, 13, 14]
Pancreatic isoamylase P3	100	100	100	100		[7]
Trypsin/ trypsinogen	89–100	78.8–82.8			87	[11, 13, 14]
Phospholipase A_2[a]	75	78			77	[15]
Phospholipase A[a]	79	79			79	[15]
Elastase 1	97–100	78.8–95.7			97.3	[10, 13, 14]
CLDL (RIA)	88–100	100				[13]
CLDL (enzymatic)	82–100	81.6–99	85	95.6		[7, 11, 12, 14, 16–18]
CLDL (ELISA)	100	100				[9]
CEH (ELISA)	100					[8]

Sensitivity is the probability of a positive test in patients with acute pancreatitis.
Specificity is the probability of a negative test in patients without acute pancreatitis.
Positive predictive value is the probability of acute pancreatitis in patients with a positive test.
Negative predictive value is the probability of not having acute pancreatitis in patients with a negative test.
Efficiency is the proportion of all results that are true results, whether positive or negative. CLDL, Colipase-dependent lipase; CEH, carboxylic ester hydrolase; RIA, radioimmunoassay; ELISA, enzyme-linked immunosorbent assay.
[a] Only patients with necrotizing pancreatitis.

used in turbidimetric tests, overcomes inhibition of serum proteins, and eliminates the variability of endogenous colipase [24].

Techniques based on antigenic properties of CLDL and CEH have been developed and used in the diagnosis of AP [9, 25–34]. Theoretically, the advantage of methods based on antigenic properties of an enzyme, in contrast to enzymatic assays, is that the enzyme protein concentration, active and inhibited forms of the enzyme, may be detected. As CLDL is secreted only from the pancreas, the radioimmunoassay should be extremely organ specific [31]. Determination of CEH and CLDL enzyme protein concentrations by enzyme-linked immunosorbent assay (ELISA) both seemingly allowed correct identification of all patients with AP (Table 1). Furthermore, the CLDL test allowed correct identification of all patients not suffering from AP [8, 9]. The specificity of the sandwich-ELISA estimating CEH protein concentrations for the diagnosis of AP has not yet been determined. All assays designed to determine pancreatic secretory enzymes show high sensitivities and specificities. Diagnostic indices of phospholipase A_2 and phospholipase A in severe pancreatitis were given by Büchler and colleagues; however, attempts to estimate diagnostic indices for severe and mild disease are usually not done [15]. Calculations of predictive values are useful in clinical practice only at rather high prevalences of AP [19]. Diagnostic indices give a relative figure of the performance of a test in the diagnosis of a specific disease which relates to the test itself, not to the individual patient.

Assays for pancreatic secretory enzymes allowing separation of patients with mild from patients with severe pancreatitis are desirable. Indeed, it has been observed that CEH protein concentrations in patients with necrotizing pancreatitis were significantly higher (concentrations related to day of admission) from the second to the tenth day after admission than those in patients with interstitial pancreatitis [8]. Furthermore, patients with NP presented with significantly higher phospholipase A_2 and phospholipase A catalytic activities (levels related to onset of pain) than did patients with AIP [15]. However, overlap of CEH protein concentrations, phospholipase A_2 and phospholipase A catalytic activities recorded daily in patients with mild and severe inflammation, restrains the use of the recordings for prognostic purposes. Persistence of high levels of these enzymes may indicate severe inflammation. Elevated levels of elastase 1, immunoreactive trypsin (IRT), and immunoreactive phospholipase A_2 have been shown in patients with AP. Serum levels of elastase 1 and IRT do not correlate to severity of inflammation [13, 35]. Elevation of elastase 1 or phospholipase A_2 in serum is not specific for pancreatitis [15, 35].

Several multiple-factor scoring systems for assessing the severity of pancreatitis and predicting its course have been developed [36]. Objective verification of AP is lacking in at least some of these. Outcomes of assays of pancreatic secretory enzymes have usually not been included in the scoring systems. Assays for pancreatic isoamylase P3 and immunological assays allowing quantitative determination of CLDL and CEH show very high sensitivites and specificites. Inclusion of data obtained from assaying pancreatic secretory enzymes and other laboratory data reflecting inflammation–e.g., CRP, in patients with an objectively verified diagnosis of AP–combined with the use of statistical methods allowing prediction of the course of the disease in the individual patient remains to be done.

References

1. Mödder U, Friedmann G, Rosenberger J (1981) Wert der Angio-CT für Stadieneinteilung, Verlaufsbeobachtung und Therapie bei akuter Pancreatitis. Fortschr Geb Rontgenstr 134:22–27
2. Lawson TL (1978) Sensitivity of pancreatic ultrasonography in the detection of pancreatic disease. Radiology 128:733
3. Thistlethwaite JR, Hill RP (1952) Serum amylase levels in experimental pancreatitis. Surgery 31:495–501
4. Spechler SJ, Schimmel EH (1985) Serum amylase in pancreatitis. Dig Dis Sci 30:92–93
5. Koehler DF, Eckfeldt JH, Levitt MD (1982) Diagnostic value of routine isoamylase assay of hyperamylasemic serum. Gastroenterology 82:887–890
6. Weaver DW, Bouwman DL, Walt AJ, Clink D, Resto A, Stephany J (1982) A correlation between clinical pancreatitis and isoenzyme patterns of amylase. Surgery 92:576–580
7. Sacchetti L, Cavalcanti E, Cerasuolo D, Oriani G, Uomo G, Rabitti PG, Laccetti M, Visconti M, Salvatore F (1989) Evaluation of pancreatic amylase immunoassay in acute pancreatitis. Clin Chim Acta 183:95–100
8. Blind PJ, Büchler M, Bläckberg L, Andersson Y, Uhl W, Beger HG, Hernell O (1991) Carboxylic ester hydrolase. A sensitive serum marker and indicator of severity of acute pancreatitis. Int J Pancreatol 8:65–73
9. Bowen M, Cooper EH, McMahon MJ (1983) The diagnosis of acute pancreatitis: enhanced sensitivity from an ELISA assay of lipase. Biomed Pharmacother 37:395–398
10. Gullo L, Ventrucci M, Pezzilli R, Platé L, Naldoni P (1987) Diagnostic value of serum elastase 1 in pancreatic disease. Br J Surg 74:44–47
11. Steinberg WM, Goldstein SS, Davis ND, Shamma'a J, Anderson K (1985) Diagnostic assays in acute pancreatitis. A study of sensitivity and specificity. Ann Intern Med 102:576–580
12. Thomson HJ, Obekpa PO, Smith AN, Brydon WG (1987) Diagnosis of acute pancreatitis: a proposed sequence of biochemical investigations. Scand J Gastroenterol 22:719–724
13. Büchler M, Uhl W, Malfertheiner P (1986) Elastase 1 in acute pancreatitis. In: Beger HG, Büchler M (eds) Acute pancreatitis. Springer, Berlin Heidelberg New York, pp 100–117
14. Ventrucci M, Pezzilli R, Gullo L, Platé L, Sprovieri G, Barbara L (1989) Role of serum pancreatic enzyme assays in diagnosis of pancreatic disease. Dig Dis Sci 34:39–45
15. Büchler M, Malfertheiner P, Schädlich H, Nevalainen TJ, Friess H, Beger HG (1989) Role of phospholipase A_2 in human acute pancreatitis. Gastroenterology 97:1521–1526
16. Patt HH, Kramer SP, Woel G, Zeitung D, Seligman AM (1966) Serum lipase determination in acute pancreatitis. Arch Surg 92:718–723
17. Clavien P-A, Robert J, Meyer P, Borst F, Hauser H, Herrmann F, Dunand V, Rohner A (1989) Acute pancreatitis and normoamylasemia. Ann Surg 210: 614–620

18. Mayer AD, McMahon MJ, Holdsworth PJ, Wilson DH, Flowers MW, Brown DA (1985) Screening for acute pancreatitis: a rapid assay for plasma lipase. Br J Surg 72:436–437
19. Goldberg DM (1990) Biochemical tests in pancreatic disease. Curr Opin Gastroenterol 6:739–749
20. Overbeek GA (1957) Fat-splitting enzymes in blood. Clin Chim Acta 2:1–8
21. Junge W, Leybold K, Kraack B (1983) Influence of colipase on the turbidimetric determination of pancreatic lipase catalytic activity. J Clin Chem Clin Biochem 21:445–451
22. Boissonnas RA (1948) Estérases. II. Purification partielle de la lipase de pancréas de porc. Helv Chim Acta 31:1577–1583
23. Blind PJ, Bläckberg L, Hernell O, Ljungberg B (1987) Carboxylic ester hydrolase: a serum marker of acute pancreatitis. Pancreas 2:597–603
24. Leybold A, Junge W (1986) Importance of colipase for the measurement of serum lipase activity. Adv Clin Enzymol 4:60–67
25. Bradshaw WS, Rutter WJ (1972) Multiple pancreatic lipases. Tissue distribution and pattern of accumulation during embryological development. Biochemistry 11:1517–1528
26. Grenner G, Deutsch G, Schmidtberger R, Dati F (1982) Hochempfindlicher Enzymimmunoassay zur Bestimmung von Human-Pankreas-Lipase. J Clin Chem Clin Biochem 20:515–519
27. Häggmark A, Cho J-W, Lamminpää K, Lundh G, Seligson U (1983) Immunochemical determination of pancreatic lipase in serum, duodenal fluid and urine in patients with pancreatic disease. Digestion 28:32–33 (abstr)
28. Jensen R (1983) Detection and determination of lipase (acylglycerol hydrolase) activity from various sources. Lipids 18:650–657
29. Royse VL (1984) Laboratory and clinical evaluation of a sensitive radioimmunoassay for lipase (Nuclipase, Nuclin Diagnostics). Clin Chem 30:1058 (abstr)
30. Jensen DM, Royse VL, Newell Bonello J, Schaffner J (1987) Use of amylase isoenzymes in laboratory evaluation of hyperamylasemia. Dig Dis Sci 32: 561–568
31. Roberts IM, Mercer D (1987) Radioimmunoassay for human pancreatic lipase in acute pancreatitis. Dig Dis Sci 32:388–392
32. Hayakawa T, Kondo T, Shibata T, Kitagawa M, Ono H, Sakai Y, Kiriyama S (1989) Enzyme immunoassay for serum lipase in the diagnosis of pancreatic lipase. Gastroenterol Jpn 24:556–560
33. Bläckberg L, Blind PJ, Ljungberg B, Hernell O (1985) On the source of bile salt-stimulated lipase in human milk: a study based on serum concentrations as determined by a sandwich enzyme-linked immunosorbent assay technique. J Pediatr Gastroenterol Nutr 4:441–445
34. Sternby B, Åkerström B (1984) Immunoreactive pancreatic colipase, lipase, phospholipase A_2 in human plasma and urine from healthy individuals. Biochim Biophys Acta 789:164–169
35. Clavien P-A, Burgan S, Moossa AR (1989) Serum enzymes and other laboratory tests in acute pancreatitis. Br J Surg 76:1234–1243
36. Williamson RCN (1984) Early assessment of severity in acute pancreatitis. Gut 25:1331–1339

Dynamic Computed Tomography of Acute Pancreatitis

P.C. FREENY[1]

Acute pancreatitis represents a spectrum of inflammatory diseases ranging from acute edematous pancreatitis to hemorrhagic or necrotic pancreatitis. As the severity of the inflammatory process increases, the associated morbidity and mortality also increase. Thus, precise diagnosis, staging, and detection of complications are important for appropriate patient management. Dynamic computed tomography (DCT) is currently the most accurate single imaging modality for diagnosis, for staging the severity of the inflammatory process, and for detection of complications of acute pancreatitis [1, 2].

Techniques of Dynamic CT

Optimal CT examination of the pancreas is performed at scan speeds of 2 s or less [1, 3, 4]. A digital radiograph is used to determine the cranial and caudal limits of the scan sequence. The entire abdomen is scanned using 5-mm collimated scans at 8-mm intervals. An oral contrast agent should be given to opacify the gastrointestinal tract, permitting differentiation of pancreatic fluid collections from loops of bowel and facilitating detection of involvement of the gastrointestinal involvement by the inflammatory process.

A 150- to 180-ml bolus of 60% contrast agent should be administered during the scanning sequence at a rate of 2.5 ml/s. Normal pancreatic parenchyma shows an increase in attenuation of 40–60 HU above baseline attenuation of normal nonenhanced parenchyma. In addition, the peripancreatic vascular structures show intense contrast enhancement, allowing detection of vascular complications associated with acute pancreatitis.

Indications for CT of Acute Pancreatitis

CT has three major roles in evaluation of patients with known or suspected acute pancreatitis: (a) initial diagnosis; (b) staging the severity of the inflammatory process; and (c) detection of complications.

[1]Department of Radiology, SB-05, University of Washington School of Medicine, Seattle, WA 98195, USA

Beger/Büchler/Malfertheiner (Eds.)
Standards in Pancreatic Surgery

Table 1. Acute pancreatitis: grade and CT severity index (from [2])

CT grade	*Score*
A	0
B	1
C	2
D	3
E	4
Add to CT score the necrosis score	
Necrosis	*Score*
None	0
One-third	2
One-half	4
>One-half	6

Diagnosis

The clinical and laboratory diagnosis of acute pancreatitis is usually staraightforward, but in some cases it may be unclear, particularly if it develops in an already critically ill, postoperative, or trauma patient. In these patients, CT can play an important diagnostic role. The CT diagnosis of acute pancreatitis is based upon a variety of morphologic changes in the gland ranging from gland enlargement, peripancreatic inflammation, fluid collections, and gland necrosis. These are discussed in detail in the following section of staging.

CT Staging of the Severity of Acute Pancreatitis

Precise staging of the severity of acute pancreatitis has important prognostic and treatment implications [2, 5–8]. Staging can be based upon clinical criteria, such as the Ranson criteria or acute physiology and chronic health evaluation (APACHE) [9, 10]. However, prospective studies have shown that clinical evaluation is able to identify only 34%–39% of patients with severe episodes of acute pancreatitis [11, 12]. More recently, several prospective studies have shown that CT performed early in the course of acute pancreatitis can better identify those patients with severe pancreatitis. This is because clinical criteria alone measure only the physiologic or systemic response of the patient, while CT can define both the extent of damage to the pancreas, particularly the presence of gland necrosis, as well as identify peripancreatic complications that subsequently can produce major sequelae, such as fluid collections, abscess formation, vascular involvement, and other complications [2, 5, 6, 13, 14].

The degree of severity of acute pancreatitis has been classified into five stages by Balthazar and co-workers [2, 5, 6] (Table 1).

Stage A: Normal Pancreas. Patients with mild, acute edematous pancreatitis may have a normal pancreatic CT in 20%–25% of cases [15]. This is

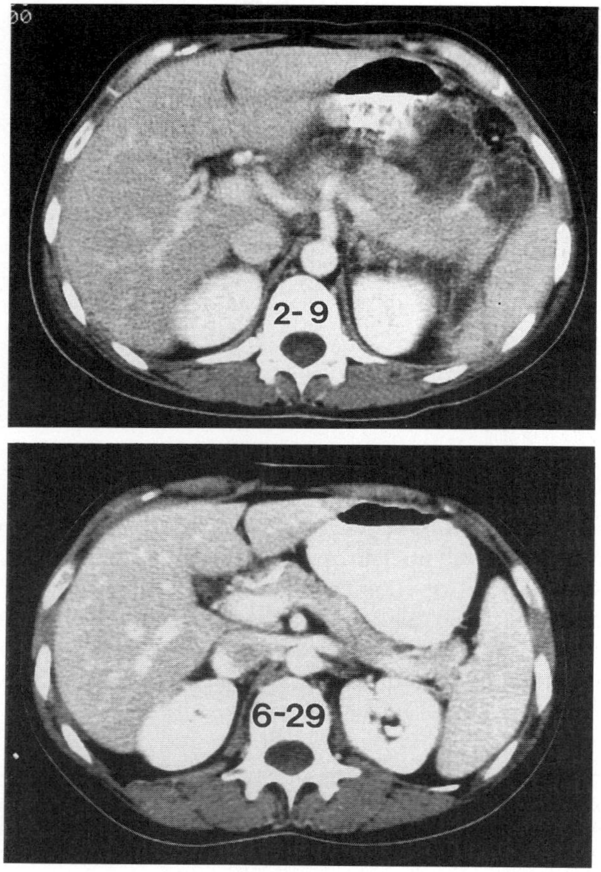

a

b

Fig. 1a,b. Acute pancreatitis, stage B. **a** DCT on 9 February in a patient with clinically mild acute pancreatitis shows a normal appearing pancreas with perhaps slight gland enlargement. **b** Subsequent DCT on 29 June shows marked reduction in gland size following resolution of episode of uncomplicated acute pancreatitis

because the inflammatory process is so mild that no fluid collections form and no changes occur in the peripancreatic soft tissues. The gland may be slightly enlarged, but without a baseline scan performed prior to the onset of the acute attack this change may be too subtle to detect (see Fig. 1).

Stage B: Focal or Diffuse Enlargement of the Gland (including contour irregularities, heterogeneous parenchymal attenuation, pancreatic duct dilatation, or small intrapancreatic fluid collections). Stage B acute pancreatitis represents a spectrum of changes ranging from gland enlargement (Fig. 1) to mild irregularities of the gland margin caused by peripancreatic

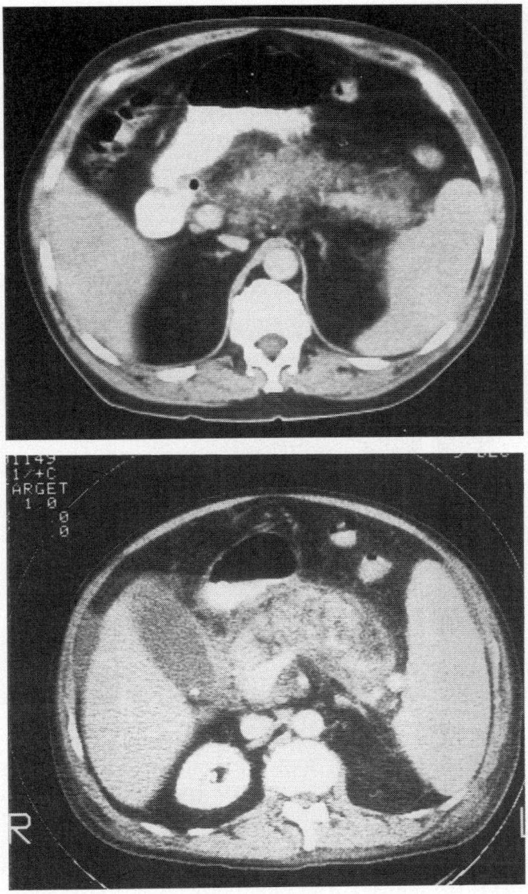

a

b

Fig. 2a,b. Acute pancreatitis, stages C and D. **a** DCT in a patient with clinically mild acute pancreatitis shows irregularity of the gland margins owing to peripancreatic inflammatory changes and inhomogenity of the parenchyma (stage C). **b** DCT in a different patient shows phlegmonous enlargement of the gland, heterogeneous parenchyma, and mild peripancreatic inflammatory changes (stage D)

soft tissue inflammation or small intrapancreatic fluid collections caused by blow-out of a small duct.

Stages C and D: Intrinsic and Extrinsic Inflammatory Changes. Stages C and D represent intrinsic gland abnormalities as described for Stage B but also include more marked peripancreatic soft tissue inflammation (Fig. 2), phlegmon formation (inflammatory enlargement of the pancreas), and peripancreatic fluid collections. These patients may progress to more severe changes, develop secondary complications, such as infection of the fluid

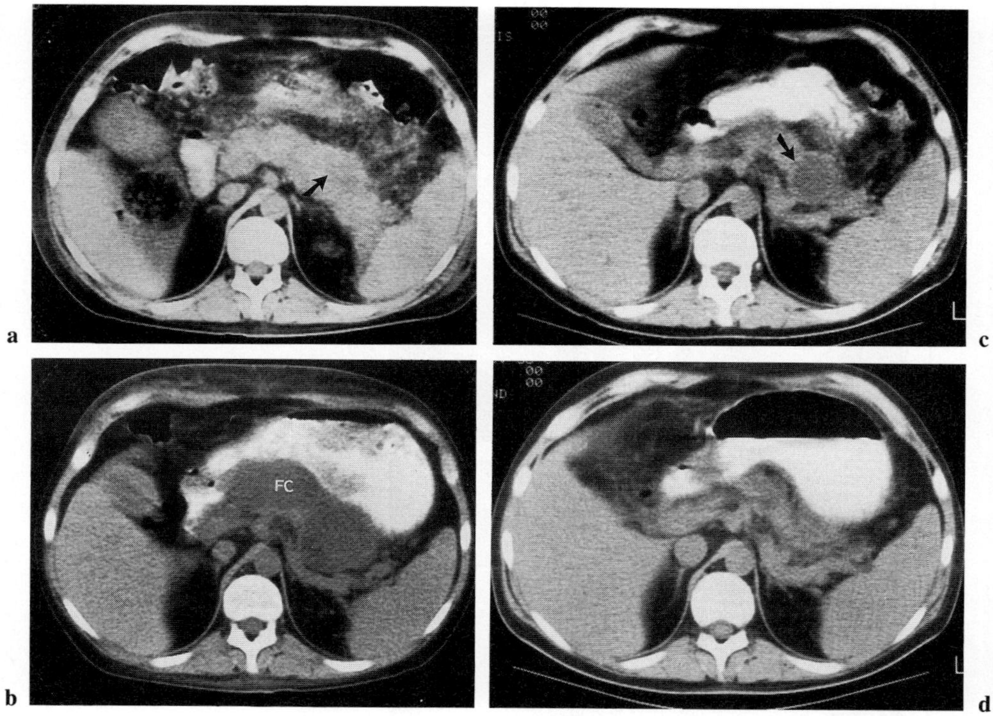

Fig. 3a–d. Acute pancreatitis, stage D. **a** DCT shows enlargement of the gland, a small intrapancreatic fluid collection (*arrow*), and peripancreatic soft tissue inflammatory changes. **b** CT 12 days later without contrast (patient was in acute renal failure) shows subsequent development of a large fluid collection (*FC*) around the pancreas. **c** CT without contrast 15 days following scan (**b**) shows only a small remaining fluid collection in the tail of the pancreas (*arrow*) and resolution of the peripancreatic inflammatory changes. **d** Final CT 8 weeks following scan (**a**) shows a normal pancreas with no remaining fluid collection

collection, or they may show progressive resolution of changes which can be demonstrated on follow-up CT (Fig. 3).

Stage E: Multiple or Extensive Extrapancreatic Fluid Collections or Abscess. This is the most severe form of acute pancreatitis and is manifested by marked intrapancreatic (fluid collections, necrosis) and peripancreatic (fluid collections, extraglandular fat necrosis) inflammatory changes, as well as frank abscess formation. These patients have significant morbidity and mortality rates and serial CT is important for following the progression of the disease and for detecting complications.

The presence of gland necrosis plays an important role in staging and is included in Balthazar's CT severity index (Table 1). It can be detected by DCT as a focal or diffuse area of diminished parenchymal contrast enhance-

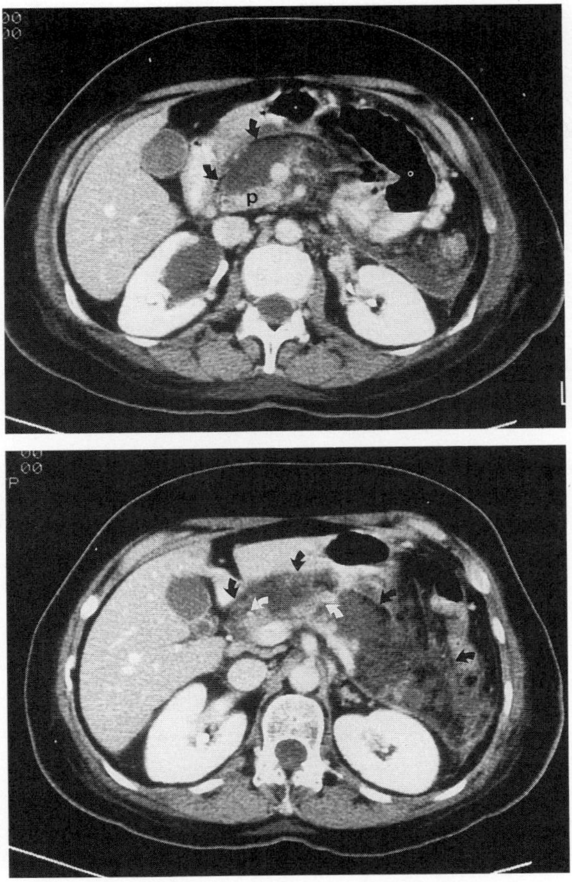

a

b

Fig. 4a,b. Acute pancreatitis, stage E (parenchymal necrosis). **a** DCT shows extensive gland necrosis in the head of the pancreas (*arrows*) with only a small volume of normally contrast-enhancing pancreas (*p*). **b** Scan at a higher level shows extensive necrosis of the body and tail of the gland (*black arrows*) with only small islands of contrast-containing parenchyma (*white arrows*)

ment (Figs. 4, 5) [13, 14]. The accuracy of CT detection of parenchymal necrosis was investigated by Beger and colleagues in a large series of patients who underwent both angiographic CT and surgery [7]. The overall accuracy for CT was 87%. The false-negative rate was 21% in patients with minor necrosis, but in cases of major or extended necrosis (>50%) the false-negative rate was only 11%. Bradley and coworkers subsequently confirmed these results and indicated that CT detection of gland necrosis has important prognostic implications [16].

Balthazar has combined the CT staging of acute pancreatitis (stages A–E) with the presence of necrosis to produce the CT severity index,

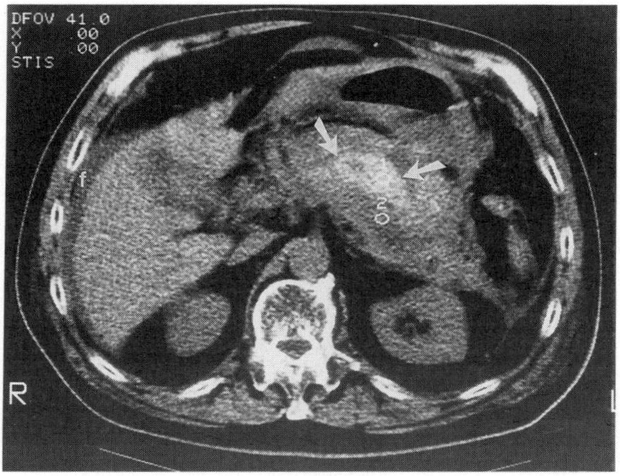

Fig. 5. Acute pancreatitis: intraparenchymal hemorrhage. CT without contrast shows enlargement of the pancreas and a central zone of increased attenuation (*arrows*) owing to hemorrhage. A small amount of free intraperitoneal fluid (*f*) surrounds the liver

Table 2. CT severity index: morbidity and mortality (from [2])

Index	Morbidity (%)	Mortality (%)
0–3	8	3
4–6	35	6
7–10	92	17

which accurately reflects the morbidity and mortality of patients with acute pancreatitis [2] (Table 1). Patients who had an index of 0 or 1 had no mortality or morbidity, while those with an index of 2 had a 4% morbidity, and those with an index of 7–10 had a 17% mortality and a 92% morbidity (Table 2).

The presence of necrosis as an isolated finding also correlated with subsequent patient morbidity and mortality [2]. Patients with no necrosis had no mortality and only 6% morbidity, while those with 50% necrosis had a 25% mortality and a 75% morbidity, and those with greater than 50% necrosis had an 11% mortality and a 100% morbidity.

CT Detection of Complications of Acute Pancreatitis

Fluid Collections. Fluid collections develop in as many as 50% or more of patients with acute pancreatitis [17]. In many cases, the collections resolve spontaneously. This can be confirmed by serial ultrasound or CT (Fig. 6).

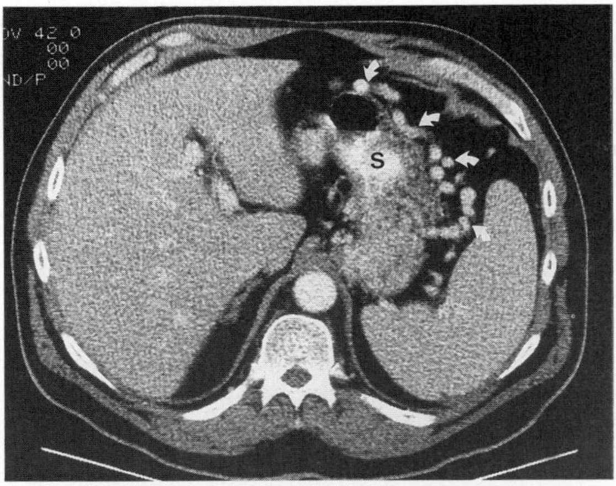

a

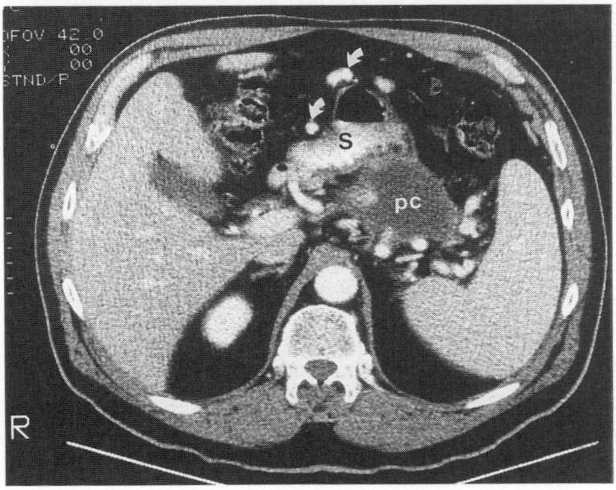

b

Fig. 6a,b. Acute pancreatitis: pseudocyst and splenic vein occlusion. **a** DCT shows contrast enhancement of multiple perigastric varices (*arrows*). **b** Scan at a lower level shows a pseudocyst (*pc*) in the tail of the pancreas and additional perigastric varices (*arrows*). *s*, Stomach

In other patients, however, the collections can persist, enlarge, become secondarily infected, or erode into contiguous structures. These persistent or enlarging collections and their secondary complications can be detected by CT and a decision regarding surgical or percutaneous drainage can be made. The presence of infection within a fluid collection can be confirmed with CT-guided fine-needle aspiration [18]. If percutaneous drainage is to be performed, CT should be obtained to define the precise anatomic relationship of the collection to surrounding structures so that the catheter can be placed safely in the appropriate location [19].

Vascular Complications. Vascular involvement by acute pancreatitis is common and can be detected accurately by DCT. Complications include erosion of pancreatic or peripancreatic arteries with acute hemorrhage (Fig. 5), formation of pseudoaneurysms, and occlusion of branches of the portal venous system with formation of varices (Fig. 6) [1, 20].

Biliary and Gastrointestinal Involvement. CT is quite accurate in detecting involvement or associated abnormalities of the biliary and gastrointestinal tract. Biliary tract abnormalities include calculi in the common bile duct, a frequent etiology of acute pancreatitis, and common bile duct obstruction. CT can demonstrate obstructive dilatation of the bile ducts and usually can define the etiology, such as stones, edema of the head of the pancreas, or pseudocyst, thus aiding in selection of appropriate treatment [21]. While both CT and contrast studies can detect abnormalities of the gastrointestinal tract caused by acute pancreatitis, CT provides the greatest amount of information [22]. The etiology of the involvement usually can be elucidated (e.g., fluid collection, pseudocyst, or direct extension of the inflammatory process) and the appropriate surgical or interventional treatment can be planned.

Summary

The ability of CT to display the precise cross-sectional anatomy of the pancreas and surrounding organs and structures has made it the most efficacious single imaging modality for evaluation of patients with acute pancreatitis. The use of DCT (automatic table incrementation, dynamic scanning mode, simultaneous intravenous infusion of a large bolus of contrast) has further extended its use for detection of parenchymal necrosis and vascular involvement. CT now plays a central role in diagnosis, prognostication (staging of severity of disease), detection of complications, and guidance for percutaneous techniques.

References

1. Freeny PC (1988) Radiology of acute pancreatitis: diagnosis, detection of complications, and interventional therapy. In: Glazer G, Ranson JHC (eds) Acute pancreatitis: experimental and clinical aspects of pathogenesis and management. Bailliere Tindall, London, pp 275–302
2. Balthazar EJ, Robinson DL, Megibow AJ, Ranson JHC (1990) Acute pancreatitis: value of CT in establishing prognosis. Radiology 174:331–336
3. Freeny PC, Lawson TL (1983) Radiology of the pancreas. Springer, Berlin Heidelberg New York, pp 169–396
4. Freeny PC (1984) Computed tomography of the pancreas. Clin Gastroenterol 13:791–818
5. Balthazar EJ, Ranson JHC, Naidich DP et al. (1985) Acute pancreatitis: prognostic value of CT. Radiology 156:767–772

6. Balthazar EJ (1989) CT diagnosis and staging of acute pancreatitis. Radiol Clin North Am 27:19–37
7. Beger HG, Maier W, Block S, Büchler M (1986) How do imaging methods influence the surgical strategy in acute pancreatitis? In: Malfertheiner P, Ditchuneit H (eds) Diagnostic procedures in pancreatic disease. Springer, Berlin Heidelberg New York, pp 54–60
8. Beger HG, Büchler M (1986) Outcome of necrotizing pancreatitis in relation to morphological parameters. In: Malfertheiner P, Ditchuneit H (eds) Diagnostic procedures in pancreatic disease. Springer, Berlin Heidelberg New York, pp 130–132
9. Ranson JHC (1982) Etiological and prognostic factors in human acute pancreatitis: a review. Am J Gastroenterol 9:633–638
10. Wilson C, Heath DI, Imrie CW (1990) Prediction of outcome in acute pancreatitis: a comparative study of APACHE II, clinical assessment and multiple factor scoring systems. Br J Surg 77:1260–1264
11. Corfield AP, Cooper MJ, Williamson RCN et al. (1985) Prediction of severity in acute pancreatitis: prospective comparison of three prognostic indices. Lancet 2:403–406
12. MacMahon MJ, Playforth MJ, Pickford IR (1980) A comparative study of methods for the prediction of the severity of attacks of acute pancreatitis. Br J Surg 67:22–25
13. Kivisaari L, Somer K, Standertskjold-Nordenstam C-G et al. (1983) Early detection of acute fulminant pancreatitis by contrast-enhanced computed tomography. Scand J Gastroenterol 18:39–41
14. Nordestgaard AG, Wilson SE, Williams RA (1986) Early computerized tomography as a predictor of outcome in acute pancreatitis. Am J Surg 152: 127–132
15. Hill MC, Barkin J, Isikoff MB, Silverstein W, Kalser M (1982) Acute pancreatitis: clinical vs. CT findings. AJR 139:263–269
16. Bradley EL III, Murphy F, Ferguson C (1989) Prediction of pancreatic necrosis by dynamic pancreatography. Ann Surg 210:495–504
17. Gonzalez AC, Bradley EL III, Clements JL Jr (1976) Pseodocyst formation in acute pancreatitis: ultrasonic evaluation of 99 cases. AJR 127:315–317
18. Gerzof SG, Banks PA, Robbins AH, Johnson WC et al. (1987) Early diagnosis of pancreatic infection by computed tomography-guided aspiration. Gastroenterology 93:1315–1320
19. Freeny PC, Lewis GP, Traverso LW, Ryan JA (1988) Infected pancreatic fluid collections: percutaneous catheter drainage. Radiology 167:435–441
20. Vujic I (1989) Vascular complications of pancreatitis. Radiol Clin North Am 27:81–91
21. Rohrmann CA Jr, Baron RL (1989) Biliary complications of pancreatitis. Radiol Clin North Am 27:93–104
22. Safrit HD, Rice RP (1989) Gastrointestinal complications of pancreatitis. Radiol Clin North Am 27:73–79

Prognosis of Acute Pancreatitis

C. NIEDERAU,[1] R. LÜTHEN, J.W. HEISE, and H. BECKER

Introduction

The diagnosis of acute pancreatitis is based on clinical symptoms and signs as well as on increases of serum concentrations of amylase or lipase. Major increases of serum pancreatic enzymes (more than three- to fivefold of the upper normal limit) almost prove the diagnosis of acute pancreatitis in particular when the patient presents with a typical clinical picture. The diagnosis may be further supported by imaging procedures such as ultrasound and computed tomography (CT). However, these imaging techniques as well as all the further laboratory and technical measurements are not needed to confirm the diagnosis but are done in order to assess the severity of pancreatitis and its prognosis.

The severity of pancreatitis varies from a mild, continuously healing edematous form to a severe necrotizing disease with complications at distant extrapancreatic organs and a mortality rate which may exceed 50%. Although there is still no specific therapy for acute pancreatitis, the improvements in supportive care may help to decrease the high mortality in necrotizing pancreatitis. Therefore, it is important to identify patients with necrotizing pancreatitis at the earliest stage possible in order to assure adequate supportive treatment. It is well known that hypovolemic shock due to sequestration of fluid into the retroperitonaeum and other third spaces is a major life-threatening condition during the first 24–48 h [2, 24]. During the early stage of necrotizing pancreatitis a variety of vasoactive and toxic compounds are released into the systemic circulation. These substances are thought to cause the pulmonary, cardiovascular, and renal complications which determine the clinical course during the first 2 weeks. The mortality seen later in the course of necrotizing pancreatitis is usually due to septic complications. Assessment of the prognosis should therefore indicate the severity of the disease and should help to identify which one of the different complications may occur.

Computed tomography (CT) is generally regarded as the gold standard for differentiation between edematous and necrotizing pancreatitis [1, 3].

[1] Department of Medicine, Gastroenterology, Heinrich-Heine-Universität Düsseldorf, Moorenstr. 5, W-4000 Düsseldorf 1, FRG

Beger/Büchler/Malfertheiner (Eds.)
Standards in Pancreatic Surgery

Table 1. Prognostic factors in scoring systems

Ranson	Imrie (Glasgow)
On admission	Within 48 h
Age > 55 years	Albumin < 32 g/l
WCC > 16 000 /mm^3	WCC > 15 000 /mm^3
LDH > 600 U/l	LDH > 600 U/l
AST > 120 U/l	AST or ALT > 100 U/l
Within 48 h	Glucose > 10 mmol/l
Hematocrit fall > 10%	Calcium > 2 mmol/l
Urea rise > 0.9 mmol/l	Urea > 16 mmol/l
Calcium < 2 mmol/l	Age > 55 years
$pO_2 < 60$ mmHg	$pO_2 < 60$ mmHg
Base deficit > 4 mEq/l	(In biliary etiology remove age factor and include transaminases only when either one is >200 U/l)
Fluid loss > 6 l	

Ultrasound is less helpful for this purpose [25]. The present analysis does not further discuss the value of CT because this topic is covered in the chapter by Freeny. Although CT is the most reliable imaging technique to identify necrosis, up to 20% of necrotizing forms may be falsely diagnosed as edematous pancreatitis by CT early after the onset of the disease [3]. Also, edematous pancreatitis may be falsely diagnosed as necrotizing pancreatitis in a considerable percentage of patients during the early stage of the disease [3]. Therefore, additional information based on clinical observations and laboratory measurements are needed to determine the severity and prognosis of acute pancreatitis.

The first widely accepted multifactorial system of grading the severity of pancreatitis was described and applied by Ranson et al. [21–23] (Table 1). This scoring system includes 11 prognostic factors, six of which are determined directly after admission. The further five laboratory and clinical factors are assessed within 24 h after admission. Thus, Ranson's score cannot be fully obtained during the first 2 days of the disease. Imrie et al. [11] have introduced a scoring system slightly modifying Ranson's grading; later they further modified their own scoring system to better evaluate the prognosis in biliary pancreatitis [19] (Table 1). Neither modification of Imrie's score (also called Glasgow score) allows assessment of the prognosis during the first 2 days after admission. This delay in characterizing the severity of pancreatitis is therefore a drawback of all the major standard scoring systems. Recently, the APACHE illness grading system (acute physiology and chronic health evaluation) [12, 16] was used to predict the outcome in acute pancreatitis [15, 26]. The original APACHE system is very complex and difficult to use in clinical routine [12, 16]. A simplified modification, the APACHE II system, utilizes 12 routinely available physiological and laboratory measurements with an additional weighing for age and preadmission health status [13]. The major drawback of the APACHE II system is the need to assess the score on multiple occasions during the course of the disease. Furthermore, the APACHE II system is still more complex and difficult to use than Imrie's or Ranson's system in clinical practice. It has been shown that only the peak of the APACHE II scores during the first 3 days after admission is superior to the older standard scoring systems [15]. Thus, the diagnostic delay using the APACHE II system is even greater than that of the older systems. The APACHE system may, however, be useful to accurately assess the prognosis of patients with a very severe course treated on intensive care units [26].

Despite the combination of CT and one of the scoring systems about 10%–15% of fatal or complicated cases of necrotizing pancreatitis cannot correctly be predicted early in the course of the disease. Therefore, investigators have tried to look for additional and better laboratory and clinical markers to predict a severe and complicated course of pancreatitis [4–8, 10, 14, 16, 18, 20–21, 23]. These laboratory signs include lactate dehydrogenase (LDH; also included in the scoring systems), phospholipase A_2 [6, 20], C-reactive protein (CRP) [4, 5, 18], α_1-antitrypsin [4, 8], α_2-macroglobulin [4, 8], serum methemalbumin [7, 17], granulocyte elastase [8], and trypsinogen-activating peptide [9]. The sensitivity of these laboratory signs for detecting pancreatic necrosis varies between 50% and 93% depending on the cutoff level used for these parameters. As yet, only measurement of LDH and to some degree also determination of CRP are used for this purpose in clinical practice. The other laboratory methods are not standardized and not available to most clinicians. It also remains to be evaluated whether one of these parameters offers significant information in addition to that obtained by the combined use of CT, clinical scoring, and CRP.

Patients and Methods

The present analysis evaluates the prognosis and the course of acute pancreatitis in 123 patients and compares the value of the standard scoring systems with the value of CT and some further laboratory measurements for prediction of severity and outcome of pancreatitis. The study analyzes the course of all patients admitted with acute pancreatitis to the Gastroenterology Unit of the Department of Medicine and of all the patients with acute pancreatitis admitted to the Department of General Surgery of the Heinrich-Heine-University of Düsseldorf. During the period 1987–1990 the present data on the medical and surgical patients with acute pancreatitis were prospectively recorded. Of the 79 patients admitted to the Department of Medicine, seven were later referred to the Department of Surgery. These patients were therefore analyzed as surgical patients. Thus, 72 of the 123 patients (58.5%) were regarded as medical patients. Including the seven patients referred from the Department of Medicine, a total of 51 patients

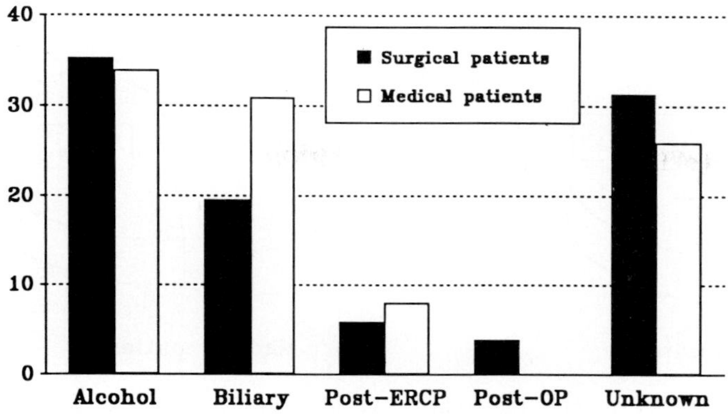

Fig. 1. Etiology of acute pancreatitis in surgical patients (*black bars*) and medical patients (*open bars*)

were analyzed as surgical patients (41.4%). The age of the surgical patients was 52.0 ± 15.1 years (mean ±SD); the age of the medical patients was slightly higher (54.2 ± 13.8 years). Of the surgical patients, 34 were men and 17 were women; of the medical patients, 43 subjects were men and 29 women.

Results

Etiology of Pancreatitis

In both the surgical and medical patients, alcohol was the leading cause of pancreatitis and accounted for about one third of all cases (Fig. 1). The biliary cause of pancreatitis was slightly more frequent in the medical patients (31%) compared with the surgical patients (19.6%). In both the Department of Medicine and the Department of Surgery between 6% and 8% of the pancreatitis cases occurred following ERCP. The etiology could not be determined in about 25%–30% of the cases in the medical and surgical groups.

Severity and Course of Pancreatitis

Pancreatitis was significantly more severe in the surgical patients compared to the medical patients both when assessed by CT or by Ranson's score (Figs. 2, 3). The majority of the medical patients showed an edemateous form of pancreatitis without major necrosis on CT. In contrast, the majority of the surgical patients presented with necrosis as assessed by CT and had a severe course as indicated by a high Ranson score (≥3 positive signs).

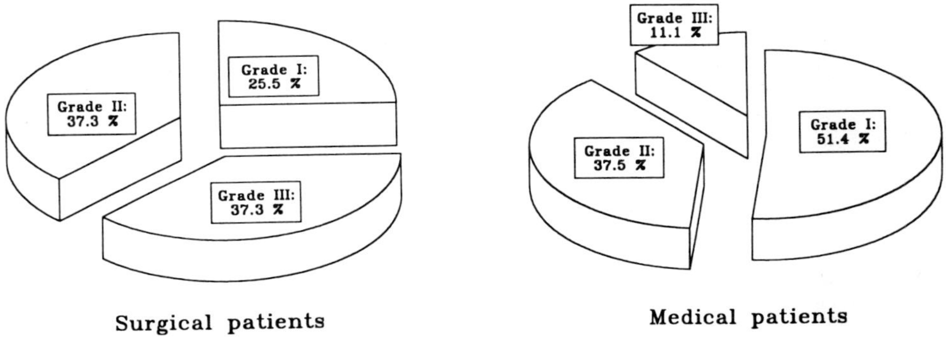

Fig. 2. CT grading of severity of acute pancreatitis. Grade 1 indicates that necrosis is absent on CT. Grade 2 indicates minor to moderate necrosis of less than one-third of the organ. Grade 3 indicates that at least one-third of the organ appeared to be necrotic on CT

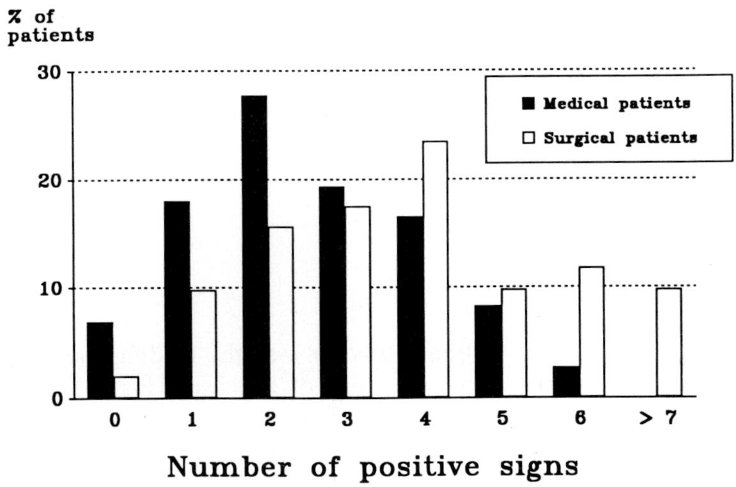

Fig. 3. Severity of pancreatitis according to Ranson's score in medical patients (*black bars*) and surgical patients (*open bars*)

Correspondingly, the mortality of 17.6% seen in the surgical group was significantly greater than the 5.6% mortality observed for the medical patients. However, when mortality was correlated with the severity of pancreatitis, there was no major difference between surgical and medical patients. In neither group was there mortality in the absence of necrosis; mortality ranged between 5% and 10% in the presence of minor to moderate necrosis and increased to approximately 25% in patients with major necrosis (Fig. 4). Mortality from biliary causes appeared to be slightly higher than

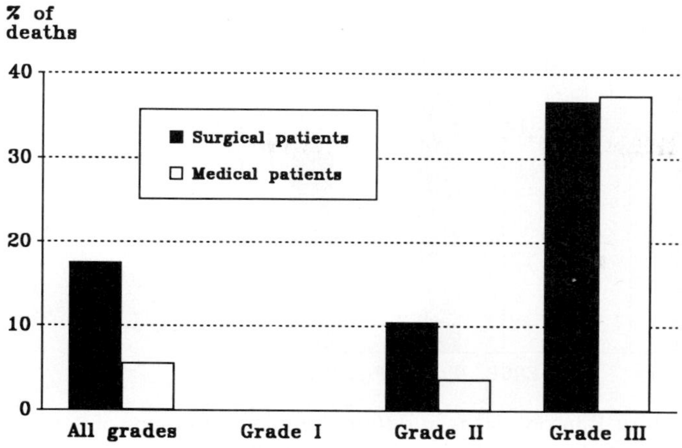

Fig. 4. Mortality according to severity of acute pancreatitis graded by CT in surgical patients (*black bars*) and medical patients (*open bars*)

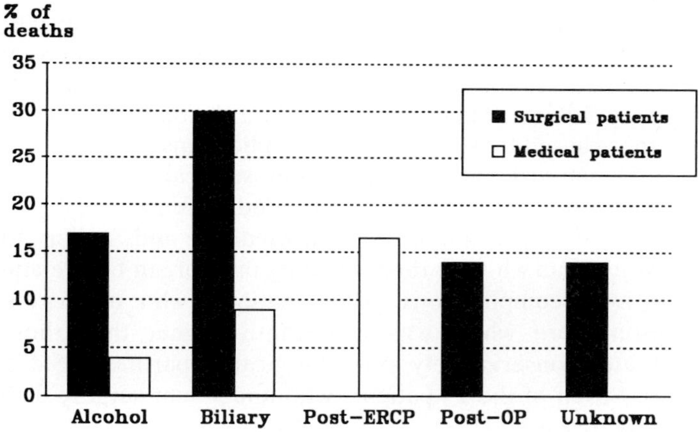

Fig. 5. Mortality from pancreatitis according to etiology in surgical patients (*black bars*) and medical patients (*open bars*)

that caused by other factors, including alcohol, both in the medical and the surgical patients (Fig. 5), although Ranson's score and CT grading were not significantly different between the various etiological groups of patients (Fig. 6).

Survival and Causes of Death

There were 13 deaths in the 123 patients – nine surgical and four medical patients. Interestingly, only 2 of the 13 deaths occurred within the 1st week

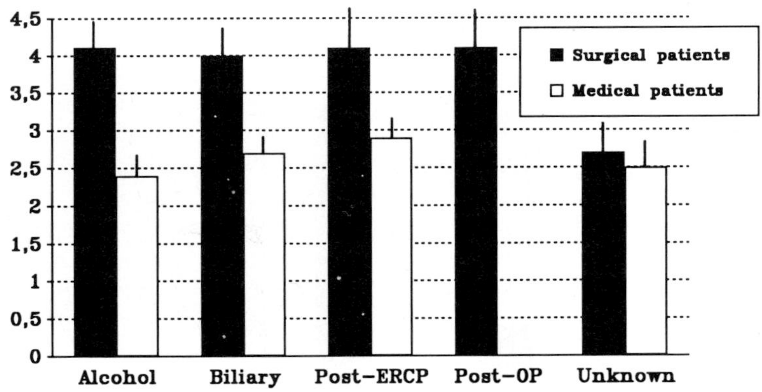

Fig. 6. Number of positive Ranson's signs in different etiological groups of patients in surgical patients (*black bars*) and medical patients (*open bars*)

after admission and there was no mortality during the first 24 h of the disease (Figs. 7, 8). All the remaining deaths were seen late in the course of pancreatitis, i.e., 4–12 weeks after admission. The two patients who died early in the course of pancreatitis both suffered from untreatable cardiovascular and pulmonary failure. Almost all of the late deaths were due to multiorgan failure often caused by severe septic complications.

Only 17 of the 51 surgical patients underwent surgical intervention. Thus, the majority of the surgical patients were treated conservatively. It is the general intention of the Departments of both Medicine and Surgery to operate only on those patients who are threatened by multiorgan failure and by severe septic or local complications. Thus, patients who underwent surgery had a Ranson score which was significantly higher than those patients who were treated conservatively in the Surgical Department (5.2 ± 1.3 versus 3.0 ± 1.6). Seven of the 17 patients who underwent surgery died during the course of the disease (41%).

Prediction of Mortality and Complications

Both CT and Ranson's score reliably predicted a severe, complicated course of pancreatitis and to a lesser degree also proved useful for prediction of a fatal outcome (Fig. 9). The grading of severity by CT was closely correlated to the number of positive Ranson's signs (Fig. 10). Mortality was closely correlated to the failure of the two organs which are most frequently affected during the course of severe pancreatitis, i.e., the kidney and the lung (Figs. 11, 12). Patients who needed intubation and mechanical ventilation had a mortality greater than 40% in both surgical and medical groups; patients who needed hemodialysis had a mortality exceeding 70%,

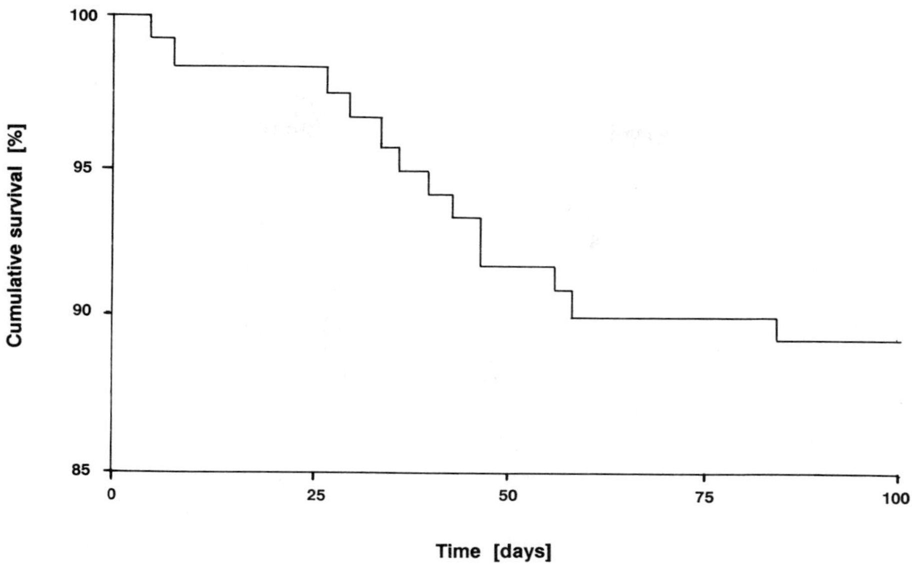

Fig. 7. Cumulative survival in patients with acute pancreatitis. There were 13 deaths among the 123 patients

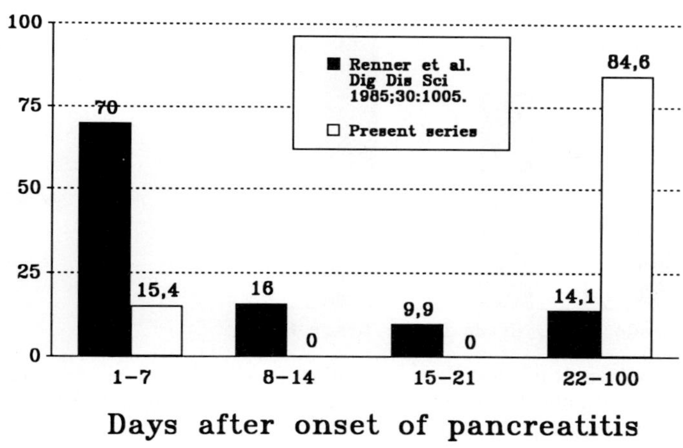

Fig. 8. Percentage of patients dying from acute pancreatitis during different periods of the disease. *Black bars*, data published by Renner et al. [24]; *open bars*, data from the present series

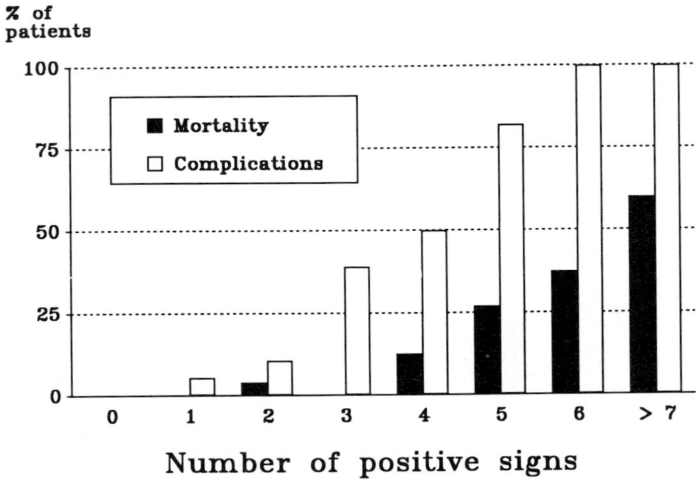

Fig. 9. Mortality and complications according to Ranson's score. *Black bars*, mortality; *open bars*, complications (renal failure, pulmonary failure, septic complications, surgery, death)

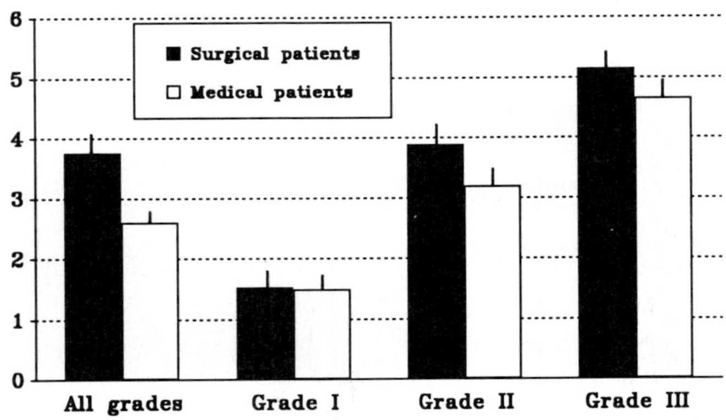

Fig. 10. Number of positive Ranson's signs according to severity of pancreatitis graded by CT in surgical patients (*black bars*) and medical patients (*open bars*)

and those who had both renal and respiratory failure had a mortality exceeding 85%.

The value of Ranson's score for the prediction of a fatal outcome or a complicated course of acute pancreatitis was further analyzed by the method of the receiver operating characteristics (Figs. 13, 14). A complicated course of pancreatitis was defined as the occurrence of at least one of the following complications: respiratory failure, renal failure, severe septic complication,

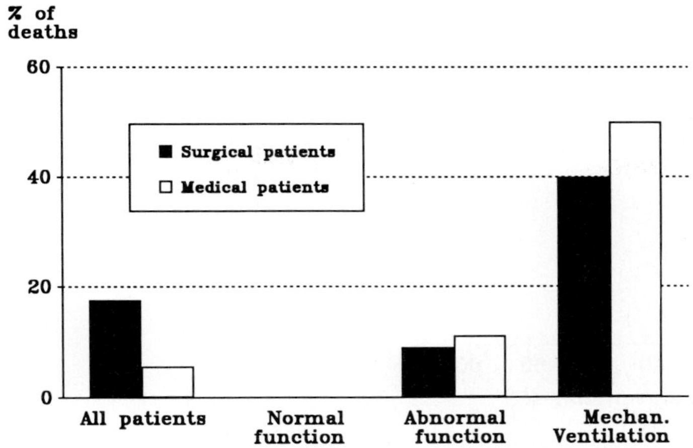

Fig. 11. Mortality from pancreatitis according to respiratory function in surgical patients (*black bars*) and medical patients (*open bars*)

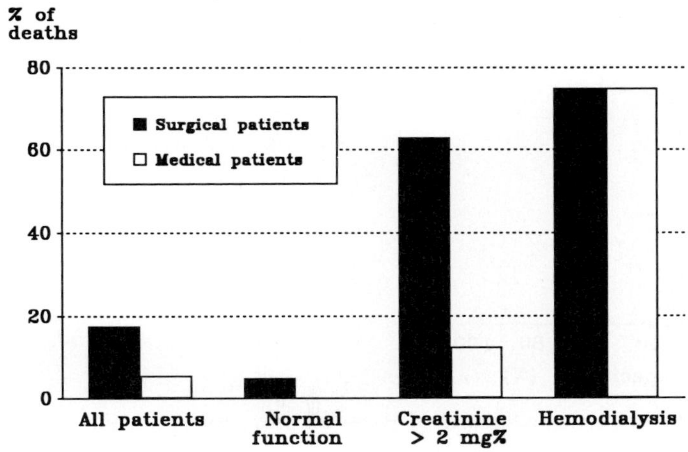

Fig. 12. Mortality from pancreatitis according to renal function in surgical patients (*black bars*) and medical patients (*open bars*)

surgery, or death. A cutoff point of at least three positive Ranson's signs identified 90% of patients or more with a complicated course of pancreatitis; however, the specificity at this cutoff level was only 60% (Fig. 13). Similarly, the cutoff level of three Ranson's signs correctly predicted 90% of the deaths; however, the specificity at this cutoff level for prediction of a fatal outcome was only 40% (Fig. 14). Therefore, an increase in the cutoff level might be helpful for prediction of mortality and probably also for prediction

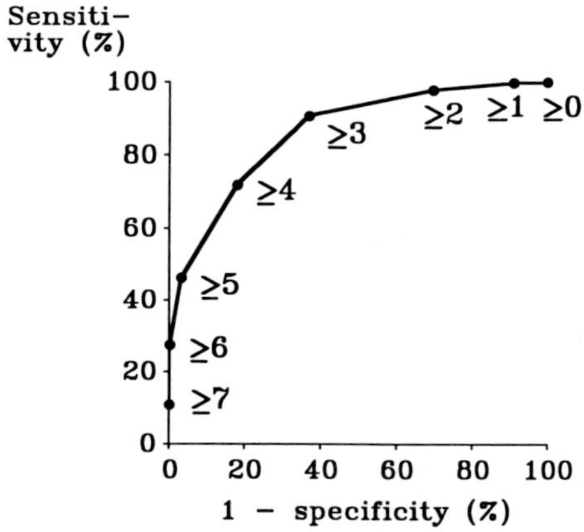

Fig. 13. Receiver operating characteristics of Ranson's score for predicting a complicated course of acute pancreatitis

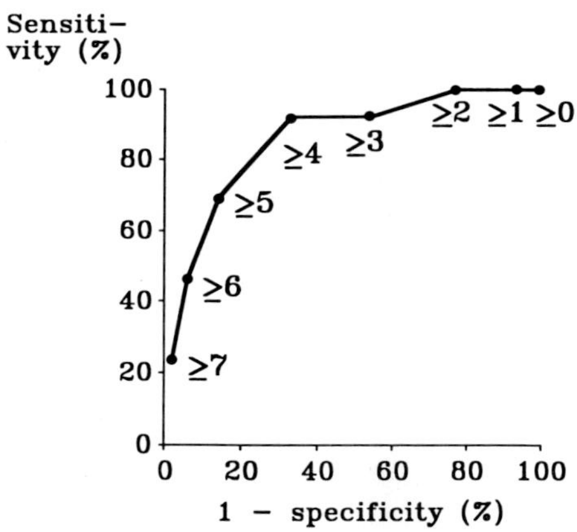

Fig. 14. Receiver operating characteristics of Ranson's score for predicting a fatal outcome

of complications. A cutoff level of at least five Ranson's signs correctly predicted 70% of the deaths with a high specificity exceeding 80% (Fig. 13). A cutoff level of at least four Ranson's signs correctly diagnosed 70% or more of the complications, with the specificity approaching 80% (Fig. 14). Thus, the cutoff level of at least four Ranson's signs appears to be appropriate for prediction of complications, and a cutoff level of at least five Ranson's points might be most helpful for prediction of a fatal outcome.

The positive predictive value at a cutoff of at least three Ranson's signs

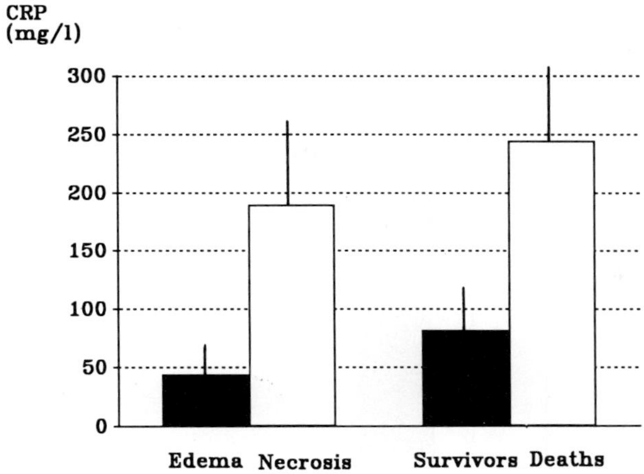

Fig. 15. CRP values versus severity and outcome of pancreatitis. CRP values were determined only in the medical patients

was only 17% for mortality and 61% for complication. The positive predictive value increased at a cutoff of at least four Ranson's signs to 25% for mortality and 71% for complications, and at a cutoff of at least five Ranson's signs to 38% for mortality and 92% for complications. The increase of the cutoff point to at least six or seven Ranson's signs increased the positive predictive values for mortality to 46% and 60%, respectively. All patients who had at least six Ranson's signs had a complicated course of pancreatitis. This type of analysis shows that the clinical grading is suited much better to predicting complications than to predicting a fatal outcome.

The additional measurement of CRP offered only slight advantage compared to the clinical grading and the CT. Nevertheless, CRP values were significantly higher in patients with pancreatic necrosis compared to those with edema. Similarly, CRP values were significantly higher in patients who died during the course of pancreatitis compared with those who survived (Fig. 15). The additional use of CRP for prediction of fatal outcome and complications did not help to increase the sensitivity at the usual cutoff level of at least three Ranson's signs. However, at this cutoff level additional measurements of CRP did increase the poor specificity of clinical scoring by about 10%. As described previously in the literature, we used a cutoff value of 120 mg/l for serum CRP.

In the present series, the age of the patients did not help to predict a fatal outcome or a complicated course when used as a single clinical characteristic. The age of the patients who died from pancreatitis was only slightly higher compared to the patients who survived the disease ($p > 0.05$ by t test; Fig. 16).

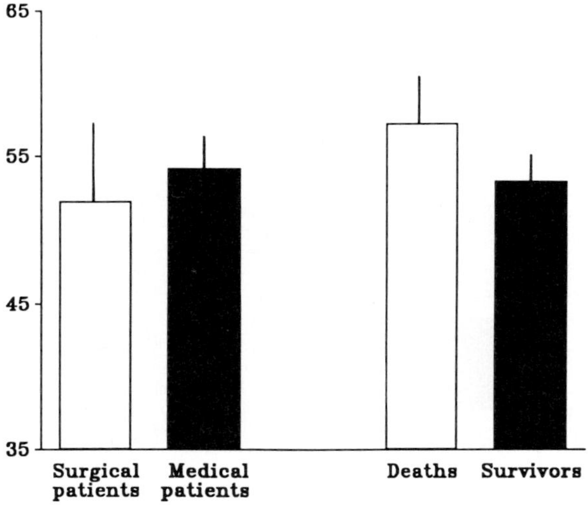

Fig. 16. Age of patients with acute pancreatitis in different groups of patients

Use of Clinical Scores Other than Ranson's Signs

The use of other clinical scores such as Imrie's score or the APACHE II system did not offer major advantages in predicting fatal outcome and complications. The one late death and a number of complications, not predicted by CT or Ranson's signs, were due to late septic complications in patients with moderate necrosis on CT and two or three positive Ranson's signs. Thus, none of the deaths and only a small number of complications not predicted by CT or Ranson's signs would have been picked up by applying other scoring systems. Additional measurements of CRP also failed to predict the one fatal outcome and the majority of complications not predicted by CT or Ranson's score.

Effects of Treatment on Prognosis of Pancreatitis

Of the 79 patients admitted to the Department of Medicine, a total of seven patients were later transferred to the Department of Surgery. Of the total number of 51 surgical patients, one third underwent laporatomy and one third peritoneal lavage. The remaining one third was treated conservatively in the Department of Surgery. Patients who underwent surgery had a high mortality of 41.2%. On the other hand, the patients who were treated conservatively in the Department of Surgery had a mortality of only 5.9%, which was virtually identical to the 5.6% mortality in the patients who were treated in the Department of Medicine.

Discussion

The most important factor for the prognosis of acute pancreatitis is the degree of necrosis. Since CT is the nonoperative gold standard to determine the degree of necrosis in acute pancreatitis [1, 3], the CT grading of severity is one of the most important prognostic factors. The value and the pitfalls of CT are discussed in the chapter by Freeny. The occurrence of pulmonary and renal failure are two other major factors which determine the outcome in acute pancreatitis. In the present series, these complications were often caused by septic complications which generally occurred at late stages of the disease. The other individual clinical characteristics including age were prognostic factors of only minor importance. However, the multifactorial clinical scoring system defined by Ranson [21–23] proved very helpful to determine a complicated course of pancreatitis. In our patients scoring systems other than the one described by Ranson did not offer major advantages. The additional use of CRP might prove useful to decrease the poor specificity of the clinical grading when a cutoff level of at least three Ranson points is used. However, CRP measurements did not significantly increase the sensitivity of CT or of the clinical grading. The number of positive Ranson's signs was less helpful for prediction of a fatal outcome. The kind of treatment did not appear as a major prognostic factor. All patients in the present series received maximal supportive care. Only those patients underwent surgery in whom severe septic complications occurred or in whom a multiorgan failure threatened to kill the patient. Accordingly, patients who underwent surgery had the most severe disease (mean Ranson's score = 5.2 ± 1.3). The patients who were treated conservatively in the Surgical Department had virtually the same mortality compared with the patients which were treated in the Department of Medicine.

The etiology of pancreatitis also appeared to be of minor importance for prediction of outcome. However, patients with biliary pancreatitis had a somewhat higher mortality compared to patients with other etiology including alcohol. This phenomenon was seen in both for the medical and surgical patients. However, the severity of biliary and alcoholic pancreatitis was very similar when graded by CT or clinical scoring.

Thus, from the present results the standard methods for prediction of prognosis are the CT (with bolus injection of contrast medium) and a clinical grading system. Ranson's score [22] was as good as Imrie's score [11, 19]. The use of one of the various laboratory markers to indicate the degree of necrosis might offer limited additional help. As yet, in most hospitals only CRP is used in clinical practice for this purpose.

In the literature, the majority of mortality from acute pancreatitis occurred at two different stages of the disease [24]. One significant part of deaths was seen in the early phase of the disease, and a considerable number of deaths even occurred during the first 24 h. A high percentage of the early deaths were caused by hypovolemic shock or untreatable cardiovascular failure [24]. The other major group of fatalities was seen during the late stages of the disease often caused by septic complications [2, 24]. This picture, which was described by several previous reports, has apparently changed during recent years. In the present series, only a few deaths were seen in the early phase of the acute pancreatitis. The great majority of fatalities occurred at late stages, i.e., between 4 and 12 weeks after admission. Almost all late deaths were associated with multiorgan failure caused by septic complications. The decrease in the percentage of early deaths might be due to improvements in supportive care and in particular due to the advances of intensive care medicine.

References

1. Balthazar EJ, Robinson DL, Megibow AJ, Ranson JHC (1990) Acute pancreatitis: values of CT in establishing prognosis. Radiology 174:331–336
2. Beger HG, Bittner R, Block S, Büchler M (1986) Bacterial contamination of pancreatic necrosis. Gastroenterology 91:433–438
3. Block S, Maier W, Bittner R, Büchler M, Malfertheiner P, Beger HG (1986) Identification of pancreas necrosis in severe acute pancreatitis: imaging procedures versus clinical staging. Gut 27:1035–1042
4. Büchler M, Malfertheiner P, Schoetensack C, Uhl W, Beger HG (1986) Sensitivity of antiproteases, complement factors and C-reactive protein in detecting pancreatic necrosis. Results of a prospective clinical study. Int J Pancreatol 1:227–235
5. Büchler M, Malfertheiner P, Uhl W, Beger HG (1987) C-reaktives Protein als Entzündungs- und Nekrosemarker in der Gastroenterologie. Med Klin 82: 180–185
6. Büchler M, Malfertheiner P, Schädlich H, Nevalainen TJ, Friess H, Beger HG (1989) Role of phospholipase A_2 in human acute pancreatitis. Gastroenterology 97:1521–1526
7. Geokas MC, Rinderknecht H, Walberg CB, Weissmann R (1974) Methemalbumin in the diagnosis of acute hemorrhagic pancreatitis. Ann Intern Med 81:483–486
8. Groß V, Schölmerich J, Leser HG, Salm R, Lausen M, Rückauer K, Schöffel U, Lay L, Heinisch A, Farthmann EH, Gerok W (1990) Granulocyte elastase in assessment of severity of acute pancreatitis. Comparison with acute phase proteins C-reactive protein, alpha$_1$-antitrypsin, and protease inhibitor alpha$_2$-macroglobulin. Dig Dis Sci 35:97–105
9. Gudgeon AM, Hurley P, Patel G, Shenkin A, Imrie CW, Heath DI, Jehanli A, Wilson C, Austen BM, Hermon-Taylor J (1990) Trypsinogen activating peptides assay in the early prediction of severity of acute pancreatitis. Lancet 335:4–8
10. Hjelmqvist B, Wattsgard C, Borgström A, Lasson A, Nyman U, Aspelin P, Ohlsson K (1989) Early diagnosis and classification in acute pancreatitis. Digestion 44:177–183
11. Imrie CW (1974) Observation in acute pancreatitis. Br J Surg 61:539–544
12. Kanus WA, Zimmermann JE, Wagner DP, Draper EA, Lawrence DE (1981) Apache – acute physiology and chronic health evaluation: a physiologically based classification system. Crit Care Med 9:591–597
13. Knaus WA, Draper EA, Wagner DP, Zimmermann JE (1985) Apache II: a severity of disease classification system. Crit Care Med 13:818–829
14. Lankisch PG, Schirren CA (1990) Increased body weight as a prognostic parameter for complications in the course of acute pancreatitis. Pancreas 5: 626–629

15. Larvin M, McMahaon MJ (1989) Apache-II score for assessment and monitoring of acute pancreatitis. Lancet ii:201–204
16. Le Gall JR, Loirat P, Alperovitch A (1984) A simplified acute physiology score for ICU patients. Crit Care Med 12:975–977
17. McMahon MJ, Playforth MJ, Pickford IR (1980) A comparative study of methods for the prediction of severity of attacks of acute pancreatitis. Br J Surg 67:22–25
18. Mayer AD, McMahon MJ, Bowen M, Cooper EH (1984) C-reactive protein: an aid to assessment and monitoring of acute pancreatitis. J Clin Pathol 27:207–211
19. Osborne DH, Imrie CW, Carter DC (1981) Biliary surgery in the same admission for gallstone-associated acute pancreatitis. Br J Surg 68:758–761
20. Poulakkainen P, Valtonen V, Paananen A, Schröder T (1987) C-reactive protein (CRP) and serum phospholipase A_2 in the assessment of the severity of acute pancreatitis. Gut 28:764–771
21. Ranson JHC, Spencer FC (1978) The role of peritoneal lavage in severe acute pancreatitis. Ann Surg 187:565–575
22. Ranson JHC, Rifkind KM, Roses DF (1974) Prognostic signs and the role of operative management in acute pancreatitis. Surg Gynecol Obstet 139:69–81
23. Ranson JHC (1979) The timing of biliary surgery in acute pancreatitis. Ann Surg 189:654–663
24. Renner IG, Savage WT, Pantoja JL, Renner VJ (1985) Death due to acute pancreatitis: a retrospective analysis of 405 autopsy cases. Dig Dis Sci 10: 1005–1018
25. Schölmerich J, Johannesson T, Brobmann G, Wimmer B, Thiedemann B, Groß V, Gerok W, Farthmann EH (1989) Die Sonographie bei akuten Pankreatitis-Diagnose, Ätiologieklärung und Prognoseabschätzung. Ultraschall 10:290–294
26. Wilson C, Heath DI, Imrie CW (1990) Prediction of outcome in acute pancreatitis: a comparative study of Apache-II, clinical assessment and multiple factor scoring systems. Br J Surg 77:1260–1264

Staging of Acute Pancreatitis

H. Röding[1]

Introduction

The staging of diseases and injuries is indispensable for evaluating therapeutic results, exchanging information among researchers, and measuring medical or surgical progress. Staging presumes the disease to be gradable according to objective or subjective criteria and related to some prospective event, and it therefore necessarily involves prognosis. Regarding the field of surgery one can note that many diseases and injuries, including acute pancreatitis, can be graded according to the degree of severity, and that the prospective event is generally either of two alternatives, either to die or to survive. If the aim is to evaluate a set of conditions by objective methods, the problem can be reduced to a correlation between quantifiable inputs and an alternative outcome or output, i.e., to establishing a dose-response relationship that expands the concept of dose beyond its conventional definition in pharmacology.

In evaluating the results of burn treatment, we developed an interest in probit analysis, elaborated by Bliss in England in 1935 and now a well-established method for calculating relationships between quantified inputs and alternative outputs. It is of value in pharmacology, toxicology, radiotherapy, burn treatment, and some microbiological problems. The surgical literature from this point of view, now encompassing several hundred examples, demonstrates that such dose-response relationships do not only exist in special fields but are a general principle in medicine, including several aspects of acute pancreatitis and its treatment.

Staging of Acute Pancreatitis

Staging of acute pancreatitis is possible by (a) clinical signs, generally combined with laboratory parameters, (b) organ-specific scales and scores, (c) imaging methods, (d) scores developed for examining the critically ill, and (e) measuring organ-system functions.

[1] Ernst von Bergmann Clinics, Dept. of Surgery, Div. of General Surgery, Charlottenstraße 72, 0-1562 Potsdam, FRG

Beger/Büchler/Malfertheiner (Eds.)
Standards in Pancreatic Surgery

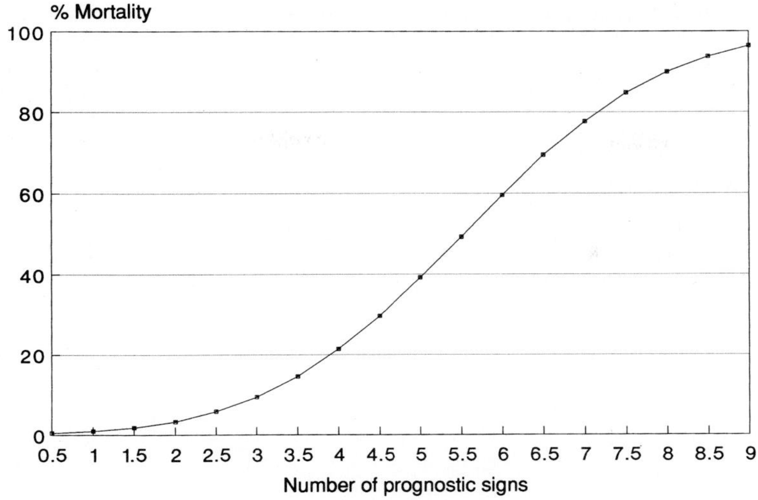

Fig. 1. Mortality by number of prognostic signs. Curve smoothed by probit method. (From Ranson 1982)

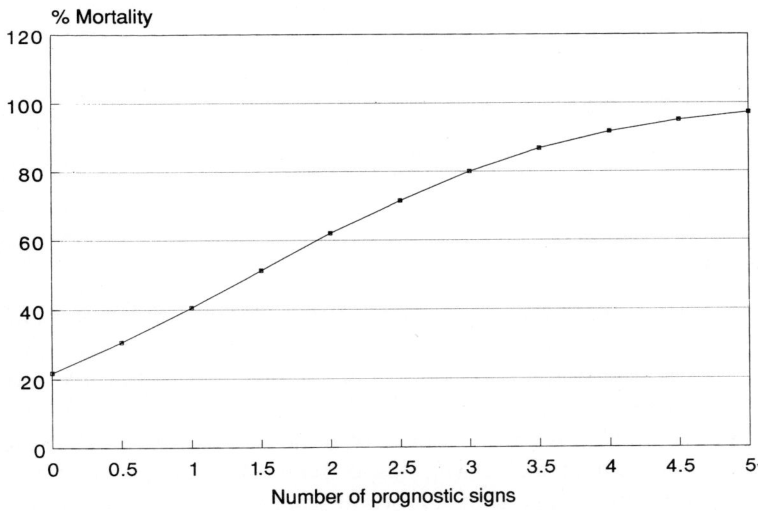

Fig. 2. Mortality by number of prognostic signs. Curve smoothed by probit method. (From Dammann et al. 1981)

Table 1. Staging based on computed tomographic criteria

<table>
<tr><th></th><th>Pérez et al. (1990)</th><th>Delaby et al. (1990)</th><th>Nordestgaard et al. (1986)</th></tr>
<tr><td>Normal pancreas</td><td>A</td><td>A</td><td>A</td></tr>
<tr><td>Enlargement</td><td>B</td><td>B</td><td rowspan="2">B</td></tr>
<tr><td>Peripancreatic inflammation</td><td>C</td><td>C</td></tr>
<tr><td>Extrapancreatic fluid (1)</td><td>D</td><td>D</td><td>C</td></tr>
<tr><td>Extrapancreatic fluid (2)</td><td>E</td><td rowspan="2">E</td><td rowspan="2">D</td></tr>
<tr><td>Gas, retropancreatic fluid</td><td>F</td></tr>
</table>

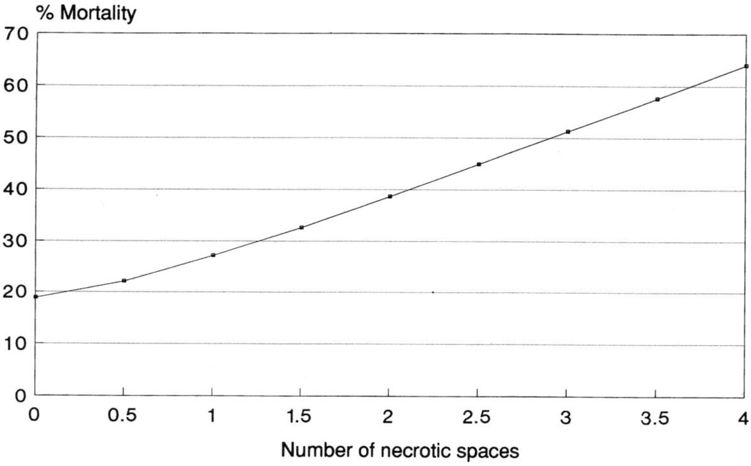

Fig. 3. Mortality in acute pancreatitis by number of necrotic spaces. (From Beger et al. 1982)

Organ Specific Scales

A number of organ specific scales have been developed in recent years. That proposed by Ranson has been widely adapted. Other scales have been put forward by Osborne, Blamey, Bank, Dammann, Fan, Imrie, and Kümmerle. Such scales all include clinical signs and results of various laboratory investigations. Figures 1 and 2 present the results of Ranson (1982) and of Dammann et al. (1981), respectively. The adaption of the curves to the results of observation by probit analysis is, in a biometric sense, ideal.

Scores Based on Imaging Procedures

According to the radiological literature staging by imaging diagnosis provides substantial standardization. Typical scores are presented in Table 1.

Table 2. Mortality by APACHE II score: personal series

APACHE II score	*n*	%	95% confidence interval
0–9	6/33	18.2	5.0–31.3
10–19	15/47	31.9	18.6–45.2
20–29	20/32	62.5	45.7–79.3
⩾30	17/18	94.4	83.9–100.0

Table 3. Mortality by APACHE II score: published reports

APACHE II score	Alberto Dougnac et al. (1989)	Lehmkuhl et al. (1986)	Sage et al. (1986)	Giangiuliani et al. (1989)
0				
	0.0%	3.0%	13.3%	
5				2%
	2.0%	5.0%		
10			16.5%	
	6.0%	10%		
15				10%
	21%	19%		
20			28.6%	
	26%	24%		
25				50%
	49%	55%		
30				
35	53%	70%	63.4%	80%
40				100%

However, the number of patients scored in this way up to now does not allow reliable calculations. Nevertheless, there is no doubt that staging by this method is in fact possible and that there is a rather strong correlation between results of imaging methods and those of organ-specific scales. Beger, for example, noted the relationship between the number of involved necrotic spaces and mortality (Fig. 3).

Scores for the Critically Ill

Staging of acute necrotizing pancreatitis is also possible by scales and scores developed for the examination and the prognosis of critically ill patients, regardless of the underlying disease. We first reported on this in 1989; however, we disagree with Larvin and McMahon (1989), who see advantages over organ-specific scores. We demonstrate here our own results from 1970 to 1990, compared with those from medical and surgical ICUs and studies on the anesthetic risk, using the APACHE II score (Tables 2, 3), HIS score (Tables 4, 5), and ASA score (Tables 6, 7). Some studies report extremely low mortality rates in the treatment of NP, but in our opinion one should not generalize from such results. Severe acute pancreatitis remains one of the most life-threatening situations in all ICUs, and therefore its results cannot be better than average.

Table 4. Mortality by HIS score: personal series

HIS score	*n*	%	95% confidence interval
0–6	6/52	11.5	2.9–20.2
7–12	28/51	54.9	41.2–68.6
13–18	17/19	89.5	75.7–100.0
19–24	7/7	100.0	–

Table 5. Mortality by HIS score: published reports

HIS score	Lehmkuhl et al. (1986)
0	
3	1.0%
6	6.0%
9	25%
12	75%
15	95%
18	100%
21	

Table 6. Mortality by ASA score: personal series

ASA score	*n*	%	95% confidence interval
2	6/40	15.0	3.9–26.1
3	22/52	42.3	28.9–55.7
4	28/36	77.8	64.0–91.6
5	2/2	100.0	–

Table 7. Mortality by ASA score: published reports

ASA score	Marx et al. (1973)	Farrow et al. (1982)	Cohen et al. (1988)	Forrest et al. (1990)
1	0.1	0.3	0.1	0.0
2	0.5	0.9	0.2	0.1
3	4.4	5.3	1.2	0.6
4	23.5	25.9	7.7	8.0
5	50.8	57.8	33.6	–

Staging by Multiorgan Failure

Finally, staging of acute pancreatitis can also be carried out by observing the function of organ systems and multiorgan failure (MOF). It is common in most surgical clinics for there to be a failure of one, two, or more organ

Table 8. Duration of MOF and number of affected organ systems (from Knaus et al. 1981)

	Duration of MOF		
	1 day	4 days	7 days
One organ system	25.6 (24.2–27.1)	34.5 (32.0–37.0)	36.2 (33.1–39.3)
Two organ systems	51.0 (48.1–53.9)	59.9 (55.8–64.0)	66.1 (61.0–71.3)
Three or more organ systems	82.3 (78.9–85.7)	95.6 (92.4–98.8)	98.1 (95.5–100.0)

systems when surgical management is impending. The findings on MOF reported by Knaus et al. (1981; Table 8) reveal relationships between age, number of failed organs, and duration of MOF, on the one hand, and mortality rate, on the other. These results are applicable to pancreatitis.

Conclusion

We can conclude with two observations. (a) Any severe, acute necrotizing pancreatitis is a challenge to the surgeon. Based on our own experiences we must confess that the policy of operative treatment does not necessarily mean a reduction in mortality to an acceptable level. We try, often in the worst situations, to ameliorate a severe course or to save a life by operative measures when conservative treatment has failed. (b) Staging of acute pancreatitis is possible by various methods, the results of which are interrelated. If staging is based on objective criteria, one must consider that this practice assumes laws of biometric probability, but not those of mathematical accuracy. Therefore staging can contribute only prognostic signs or impressions. Characteristic of any prognosis remains the fact that we cannot know whether it is correct or not at the time it is made. Therefore any result of staging which indicates a very poor prognosis must never allow therapeutic nihilism or the interruption of intensive surgical and medical care.

References

Alberto Dougnac L, Domingo Arriagada M, Andresen HM et al. (1989) Sistemas de evaluacion de gravedad: APACHE, SAPS. Experienca nacional en una unidad de terapia intensiva medica. Rev Med Chil 117:1357–1362

Beger HG, Block S, Krautzberger W, Bittner R (1982) Die nekrotisierende Pankreatitis. Chirurg 53:784–789

Cohen MM, Duncan PG, Tate RB (1988) Does anesthesia contribute to operative mortality? JAMA 260:2859–2863

Dammann HG, Döpner M, von Wichert P, Harders H (1981) Die Beurteilung der Frühprognose der akuten Pankreatitis. Zenttalbl Chir 106:154–160
Delaby J, Rieux D, Coppo B et al. (1990) Pancréatites aigues: valeur pronostique de la tomodensitomètrie précoce couplée aux criterés de Ranson et son ròle dans la surveillance de évolution. Gastroenterol Clin Biol 14:209–216
Demmy TL, Burch JM, Feliciano DV, Mattox KL, Jordan GL (1988) Comparison of multiple-parameter prognostic systems in acute pancreatitis. Am J Surg 156:492–496
Farrow SC, Fowkes FGR, Lunn JN, Robertson I, Samuel P (1982) Epidemiology in anaesthesia. II. Factors affecting mortality in hospital. Br J Anaesth 54:811–817
Forrest JB, Rehder K, Goldsmith CH et al. (1990) Multicenter study of general anesthesia. Anesthesiology 72:252–268
Giangiuliani G, Mancini A, Gui D (1989) Validation of a severity of illness score (APACHE II) in a surgical intensive care unit. Intensive Care Med 15:519–522
Knaus WA, Zimmermann JE, Wagner DP, Draper EA, Lawrence DE (1981) APACHE – acute physiology and chronic health evaluation: physiologically based classification system. Crit Care Med 9:591–597
Larvin M, McMahon M (1989) APACHE-II score for assessment and monitoring of acute pancreatitis. Lancet ii:201–205
Lehmkuhl P, Lips U, Pichlmayr I (1986) Der Hannover Intensive Score (HIS) als neues Klassifikationssystem zu Verlaufskontrollen und Prognosestellung bei Intensivpatienten. Med Klin 81:235–240
Marx GF, Matea CV, Orkin LR (1973) Computer analysis of postanaesthetic deaths. Anasthesiology 39:54–58
Nordestgaard AG, Wilson SE, Williams RA (1986) Early computerized tomography as a predictor of outcome in acute pancreatitis. Am J Surg 152:127–132
Pérez C, Llauger J, Andreu J, Palmer J, Puig J (1990) Acute pancreatitis: value of CT as a predictor of outcome. Eur J Radiol 10:118–123
Ranson JHC (1982) Etiological and prognostic factors in human acute pancreatitis: a review. Am J Gastroenterol 77:633–638
Röding H (1985) Prognosen chirurgischer Erkrankungen und Schädigungen. Barth, Leipzig
Röding H (1987) Dosis-Wirkungs-Beziehungen in der klinischen Medizin: Zufälligkeit oder Prinzip? Z Klin Med 42:2159–2166
Röding H, Krenzien J, Röding T (1989) Acute pancreatitis-physiologic impairment and outcome 33rd World-Congress of Surgery, 10–16 Sept 1989, Toronto
Sage WM, Rosenthal MH, Silverman JF (1986) Is intensive care worth it? An assessment of input and outcome for the critically ill. Crit Care Med 14:777–782
Takada T, Yasuda H, Uchiyama K, Hasegawa H, Shikata J, Nagai J (1988) CT score and the severity of acute pancreatitis. Int Surg 73:94–98

Is Differentiation of Haemorrhagic from Oedematous Acute Pancreatitis of Clinical Importance?

P. Curley[1] and M.J. McMahon[1]

Introduction

The presence of "prune juice" fluid in the peritoneal cavity predicts severe acute pancreatitis with a specificity of more than 80% and a sensitivity of about 60% [1]. This test is invasive, has the potential to cause visceral perforation and is not routinely used to formulate a prognosis in patients with acute pancreatitis. Nevertheless, if it is carefully performed, the risk of misadventure is small and with the possible exception of the APACHE II score [2, 3], it provides the best indication of an impending severe attack when the patient is admitted to hospital. However, since it remains to be proven that introduction of intensive therapy at the time of the development of prognostic indicators of a severe attack can influence outcome or attenuate severity, it is difficult – in our opinion – to justify the routine use of peritoneal lavage in patients with acute pancreatitis. We continue to use lavage in patients who have clinical evidence of a severe attack because it may show that the diagnosis of acute pancreatitis is erroneous [4].

"Prune juice" peritoneal fluid is the hallmark of "haemorrhagic", as opposed to "oedematous", acute pancreatitis. The dark, characteristic colour is believed to be derived largely from methaemalbumin [5–7], and it is usually assumed that there is associated tissue necrosis in or around the pancreas. Whilst it is known that "prune juice" predicts physiological instability and perhaps hypotension and multiple organ failure, it is not known to what extent it predicts the presence of significant pancreatic or peripancreatic necrosis and, in turn, the need for percutaneous drainage or operative intervention for necrosis, abscess or pseudocyst during the patient's hospital course.

We have analysed 556 attacks of acute pancreatitis to assess the ability of "haemorrhagic" pancreatitis to predict local pancreatic rather than systemic complications.

[1] University Department of Surgery, General Infirmary, Leeds England

Beger/Büchler/Malfertheiner (Eds.)
Standards in Pancreatic Surgery

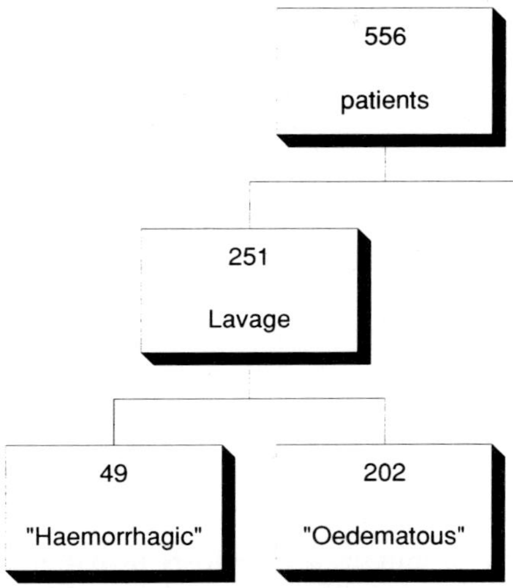

Fig. 1. Breakdown of 556 patients with acute pancreatitis assessed between 1982 and 1988

Methods

A Seldinger technique was used (Arrow peritoneal dialysis catheter) for peritoneal lavage. Following bladder emptying, a 0.5-cm midline skin incision was made and the trocar introduced obliquely below the umbilicus towards the pelvis. Volume and colour of free peritoneal fluid were recorded, and lavage with 1 l warmed normal saline was performed. Aspiration of dark peritoneal fluid or a lavage return fluid of midstraw colour or darker was defined as "haemorrhagic" acute pancreatitis [8]. Development of pancreatic collections was confirmed at laparotomy, by ultrasound or CT scan, or at post-mortem examination.

Between 1982 and 1988, 556 patients with acute pancreatitis were assessed. Of these, 305 had mild attacks and did not undergo peritoneal lavage. Of the 251 patients lavaged, 49 had haemorrhagic pancreatitis (Fig. 1).

Patients

Of the 251 patients studied, 130 were female and 121 were male. There was a slight preponderance of men in the "haemorrhagic" group and of women in the "oedematous" group (Table 1). Biliary induced attacks accounted for 57% of all attacks, but for almost 60% of "oedematous" attacks (Fig. 2). The mean age was approximately 60 years in both groups, as previously reported in our patient population. The delay from admission to peritoneal lavage was slightly longer in the "haemorrhagic" group.

Table 1. Clinical data of 251 patients with acute pancreatitis who underwent lavage

	Haemorrhagic	Oedematous
n	49	202
M:F	29:20	92:110
Gallstones	24 (49%)	120 (59%)
Alcohol	10 (20%)	37 (18%)
Idiopathic	15 (31%)	45 (23%)
Age (years)	60.22 ± 12.5	59.09 ± 18.5
Onset to lavage (hours)	33.7 ± 23.6	26.99 ± 22.9

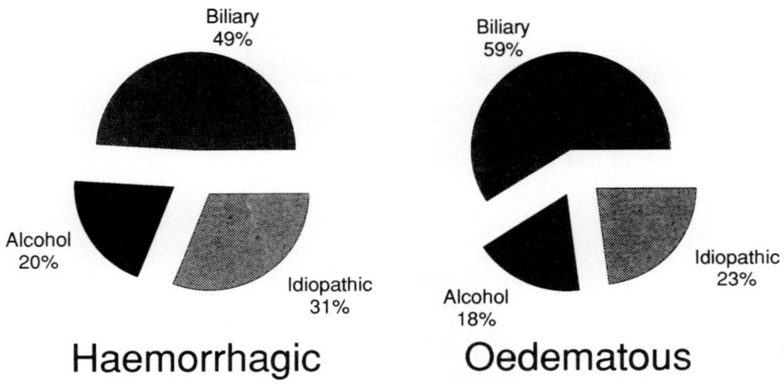

Fig. 2. Aetiology of pancreatic attacks among the 251 patients who underwent lavage

Results

Multiple Organ Failure

Twenty-two percent of "haemorrhagic" attacks and 1.5% of "oedematous" attacks were associated with the development of multi-organ failure.

Pancreatic Collection

Thirty-five percent of "haemorrhagic" attacks were associated with the development of a pancreatic collection while only 3.5% of "oedematous" attacks progressed to this complication (Fig. 3). Following development of a collection, outcome was poor in both groups (Fig. 4).

Mortality

Of the "haemorrhagic" group 33% died, compared with 5% of the "oedematous" group.

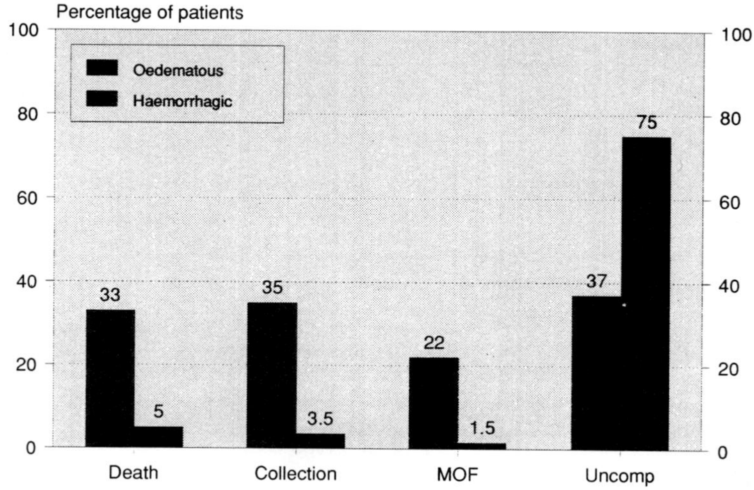

Fig. 3. Outcome of disease in 251 patients lavaged

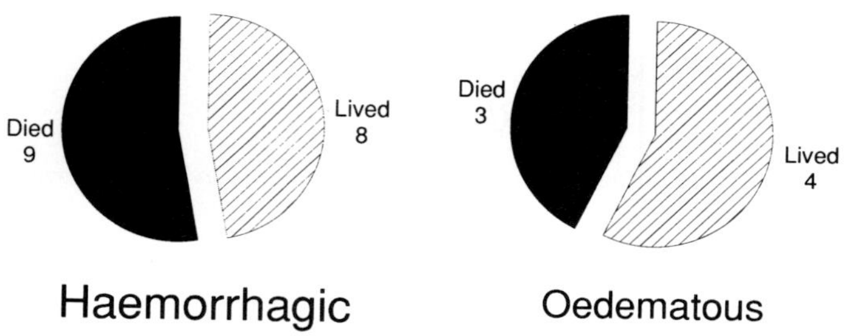

Fig. 4. Mortality from pancreatic collections among patients with haemorrhagic and oedematous attacks

Despite the higher incidence of morbidity and mortality in the haemorrhagic group, over one third of all such attacks were associated with an uneventful course. The fact that over 60% of attacks of "haemorrhagic" pancreatitis did not develop a pancreatic collection is of interest, since such collections are frequently the sequelae of pancreatic/peripancreatic necrosis. Since there is growing evidence that early intervention in infected pancreatic necrosis is an important treatment strategy, aimed at decreasing the mortality from severe acute pancreatitis, the potential for introducing infection via peritoneal lavage should not be overlooked. The poor correlation between "haemorrhagic" pancreatitis and the development of the complications of pancreatic necrosis in this group of patients strongly suggests that while "haemorrhagic" fluid does indicate the presence of a more severe attack, it is of little value in planning treatment strategies.

Discussion

Haemorrhagic acute pancreatitis is associated with a poor prognosis compared with the oedematous form of the condition. The toxic effects in haemorrhagic pancreatitis are mainly systemic in nature, and aggressive fluid therapy can prevent the circulatory collapse and high early mortality associated with it. However, the major cause of mortality currently is the development of sepsis associated with pancreatic necrosis and the development of pancreatic collections in a necrotic gland. Our results clearly indicate that such complications are seen in only one third of all attacks of haemorrhagic pancreatitis but that they are associated with a mortality of greater than 50%. Although haemorrhagic pancreatitis is associated with a worse prognosis than the oedematous form of the disease, most reports have concentrated on the systemic effects of vasoactive agents absorbed from the peritoneum during such an attack. With advances in intensive care medicine and invasive monitoring, early development of multi-organ failure due to hypovolaemic shock is now much less common than it used to be. Therefore, unless the presence of haemorrhagic peritoneal fluid can predict the presence of pancreatic necrosis and the development of pancreatic collections or sepsis, its value in predicting outcome is limited.

The toxic effects of "haemorrhagic" peritoneal fluid have been extensively studied. The level of absorbed systemic methaemalbumin correlates with outcome in a given attack of pancreatitis [9] and it is known that intravenous administration of haemorrhagic peritoneal fluid in an animal model is associated with a mortality of up to 80% [10, 11].

However, there are a number of putative mediators of this toxic effect other than methaemalbumin. Activated pancreatic enzymes such as trypsin are absorbed via the peritoneal surface and the pancreatic lymphatics [12] and are of known toxicity. Prostaglandin E_2 may also play a role [13]. In addition, yet unidentified vasoactive compounds may be involved in the haemoconcentration, third space losses and circulatory collapse, previously the most common cause of death in acute pancreatitis [14]. This evidence laid the foundation for the use of peritoneal lavage as a therapeutic modality in severe acute pancreatitis. As early as 1965, Wall reported the use of antiprotease peritoneal lavage as a therapeutic modality in acute pancreatitis [15]. Since then, a number of clinical trials have been reported with mixed effects (Table 2) [16–22]. Removal of toxic metabolites from the peritoneum may avoid absorption to the systemic circulation, and hence be associated with a lower incidence of hypotension and its sequelae. However, on the whole the results of therapeutic peritoneal lavage have been disappointing.

Any beneficial effects were limited to particular groups of patients [17] or affected only early mortality [21]. The generally disappointing results of

Table 2. Results of various clinical trials of lavage reported in the literature

Reference	Protocol	No. of patients	Benefit	Fluid	Design
Mayer et al. [16]	2 l/h × 3	91	No	Dialysis fluid	Randomised
Stone and Fabian [17]	0.5 l/h × 1	70	Yes	Dialysis fluid	Randomised
Reynaert et al. [18]	1 l/h × 4.5[a]	53	No	Dialysis fluid	Retrospective
Ihse et al. [19]	1 l/h × 4	39	No	Dialysis fluid	Randomised
Cooper et al. [20]	2 l/h × 72	23	No	Dialysis fluid	Randomised
Ranson and Spencer [21]	2 l/h × 2	103	Yes[b,c]	Dialysis fluid	Retrospective
Ranson and Berman [22]	2 l/h × 2 vs 2 l/h × 7	29	Yes[d]	Dialysis or hypertonic dextrose	Randomised

[a] Mean duration of lavage.
[b] Alcohol and postoperative cases only.
[c] Decreased early mortality only.
[d] Short lavage vs long lavage: Mortality 20% vs 0%.
Pancreatic sepsis 40% vs 0%.

peritoneal lavage in human beings are in stark contrast to those seen in animal studies [23, 24]. This may be explained by the fact that peritoneal lavage simply prevents absorption of the vasoactive compounds described above and has little or no effect on the development of pancreatic necrosis and sepsis, which are now the most common causes of death in this condition [25]. Since the supportive measures available nowadays are superior to those of 10 years ago, fewer patients die of early hypotension in hospital and hence the need for specific measures directed against toxic peritoneal fluid is less pressing.

Conclusion

Use of peritoneal lavage has been advocated for two reasons: to avoid misdiagnosis, and to differentiate between haemorrhagic and oedematous pancreatitis. The latter has previously been important as a marker of severity and as a prognostic index early in the course of an attack. The advent of the APACHE II scoring system has superseded the need for an interventional prognostic index, and attention has turned to the efficacy of peritoneal lavage as a therapeutic modality. The evidence presented here suggests that the presence of haemorrhagic pancreatitis correlates poorly with the development of local pancreatic complications; hence, peritoneal lavage is unlikely to influence the course of an attack in which such a complication is destined to supervene.

References

1. Steinberg WM (1990) Predictors of severity of acute pancreatitis. Gastrointest Clin North Am 19:849–861
2. Knaus WA, Draper EA, Wagner DP, Zimmerman JE (1985) APACHE II: a severity of disease classification system. Crit Care Med 13:818–829
3. Larvin M, McMahon MJ (1989) APACHE II score for assessment and monitoring of acute pancreatitis. Lancet 1:201–204
4. Bradley JA, Bradley P, McMahon MJ (1981) Diagnostic peritoneal lavage in acute pancreatitis – the value of microscopy of the lavage fluid. Br J Surg 68:245–246
5. Goodhead B (1970) Significance of methaemalbuminaemia in acute abdominal emergencies. Arch Surg 101:376–378
6. Silver VE, Wulsin JH, Carter BN (1955) Important clinical factors of acute pancreatitis. Surg Gynecol Obstet 100:357–365
7. Geokas MC, Rinderknecht H, Walberg CB, Weissman R (1974) Methaemalbumin in the diagnosis of acute haemorrhagic pancreatitis. Ann Intern Med 81:483–486
8. McMahon MJ, Playforth MJ, Pickford IR (1980) A comparative study of methods for the prediction of severity of attacks of acute pancreatitis. Br J Surg 67:22–25
9. Geokas MC, Rinderknecht H, Brodrick JW, Largman C (1978) Studies on the ascitic fluid of acute pancreatitis in man. Dig Dis 23:182–188
10. Pullos T, Frey CF, Zaiss C (1982) Toxicity of ascitic fluid from pigs with haemorrhagic pancreatitis. J Surg Res 33:136–139
11. Frey CF, Wong HN, Hickman D, Pullos T (1982) Toxicity of haemorrhagic ascitic fluid associated with haemorrhagic pancreatitis. Arch Surg 117:401–404
12. Mayer AD, Airey M, Hodgson J, McMahon MJ (1985) Enzyme transfer from pancreas to plasma during acute pancreatitis. The contribution of ascitic fluid and lymphatic drainage of the pancreas. Gut 26:876–881
13. Farias LR, Frey CF, Holcroft JW, Gunther R (1985) Effect of prostaglandin blockers on ascites fluid in pancreatitis. Surgery 98:571–578
14. Ellison EC, Pappas TN, Johnson JA, Fabin PJ, Carey LC (1981) Demonstration and characterisation of the haemoconcentrating effect of ascitic fluid that accumulates during haemorrhagic pancreatitis. J Surg Res 30:241–248
15. Wall AJ (1965) Peritoneal dialysis in the treatment of severe acute pancreatitis. Med J Aust 2:281–283
16. Mayer AD, McMahon MJ, Corfield AP, Cooper MJ et al. (1985) Controlled clinical trial of peritoneal lavage for the treatment of severe acute pancreatitis. N Engl J Med 312:399–404
17. Stone HH, Fabian TC (1980) Peritoneal dialysis in the treatment of acute alcoholic pancreatitis. Surg Gynecol Obstet 150:878–882
18. Reynaert MS, Bshouty ZH, Otte JB, Kestens PJ et al. (1985) Percutaneous peritoneal dialysis as an early treatment of acute necrotic haemorrhagic pancreatitis. Intensive Care Med 11:123–128
19. Ihse I, Evander A, Holmberg JT, Gustafson I (1986) Influence of peritoneal lavage on objective prognostic signs in acute pancreatitis. Ann Surg 204:122–127
20. Cooper MJ, Williamson RCN, Pollock AV (1982) The role of peritoneal lavage in the prediction and treatment of severe acute pancreatitis. Panc Soc Proc: 422–427
21. Ranson JHC, Spencer FC (1978) The role of peritoneal lavage in severe acute pancreatitis. Ann Surg 187:565–573
22. Ranson JHC, Berman RS (1990) Long peritoneal lavage decreases pancreatic sepsis in acute pancreatitis. Ann Surg 211:708–718
23. Rosato EF, Mullis WF, Rosato FE (1973) Peritoneal lavage therapy in haemorrhagic pancreatitis. Surgery 74:106–115

24. Bolooki H, Gliedman ML (1968) Peritoneal dialysis in treatment of acute pancreatitis. Surgery 64:466–471
25. Wilson C, Imrie CW, Carter DC (1988) Fatal acute pancreatitis. Gut 29:782–788

Bacterial Infection and the Role of Fine Needle Aspiration

W. Uhl, M. Büchler, B. Rau, and H.G. Beger[1]

There is general agreement among clinicians and pancreatologists that pancreatic infection is the most important causal factor of lethal outcome in human acute pancreatitis today [1–3]. Bacterial contamination of pancreatic necrosis has been demonstrated in 40%–70% of patients suffering from necrotizing pancreatitis [4–8], and it has been shown that the frequency of positive cultures increases directly with the duration and extent of necrosis. The necroses in 24% of patients with necrotizing pancreatitis operated on during the first week after hospitalization showed bacterial contamination. This percentage increased to 36% in the second week and to 72% in the third week; thereafter a decrease was found to 32% [9]. Bacterial contamination of pancreatic necrosis occurs early and frequently, as verified by Bassi in a similar study and by Gerzof with the aid of computed tomography (CT)-guided fine needle aspiration and Gram staining [5, 6].

An analytical review of the literature yielded a 100%-mortality rate in infected necrosis if patients were treated conservatively without surgical drainage [10–13]. From the surgeon's point of view, there is an absolutely clear indication for an adequate surgical therapy or interventional drainage procedure if necrotizing pancreatitis is shown to be infected [14–16].

The bacteria commonly found in infected necroses of necrotizing pancreatitis are shown in Table 1; these data were calculated from three prospective studies [4–6]. In most cases, the infection is caused by a single organism of gram-negative germs which originates from the digestive tract. The most frequent germ is *Escherichia coli*, which is found in about 26%. The pathophysiological pathway for these bacteria may be either translocation, infected bile, or hematogenous or lymphatic spread [17, 18].

Patients

Between May 1982 and May 1991, 201 patients with necrotizing pancreatitis were treated, representing 18% of all patients with acute pancreatitis hospitalized at the University Hospital of Ulm, FRG (Table 2). Of those,

---

[1] Department of General Surgery, University of Ulm, Steinhövelstraße 9, W-7900 Ulm, FRG

Beger/Büchler/Malfertheiner (Eds.)
Standards in Pancreatic Surgery

Table 1. Bacteria found in infected necroses[a]

Bacteria	Percentage
E. coli	25.9
Pseudomonas spp.	15.9
Staphylococcus aureus	15.3
Klebsiella spp.	10.1
Proteus spp.	10.1
Streptococcus faecalis	4.4
Enterobacter	2.5
Other anaerobes	15.8
	100.0

[a] Calculated from three studies [4–6].

Table 2. Classification of 1099 patients with acute pancreatitis[a]

	No. of patients	Frequency (%)
Acute interstitial-edematous pancreatitis	812	74.0
Acute necrotizing pancreatitis	201	18.0
Pancreatic abscess	26	2.4
Pancreatic pseudocyst	60	5.5

[a] All patients hospitalized at the Departments of Surgery and Gastroenterology, University of Ulm, FRG between May 1982 and May 1991.

133 patients were male and 68 female, and the mean age was calculated to be 52 years (range 18–89 years). The etiological factors were alcohol overindulgence in 95 patients (47%), biliary tract disease in 61 patients (30%), and idiopathic or other reasons in the remaining 45 cases (23%). The mean Ranson score was 4.3, ranging from 1 to 10 prognostic criteria. Forty-two patients were treated conservatively, and their condition improved after treatment in a mean of 12.3 days (range 1–110 days).

Algorithm for Clinical Decision-Making in Acute Pancreatitis

Since 1984 we have introduced a new approach to patients with acute pancreatitis at our hospital, based on the above-mentioned increase in experience and knowledge (Fig. 1). After acute pancreatitis has been diagnosed and after differentiating between edematous and necrotizing pancreatitis using necrosis indicators such as C-reactive protein (CRP) [19, 20], antiproteases [21], and recently polymorphonuclear (PMN) elastase [22, 23], contrast-enhanced CT scanning [24–27] is performed to evaluate the extent of pancreatic parenchymal and extrapancreatic spread of fatty tissue necrosis. Thereafter, a fine needle puncture and aspiration of fluid collec-

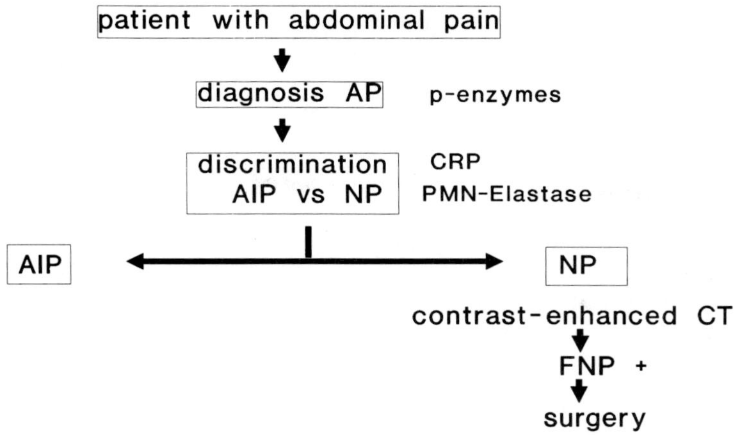

Fig. 1. Algorithm for clinical decision-making in acute pancreatitis. *AP*, acute pancreatitis; *AIP*, acute interstitial–edematous pancreatitis; *NP*, acute necrotizing pancreatitis; *FNP*, fine needle puncture; *CRP*, C-reactive protein; *PMN*, polymorphonuclear; *CT*, computed tomography

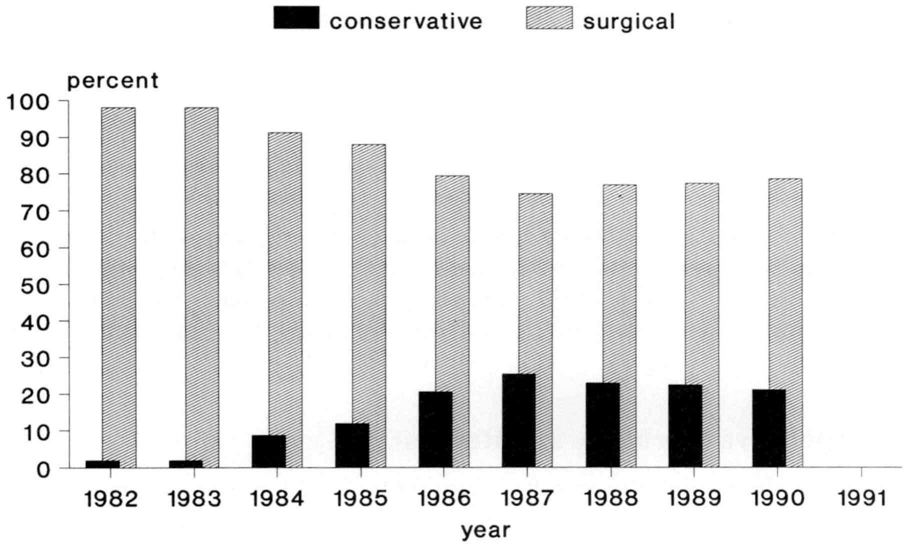

Fig. 2. Necrotizing pancreatitis. Conservative (*black bars*) and surgical (*hatched bars*) treatment in 201 patients hospitalized at the University Hospital Ulm, FRG, between May 1982 and December 1990

Table 3. Preoperative morbidity in 201 patients with necrotizing pancreatitis[a]

	Infected (n = 69)	Sterile (n = 132)
Pulmonary insufficiency (%)[b]	74	47
Renal insufficiency (%)[c]	45	22
Shock (%)[d]	29	13
Sepsis (%)[e]	43	8
Metabolic disorders (%)[f]	52	28
Mean Ranson score (range)	4.3 (1–10)	3.1 (1–10)
Extent of necrosis		
<30% (%)	35	45
>30%–<50% (%)	41	29
>50% (%)	24	26

[a] All patients hospitalized between May 1982 and May 1991 at the Departments of Surgery and Gastroenterology at the University of Ulm, FRG.
[b] pO_2 <60 mmHg.
[c] Serum creatinine >240 μmol/l.
[d] Pulse rate >100 bpm and systolic blood pressure <80 mmHg for more than 10 min.
[e] Leukocytes >12 g/l or <4 g/l; platelets <100 g/l; rectal temperature >38.5°C; positive blood culture; metabolic acidosis, base excess >−4 mmo/l.
[f] Hyperglycemia, blood glucose >8.4 mmol/l; hypocalcemia, calcium <2.0 mmol/l; coagulation disorders, prothrombin time <70% or partial thromboplast time >45 s.

tion or necrosis is performed under local anesthesia and with ultrasound guidance. The aspirates are examined for Gram's stain, and culture and enzyme activities. Since 1987 our percentage of patients suffering from necrotizing pancreatitis and treated conservatively has remained almost constant at 20% (Fig. 2).

Preoperative Morbidity and Results

Table 3 shows the preoperative morbidity in the group of necrotizing pancreatitis with infected (n = 69) versus sterile (n = 132) necrosis. The overall infection rate, as determined during operation, was 44% (69/159), thereby confirming our previous results [4]. The time intervals between hospital admission and surgical intervention were a mean of 6.6 days (range, 0.2–25) and 2.8 days (range, 0.1–9) in infected and sterile neroses, respectively. The presence of pulmonary and renal insufficiency, shock, sepsis, and metabolic disorders prior to surgery were 74%, 45%, 29%, 43%, and 52% in infected necrosis and 47%, 22%, 13%, 8%, and 28% in sterile necrosis, respectively. The mean Ranson score was higher in patients with infected

Table 4. Results of operative management in 159 patients with necrotizing pancreatitis[a]

	Infected ($n = 69$)	Sterile ($n = 90$)
Mean interval from onset of symptoms to surgery in days (range)	22 (1.2–88)	10.6 (1–93)
Mean duration of hospital stay in days (range)	65 (1–238)	41 (4–162)
Mean duration of lavage in days (range)	32 (1–95)	36 (3–109)
Number of reoperations	22[b]	39[c]
Number of reoperations per patient (range)	3.2 (1–9)	1.7 (1–4)
Mortality (%)	17.3[d]	10.0[e]

[a] All patients hospitalized between May 1982 and May 1991 at the Departments of Surgery and Gastroenterology, University of Ulm, FRG.
[b] 32%. [c] 43%. [d] $n = 12$. [e] $n = 9$.

necrosis than in those with sterile necroses (4.3 versus 3.1). On contrast-enhanced CT scanning, the necrosis extended more frequently over more than 30% of the pancreas in infected necrosis than in the bacteria-negative group (65% versus 55%).

Table 4 compares the results in patients with infected and sterile necrosis undergoing surgery. The time interval between the onset of symptoms of acute pancreatitis and surgical intervention and the duration of hospital stay were significantly higher in patients with infected necrosis than in those with sterile necrosis (22 versus 11 days and 65 versus 41 days, respectively). The duration of lavage was approximately equal in both groups. The reoperation rate was 32% in infected necrosis and 43% in sterile necrosis, but the reoperation rate per operated person was twice as high in infected necrosis. In infected necrosis, the reasons for reoperations were abscess formation (33%), persisting sepsis (26%), bleeding (23%), and an ongoing necrotizing process confirmed by contrast-enhanced CT scans (13%), whereas in the bacteria-negative group the respective percentages were 15%, 17%, 15%, and 41%. The mortality rate was higher in the bacteria-postive group than in the bacteria-negative group (17% versus 10%).

Fine Needle Puncture and Aspiration

The results of fine needle aspiration in patients examined between May 1990 and May 1991 is given in Table 5. Fine needle puncture and aspiration was

Table 5. Fine needle puncture and aspiration in 28 patients with necrotizing pancreatitis[a]

	Type of treatment	
	Surgical (n = 21)	Conservative (n = 7)
Hemorrhagic aspirate (%)	33	14
Enzyme activity (%)	81	57
Infection (%)	43	0

[a] All patients hospitalized between May 1990 and May 1991 at the Departments of Surgery and Gastroenterology, University of Ulm, FRG.

performed with ultrasound guidance with a 21-gauge needle after local anesthesia. The aspirates were examined for color, Gram's stain, and culture and enzyme activities. Twenty-eight patients suffering from necrotizing pancreatitis were hospitalized during this period; 21 were treated surgically and seven conservatively. Hemorrhagic ascites was found in 33% of patients treated surgically and in 14% of those undergoing conservative treatment. The preoperatively proven infection rate was 43% in the patients treated surgically. All patients tolerated this procedure well, and no complications were seen.

Summary

There is no doubt that bacterial infection is the most important risk factor in acute necrotizing pancreatitis [1–3]. Therefore, thorough screening for bacterial infection is of utmost importance, and fine needle aspiration is a reliable and harmless procedure to determine whether there is bacterial contamination of the necroses [5, 28]. Patients with necrotizing pancreatitis and clinical signs of bacterial infection should undergo fine needle aspiration. A bacterial infection in necrotizing pancreatitis is the best indicator for surgical intervention.

In sterile necrosis, there are some problems in deciding which patients should undergo surgery. Precise criteria for shifting from intensive conservative care to surgery are mandatory in the bacteria-negative group of necrotizing pancreatitis, in order to be able to assess the benefits of early operative management with regard to the remote complications of severe acute pancreatitis and the prevention of abdominal sepsis. Some patients with sterile necrotizing pancreatitis can be treated conservatively [29], but the group of more severely ill patients who are nonresponsive to intensive care treatment are candidates for surgical management [30]. Clear definitions are mandatory for these patients.

In this context, a further problem is prophylactic treatment with antibiotics [31]. From the clinician's point of view, the question must be raised as to what kinds of patients with acute pancreatitis need antibiotic treatment. In three prospective controlled trials, antibiotics were not helpful in improving patients' prognosis [32–34]. But in none of these studies, on the one hand were antibiotics used which enter the pancreas and, on the other hand, the authors did not recruit patients where a risk of pancreatic infection existed.

Patients with necrotizing pancreatitis should be treated with antibiotics from the beginning, because of the known 40%–70% risk of bacterial contamination of the necroses. First-choice drugs are antibiotics; firstly those which are able to penetrate into the pancreas, and secondly those which have a high efficiacy factor locally [31].

References

1. Buggy BP, Nostrant TT (1983) Lethal pancreatitis. Am J Gastroenterol 78:810–814
2. Allardyce DB (1987) Incidence of necrotizing pancreatitis and factors related to mortality. Am J Surg 154:295–299
3. Beger HG, Büchler M (1986) Decision-making in surgical treatment of acute pancreatitis: operative or conservative management of necrotizing pancreatitis? Theor Surg 1:61–68
4. Beger HG, Krautzberger W, Bittner R, Büchler M, Block S (1986) Bacterial contamination of pancreatic necrosis. A prospective clinical study. Gastroenterology 91:433–438
5. Gerzof SG, Banks PA, Robbins AH, Johnson WC, Spechler SJ, Wetzner SM, Snider JM, Langevin RE, Jay ME (1987) Early diagnosis of pancreatic infection by computed tomography-guided aspiration. Gastroenterology 93:1315–1320
6. Bassi C, Falconi M, Girelli R, Nifosi F, Elio A, Martini N, Pederzoli P (1989) Microbiological findings in severe pancreatitis. Surg Res Comm 5:1–4
7. Jones CE, Polk HC, Fulton RL (1975) Pancreatic abscess. Am J Surg 129:44–47
8. Becker JM, Pemberton JH, DiMagno EP, Ilstrup DM, McIlrath DC, Dozois RR (1984) Prognostic factors in pancreatic abscess. Surgery 96:455–460
9. Beger HG, Büchler M, Bittner R, Block S, Nevalainen T, Roscher R (1988) Necrosectomy and postoperative local lavage in necrotizing pancreatitis. Br J Surg 75:207–212
10. Malangoni MA, Richardson JD, Shallcross JC, Seiler JG, Polk HC (1986) Factors contributing to fatal outcome after treatment of pancreatic abscess. Ann Surg 203:605–613
11. Evans FC (1969) Pancreatic abscess. Am J Surg 117:537–540
12. Cramer SI, Tan EGC, Warren KW, Braasch JW (1975) Pancreatic abscess: a critically analysis of 113 cases. Am J Surg 129:426–431
13. Bradley EL, Fulenwider JT (1984) Open treatment of pancreatic abscess. Surg Gynecol Obstet 159:509–513
14. Gerzof SG, Robbins AJ, Johnson WC, Birkett DH, Nabseth DC (1981) Percutaneous catheter drainage of abdominal abscess: a five year experience. N Engl J Med 305:653–657
15. van Sonnenberg E, Wing VW, Casola G, Nakamoto SK, Mueller PR, Ferrucci JT, Halasz NA, Simeone JF (1984) Temporizing effect of percutaneous drainage of complicated abscesses in critically ill patients. AJR 142:821–826

16. Warshaw AL (1974) Inflammatory masses following acute pancreatitis. Surg Gynecol Obstet 139:69–81
17. Wells CL, Rotstein OD, Pruett TL, Simmons RL (1986) Intestinal bacteria translocate into experimental intra-abdominal abscesses. Arch Surg 121:102–106
18. Lange JF, van Gool J, Tytgat GNJ (1985) The protective effect of a reduction in intestinal flora on mortality of acute haemorrhagic pancreatitis in the rat. Hepatogastroenterology 34:28–30
19. Büchler M, Malfertheiner P, Schoetensack C, Uhl W, Beger HG (1986) Sensitivity of antiproteases, complement factors and C-reactive protein in detecting pancreatic necrosis. Results of a prospective clinical study. Int J Pancreatol 1:227–235
20. Büchler M (1991) Objectivation of the severity of acute pancreatitis. Hepato-Gastroenterol 38:101–108
21. Mc Mahon MJ, Bowen M, Mayer AD, Cooper EH (1984) Relationship of α2-macroglobulin and other antiproteases to the clinical features of acute pancreatitis. Am J Surg 147:164–169
22. Uhl W, Büchler M, Malfertheiner P, Martini M, Beger HG (1991) PMN-Elastase in comparison with CRP, antiproteases and LDH as indicators of necrosis in human acute pancreatitis. Pancreas 6:253–259
23. Gross V, Schölmerich J, Leser HG (1989) Wertigkeit von Leukozytenelastase, C-reaktiven Protein und Proteaseninhibitoren für die Prognose der akuten Pankreatitis. Klin Wochenschr 67:237 (abstract)
24. Schröder T, Kivilaakso E, Lempinen M (1984) A new method for the diagnosis of acute hemorrhagic necrotising pancreatitis using contrast-enhanced CT. Gastrointest Radiol 9:27–30
25. Block S, Maier W, Clausen C, Bittner R, Büchler M, Malfertheiner P, Beger HG (1986) Identification of pancreas necrosis in severe acute pancreatitis. Gut 27:1035–42
26. Balhazar EJ (1989) CT diagnosis and staging of acute pancreatitis. Rad Clin North Am 27:19–37
27. Bradley EL, Murphy F, Ferguson C (1989) Prediction of pancreatic necrosis by dynamic pancreatography. Ann Surg 210:495–504
28. Gerzof SG, Banks PA, Robbins AH (1984) Role of guided percutaneous aspiration in early diagnosis of pancreatic sepsis. Dig Dis Sci 29:950 (abstract)
29. Büchler M, Malfertheiner P, Uhl W, Beger HG (1988) Conservative treatment of necrotizing pancreatitis in patients with minor pancreatic necrosis. Pancreas 3:592 (abstract)
30. Beger HG, Uhl W (1990) Severe acute pancreatitis. II: The surgical approach. Clin Int Care 1:223–227
31. Büchler M, Malfertheiner P, Frieß H, Bittner R, Vanek E, Schlegel P, Beger HG (1989) The penetration of antibiotics into human pancreas. Infection 17: 20–25
32. Craig RM, Dordal E, Myles L (1975) The use of ampicillin in acute pancreatitis. Ann Int Med 83:831–832
33. Howes R, Zuidema GD, Cameron JL (1975) Evaluation of prophylactic antibiotics in acute pancreatitis. J Surg Res 18:197–200
34. Finch WT, Sawyers JL, Schenkers S (1976) A prospective study to determine the efficacy of antibiotics in acute pancreatitis. Ann Surg 183:667–671

Conservative Treatment of Acute Pancreatitis

J.H. GRENDELL[1]

Introduction

In the practice of medicine, the definition of "conservative" is often subject to as many and varied interpretations as it is in the field of politics. For the purpose of this discussion, conservative treatment of acute pancreatitis is considered to encompass all therapeutic measures except (a) operative procedures, (b) therapeutic endoscopy, (c) percutaneous placement of drainage catheters, and (d) peritoneal dialysis for indications other than renal failure. It is crucial to distinguish between conservative treatment and nonaggressive treatment. The conservative management of severe acute pancreatitis is quite vigorous and aggressive, focusing on provision of necessary supportive care and early recognition and treatment of any complications.

The great majority of patients with acute pancreatitis recover with conservative treatment alone. Indeed a strong case can be made that conservative treatment should be the initial form of treatment in patients with even the most severe forms of acute pancreatitis for the following reasons: (a) There is no unequivocal evidence from prospective, randomized controlled trials that surgical, endoscopic, or radiologic interventions are beneficial in acute pancreatitis except to treat complications of the disease or, possibly, to mitigate the adverse effects of persistent impaction of a gallstone in the region of the duodenal papilla [1]. (b) All predictors of prognosis are of limited applicability when applied to the individual patient [2].

Accepted Elements of Conservative Treatment

The elements of conservative treatment vary from center to center and even from patient to patient in the same center because of the highly variable nature of the disease. Some of the more widely accepted and employed methods are considered below. However, the popularity of a particular

[1] Gastroenterology Section (111B), San Francisco VA Medical Center, 4150 Clement Street, San Francisco, CA 94121, USA

Beger/Büchler/Malfertheiner (Eds.)
Standards in Pancreatic Surgery

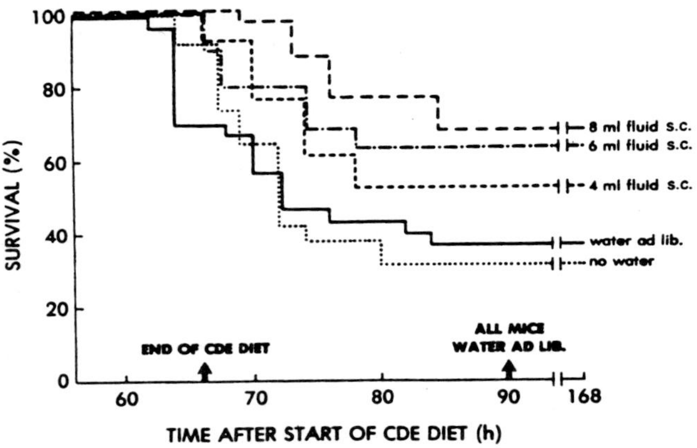

Fig. 1. Effect of parenteral hydration with an electrolyte solution (Plasmalyte) in mice with severe, necrotizing acute pancreatitis produced by feeding a choline-deficient, ethionine-supplemented (*CDE*) diet. Hydration and electrolyte replacement resulted in a dose-related doubling of survival compared to animals receiving no water or water ad libitum. (From [7], reprinted with permission)

aspect of therapy should not be confused with proof of effectiveness, which is wanting for most elements of conservative treatment just as it is for "nonconservative" forms of treatment.

Clinical and Physiologic Monitoring

This may range from simple assessment of physical findings, vital signs, and urine output to insertion of radial and pulmonary artery catheters for measurement of blood pressure, arterial blood gas, cardiac index, and pulmonary capillary wedge pressure. The extent and frequency of such monitoring must of course be tailored to the individual patient's condition.

Bed Rest, No Oral Intake

Patients with moderate or severe acute pancreatitis generally are more comfortable if kept at bed rest and without oral intake. Early refeeding has been proposed to predispose to reactivation of acute pancreatitis and increased morbidity [3], although this has not been evaluated in a clinical trial.

Nasogastric Suction

Although prospective, randomized studies showed no improvement in outcome in patients with milder forms of alcoholic pancreatitis [4–6], nasogastric suction remains very useful in more severe disease for the relief of symptomatic nausea, vomiting, and abdominal distension.

Fluid Resuscitation, Electrolyte Replacement

This is the *most* important aspect of the early treatment of patients with severe acute pancreatitis. These patients must be regarded as having a potentially severe chemical burn of the body's "inner surface" and treated accordingly. Studies in an animal model of severe, necrotizing acute pancreatitis have demonstrated a doubling in survival attributable solely to vigorous rehydration and electrolyte replacement (Fig. 1) [7].

Replacement of Blood Products, Oxygen, Ventilatory Support, Dialysis for Renal Failure

Indications for use of these important supportive measures in acute pancreatitis are similar to those for their use in other severe acute diseases.

Prophylaxis of Stress Gastritis

This is an important concern especially in the patient with associated sepsis or multisystem organ failure. Although H_2 antagonists administered intravenously and sucralfate or antacids given through a nasogastric tube have all been shown to reduce the risk of bleeding from stress gastritis, ventilated patients should be treated with either H_2 antagonists or sucralfate because of a lower risk of developing nosocomial pneumonia compared to that of antacid-treated patients [8, 9].

Nutritional Support

Many patients with more severe acute pancreatitis are unable to eat for prolonged periods of time. In addition, avoidance of meal-stimulated pancreatic secretion is frequently a goal of therapy. Therefore total parenteral nutrition is often employed. This should be instituted when a patient appears unlikely to be able to tolerate oral or enteral feeding for at least 1 week (this is correlated with a Ranson score of $\geqslant 3$ [10]). Although concerns have been raised about possible deleterious effects of lipid emulsions [11], these seem to be well-tolerated by most patients who do not have a genetic tendency to develop hypertriglyceridemia [10]. However, a high incidence of glucose intolerence has been reported [10]. Although failure to achieve positive nitrogen balance is associated with a poor prognosis, early institution of total parenteral nutrition has not been convincingly shown to improve survival or to reduce complications in acute pancreatitis [10, 12].

Antibiotics

There is little question that antibiotics should be administered to patients with acute pancreatitis if bacterial infection is present or strongly suspected. It should be noted that the prophylactic use of antibiotics has not been shown to be beneficial in prospective studies [13, 14]; however, these studies have primarilly involved patients with mild alcoholic pancreatitis. There is a strong need for prospective, randomized controlled trials in patients with more severe pancreatitis, especially when related to gallstones.

Vigorous Surveillance for Potential Complications

In particular the increasing use of computed tomography and guided-needle aspiration has facilitated the diagnosis and treatment of infected necrosis/ pancreatic abscess and of infected pancreatic pseudocysts [15, 16]. This is a key aspect of conservative treatment later (after 1 week) into the course of moderate or severe acute pancreatitis.

Proposed Elements of Conservative Therapy Without Benefit in Prospective Trials or Having Limited Clinical Experience

Protease Inhibitors

In theory the inactivation of pancreatic proteases such as trypsin would appear to be a promising therapeutic approach. In practice, however, the serine protease inhibitors (aprotinin, gabexate, camostate) keep getting better, although the results of clinical trials do not [17, 18].

Inhibitors of Pancreatic Secretion or Function

Prospective clinical studies have so far failed to demonstrate a benefit for any of the inhibitors of pancreatic secretion or function (H_2 antagonists, anticholinergics, glucagon, calcitonin, somatostatin) [19]. It is not surprising that inhibitors of pancreatic secretion have not improved the outcome in this disease because acute pancreatitis itself produces a "secretory block" in both experimental models (Fig. 2) [20] and, probably, in clinical disease [21].

Other Investigational Forms of Therapy

Because of the very limited experience with other investigational forms of therapy (e.g., indomethacin, prostaglandins, plasmapheresis) clinical trials are needed to assess their potential value, if any, in acute pancreatitis.

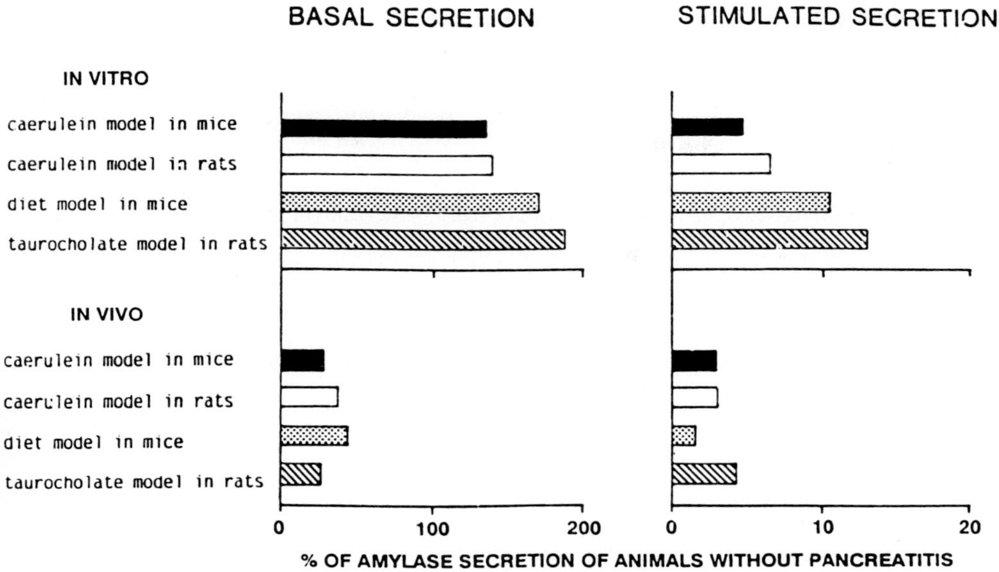

Fig. 2. In a variety of experimental models of acute pancreatitis, both in vitro and in vivo stimulated pancreatic enzyme secretion are markedly reduced. This finding and supporting data from clinical observations [20] suggest the presence of a "secretory block" during the development of acute pancreatitis. (From [19], reprinted with permission)

When Is Conservative Treatment Alone Not Enough?

Not all patients with moderate or severe acute pancreatitis respond to conservative care alone. Established indications for proceeding to additional measures are (a) some major complications of acute pancreatitis such as infected necrosis/abscess, hemorrhage from a pseudoaneurysm, or symptomatic pseudocysts [22]; and (b) severe gallstone pancreatitis (proven or suspected) with failure of the patient to improve or at least stabilize despite 24–36 h of appropriate conservative treatment [1].

The use of additional measures beyond conservative therapy has been proposed for other indications, but the value of such measures remains to be established. Such additional potential indications include (a) severe acute pancreatitis with continued clinical deterioration of the patient in the setting of "sterile necrosis" (for: [23]; against: [24]); and (b) failure of acute pancreatitis to resolve completely despite a prolonged trail of conservative treatment [25].

References

1. Neoptolemos JP, Carr-Locke DL, London NJ, Bailey IA, James D, Fossard DP (1988) Controlled trial of urgent endoscopic retrograde cholangiopancreatography versus conservative treatment for acute pancreatitis due to gallstones. Lancet 2:979–983
2. Steinberg WM (1990) Predictors of severity of acute pancreatitis. Gastroenterol Clin N Am 19:849–861
3. Ranson JHC, Spencer FC (1978) The role of peritoneal lavage in severe acute pancreatitis. Ann Surg 187:565–575
4. Loiudice TA, Lang J, Mehta H, Banta L (1984) Treatment of acute alcoholic pancreatitis: the roles of cimetidine and nasogastric suction. Am J Gastroenterol 79:553–558
5. Sarr MG, Sanfey H, Cameron JL (1986) Prospective randomized trial of nasogastric suction in patients with acute pancreatitis. Surgery 100:500–504
6. Bradley EL III, Hall JR, Lutz J, Hamner L, Lattouf O (1983) Hemodynamic consequences of severe pancreatitis. Ann Surg 198:130–133
7. Niederau C, Crass RA, Silver G, Ferrell LD, Grendell JH (1988) Therapeutic regimens in acute experimental hemorrhagic pancreatitis. Effects of hydration, oxygenation, peritoneal lavage, and a potent protease inhibitor. Gastroenterology 95:1648–1657
8. Driks MR, Craven DE, Celli BR, Manning M, Burke RA, Garvin GM, Kunches LM, Farber HW, Wedel SA, McCabe WR (1987) Nosocomial pneumonia in intubated patients given sucralfate as compared with antacids or histamine type 2 blockers. The role of gastric colonization. N Engl J Med 317:1376–1382
9. Tryba M (1985) Risk of acute stress bleeding and nosocomial pneumonia in ventilated intensive care unit patients: sucralfate versus antacids. Am J Med 83 [Suppl 3B]:117–124
10. Kalfarentzos FE, Karavias DD, Karatzas TM, Alevizatos BA, Androulakis JA (1991) Total parenteral nutrition in severe acute pancreatitis. J Am Coll Nutr 10:156–162
11. Latifi R, McIntosh JK, Dudrick SJ (1991) Nutritional management of acute and chronic pancreatitis. Surg Clin N Am 71:579–595
12. Goodgame JT, Fischer JE (1987) Parenteral nutrition in the treatment of acute pancreatitis: effect on complications and mortality. Ann Surg 186:651–658
13. Howes R, Zuidema GD, Cameron JL (1975) Evaluation of prophylactic antibiotics in acute pancreatitis. J Surg Res 18:197–200
14. Finch WT, Sawyers JL, Schenker S (1976) A prospective study to determine the efficacy of antibiotics in acute pancreatitis. Ann Surg 183:667–671
15. Jeffrey RB Jr, Grendell JH, Federle MP, Meyer AA, Wing VW, Wall SD, Shea WJ (1987) Improved survival with early CT diagnosis of pancreatic abscess. Gastrointest Radiol 12:26–30
16. Gerzof SG, Banks PA, Robbins AH, Johnson WC, Spechler SJ, Wetzner SM, Snider JM, Langevin RE, Jay ME (1987) Early diagnosis of pancreatic infection by computed tomography-guided aspiration. Gastroenterology 93:1315–1320
17. Medical Research Council Multicentre Trial (1980) Morbidity of acute pancreatitis. The effect of aprotinin and glucagon. Gut 21:334–349
18. Büchler M, Malfertheiner P, Uhl W, Stockmann F, Schölmerich J, Adler G, Rolle K, Ditschuneit H, Beger HG (1990) The German multicenter double blind randomized study of gabexate-mesilate (4 g/day i.v.) in acute pancreatitis. Gastroenterology 98:A124 (Abstract)
19. Niederau C, Niederau M, Lüthen R, Strohmeyer G, Ferrell LD, Grendell JH (1990) Pancreatic exocrine secretion in acute experimental pancreatitis. Gastroenterology 99:1120–1127
20. Mitchell CJ, Playforth M, Kelleher J, McMahon MJ (1983) Functional recovery of the exocrine pancreas after acute pancreatitis. Scand J Gastreonterol 18:5–8

21. Grendell JH, Egan J (1987) Acute pancreatitis. West J Med 146:598–602
22. Forsmark CE, Grendell JH (1991) Complications of pancreatitis. Seminars in Gastrointestinal Disease 2:165–170
23. Beger HG, Büchler M, Bittner R, Oettinger W, Block S, Nevalainen T (1988) Necrosectomy and postoperative local lavage in patients with necrotizing pancreatitis: results of a prospective clinical trial. World J Surg 12:255–262
24. Bradley EL III, Allen K (1991) A prospective longitudinal study of observation versus surgical intenvention in the management of necrotizing pancreatitis. Am J Surg 161:19–25
25. Rutledge PL, Warshaw AL (1988) Persistent acute pancreatitis. A variant treated by pancreatoduodenectomy. Arch Surg 123:597–600

Intensive Care Therapy in Acute Pancreatitis

H. Wiedeck[1] and B. Stein

The clinical course of acute pancreatitis (AP) varies from a mild self-limiting condition to an extremely severe disease with multiple organ failure and a high mortality rate. The reported incidence of the necrotizing or hemorrhagic form varies between 5% to 10% of all cases of acute pancreatitis [1].

The dimension of organ dysfunctions in acute pancreatitis – especially the necrotizing form – differs a lot in the literature. However there is correspondence suggesting that respiratory dysfunction is the most frequent organ failure in patients with AP followed by renal and cardiovascular failure (Table 1).

Pulmonary Changes and Ventilatory Support

The pulmonary dysfunctions listed in Table 2 are caused by mechanical restriction of pulmonary distention due to the known intestinal atony which leads to an elevation of the diaphragm followed by atelectasis. Pleural effusions with high concentrations of pancreatic enzymes often develop [11].

Pancreatitis has been identified as one etiologic factor in acute respiratory distress syndrome (ARDS). There are some clinical and animal studies that record ARDS in AP as a sequel of pulmonary edema caused by increased permeability of the capillary endothelium and the presence of leucocytes, lysosomal enzymes, oxygen radicals and microembolisms [2, 5, 8, 9].

A raised intrapulmonary right-to-left shunt leads to hypoxemia. Prostacyclin may be involved, neutralizing the hypoxemic vasoconstriction of the pulmonary vessels. In the later course of the disease pulmonary hypertension may become a limiting factor because of increased right ventricular strain.

Another pulmonary dysfunction concerns the surfactant. The question of whether increased levels of phospholipase A_2 destroy the surfactant and lead to pulmonary dysfunction in AP has been discussed ever since publica-

[1] Universitätsklinik für Anästhesiologie, Klinikum der Universität Ulm, Steinhövelstraße 9, W-7900 Ulm (Donau), FRG

Beger/Büchler/Malfertheiner (Eds.)
Standards in Pancreatic Surgery

Table 1. Frequency of organ dysfunction in acute pancreatitis

Dysfunction	Frequency (%)
Respiratory	20–70
Renal	6–18
Circulatory	1–60

Table 2. Causes of respiratory dysfunction in acute pancreatitis

Mechanical restriction
elevated diaphragm
atelectasis
pleural effusion
Dysfunction of gas exchange, alterations of pulmonary perfusion
increased capillary permeability with pulmonary edema
increased intrapulmonary right-to-left shunt
Dysfunction of surfactant
increased levels of phospholipase A_2?

Table 3. Diagnosis and therapy for respiratory dysfunction in acute pancreatitis

Diagnosis
auscultation, percussion
chest X-ray
blood gas analysis
pulmonary compliance
shunt, pulmonary capillary wedge pressure
Therapy
well-balanced fluid control
aspiration of the pleural cavity
physical therapy
mechanical ventilation with positive end-expiratory pressure

tion of the study by Zieve and Vogel [12], but this effect still has to be proved in patients.

Proceeding from the pulmonary dysfunction described above, the indication for mechanical ventilation is generous. Since detection of dysfunction depends on diagnostic techniques (Table 3) we presume high pulmonary risk until the contrary has been proved.

We routinely apply mechanical ventilation with a positive end-expiratory pressure (PEEP). If pulmonary function deteriorates, PEEP is increased and the ratio of inspiration to expiration is inversed to reach an FIO_2 of less than 0.5. Physiotherapy and changing of the patient's position are of prime

Table 4. Dysfunction of the cardiovascular system

Cause
loss of volume
decreased systemic vascular resistance
Diagnosis
central venous pressure
Swan-Ganz catheter
for: cardiac output
pulmonary capillary wedge pressure
systemic vascular resistance
Therapy
volume replacement
catecholamines

importance. A well-balanced fluid control is essential. Aspiration of the pleural cavity is only performed if we expect more than 500 ml of fluid.

Dysfunction of the Cardiovascular System

Severe pancreatitis leads to systemic effects which predominantly reveal themselves by hemodynamic alterations (Table 4). The initial loss of volume and fluid are often underestimated.

The investigations by Oettinger et al. [10] could show that the hemodynamic pattern, characterised by significant elevation in cardiac index, reduction in total peripheral resistance and considerable increase of pulmonary right-to-left shunt bears a remarkable resemblance to what is found in early septic shock [6]. Therefore careful cardiovascular monitoring is required. Central venous and arterial cannulation as well as a pulmonary artery catheter are mandatory. In the therapeutic management of circulatory dysfunction volume and fluid administration is essential. If volume and fluid replacement is not successful in producing an adequate mean arterial blood pressure we use catecholamines, preferring norepinephrine if systemic vascular resistance is low.

Renal Dysfunction

The early hemodynamic changes in AP described above often lead to renal dysfunction if not adequately treated. In the later course of the disease septic complications are the main reason for renal dysfunction (Table 5). Therefore diagnostic parameters, such as urine output and laboratory tests as listed in Table 6, are of great importance.

The therapeutic consequences include sufficient fluid and volume replacement with regard to central venous pressure and pulmonary capillary wedge pressure. The use of dopamine in a dosage of 1–5 μg/kg per min to

Table 5. Causes of renal dysfunction in acute pancreatitis

Hypovolemia caused by
shock
fluid loss into third space
Sepsis, septic shock

Table 6. Diagnosis and therapy for renal dysfunction in acute pancreatitis

Diagnosis
urine output
laboratory tests
serum creatinine
serum urea
electrolytes
osmolarity
Therapy
volume and fluid replacement
improvement of renal perfusion
diuretics
hemodialysis/hemofiltration

improve renal perfusion could be helpful. The value of stimulating decreased renal function by diuretics with regard to the duration of acute renal failure and the outcome of the patients is still discussed.

In our intensive care unit the indication for hemodialysis or hemofiltration is generous especially when pulmonary function deteriorates. Whether early hemofiltration improves the outcome of patients with AP by elimination of toxic peptides and other mediators is not yet clear [3].

Nutritional Therapy

The severely catabolic state of patients with AP requires adequate nutritional support. The preferred route for the administration of nutrients in patients with AP is still the parenteral, although there are surprisingly few data on this field [4]. Beaulieux was one of the first who reported favorable results of enteral feeding by jejunostomy in 11 patients with severe AP in 1981. We therefore investigated in a prospective study on 27 patients with AP the metabolic consequences of parenteral and enteral nutritional therapy (unpublished data).

As known from the literature we found hyperglycemia in all patients irrespective of nutritional therapy, but compared to the parenteral group the enterally fed patients showed a significantly lower glucose concentration in serum. We could not find an amino acid pattern specific to the disease as described by Hölbling and co-workers [7]. With respect to the urea production rate the enterally fed patients showed a better utilization of the administered amino acids.

We therefore conclude that patients with AP can profit by enteral feeding if adequate metabolic monitoring is guaranteed.

References

1. Banks PA (1979) Pancreatitis. Plenum, New York
2. Barie PS, Tahamont MV, Malik AB (1982) Prevention of increased pulmonary vascular permeability after pancreatitis by granulocyte depletion in sheep. Am Rev Respir Dis 126:904–908
3. Barzilay E, Kessler D, Berlot G, Gullo A, Geber D, Zeev JB (1989) Use of extracorporeal supportive techniques as additional treatment for septic-induced multiple organ failure patients. Crit Care Med 17:634–637
4. Beaulieux J, Boulez J, Peix JL, Donne R (1981) La nutrition enterale par jejunostomie d'alimentation au cours des pancreatites aigues graves. Chirurgie 107:59
5. Garcia-Szabo RR, Malik AB (1984) Pancreatitis-induced increase in lung vascular permeability. Am Rev Respir Dis 129:580–583
6. Hess ML, Hastillo A, Greenfield LJ (1981) Spectrum of cardiovascular function during gram-negative sepsis. Prog Cardiovasc Dis 23:279–298
7. Hölbling N, Roth E, Karner J, Zöch G, Funovics J (1981) Change of free amino acid metabolism in acute necrotizing pancreatitis. Eur Surg Res 13:34
8. Lee BC et al. (1981) Effect of acute pancreatitis on pulmonary transvascular fluid and protein exchange. Am Rev Respir Dis 123:618–621
9. Murphy D et al. (1976) The mechanism of acute respiratory insufficiency in acute pancreatitis. Br J Surg 63:669
10. Oettinger W, Walter G, Jensen U, Beyer A, Peskar BA (1983) Endogenous prostaglandin F_{22} in the hyperdynamic state of severe sepsis in man. Br J Surg 70:237–239
11. Ranson JHC et al. (1974) Respiratory complications in acute pancreatitis. Am Surg 179:557–566
12. Zieve L, Vogel WC (1961) Measurement of lecithinase A in serum and other body fluids. J Lab Clin Med 57:586–599

Endoscopic Treatment of Biliary Acute Pancreatitis

D.L. CARR-LOCKE[1]

Etiology

Gallstones and alcohol represent the most common etiologic factors associated with over 80% of the cases of acute pancreatitis. There is an extensive list of other associated conditions (see Table 1), with approximately 10% of cases falling into the idiopathic category if a thorough investigation is carried out [1–4]. Gallstones are the most common single cause of acute pancreatitis in the United Kingdom [2, 5–7] and in certain parts of North America [8–10].

The clinical course of acute pancreatitis is variable and several established criteria are used to predict prognosis. Acute pancreatitis may progress to coagulative necrosis with resultant necrotizing pancreatitis, and hemorrhagic pancreatitis develops if there is rupture of blood vessels. As the blood dissects along tissue planes a bluish discoloration in the periumbilical area (Cullen's sign) or in the flank area (Grey Turner's sign) may become apparent. Abscess and pseudocyst formation, extension into adjacent viscera and spaces, exudative effusions, and systemic manifestations including adult respiratory distress syndrome, disseminated intravascular coagulation, distant fat necrosis, hypovolemia, and shock are all components of the spectrum of severe complications of the disease [3–14].

Pathogenesis

In 1901, Opie [15] reported on a patient who died of pancreatitis; an autopsy revealed a small stone impacted at the ampulla of Vater. The stone was small enough to be in the common channel communicating with the common bile duct and the pancreatic duct. Opie reasoned that this allowed reflux of bile into the pancreatic duct, and in subsequent experimentation he produced hemorrhagic pancreatitis by injecting bile into the pancreatic duct. In retrospect, the pressure of injecting fluid into the pancreatic duct may have been equally responsible. The role of infected bile in the pathogenesis

[1] Brigham and Women's Hospital, Dept. of Endoscopy, 75, Francis Street, Boston, MA 02115, USA

Beger/Büchler/Malfertheiner (Eds.)
Standards in Pancreatic Surgery

Table 1. Factors/conditions associated with acute pancreatitis

Cholelithiasis/choledocholithiasis
Ethanol
Medication (L-asparaginase, sulfonamidies, tetracyclines, furosemide, ddI chlorothiazides, estrogens, etc.)
Hyperlipoproteinemia
Hypercalcemia
Familial/hereditary
Traumatic
Postoperative (cardiopulmonary bypass, abdominal operations including biliary and gastric)
Pregnancy
ERCP
Pancreatic duct obstruction (tumor, stricture, choledochocele)
Pancreas divisum
Vascular (arteritis, embolic)
Infectious (viral: mumps, coxsackie; intraductal parasites; *Mycoplasma pneumoniae*)
Scorpion bite

of pancreatitis remains to be determined. The 'obstructive' theory has been supported by observation of operative cholangiography in patients with a history of pancreatitis; reflux of contrast into the pancreatic duct was demonstrated in about 60% of patients compared with 15% of controls, and a common channel of 5 mm or more was found in 72% of pancreatitis cases compared with only 20% of control subjects [16, 17]. Gallstones are recovered in the feces in 85%–95% of acute pancreatitis cases compared with 10% recovered in patients with symptomatic cholelithiasis without pancreatitis [18]. In patients with acute pancreatitis undergoing urgent operative intervention an incidence of common bile duct (CBD) stones as high as 63%–78% has been reported, compared with patients undergoing delayed operative procedures who have a 3%–33% incidence of CBD stones [8, 10, 18–23].

An alternative hypothesis of an incompetent or lax sphincter of Oddi, facilitating reflux of "activating" duodenal contents containing lysolecithin, bacterial toxin, and enterokinase into the pancreatic duct, has been thought to be present in patients prone to acute pancreatitis. This may be explained by previous gallstone passage, which can be sometimes identified at the time of ERCP on the basis of a patulous papilla [24].

Elements of both "obstructive" and "reflux" theories seem plausible; indeed, both obstruction at, and the passage of a stone through, the sphincter of Oddi may initiate an attack of acute pancreatitis.

Prediction of Severity and Outcome

The majority of patients with acute pancreatitis fully recover within a week or so of the attack with conservative management alone. A mortality of

Table 2. Ranson's criteria in acute pancreatitis – factors to predict severity of outcome [9]

At admission or diagnosis
Age over 55
WBC ⩾16 000/mm^3
Blood glucose ⩾100/dl
Serum LDH ⩾350 IU/l
Serum ALT (SGOT) ⩾250 IU/l
During initial 48 h
Hematocrit fall ⩾10%
BUN rise ⩾5 mg/dl
Serum calcium ⩽8 mg/dl
PaO_2 ⩽60 mmHg
Base deficit ⩾4 mEq/l
Fluid sequestration ⩾6 l
A mild attack: 0–2 factors present
A severe attack: 3–11 factors present

Table 3. Modified Glasgow criteria to predict severity of outcome of acute pancreatitis within the first 48 h [32, 33][a]

Age ⩾55 years
WBC ⩾15 000/mm^3
Serum glucose ⩾180 mg/dl (no previous Hx of diabetes)
Serum urea ⩾96 mg/dl (no response to i.v. fluids)
PaO_2 ⩽60 mmHg (no O_2 by mask for 15 min)
Serum Ca ⩽8 mg/dl
LDH ⩾600 IU/l
Serum albumin ⩽3.2 gm/dl

[a] Patient falls in mild attack category with 0–2 criteria, in severe attack category with 3–8 criteria.

about 10% is reported in unselected clinical series, but the true figure is closer to 20% if those additional cases diagnosed at postmortem are included [2, 6, 7, 25, 26]. Stratifying patients into mild and severe categories is helpful in directing appropriate management. This stratification also allows direct comparison between groups studied at different institutions and comparison between different treatment modalities. Ranson developed an 11-factor system to predict severity (see Table 2) [4].

Imrie et al. proposed a more simplified 8-factor system [27, 28]. A modified Glasgow System (see Table 3) is now widely used and includes age greater than 55 years, but not transaminases greater than 200 IU/l. This change was made after several recent reports – including one from Glasgow [5] and an independent study from Leicester [29] – confirmed the statistical significance of age in relation to outcome but not to the level of transaminases. The validity of these systems is now accepted and they are widely used to stratify patients [30]. Additional methods of predicting severity, such as Apache II scores, C-reactive protein concentrations, and others, are currently under assessment.

Clinical Assessment and Initial Management

Initial stabilization of the patient and assessment of the severity of the attack of acute pancreatitis to anticipate the potential systemic complications are important. Supportive measures including i.v. fluids, monitoring of arterial blood gases, chest X-ray, plain abdominal film with the patient upright to rule out free air from a perforated abdominal viscus, and serial physical examination of the abdomen are crucial. Nasogastric suction should be considered when severe nausea and vomiting occur or when ileus is present. Adequate analgesia can be safely administered once the etiology of the abdominal pain is identified. Narcotic analgesia can be safely administered despite the theoretical concern of inducing spasm of the sphincter of Oddi. Controversy regarding the routine use of antibiotics still exists [31]. Interventions to modify an acute attack of pancreatitis include consideration of ERCP and endoscopic sphincterotomy with stone extraction if choledocholithiasis is present, peritoneal lavage, or surgical intervention.

Identifying those patients who have gallstones is one of the most difficult problems. Ultrasonography during the acute phase of an attack can detect only about 60% of cases of acute pancreatitis that are subsequently shown to involve gallstones [30]. CT scanning has a low sensitivity and specificity for the detection of choledocholithiasis. Radionuclide biliary scanning is of no value in distinguishing those patients with gallstones from those without during the acute phase of pancreatitis [32, 33]. Biochemical predictive tests are of value, and the simple finding of raised bilirubin on admission greater than 40 μmol/l (3 mg/dl) has a sensitivity of 83% for bile duct stones [34].

Urgent Treatment

Early surgical intervention in cases of acute gallstone pancreatitis to prevent progression of the current attack to a more severe case and to reduce the chance of a recurrent attack [35] has been challenged due to the high risk of surgical morbidity and mortality. The application of ERCP was also thought to be too risky because of the possibility of aggravating the pancreatitis. The majority of cases of acute pancreatitis fall into the mild category and respond to conservative management alone [32, 33, 36].

Those cases predicted to be severe by either Ranson or Glasgow criteria cause the greatest amount of controversy. Common bile duct stones are found in 30%–60% of patients who die from gallstone-associated pancreatitis, but these stones are not always impacted in the ampulla or sitting in the common channel [6, 26]. Evaluation of the surgical literature on the treatment of gallstone-associated pancreatitis remains difficult, because patients have not usually been stratified into mild or severe cases and historical controls are often used to compare results [37]. Acosta et al. [38] reported only 1/46 deaths (2.9%) in a group treated by urgent surgical intervention as compared with 14/86 deaths (16%) of the historical control group, and Stone et al. [21] undertook a randomized prospective study, with 1/36 (2.8%) deaths for urgent surgery and 2/29 (5.9%) for early or delayed surgery, but in neither study was there any differentiation between mild and severe cases. Ranson urged nonoperative intervention after experiencing a high mortality for surgery during the acute phase of gallstone pancreatitis [23]. In this series, although groups were stratified by severity, the comparison was not appropriate owing to the mean prognostic score of 5.4 in those who underwent urgent surgery compared with 3.5 in those treated conservatively. Those who died after surgery had a higher severity score than those who survived surgery. This problem of nonstratification for severity has been seen in other studies with similar design flaws [8, 28, 35]. In the most recent prospective randomized surgical study [39], Kelly and Wagner demonstrated a very high mortality of 48% in patients with predicted severe attacks operated upon early compared with a still unacceptable 11% mortality for those operated upon later. By contrast, those patients with low Ranson scores carried mortalities of 3.3% and 0% respectively. Thus, surgical opinion would point toward avoidance of biliary surgery during the acute phase of pancreatitis, but a safer nonsurgical method might achieve the advantages of clearing the bile duct of stones without the complications inherent in open surgery in these very ill patients.

ERCP and Endoscopic Sphincterotomy

The initial application of ERCP and endoscopic sphincterotomy (ES) in acute gallstone-associated pancreatitis began with sporadic case reports from various centers around the world [40–48]. The fear of complications of ES, including exacerbation of pancreatitis, cholangitis, hemorrhage, and perforation, was not realized. All authors commented on how rapidly some patients improved with establishment of effective drainage and normalization of laboratory values [40–48]. Although encouraging, these reports were deficient in terms of methods, patient selection, timing of ES in relationship to attack, stratification of patients, and standardization of reporting complications.

The Leicester group published the first and, to date, only prospective randomized controlled trial of urgent ERCP and ES versus conservative treatment for acute pancreatitis due to gallstones [49]. They randomized 121 patients with gallstone pancreatitis either to receive conventional conservative treatment or to undergo urgent (within 72 h) ERCP with ES, and stone extraction only in those whose ERCP showed stones in the CBD. From a total of 223 consecutive patients admitted, the 121 were selected on the basis of urgent findings of ultrasonography performed within 24 h and/or biochemical prediction based on a validated system [49]. Patient stratification was based on the modified Glasgow criteria.

There were 59 patients randomized to ERCP, with successful cholangiography in 80% of the group classified as severe and in 94% in the group classified as mild. An effort was made not to inject the pancreatic duct, and if the pancreatic duct was injected, the injection was immediately stopped. The pancreatic duct filled, often incompletely, in 50% of the severe group and 90% of the mild group. Undue manipulation of the ampulla was avoided. Common bile duct stones were found in 63% of the predicted severe group and only 26% of those with predicted mild attacks. Notably, the CBD diameter was greater in those patients predicted to be in the severe category.

This study had four important findings: (a) ERCP can be safely performed in acute pancreatitis by an experienced endoscopist. (b) There was a significant reduction in major complications of acute pancreatitis due to stones following ERCP, ES, and stone extraction (12% morbidity compared with 61% morbidity in the conventional group). (c) This significant reduction in morbidity was also apparent in those with predicted severe attacks. (d) Urgent sphincterotomy nearly halved the hospital stay for those with severe attacks (median 9.5 days versus 17 days).

A statistical difference in mortality was not demonstrated in this trial, but none was anticipated given the size of the group studied. It is notable that of the three patients in the conventional group with confirmed gallstones who died, one at was found postmortem to have a stone impacted at the ampulla of Vater. This study provided a rational basis for the application of ERCP/ES and stone extraction in cases of acute pancreatitis associated with gallstones. The increasing evidence of coexistent cholangitis may give added reason for rapid improvement after endoscopic bile duct clearance [50]. The lower morbidity and mortality of ERCP/ES compared with those of surgical decompression may be due to the fact that outcome of ES, unlike that with general anesthesia and surgery, is independent of associated medical risk factors [34, 50, 51].

References

1. Steer ML (1989) Classification and pathogenesis of pancreatitis. Surg Clin North Am 69:467–480
2. Goodman AJ, Neoptolemos JP, Carr-Locke DL et al. (1985) Detection of gallstones after acute pancreatitis. Gut 26:125–132
3. Corfield AP, Cooper MJ, Williamson RCN (1985) Prediction of severity in acute pancreatitis: a prospective comparison of the prognostic indices. Lancet 2:403–407

4. Ranson JHC (1982) Etiologic and prognostic factors in human acute pancreatitis: a review. Am J Gastroenterol 77:633–638
5. Blamey SL, Imrie CW, O'Neill J et al. (1984) Prognostic factors in acute pancreatitis. Gut 25:1340–1346
6. Corfield AP, Cooper MJ, Williamson RCN (1985) Acute pancreatitis: a lethal disease of increasing incidence. Gut 26:724–729
7. MRC Multicentre Trial (1977) Death from acute pancreatitis. Lancet 2:632–635
8. Kelly TR (1980) Gallstone pancreatitis. The timing of surgery. Surgery 88: 345–349
9. Acosta JM, Peligrini CA, Skinner DB (1980) Etiology and pathogenesis of acute biliary pancreatitis. Surgery 88:118–125
10. Dixon JA, Hillam JD (1970) Surgery treatment of biliary tract disease associated with acute pancreatitis. Am J Surg 120:371–375
11. Frey CF, Bradley EL III, Beger HG (1988) Progress in acute pancreatitis. Surg Gynecol Obstet 167:282–286
12. van Sonnenberg E, Casola G, Varney RR et al. (1989) Imaging and interventional radiology for pancreatitis and its complications. Radiol Clin North Am 27:65–72
13. Steiner E, Mueller PR, Hahn PF et al. (1988) Complicated pancreatic abscesses: problems in interventional management. Radiology 167:443–446
14. Ranson JHC, Balthazar E, Caccavale R et al. (1985) Computed tomography and the prediction of pancreatic abscess in acute pancreatitis. Ann Surg 201:656–665
15. Opie EL (1901) The etiology of acute hemorrhagic pancreatitis. Johns Hopkins Hosp Bull 121:182–188
16. Cuschieri A, Hughes JH (1973) Pancreatic reflux during operative choledochography. Br J Surg 60:933–936
17. Kelly TR (1976) Gallstone pancreatitis: pathophysiology. Surgery 80:488–492
18. Armstrong CP, Taylor TV, Jeacock J et al. (1985) The biliary tract in patients with acute gallstone pancreatitis. Br J Surg 72:551–555
19. Acosta JM, Ledesma CL (1974) Gallstone migration as a cause of acute pancreatitis. N Engl J Med 290:484–487
20. Kelly TR, Swaney PE (1982) Gallstone pancreatitis: the second time around. Surgery 92:571–575
21. Stone HH, Fabian TC, Dunlop WE (1981) Gallstone pancreatitis: biliary tract pathology in relation to time of operation. Ann Surg 194:305–310
22. Paloyan D, Simonowitz D, Skinner DB (1975) The timing of biliary tract operations in patients with pancreatitis associated with gallstones. Surg Gynecol Obstet 141:737–739
23. Ranson JHC (1979) The timing of biliary surgery in acute pancreatitis. Ann Surg 189:654–662
24. Cuschieri A, Cumming JGR, Wood RAB et al. (1983) Evidence for sphincter dysfunction in patients with gallstone-associated pancreatitis. Effect of ceruletide in patients undergoing cholecystectomy for gallbladder disease and gallstone-associated pancreatitis. Br J Surg 71:885–888
25. Mayer AD, McMahon MJ, Benson EA et al. (1984) Operations upon the biliary tract in patients with acute pancreatitis: aims, indications and timing. Ann R Coll Surg Engl 66:179–183
26. DeBolla AR, Obeid ML (1984) Mortality in acute pancreatitis. Ann R Coll Surg Engl 66:184–186
27. Imrie CW, Banjamin IS, Ferguson JC (1978) A single-centre double-blind trial of Trasyol therapy in primary acute pancreatitis. Br J Surg 65:337–641
28. Obsorne DH, Imrie CW, Carter DC (1981) Biliary surgery in the same admission for gallstone-associated acute pancreatitis. Br J Surg 68:758–761
29. Leese T, Shaw D (1988) Comparison of three Glasgow multifactor prognostic scoring systems in acute pancreatitis. Br J Surg 75:460–462

30. Williamson RCN (1984) Early assessment of severity in acute pancreatitis. Gut 25:1331–1339
31. Beger HG, Bittner R, Block S et al. (1986) Bacterial contamination of pancreatic necrosis. A prospective clinical study. Gastroenterology 91:433–438
32. Neoptolemos JP, Hall AW, Finlay DF et al. (1984) The urgent diagnosis of gallstones in acute pancreatitis: a prospective study of three methods. Br J Surg 71:230–233
33. Neoptolemos JP, Fossard DP, Berry JM (1983) A prospective study of radionuclide biliary scanning in acute pancreatitis. Ann R Coll Surg Engl 65:180–182
34. Neoptolemos JP, London N, Bailey I et al. (1987) The role of clinical and biochemical criteria and endoscopic retrograde cholangiopancreatography in the urgent diagnosis of common bile duct stones in acute pancreatitis. Surgery 100:732–742
35. Tondelli P, Stutz K, Harder F et al. (1982) Acute gallstone pancreatitis: best timing for biliary surgery. Br J Surg 69:709–710
36. Fan ST, Choi TK, Lai CS et al. (1988) Influence of age on the mortality from acute pancreatitis. Br J Surg 75:463–466
37. Ranson JHC (1990) The role of surgery in the management of acute pancreatitis. Ann Surg 211:382–393
38. Acosta JM, Rossi R, Galli OMR et al. (1978) Early surgery for acute gallstone pancreatitis: evaluation of a systematic approach. Surgery 83:367–370
39. Kelly TR, Wagner DS (1988) Gallstone pancreatitis: a prospective randomized trial of the timing of surgery. Surgery 104:600–605
40. Roesch W, Demling L (1982) Endoscopic management of pancreatitis. Surg Clin North Am 62:845–852
41. Classen M, Ossenberg W, Wurbs D et al. (1978) Pancreatitis: an indication for endoscopic papillotomy? Endoscopy 10:223 (abstr)
42. Van Spuy DS (1981) Endoscopic sphincterotomy in the management of gallstone pancreatitis. Endoscopy 13:25–26
43. Safrany L (1982) Controversies in acute pancreatitis. In: Hollender LF (ed) Controversies in acute pancreatitis. Springer, Berlin Heidelberg New York, pp 214–218
44. Schott B, Neuhaus B, Portacarrero G et al. (1982) Endoskopische Papillotomie bei akuter bilaren Pankreatitis. Klinikarzt 11:52–54
45. Kautz G, Kohaus H, Keferstein R-D et al. (1982) Zur Pathogenese und endoskopischen Therapie der akuten bilaren Pankreatitis. Klinikarzt 11: 1202–1212
46. Riemann von JF, Lux G (1984) Therapeutische Strategie bei der akuten Pankreatitis. 1. Fortschr Med 102:179–182
47. Rosseland AR, Solhaug JH (1984) Early or delayed endoscopic papillotomy (EPT) in gallstone pancreatitis. Ann Surg 199:165–167
48. Neoptolemos JP, London N, Slater ND et al. (1986) A prospective study of ERCP and endoscopic sphincterotomy in the diagnosis and treatment of gallstone acute pancreatitis. Arch Surg 121:697–702
49. Neoptolemos JP, Carr-Locke DL, London NJ (1988) Controlled trial or urgent endoscopic retrograde cholangiopancreatography and endoscopic sphincterotomy versus conservative treatment for acute pancreatitis due to gallstones. Lancet 2:979–983
50. Neoptolemos JP, Davidson BR, Vallance D et al. (1988) The role of duodenal bile crystal analysis in the investigation of "idiopathic" pancreatitis. Br J Surg 75:450–453
51. Neoptolemos JP (1988) The urgent diagnosis and treatment of biliary (gallstone associated) acute pancreatitis. Hunterian Lecture: Royal College of Surgeons of England, London, September

Percutaneous Drainage of Severe Complications of Pancreatitis

E. vanSonnenberg[1]

Introduction

Percutaneous needling and catheterization guided by radiologic imaging have become well-accepted and valuable adjuncts for the treatment of complications of pancreatitis. Diagnostic aspiration of pancreatic collections has value in establishing the presence of infection. Catheter drainage is a safe and efficacious method to treat infected and noninfected pancreatic pseudocysts. Percutaneous drainage usually is beneficial with pancreatic abscess as well (Fig. 1). Pancreatic necrosis can be quite problematic, and pancreatic phlegmon is generally not in the purview of catheter drainage. This article will focus on the indications, problems, and role of catheter drainage for the severe complications of pancreatitis – pseudocyst, abscess, and necrosis.

Imaging Preceding Radiologic Intervention

Computed tomography (CT) is the modality of choice to image complications of pancreatitis. While ultrasound may demonstrate the pancreas, there commonly are impediments to a complete sonographic examination of the pancreas. However, ultrasound does provide important information about whether or not the bile duct is obstructed, whether or not there are gall-bladder stones, and the status of the liver. However, to best visualize the pancreas and the inflammatory response that is evolving, CT is preferable.

The technique for imaging with CT should involve a few scans through the pancreas initially without contrast to determine whether there is hemorrhagic pancreatitis. If so, high-density material is seen on the non-contrast scans. Percutaneous drainage has no role in this situation.

With intravenous contrast, scans should be obtained at 1-cm intervals through the upper abdomen and at 1.5-cm intervals through the pelvis. Since pancreatic inflammatory changes can be quite extensive and extend into the supradiaphragmatic region, correlation should be made with a chest

[1] Departments of Radiology and Medicine, University of California, San Diego Medical Center, 225 Dickinson Street, San Diego, CA 92103, USA

Beger/Büchler/Malfertheiner (Eds.)
Standards in Pancreatic Surgery

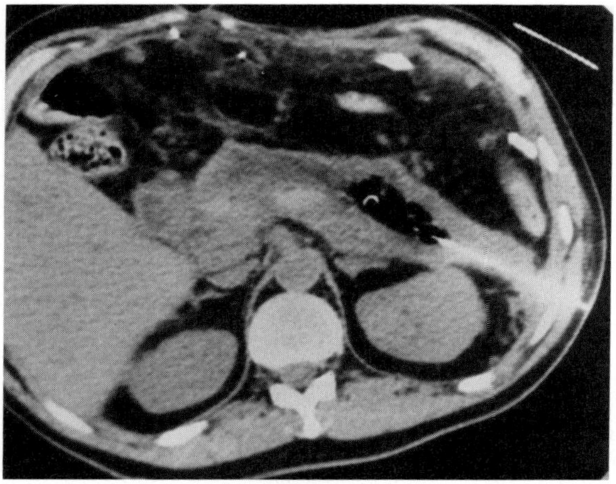

Fig. 1. Percutaneous drainage of pancreatic abscess in a patient with persistent sepsis after several operations

X-ray; if there are signs of mediastinal and pleural disease, scans can be extended into the chest to further delineate these abnormalities – parenchymal disease, pleural effusion, mediastinal pseudocyst.

Intravenous contrast provides information on the integrity of the pancreas, on the density of the inflammatory response, and on the "drainability" of the pancreatic and peripancreatic abnormalities [2, 3]. Contrast enhancement within the inflammatory mass signifies tissue that is likely to be phlegmon and therefore is not amenable to catheter drainage. Conversely, areas within the inflammation that do not enhance and are low density either represent edema, noninfected fluid, abscess, or necrosis (Fig. 2). Edema does not need to be drained, and thick necrotic tissue cannot be drained with a catheter. However, both necrosis in the form of low or medium viscosity brownish fluid and frank pus from an abscess can be drained with a catheter. Differentiating abscess from necrosis is not always possible by the CT scan alone. Needle aspiration or a trial of catheter drainage may be necessary to assess drainability in this situation.

Both infected and noninfected pseudocysts may be drained effectively with a catheter [4–6]. By imaging, pseudocysts are discrete, usually with a definable wall, and generally are unilocular (but may have septa). Although most commonly located in the pancreatic bed or lesser sac, the pseudocysts can be in remote sites such as intrahepatic, intrasplenic, or in the mediastinum, flanks, or groin. All these areas are all well visualized by CT.

Cystic tumors in the pancreas must be differentiated from pancreatic fluid collections. Usually these tumors have some nodularity or eccentric thickening of the wall. Calcification also occurs in 10%–20% of these tumors.

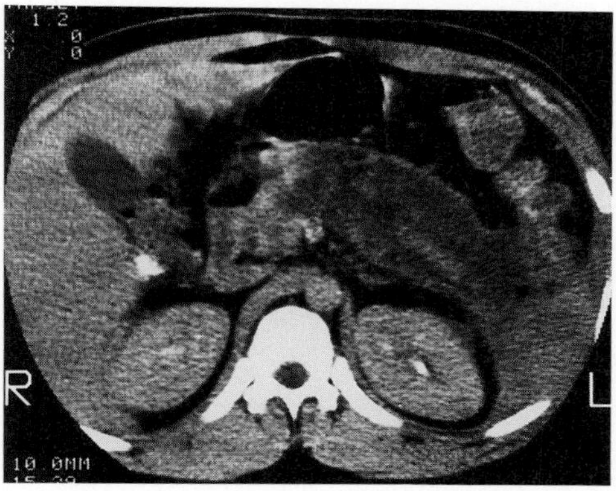

Fig. 2. After intravenous contrast administration, CT scan through the pancreatic bed reveals no definable pancreatic tissue. This appearance indicates necrotic, destroyed pancreas. (Reprinted from [1])

With chronic alcoholic pancreatitis, punctate calcifications commonly are seen within the pancreas. These type of calcifications are not seen with other forms of pancreatitis such as gallstone pancreatitis, traumatic pancreatitis, or drug-induced pancreatitis. The rare condition of hereditary pancreatitis also can result in intrapancreatic calcifications.

Diagnostic Aspiration

Fine needle insertion into a pancreatic or peripancreatic collection serves numerous purposes. Most important is to obtain a specimen for culture and sensitivity. While gram-positive and gram-negative organisms are found commonly, Candida and other yeast also are seen on occasion [7, 8]. The fluid that is extracted by fine needle aspiration determines drainability – pus is an indication for catheter drainage, brownish material indicates necrosis and possible drainage, and bloody material or lack of aspiration means that catheter drainage would be ineffective and is inappropriate.

A fine needle inserted into a pancreatic collection also serves as a localizing marker for subsequent catheter insertion. This method is termed the tandem trocar technique. On occasion, it may be necessary to insert a 20- or 18-G needle, either to obtain a specimen or to perform a biopsy if 22-G needle aspiration has been unsuccessful in extracting fluid. Biopsy of a phlegmon or necrosis may yield a bacterial diagnosis (Fig. 3).

Percutaneous Drainage of Pancreatic Pseudocysts

Pancreatic pseudocysts can be drained effectively by percutaneous catheters. The indications differ depending on whether or not the pseudocyst is

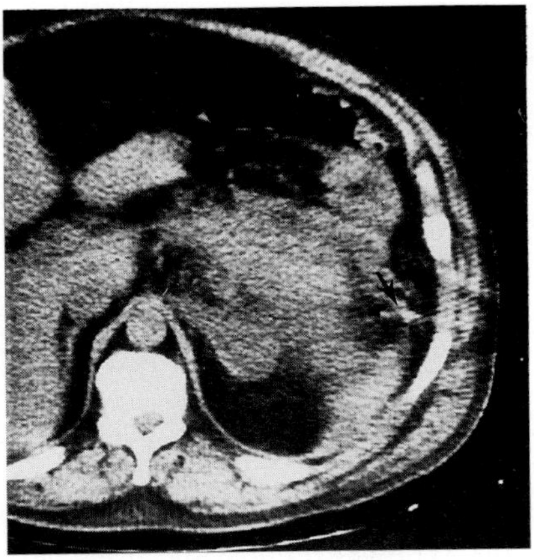

Fig. 3. Aspiration of a pancreatic phlegmon with a 20-gauge needle establishes diagnosis of infection with *E. coli*. CT shows high-density material in this phlegmon located in the tail of the pancreas; no gas is visible. Aspiration with a 22-gauge needle (*arrow*) was unsuccessful due to tissue viscosity. Surgical exploration and débridement were prompted by the diagnosis of infection. (Reprinted from [3])

infected. Infected discrete pseudocysts must be drained emergently (Fig. 4). Noninfected pseudocysts are not drained unless they are causing pain or obstruction or are enlarging over time.

One catheter usually suffices to drain a pancreatic pseudocyst. The catheter needs to remain in place until drainage ceases and communication to the pancreatic duct seals off. Intramuscular administration of octreotide may be a beneficial adjunct to drainage in cases with persistent clear drainage ("pancreatic fistula").

Patients with percutaneous catheters must be followed carefully on the ward by radiologists. Minor problems may arise that need attention; these include catheter clogging, leakage, migration, and wound infection. With appropriate attention, drainage should proceed efficiently. Cure occurs in up to 85% for noninfected pseudocysts and in over 90% for infected pseudocysts [3–6]. Occasionally a catheter may need to be exchanged; this can be done in the radiology suite without much difficulty.

The preferred route for pancreatic pseudocyst drainage is direct retroperitoneal or transperitoneal. Transgastric drainage is advocated by some authors [9], but benefits to this approach are unproven. However, where no other route is available (i.e., the pseudocyst is shielded), a transgastric, transenteric, transhepatic, or surgical approach must be utilized. While a transgastric double-J catheter provides complete internalization, the catheter cannot be exchanged easily, cannot be injected, and may migrate.

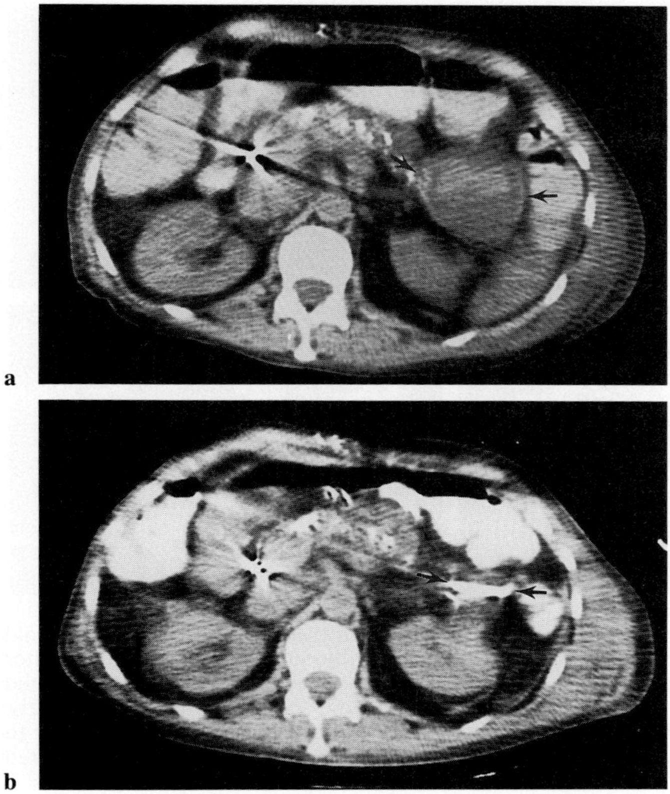

Fig. 4a,b. Successful drainage of an infected pseudocyst in the tail of the pancreas. This patient was semicomatose, had a temperature of 105°C, and a white blood cell count of 26000. **a** CT scan demonstrates a low-density mass (*arrows*) with higher-density tissue (pancreas?) within. No gas is seen to suggest infection. Chronic pancreatitis with calcification is evident. Aspiration with a 20-gauge needle revealed frank pus. **b** A 12-F sump catheter (*arrow*) has evacuated the collection (70 ml) that grew *E. coli* and *Staphylococcus aureus* (note severe left flank wall infection as well). The catheter was removed on the sixth day with no evidence of recurrence. (Reprinted from [3])

Drainage of Pancreatic Abscess

Pancreatic abscess usually is extensive and frequently multiseptated or multiloculated. Consequently, to adequately drain collections such as these, use of multiple catheters is the rule. Drainage is performed exclusively with CT guidance. Catheters that are used vary from 12–16 Fr initially. Sump systems are used routinely. Occasionally, larger bore catheters such as Malecots or Salem sumps up to 30 Fr may be inserted by the exchange

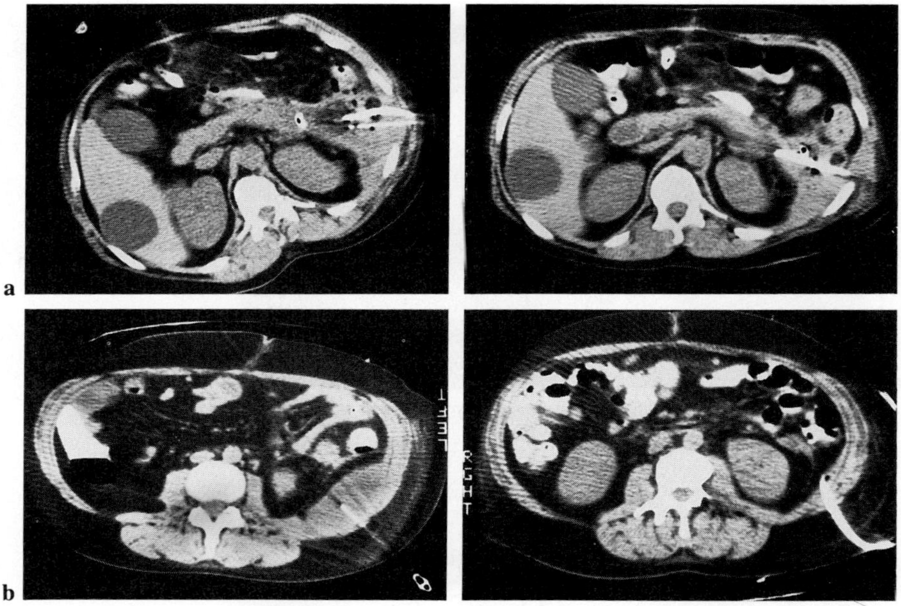

Fig. 5a–d. Percutaneous drainage cures complicated pancreatic abscess. 32-year-old woman with a temperature of 104°C and a white blood cell count of 35,000 after operation for pancreatic abscess. **a** CT scan demonstrates 5-cm multiloculated abscess in the tail of the pancreas. A 22-gauge needle and 12-F sump catheter have been placed in the abscess. Note the surgical drain outside the abscess, anterior to the pancreas. There is an incidental hepatic cyst. **b** The pancreatic abscess dissected caudally. At the lower level, pus was extracted through a 20-gauge needle, and a 12-F sump catheter was placed after needle localization. **c** CT scan 2 weeks later reveals marked improvement. **d** Lower abscess has resolved at 3 weeks on follow-up CT scan. The patient recovered and left the hospital after 28 days of catheter drainage. (Reprinted from [3])

technique. Initial catheter insertion usually is done by trocar technique, similar to drainage of most abscesses.

Cure of these abscesses by percutaneous drainage varies from 35% to 100% [3, 11, 12]. Problems that limit drainage include the presence of necrotic tissue that cannot be evacuated through a catheter, multiloculations, and extensiveness of disease.

Not infrequently, an operation for debridement will need to be performed after initial percutaneous drainage. Conversely, if surgery is undertaken initially, it is common to utilize percutaneous drainage subsequently to treat residual purulent collections (Fig. 5). This combined approach is curative in many cases.

Percutaneous Management of Pancreatic Necrosis

When pancreatic inflammation has progressed to solid tissue necrosis, percutaneous drainage will not be effective. When thick organized material occurs in the pancreatic and peripancreatic bed, this can only be removed surgically. Operative "necrosectomy" is indicated in this circumstance, and frequently multiple operations are required.

On the other hand, when necrosis is in the form of lysed fluid, catheter drainage can be successful. Commonly, one finds brownish fluid interspersed with debris. CT demonstrates low-density material in these cases.

The findings of necrosis on CT include glandular swelling and progressive, low-density areas within the pancreas. The necrotic areas do not enhance with intravenous contrast. The internal contents often are inhomogeneous, and ring-like contrast enhancement may be seen. Gas in a collection is not pathognomic for infection, and the presence or absence of infection cannot be distinguished by the CT scan (7). The presence of nonenhancement of the pancreas on bolus CT examination bodes for more complications, a stormier course for the patient, and a higher mortality [2, 13].

With percutaneous drainage, catheters must be irrigated frequently, sump systems are beneficial, and large-bore tubes are essential. Multiple catheters are the rule, usually entering from various sites – anteriorly into the head region and via the flanks, both transperitoneally and retroperitoneally.

Results of drainage of pancreatic necrosis reveal a beneficial temporizing effect in many patients [14]. Cure may be achieved if the necrotic material is not too viscous and if an adequate number of drainage catheters has been inserted.

Follow-up CT usually is essential. This is both to monitor the adequacy of drainage and to ascertain whether undrained collections remain. CT with intravenous contrast reveals the amount of viable pancreas after surgery or percutaneous drainage. Necrosis with phlegmon is associated with a higher rate of morbidity and mortality than phlegmon alone [13].

Acknowledgement. Thanks to Mrs. Peggy Chambers for preparation of the manuscript.

References

1. Anderson N, vanSonnenberg E, Casola G, Varney RR (1989) Radiologic imaging and intervention for pancreatic inflammatory disease. In: Thompson WM (ed) Common problems in gastrointestinal radiology. Yearbook, Chicago, pp 601–619
2. Balthazar EJ (1989) CT diagnosis and staging of acute pancreatitis. Radiol Clin N Am 27:29–37

3. vanSonnenberg E, Wittich GR, Casola G, Stauffer AE, Polansky AD, Coons HG, Cabrera OA, Gerver PS (1985) Complicated pancreatic inflammatory disease: diagnostic and therapeutic role of interventional radiology. Radiology 155:335–340
4. Torres WE, Evert MB, Baumgartner BR, Bernardino ME (1986) Percutaneous aspiration and drainage of pancreatic pseudocysts. AJR 147:1007–1009
5. vanSonnenberg E, Wittich GR, Casola G, Brannigan TC, Karnel F, Stabile BE, Varney RR, Christensen R (1989) Percutaneous drainage of infected and noninfected pancreatic pseudocysts: experience in 101 cases. Radiology 170: 757–761
6. Gerzof SG, Johnson WC, Robbins AH, Spechler SJ, Nabseth DC (1984) Percutaneous drainage of infected pancreatic pseudocysts. Arch Surg 119: 888–893
7. Hill MC, Cach JL, Barkin J, Isikoff MB, Morse B (1983) The role of percutaneous aspiration in the diagnosis of pancreatic abscess. AJR 141: 1035–1038
8. White EM, Wittenberg J, Mueller PR, Simeone JF, Butch RJ, Warshaw AL, Neff CC, Nardi GL, Ferrucci JT Jr (1986) Pancreatic necrosis: CT manifestations. Radiology 158:343–346
9. Sacks BA, Greenberg JJ, Porter DH, Capobianco A, Painter M, Kim R, Orron DE, Kim D (1989) An internalized double-J catheter for percutaneous transgastric cystogastrostomy. AJR 152:523–526
10. vanSonnenberg E, Casola G, Varney RR, Wittich GR (1989) Imaging and interventional radiology for pancreatitis and its complications. Radiol Clin N Am 271:65–72
11. Karlson KB, Martin EC, Fankuchen EI, Mattern RF, Schultz RW, Casarella WJ (1982) Percutaneous drainage of pancreatic pseudocysts and abscesses. Radiology 142:619–624
12. Freeny PC, Lewis GP, Traverso LW, Ryan JA (1988) Infected pancreatic fluid collections: Percutaneous catheter drainage. Radiology 167:435–441
13. Balthazar EJ, Robinson DL, Megibow AJ, Ranson JHC (1990) Acute pancreatitis: Value of CT in establishing prognosis. Radiology 174:331–336
14. vanSonnenberg E, Wing VW, Casola G, Coons HG, Nakamoto SK, Mueller PR, Ferrucci JT, Halasz NA, Simeone JF (1984) Temporizing percutaneous drainage of complicated abscesses in critically ill patients. AJR 142:821–826

Indications for Surgery: The Internist's View

P.A. BANKS[1]

There are many indications for intervention in acute pancreatitis, including trauma to the pancreas, impacted gallstone, complications of pseudocyst, pancreatic abscess, infected necrosis, and possibly sterile necrosis. Most of these have been covered elsewhere. I would like to focus on infected necrosis and sterile necrosis.

There is general agreement that infected necrosis requires surgical débridement [1, 2]. In our experience, guided percutaneous aspiration has proven to be a safe, accurate method for distinguishing pancreatic infection from severe sterile pancreatitis [3, 4]. Among 72 patients strongly suspected of harboring pancreatic infection because they had evidence of severe pancreatitis on CT scan (grade D or E according to the Balthazar criteria) [5] and also exhibited severe clinical toxicity (high fever and leukocytosis), CT-guided percutaneous aspiration correctly identified the 39 patients with pancreatic infection. The prior use of antibiotics did not diminish our ability to distinguish sterile from infected pancreatitis. All but one Gram stain from infected aspirates were positive (all infected aspirates were confirmed by culture). Hence, Gram staining was of great value in the immediate recognition of pancreatic infection. Others have also found that CT-guided percutaneous aspiration is reliable in diagnosing pancreatic infection [6–8].

We further found that 51% of pancreatic infections (20 of 39 patients) took place within the first 2 weeks of illness. In the experience of Beger and his associates [9], 30% of infections occurred during the first 2 weeks of illness. Hence, pancreatic infection may occur early in acute pancreatitis, and guided percutaneous aspiration should be performed as soon as there is clinical suspicion of infection.

Aided by bacteriologic information provided by guided percutaneous aspiration, we should be able to diagnose infected necrosis of the pancreas at an early stage. Early surgical débridement is an important factor in the improved survival of patients with infected necrosis [10].

When we looked carefully at our results with guided percutaneous aspiration for the purpose of distinguishing sterile from infected necrosis at

[1] Brigham and Women's Hospital, GI Suite ASBII-2, 75 Francis Street, Boston, MA 02115, USA

Beger/Büchler/Malfertheiner (Eds.)
Standards in Pancreatic Surgery

several hospitals in Boston, we were impressed that the clinical toxicity of patients who proved to have sterile necrosis was similar to that of patients with infected necrosis [3, 4]. This is not to say that all patients with sterile necrosis have clinical toxicity, or that all patients with sterile necrosis should receive guided percutaneous aspiration. Only those patients with necrotizing pancreatitis who were experiencing clinical toxicity were subjected to guided percutaneous aspiration. Our experience does indicate that when necrotizing pancreatitis is associated with clinical toxicity, it is impossible to distinguish sterile necrosis from infected necrosis without guided percutaneous aspiration.

We were also impressed that the mortality of patients with sterile necrosis who had clinical toxicity (and who therefore had received guided percutaneous aspiration to exclude pancreatic infection) was somewhat higher than that of patients with infected necrosis 23% vs. 10%) [3, 4]. This does not imply that the mortality of sterile necrosis in general is higher than that of infected necrosis. The mortality of sterile necrosis is usually lower than that of infected necrosis [9–11]; however, when sterile necrosis is associated with clinical toxicity, in our experience the mortality has been high.

There is reason to suspect that the mortality of sterile necrosis associated with clinical toxicity is indeed higher than is generally appreciated. First, in the only published report on the mortality of sterile necrosis associated with systemic complications, mortality ranged from 16% to 22% [11]. In particular, patients with sterile necrosis with a sepsis-like picture experienced a mortality of 22% [10].

Second, among reports of patients with severe pancreatitis who experienced systemic complications, including respiratory failure, shock, renal failure, or a sepsis-like picture, average mortality in published reports has been 32% (range 9.4%–56%) [11–24]. These reports did not provide information as to whether patients had sterile or infected necrosis.

Third, when death occurs in necrotizing pancreatitis and there is no bacteriologic information provided by guided percutaneous aspiration, surgery, or autopsy, it remains unclear whether the patient died of sterile or infected necrosis.

Finally, the criteria that are utilized for the purpose of designating whether patients have either sterile or infected necrosis may differ from institution to institution. For example, in one published report [25], patients with sterile necrosis who underwent surgical débridement and then developed pancreatic infection during the postoperative period were listed as having infected necrosis rather than sterile necrosis. In my view, patients who are bacteriologically sterile at the time of the first intervention should be classified as having sterile necrosis even if pancreatic infection ensues as a result of surgery.

In view of our high mortality in sterile necrosis associated with clinical toxicity, we have sought to identify factors that might predict a fatal outcome. Diagnosis of pancreatic necrosis was confirmed by CT scan with i.v. contrast with the bolus technique and/or by findings at surgery or autopsy. Pancreatic infection was excluded by negative Gram stain and culture of aspirates obtained percutaneously and/or negative culture and tissue Gram stain obtained at surgery. All patients were considered to have clinical toxicity if they experienced one or more systemic complications (respiratory insufficiency, shock, renal failure, or a sepsis-like picture).

Based on these criteria, we have identified 26 patients with severe sterile necrosis at St. Elizabeth's Hospital of Boston during the past 5 years. Of these 26 patients, ten had a fatal outcome.

Possible prognostic factors that were evaluated included age, sex, etiology, data at admission (including delay of admission, vital signs, laboratory tests, admission first to outside hospital), body mass index (BMI), Ranson's scores, APACHE-II scores at admission and at 48 h, and presence of one or more complications: cardiovascular (systolic blood pressure less than 80 mmHg for 15 min); respiratory (PO_2 less than 60 mmHg requiring oxygen therapy for greater than 24 h); renal (serum creatinine greater than 1.4 mg% during the hospitalization); sepsis-like picture (temperature greater than 38.5°C and white blood count greater than 20 000 mm^3); coagulopathy; and GI bleeding requiring transfusion. Other factors included number of complications, timing of complications, CT appearance, and surgical therapy (compared with medical therapy, timing of urgent surgery, and APACHE-II scores on the day of surgery).

The factors that proved to be of prognostic significance ($p < 0.05$) in the 16 patients who lived compared with the ten who died included BMI (25.2 vs. 28.9), Ranson's scores (4.6 vs. 6.3), APACHE-II scores at admission (6.9 vs. 13), APACHE-II scores at 48 h (8.9 vs. 16.5), the presence of shock (12.5% of patients who lived vs. 90% of patients who died), and the number of complications (mean 2.7 vs. 3.9). No other factors achieved statistical significance. Eight of 11 patients with four or more complications died; all eight patients with two or less complications survived. Almost all complications occurred within the first 14 days of illness. The timing of complications did not have prognostic significance in those who lived versus those who died. Patients who survived were operated on approximately 33 days from the onset of symptoms; those who died were operated on 21 days after the onset ($p > 0.05$). Deaths occurred an average of 30 days after the onset of symptoms. The amount of necrosis did not correlate with a fatal outcome.

We concluded that in severe sterile necrosis, factors that correlated with a fatal outcome were obesity, high Ranson's scores, high APACHE-II scores at admission and at 48 h, the presence of shock, and multiple systemic complications. Since systemic complications usually took place within the first 2 weeks of illness, efforts directed toward improving survival of patients with severe sterile necrosis must be made during this time period.

While this study does not specifically address the question of whether surgery in particular offers an advantage when compared with medical treatment, the experience of Beger and his associates strongly suggests that in severe sterile pancreatitis associated with organ failure there is a role for early surgery [10, 11]. An opposing view has been taken by Bradley [26], who has managed 11 patients with severe sterile necrosis nonoperatively without a fatality. Additional information is required to clarify whether patients in his report had prognostic factors that would be predictive of a nonfatal outcome, such as the absence of shock and lower APACHE-II scores.

The results of the present study suggest to me that patients with severe sterile necrosis who have unfavorable prognostic factors that predict a fatal outcome, including high Ranson's scores, high APACHE-II scores, and organ failure, should be seriously considered for surgical débridement within the first 2 weeks of illness.

References

1. Banks PA, Gerzof SG, Chong FK et al. (1990) Bacteriologic status of necrotic tissue in necrotizing pancreatitis. Pancreas 5:330–333
2. Banks PA (1991) Infected necrosis: morbidity and therapeutic consequences. Hepatogastroenterology 38:116–119
3. Gerzof SG, Banks PA, Robbins AH, Johnson WC, Spechler SJ, Wetzner SM, Snider JM, Langevin RE, Jay ME (1987) Early diagnosis of pancreatic infection by CT-guided aspiration. Gastroenterology 93:1315–1320
4. Banks PA, Gerzof SG, Robbins AH, Johnson WC, Spechler SJ, Wetzner SM, Snider JM, Langevin RE, Jay ME (1988) Diagnosis of pancreatic infection by CT-guided aspiration: an update. American Pancreatic Association, Chicago, October 1988. Pancreas 3:590
5. Balthazar EJ, Robinson DL, Megibow AJ, Ranson JHC (1990) Acute pancreatitis: value of CT in establishing prognosis. Radiology 174:331–336
6. Crass RA, Meyer AA, Jeffrey RB et al. (1985) Pancreatic abscess: impact of computerized tomography on early diagnosis and surgery. Am J Surg 150: 127–131
7. Hiatt JR, Fink AS, King W III, Pitt HA (1987) Percutaneous aspiration of peripancreatic fluid collections: a safe method to detect infection. Surgery 101:523–530
8. Stiles GM, Berne TV, Thommen VD et al. (1990) Fine-needle aspiration of pancreatic fluid collections. Am Surg 56:764–768
9. Beger HG, Bittner R, Block S et al. (1986) Bacterial contamination of pancreatic necrosis. Gastroenterology 91:433–438
10. Beger HG, Buchler M, Bittner R et al. (1988) Necrosectomy and post-operative local lavage in necrotizing pancreatitis. Br J Surg 75:207–212
11. Roscher R, Beger HG (1987) Bacterial infection of pancreatic necrosis. In: Beger HG, Buchler M (eds) Acute pancreatitis. Springer, Berlin Heidelberg New York, pp 314–317
12. Leese T, Shaw D, Holliday M (1988) Prognostic markers in acute pancreatitis: can pancreatic necrosis be predicted? Ann R Coll Surg Engl 70:227–231
13. Demmy TL, Burch JM, Feliciano DV, Mattox KL (1988) Comparison of multiple-parameter prognostic systems in acute pancreatitis. Am J Surg 156: 492–496
14. Gudgeon AM, Heath DI, Hurley P et al. (1990) Trypsinogen activation peptides assay in the early prediction of severity of acute pancreatitis. Lancet 1(335):4–8
15. Buchler M, Malfertheiner P, Schadlich H et al. (1989) Role of phospholipase A_2 in human acute pancreatitis. Gastroenterology 97:1521–1526

16. Choi TK, Lai ECS, Wong J (1989) Prediction of severity of acute pancreatitis: an alternative approach. Gut 30:1591–1595
17. Corfield AP, Williamson RCN, McMahon MJ et al. (1985) Predictions of severity in acute pancreatitis: prospective comparison of three prognostic indices. Lancet 2:403–407
18. Gross V, Scholmerich J, Leser HG et al. (1987) Leukocyte elastase as a marker for severity of acute pancreatitis. Gastroenterology 96:A186
19. Larvin M, Chalmers AG, McMahon MJ (1990) Dynamic contrast-enhanced computed tomography: a precise technique for identifying and localising pancreatic necrosis. Br Med J 300:1425–1428
20. Larvin M, McMahon MJ (1989) APACHE-II score for assessment and monitoring of acute pancreatitis. Lancet 2:201–204
21. Clavien PA, Hauser H, Meyer P et al. (1988) Value of contrast-enhanced computerized tomography in the early diagnosis and prognosis of acute pancreatitis. Am J Surg 155:457–466
22. London NJM, Neoptolemos JP, Lavelle J et al. (1989) Serial computed tomography scanning in acute pancreatitis: a prospective study. Gut 30:397–403
23. Wilson C, Heath DI, Imrie CW (1990) Prediction of outcome in acute pancreatitis: a comparative study of APACHE-II, clinical assessment and multiple-factor scoring systems. Br J Surg 77:1260–1264
24. Bank S, Wise L, Gersten M (1983) Risk factors in acute pancreatitis. Am J Gastroenterol 78:637–640
25. Wilson C, McArdle S, Carter DC et al. (1988) Surgical treatment of acute necrotizing pancreatitis. Surgery 75:1119–1123
26. Bradley EL III, Allen K (1991) A prospective longitudinal study of observation versus surgical intervention in the management of necrotizing pancreatitis. Am J Surg 161:19–24

Indications for Surgery: The Surgeon's View

C.W. Imrie[1]

Indications for Surgery in Acute Necrotizing Pancreatitis

Among patients with severe acute pancreatitis, who represent approximately 20%–25% of all patients diagnosed with this disease, a proportion will come to surgery early in the first admission. This specifically excludes patients in whom the rarity of a diagnostic laparotomy is required. Within the severe group a minority will meet the indications for surgical intervention, provided the best possible conservative management is given. This minority group comprises between 4% and 17.5% of all patients [1, 2].

The major indications for surgical intervention are:

1. Sepsis in or around the pancreas
2. Failure to improve after 72h intensive care therapy, especially if combined with objective evidence of areas of poor or zero vascular perfusion of the pancreas

To obtain information prior to planned urgent surgical intervention, angiogram-enhanced computed tomography (CT) is crucial [3–6]. CT may also be of great help in localization of focal areas of sepsis. Seriously ill patients with acute pancreatitis should be moved to hospitals with the appropriate type of CT scanner and clinicians with expertise and major interest in this area.

The Proof of Peripancreatic/Pancreatic Sepsis

The presence of sepsis in this area may be strongly implied without imaging equipment in the patient who has a clinical and biochemical diagnosis of acute pancreatitis and in whom pyrexia persists without evidence of respiratory or urinary tract infection and in the absence of any intravenous line sepsis. Positive blood cultures can be most helpful, but often such patients are empirically put on wide-spectrum antibiotic therapy, and the failure of such a measure to lower the temperature is also a pointer to the need for surgical intervention.

[1] Royal Infirmary, Surgical Unit – Main Building, Glasgow G4 0SF, UK

Beger/Büchler/Malfertheiner (Eds.)
Standards in Pancreatic Surgery

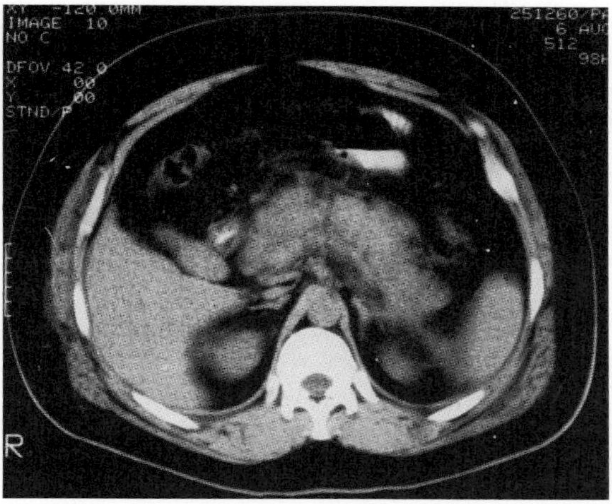

Fig. 1. CT scan of 30-year-old male patient 72 h after admission with severe acute pancreatitis. This shows marked pancreatic swelling throughout the gland

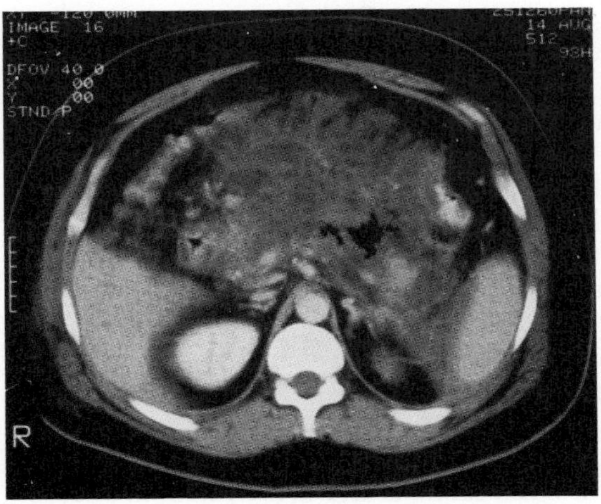

Fig. 2. The same patient 8 days later with development of focal abscess formation around the pancreas indicated by the black gas shadows on the anterior surface of the distal pancreas. A short time after this scan was taken surgical intervention was performed with a good result

Straight abdominal X-ray with the patient in an erect position may outline small bubbles of gas, especially in patients who have been ill for more than a week, but on occasion, gas-producing organisms can be detected at an earlier time by means of CT. A more typical situation is depicted in Figs. 1 and 2, where the initial scan shows evidence of widespread disruption associated with severe acute pancreatitis, gross pancreatic swelling and loss of tissue planes. Some 8 days later free gas in the peripancreatic area is noted, and this, combined with clinical deterioration and the classical signs of sepsis, makes surgical intervention the major clinical option, although in some old and frail patients, the percutaneous placement of small sump drains of the van Sonnenberg type may be an alternative therapy. These drains have a standard size of 7 FG and have a sump facility which allows for wash-through and aspiration.

Without access to a high-quality CT scanner we found in an earlier study [1] that the presence of a deteriorating clinical condition despite full high dependency or intensive care therapy is associated with the most extensive macroscopic necrosis in and around the pancreas. It is now my belief that surgery was delayed, or even withheld, because of the lack of objective evidence to indicate a requirement for surgical intervention in the absence of a high-quality CT scanner.

The Detection of Poor Vascular Perfusion

Poor vascular perfusion is best detected by angiogram-enhanced CT, and it is to the credit of progressive radiologists such as Freeny [3] that fewer and fewer patients come before a CT scan procedure to examine the pancreas, primarily without the intention of moving on to angiogram-enhanced CT. The difference in what can be obtained with and without angiogram enhanced. CT scan is indicated in Figs. 3 and 4. The presence of partial or complete failure to perfuse areas of the pancreas in the patient with a poor clinical status, especially one who has failed to improve after 72 h respiratory intensive care, warrants, I am convinced, full surgical intervention with digital necrosectomy of peripancreatic necrosis and any macroscopic pancreatic necrosis. The patient who is improving may demonstrate a disturbing CT scan: this should be monitored but never taken as a sole indicator for intervention.

Following digital necrosectomy, which may be aided by the gentle use of de Bakey forceps, peroperative warm saline lavage is indicated; in addition, it is my increasingly firm conviction that *cholecystectomy should be performed* in all patients who are reasonably likely to have tiny stones in the gallbladder, as well as those who have proven larger stones. The object of this is obviously to minimize the risk of further attacks of acute pancreatitis, and the failure to outline such stones by imaging methods, including ultrasound and ERCP, should not deter the surgeon. Examples of two patients whose gallbladders had been considered free from stones on ultrasound scanning are given in Figs. 5 and 6. Peroperative cholangiography should also be performed unless an ERCP [6] has been carried out immediately beforehand. In this latter circumstance the duct may well have been cleared, and no patient should leave the operating room with stones or biliary sand remain-

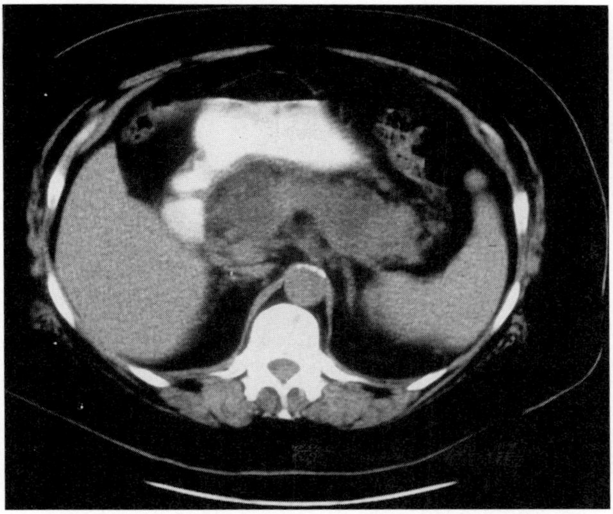

Fig. 3. Routine CT scan of 63 year old female (gallstone) patient at 11 days after onset of disease

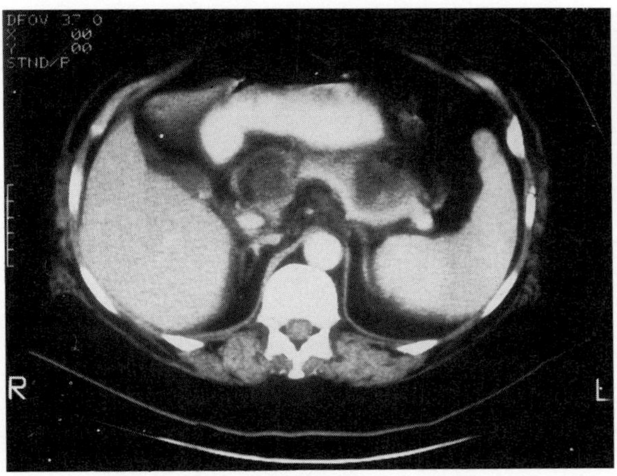

Fig. 4. Same patient at same time 4 level of scan showing benefit of angiogram enhancement to outline 2 areas of very poor perfusion (necrosis) of pancreas found in head and tail at operation

ing anywhere in the biliary tree. At the time of necrosectomy generous use of saline washing is recommended, and, if bleeding is difficult to control, packing the abdomen with cotton packs (enclosed in paraffin gauze to minimize adherence) should be preferred to the use of lavage tubes then and later.

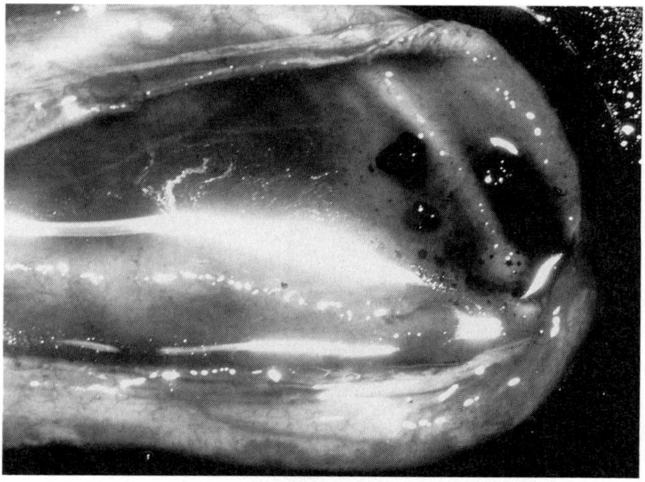

Fig. 5. Gallstones "missed" on 3 ultrasound scans in 21 year old male patient with severe AP and infected necrosis

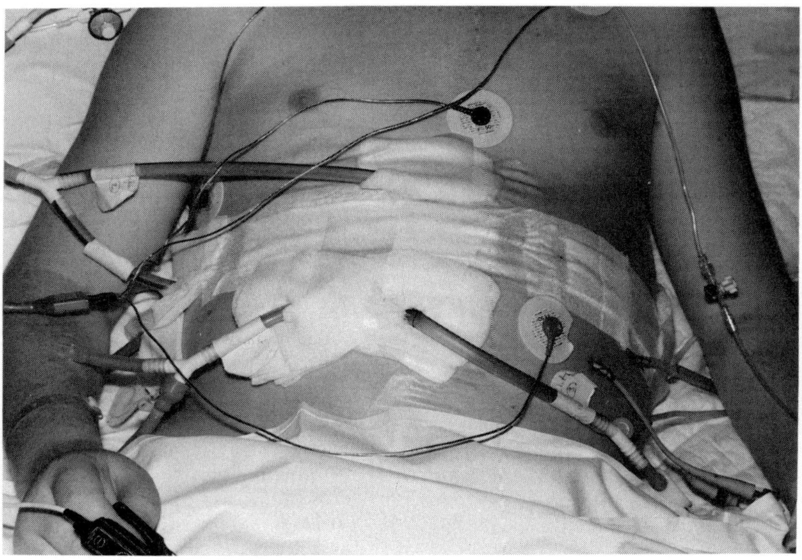

Fig. 6. Post operative patient with multiple inflow and outflow lavage tubes plus small Foley catheter used for feeding jejunostomy

The Timing of Surgical Intervention

Many experts consider it most desirable to allow the septic process to localize so that interventional procedures may be helped by good demarcation of the affected area, by the body's defence processes "walling off" the septic process. This is a laudable approach and will usually necessitate waiting at least 10 days from admission, but rigid adherence to this policy can be counterproductive to certain patients who develop extensive necrosis within the first few hours of illness with subsequent contamination as early as the 3rd day of illness. Indeed, Beger and his group in Ulm have, in an uncontrolled study, shown that some patients require surgical intervention 72 h from onset of disease.

There is therefore no such thing as the "optimum timing" for all patients with severe acute pancreatitis; rather, therapy must heed to the individual needs and objective evidence in each patient.

The role of *percutaneous needle aspiration* of fluid in and around the pancreas, guided by ultrasound and CT, may well have been overemphasized in the recent past [7]. However, this can be a very valuable technique because of the accuracy of "negative aspiration", as well as the positive results [7].

Do Prognostic Criteria Have a Role?

It has been shown by various groups of clinicians that the patients with the most severe disease tend to have much higher levels of APACHE II score (in the range 12–30) [8, 9], C-reactive protein (over 150 mg/l), [10, 11] PMN elastase [12, 13] and trypsinogen activation peptide [14]. The Ulm group have published a comparison of C-reactive protein, CT and levels of α_2-macroglobulin for accurately detecting acute necrotizing pancreatitis [4]. Elevations of C-reactive protein proved slightly more accurate than CT, which in turn was more accurate than the lowered levels of α_2-macroglobulin [15]. Most recently, PMN elastase elevations in blood have clearly related to outcome [12, 13]. Despite this evidence it is highly improbable that any surgeon would consider the altered levels of any blood or urinary biochemical measure to be an indicator of the requirement for surgical intervention. However, the presence of high levels of these substances does indicate a greater likelihood of the presence of extensive necrosis. In particular, should trypsinogen activation peptide become commercially available as a measure of severity of pancreatitis, then those patients with the greatest change in this peptide would require the closest scrutiny. This is probably the most important role of the new markers of severity of acute pancreatitis: the fact that the most marked changes alert the clinician to the need to perform angiogram-enhanced CT frequently (every 48 h). The real place of such biochemical measurements in the future will require to be assessed in prospective studies alongside imaging modalities [12]. It is possible for gross changes to be significantly related to the presence of necrosis, and this, together with an unsatisfactory clinical state, would represent a pointer to the requirement for surgical intervention. All surgeons would be much happier to have the morphological details which can be obtained by CT, as this helps not only in the dissection in and around the pancreas, but also in the extension of dissection along the paracolic gutters.

It is worthy of mention that continuation of tube lavage postoperatively (usually at rate of 0.5–1.0 l/h) necessitates the placing of a large number of inflow and outflow drains. The number will depend on the size of the patient and the extension of the septic process, but as a general guideline, a total of between 6 and 8 drains is advocated. It is important that soft plastic drains are used and not rigid plastic, because this has a greater propensity to cause pancreatic and bowel fistulae. The reappearance of clinical or other signs of sepsis after the initial procedure must be monitored, as approximately 25% of patients need more than one operation [2].

In centres which have changed to per- and postoperative lavage as their objective after necrosectomy, improved results have been obtained [16, 17]. However, in some of the worst cases only packing may be initially applicable owing to venous ooze [17–19]. There is then the choice between continuing regular changes of the packs and converting to a closed lavage system. Finally, the surgical therapy may be by a retroperitoneal approach alone, provided the infected and/or necrotic tissue is focal to the left of the midline [20].

Types of Abscess Formation

In the early stages of severe acute pancreatitis it is most usual to find that the septic process is not well localized and that it has spread in the peripancreatic and other retroperitoneal areas, thus representing a diffuse septic process, in contrast to the focal thick-walled abscess which tends to present much later in the disease. In order to emphasize the difference in the therapeutic potential and likely results, as well as the type of surgery required, it would be preferable to label the *focal abscess as type 1* and the *diffuse sepsis as type 2*. Indeed, the focal lesion may be most satisfactorily treated by percutaneous drains carefully placed with the aid of ultrasound or CT as an alternative to surgical intervention. Both of these methods should be associated with excellent results, whereas even in the best hands there will be higher morbidity and mortality associated with drainage of type 2 sepsis. In these patients it is worthwhile for the surgeon to insert a feeding jejunostomy into the proximal jejunum at the time of the operation to remove the septic process, as this is a more physiological way of feeding the patient in the postoperative period than intravenous nutrition. Figure 6 illustrates a patient with multiple soft plastic sump drains undergoing postoperative lavage, with a fine 10-FG Foley catheter used as a feeding jejunostomy tube. Even finer tubes are preferred by some surgeons, but they tend to clog up more easily with the rather viscous feeds.

The source of sepsis is still uncertain, and it is possible that the bacteria migrate from an infected biliary tree along the pancreatic duct and thereby into the ischaemic areas of pancreas and beyond. An alternative explanation is that bacteria migrate through the posterior wall of the compromised transverse colon in these patients.

The Place of Antibiotic Therapy

Many patients will have been tried on broad-spectrum antibiotic therapy prior to the decision to undertake surgery, and it is usual to continue such antibiotics through the initial 48–72 h of the post-operative period. By this time much more information will be available which should allow a much more specific antibiotic policy to be pursued; in those patients who have undergone percutaneous aspiration preoperatively, the information will be available at an earlier time.

When antibiotics have been withheld, then it is wise to choose antibiotics with proven good tissue penetration of the pancreas, e.g. mezlocillin, although little can go wrong with "blunderbuss" antibiotic cover at this time, utilizing gentamicin, ampicillin and metronidazole. Others prefer cefotaxime or cefuroxime with metronidazole, but it should be stated that there is no good evidence that more expensive antibiotic therapy is of any greater benefit for the patient.

Other Surgical Measures

Some patients may have an obviously compromised transverse colon and thus require localized colectomy at the time of the surgical procedure for treatment of intra-abdominal sepsis. The safest procedure is then to bring out widely separated colostomies in the right and left upper quadrants of the abdomen with the intention of rejoining the colon at a future date.

Most fistulas connecting to the pancreas or bowel will close without direct intervention if rigid drainage tubes are avoided or removed and intravenous nutrition is given. Octreotide, given in a dose of 100 μg every 8 h subcutaneously, can also be helpful in promoting fistula closure.

References

1. Wilson C, McCardle CS, Carter DC, Imrie CW (1988) Surgical treatment of acute necrotizing pancreatitis. Br J Surg 75:1119–1123
2. Beger HG, Buchler M, Bittner R et al. (1988) Necrosectomy and postoperative local lavage in necrotizing pancreatitis. Br J Surg 75:207–212
3. Freeny PC (1982) Radiology of the pancreas. Springer, Berlin Heidelberg New York

4. Kivisaari L, Somer K, Standertskjoeld-Nordenstam CG (1983) Early detection of acute fulminant pancreatitis by contrast enhanced computed tomography. Scand J Gastroenterol 18:39–41
5. London NJM, Neoptolemos JP, Lavelle JM et al. (1989) Contrast enhanced abdominal computerised tomography scanning and prediction of severity of acute pancreatitis: a prospective study. Br J Surg 76:268–272
6. London NJM, Leese T, Lavelle JM et al. (1991) Rapid-bolus contrast-enhanced dynamic computed tomography in acute pancreatitis: a prospective study. Br J Surg 78:1452–1456
7. Gerzof SG, Banks PA, Robbins AH et al. (1987) Early diagnosis of pancreatic infection by computed tomography-guided aspiration. Gastroenterology 93:1315–1320
8. Larvin M, McMahon MJ (1989) APAGHE II score for assessment and monitoring of acute pancreatitis. Lancet ii:201–205
9. Wilson C, Heath DI, Imrie CW (1990) Prediction of outcome in acute pancreatitis: a comparative study of APACHE II clinical assessment and multiple factor scoring systems. Br J Surg 7:1260–1264
10. Puolakkainen P, Valtonen V, Paananen A, Schroder T (1987) C-reactive protein (CRP) and serum phospholipase A2 in the assessment of the severity of acute pancreatitis. Gut 28:764–771
11. Wilson C, Heads A, Shenkin A, Imrie CW (1989) C-reactive antiproteases and complement factors as objective markers of severity in acute pancreatitis. Br J Surg 76:177–181
12. Uhl W, Buchler M, Malfertheiner P et al. (1991) PMN elastase in comparison with CRP, antiproteases, and LDH as indicators of necrosis in human acute pancreatitis. Pancreas 6:253–259
13. Dominquez-Munoz JE, Carbello F, Garcia MJ et al. (1991) Clinical usefulness of polymorphonuclear elastase in predicting the severity of acute pancreatitis: results of a multicentre study
14. Gudgeon M, Heath DI, Hurley P et al. (1990) Trypsinogen activation peptides assay in the early severity prediction of acute pancreatitis. Lancet 335:4–8
15. Buchler M, Malfertheiner P, Beger HG (1986) Correlation of imaging procedures, biochemical parameters and clinical stage in acute pancreatitis. In: Malfertheiner P, Ditschuneit H (eds) Diagnostic procedures in pancreatic disease. Springer, Berlin Heidelberg New York
16. Pederzoli P, Bassi C, Vesentini S et al. (1990) Necrosectomy by lavage in the surgical treatment of severe necrotising pancreatitis. Results in 263 patients. Acta Chir Scand 156:775–780
17. Stanton R, Frey C (1990) Comprehensive management of acute necrotising pancreatitis and pancreatic abscess. Arch Surg 125:1269–1275
18. Bradley EL (1987) Management of infected necrosis by open drainage. Ann Surg 206:542–550
19. Waclawiczek HW, Heinerman M, Chmelizek F, Boeckl O (1991) Interdisciplinary management in necrotising pancreatitis. In: Waclawiczek HW, Boeckl O, Pauser G (eds) The open packing laparostomy. Springer, Berlin Heidelberg New York
20. Fagniez JP, Rotman N, Cracht M (1989) Direct retroperitoneal approach to necrosis in severe acute pancreatitis. Br J Surg 76:276–267

Treatment of Microcirculation Disorders of the Pancreas in Acute Pancreatitis

E. KLAR[1]

The prognosis of acute pancreatitis is determined by the extent of pancreatic necrosis. Thus, the main effort of conservative therapy must be directed at avoiding the development of tissue destruction or at limiting progression once necrosis has been established. There is experimental and clinical evidence that the impairment of pancreatic microcirculation plays a major role in the pathogenesis of acute pancreatitis [26]. Two different mechanisms must be distinguished: secondary pancreatic ischemia induced by the impairment of systemic hemodynamics and the disturbance of pancreatic microcirculation, which also takes place despite stable macrohemodynamics.

Secondary Ischemia of the Pancreas

The intact pancreas seems to be relatively resistant to total ischemia. Complete arterial obstruction for 1h causes reversible functional and histologic changes [10], and ischemia of 2h results in mild hemorrhage [43]. However, arterial occlusion of only 15min can induce necrotizing pancreatitis if superimposed on pancreatic edema [53]. Ischemia seems to sensitize the acinar cell to degradation by activated enzymes since the same changes were observed even if ischemia was induced prior to the induction of edematous pancreatitis.

There is also clinical evidence for the pathogenetic connection between splanchnic hypoperfusion and acute pancreatitis. In patients dying after oligemic shock a significantly higher incidence of acute pancreatitis or pancreatic necrosis was demonstrated in the presence of concomitant renal tubular necrosis, indicating the severity of shock compared with patients without accompanying renal changes [59]. In addition, acute pancreatitis following cardiopulmonary bypass operations seems to be correlated to intraoperative splanchnic hypoperfusion, the severity of the disease being increased by postoperative hypotension [20].

[1] Chirurgische Klinik der Universität Heidelberg, Im Neuenheimer Feld 110, W-6900 Heidelberg, FRG

Beger/Büchler/Malfertheiner (Eds.)
Standards in Pancreatic Surgery

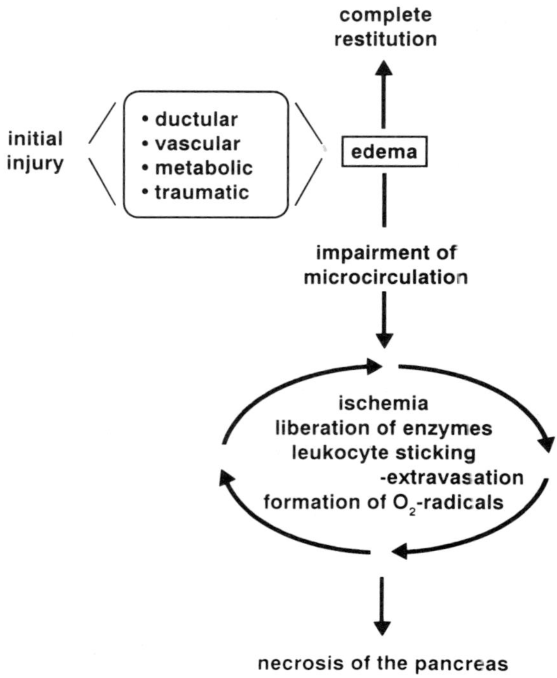

Fig. 1. Impairment of pancreatic microcirculation as one main mechanism for the progression of edematous pancreatitis to pancreatic necrosis

Primary Ischemia of the Pancreas

Regardless of the etiology, in most cases of acute pancreatitis the very early stage is characterized by pancreatic edema. In 90% of patients a complete restitution takes place [13]. The mechanisms responsible for the transition from edematous to necrotizing pancreatitis are not fully understood. However, there is increasing evidence suggesting a primary impairment of pancreatic microcirculation to play a pathogenetic key role (Fig. 1). A vicious circle is triggered consisting of further liberation of enzymes, formation of oxygen radicals, leukocyte sticking and extravasation.

An alteration in pancreatic microcirculation during acute pancreatitis is well documented in the literature, most of the studies using indirect methods for the quantification (Table 1). A constriction of arterioles was detected 3 h after induction of biliary pancreatitis by injecting polyvinyl chloride and india ink gelatin into the pancreaticoduodenal artery [45, 50]. A reduction of pancreatic blood flow could be demonstrated by the rubidium-86 clearance technique [18, 44] and was further substantiated with electromagnetic flow meters and radioactive microspheres [9, 27]. In most of the studies the

Table 1. Survey of previous studies on pancreatic microcirculation during acute pancreatitis (from [26])

Author	Species	Methods	Time after induction of pancreatitis	Findings
Thal [56]	Rabbit	Intravital observation	5 min	Spasm of interlobular vessels
			15 min	Capillary stasis
			20 min	Hemorrhage
			3 h	Similar changes
Papp et al. [44]	Dog	Rubidium-86 extraction	24 h	Decrease in pancreatic blood flow, MAP and CO (disproportionate)
Anderson et al. [6]	Dog	Intra-arterial methylene blue	1 h	Increase in capillary permability (histology)
Anderson and Schiller [5]	Dog	Intra-arterial india ink (histology)	30 min	Reduction in arterial perfusion (histology)
Goodhead [18]	Dog	Rubidium-86 extraction	20 h	Pancreatic blood flow increased in edematous, decreased in hemorrhagic pancreatitis; disproportionate reduction in CO and MAP
Papp et al. [45]	Dog	Intra-arterial india ink and polyvinyl chloride	3 h 12 h	Vasoconstriction of arteries and intralobular arterioles; no capillary filling, AV shunts (histology)
Pissiotis et al. [46]	Dog	Venous outflow	10 min–6 h	Decrease in pancreatic blood flow and BP (proportion?)
Schiller and Anderson [50]	Dog	Intra-arterial silicone rubber	24 h	Constriction of intra- and interlobular arterioles; vasodilatation in less affected areas (histology)
Donaldson et al. [15]	Dog	Arterial flow probe	15 min–3 h	Decrease in pancreatic blood flow (disproportionate)
Becker et al. [9]	Dog	Flow probe, radioactive microspheres, 15 μm	30 min–2 h	Decrease in pancreatic blood flow, MAP and CO (disproportionate)
Knol et al. [27]	Dog	Flow probe, radioactive microspheres, 15 μm	1–4 h	Decrease in pancreatic blood flow and CO (disproportionate), no change in shunt perfusion
Klar et al. [24]	Rabbit	Intravital microscopy	30 min–3 h	Decrease in capillary perfusion

BP, blood pressure; CO, cardiac output; MAP, mean arterial pressure; AV, arteriovenous.

degree of pancreatic hypoperfusion was disproportionately greater than the decrease in cardiac output at comparable intervals. Oxygen consumption dropped at the same time in conjunction with a constant arteriovenous difference of oxygen [14], suggesting arteriovenous shunting. However, the presence of arteriovenous shunts has never been ascertained functionally [27] despite some histologic evidence [45]. We therefore developed a model for the direct quantification of pancreatic microcirculation in rabbits, using intravital microscopy.

Analysis of the Pancreatic Microcirculation and Histology in Rabbits

Method

The model has been described in detail elsewhere [24]. In brief, anesthesia was induced and maintained with sodium pentobarbital. The duodenal loop was exposed, together with the intramesenterically located pancreas, via a right lateral laparotomy and immobilized on a plexiglas stage. Biliary pancreatitis was induced by retrograde injection into the pancreatic duct of a mixture of sodium taurocholate, trypsin, and autologous blood at a maximum pressure of 40 mmHg. FITC dextran 70 was given intravenously to improve the contrast between the capillary wall, adjacent tissue, and blood cells. To assess the number of perfused capillaries per observation site, video recordings of intravital microscopy were obtained from selected areas measuring $361 \times 241\,\mu m$ prior to and 3 and 12 h after induction of pancreatitis. These regions were identified within the exteriorized pancreas on the basis of tissue transparency and visibility of the capillary network in the periphery of the pancreatic lobules and used for analysis throughout the study. To avoid artifacts due to long-term exposure, the exposed pancreas was inserted into the abdominal cavity 3 h after the induction of pancreatitis and reexposed at 12 h.

At the end of the experiment the corresponding part of the pancreas which had been assessed by intravital microscopy was fixed with formalin and later subjected to morphometric evaluation at a magnification of 400:1, corresponding to 3000 visual fields per pancreas.

In 9 of 18 animals isovolemic hemodilution was performed by the exchange of 10.0 ± 1.3 ml/kg whole blood for the identical volume of dextran 60 (Macrodex 6%, Schiwa, Glandorf, FRG) in steps of 2 ml 30 min after the induction of pancreatitis to reduce the arterial hematocrit by 25% of the initial value.

Special care was taken to maintain mean arterial pressure, central venous pressure, and heart rate at a constant level. In all animals 8.5 ml/kg Ringer's solution was administered per hour as basic fluid therapy.

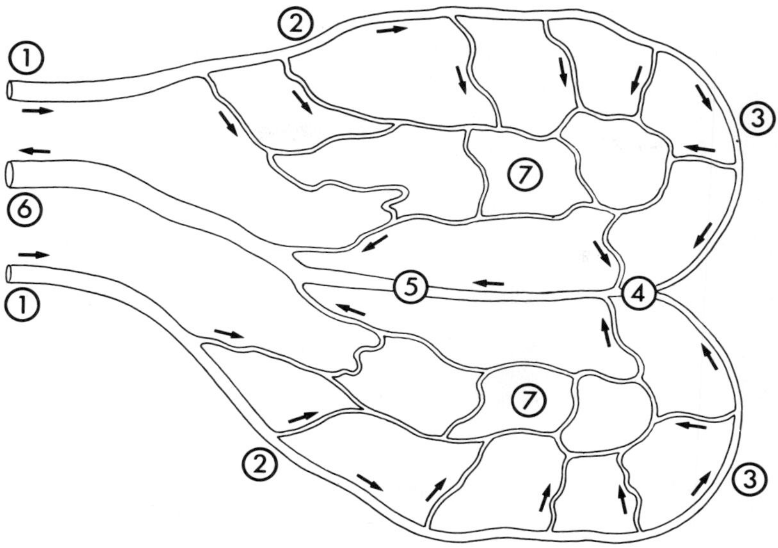

Fig. 2. The microangioarchitecture of a pancreatic lobule in the rabbit. *1*, Intralobular arteriole; *2*, terminal arteriole; *3*, "preferential pathway;" *4*, postcapillary venule; *5*, collecting venule; *6*, intralobular venule; *7*, capillary network. (From [24])

Results and Discussion

The description of the normal microvascular architecture of the pancreas was based on the assessment of flow direction, vessel diameter, and branching pattern. A preferential pathway was defined by the topical application of noradrenaline (Fig. 2). On average these preferential channels were found to be only 9.2 μm in diameter. Obviously, these small functional shunts were not detected by the 15-μm microspheres used in other studies to detect shunting in acute pancreatitis [27].

Pathogenesis of Capillary Stasis in Acute Pancreatitis

Vasoconstriction is likely to play a part in the pathogenesis of acute pancreatitis since edematous pancreatitis could be converted to hemorrhagic necrosis in cats by electric stimulation at the hypothalamus to increase sympathetic activity [16]. Conversely, the evolution of necrosis form pancreatic edema could be suppressed by postganglionic sympathectomy [17].

Direct injury to the capillary wall by the vasotoxic effect of taurocholate and trypsin seems to be exerted via the interstitial route, resulting in endothelial detachment and intravascular coagulation [3, 12]. By means of

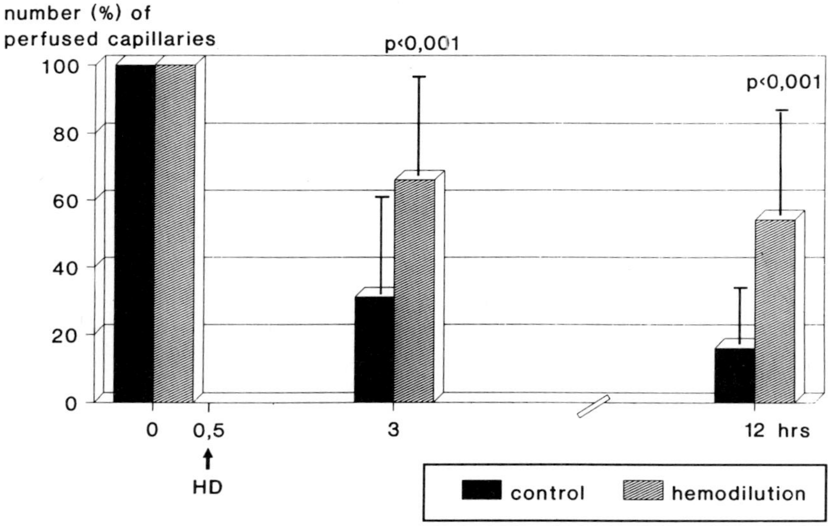

Fig. 3. Number of perfused capillaries per observation site (percentage of initial value; mean ± SD) Stabilization of capillary flow by isovolemic hemodilution (*HD*) 30 min after induction of pancreatitis (0). Progressive reduction of microvessel perfusion in the untreated control group. Investigated capillaries: HD, n = 2160; control, n = 1920

electron microscopy Bockman et al. [11] demonstrated that a rupture of the ductoacinar junction occurs during the induction of biliary pancreatitis even if the intraductal injection is performed at a low pressure of 40 cm H_2O. Low-flow conditions are further precipitated by hemoconcentration due to a massive increase in permeability during the initial phase of biliary pancreatitis [24].

Pancreatic capillary perfusion is further impaired by an increase in interstitial pressure as a consequence of obstructed lymph drainage [2]. Erythrocytes originating from pancreatic interstitial hemorrhages were shown to enter the microlymphatics [6].

Oxygen radicals induce lipid peroxidation leading to a disintegration of cell membranes, also affecting the capillary endothelium. In addition, margination of granulocytes is precipitated, further impairing pancreatic microperfusion [52].

Isovolemic Hemodilution with Dextran 60: Effect and Mode of Action

Nonhemodiluted animals exhibited a progressive reduction in pancreatic capillary perfusion beginning 30 min after induction of acute pancreatitis with blood flow in only 16% of the capillaries at 12 h. In the animals subjected to isovolemic hemodilution with dextran 60 perfusion was sustained

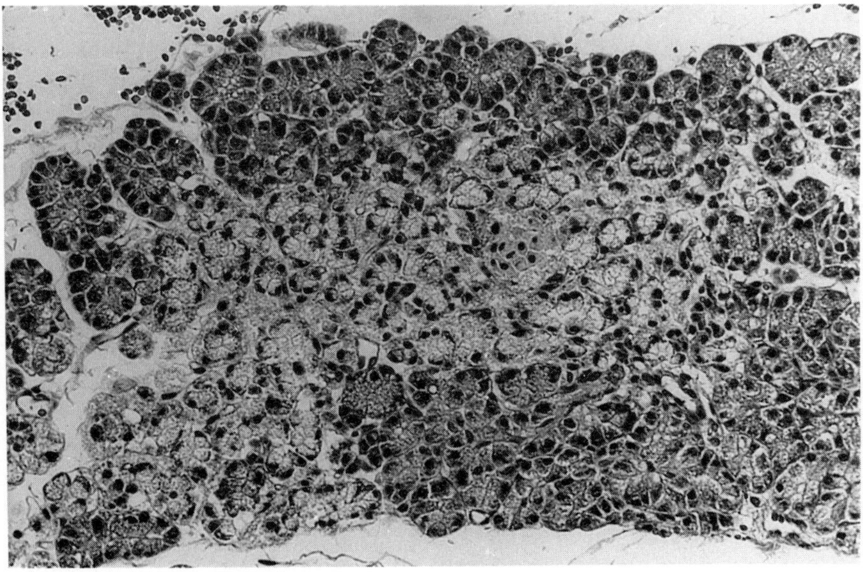

Fig. 4. Control rabbit pancreas 12 h after induction of biliary pancreatitis. Area of cytoplasmic vacuolization of acinar cells surrounded by normal acini. (H&E ×228)

in 54% of the capillaries throughout the whole period (Fig. 3). In both groups fluid administration was adjusted to maintain central venous pressure to avoid unspecific hemodynamic effects due to changes in intravascular volume.

The direct correlation of microcirculation and histology of the pancreas in our study demonstrates that an improvement of pancreatic microcirculation during acute pancreatitis results in a significant reduction of interstitial edema and cell vacuolisation (Fig. 4) (E. Klar, submitted for publication). These changes represent potentially reversible tissue damage [61] characterizing the perinecrotic zone of parenchymal injury.

Intentional normovolemic hemodilution as induced by isovolemic exchange of whole blood with colloid solutions is a recognized therapeutic procedure for treatment of microcirculatory disorders in ischemic diseases [40, 48, 54]. Following normovolemic hemodilution, characteristic hemodynamic changes in the macro- as well as microcirculation are induced which compensate for the acute reduction of red cell concentration and thereby oxygen content of the arterial blood [22, 30, 32, 34–37, 39, 41, 42, 51, 55, 58].

A disproportionate decrease in blood viscosity following a linear reduction in hematocrit is considered as the key mechanism [36] influencing the main determinants of whole blood viscosity: red cell–red cell interaction and red cell–protein interaction [34]. The fall in blood viscosity gives rise to an increased venous return and a reduction in afterload resulting in an enhanced stroke volume [32, 37, 55].

Additional effects, not apparent from the described macrohemodynamic changes allow compensation for the reduced oxygen content of blood mainly by the increase in red cell velocity in the microvessels [41] and through the enhancement of flow motion in the capillaries [30, 42, 58]. Following hemodilution, less oxygen is lost by the red blood cells due to a shorter transit time, hence a greater amount of oxygen is available at the level of the capillaries [41], where a higher extraction of oxygen is recorded at low hematocrit values [32]. Maintenance of the mean tissue PO_2 has been demonstrated at a hematocrit range between 42% and 19% in various organs, including the pancreas [39]. In our model isovolemic hemodilution was induced to achieve a stepwise reduction in systemic hematocrit to 28%–30%, because this range is considered the optimal compromise between fluidity and oxygen content of the blood [33]. The described compensatory mechanisms are most pronounced in ischemic tissue areas counteracting low flow velocity, margination of leukocytes [23], and capillary stasis [21].

The choice of the most suitable diluent to perform isovolemic hemodilution is dependent upon the fact that even small and temporary reductions in intravascular volume prevent the compensatory increase in cardiac output and thus abolish the positive effect on the macro- and microhemodynamics. In general, the volume-sustaining capacity of crystalloids is inferior to colloids, and the colloid osmotic pressure of the plasma cannot be maintained by crystalloids [38]. The risk of a hazardous shift in blood volume is accentuated by the increase in vascular permeability in the early stage of acute biliary pancreatitis, encountered in our study and before by Sanfey [49]. Among the available colloids dextran 60/70 seems particularly suitable in acute pancreatitis due to its intravascular persistence of 6 h and its additional antithrombotic properties, unique characteristics compared as to hydroxyethyl starch and gelatin [1, 7, 8, 19].

Furthermore, it has been demonstrated that postischemic leukocyte–endothelium interaction in the skeletal muscle can be prevented by prophylactic hemodilution with dextran 60 [57] more effectively as compared to hydroxyethyl starch [31], supporting our previous findings in the pancreas based on electron microscopy (Fig. 5).

In previous studies, dextran was administered as a continuous infusion, whereby dilution of blood occurred slowly, and the therapeutic effect was inevitably delayed [4, 6, 15, 29, 60]. Since microcirculatory impairment takes place within 3 h after the induction of acute pancreatitis, isovolemic hemodilution allowing for an instantaneous drop in blood viscosity is considered the therapy of choice. With this technique the unspecific effect of volume expansion, which has made the interpretation of historic studies difficult, is reliably avoided. In our study, hemodilution was performed 30 min after induction of acute biliary pancreatitis because in untreated

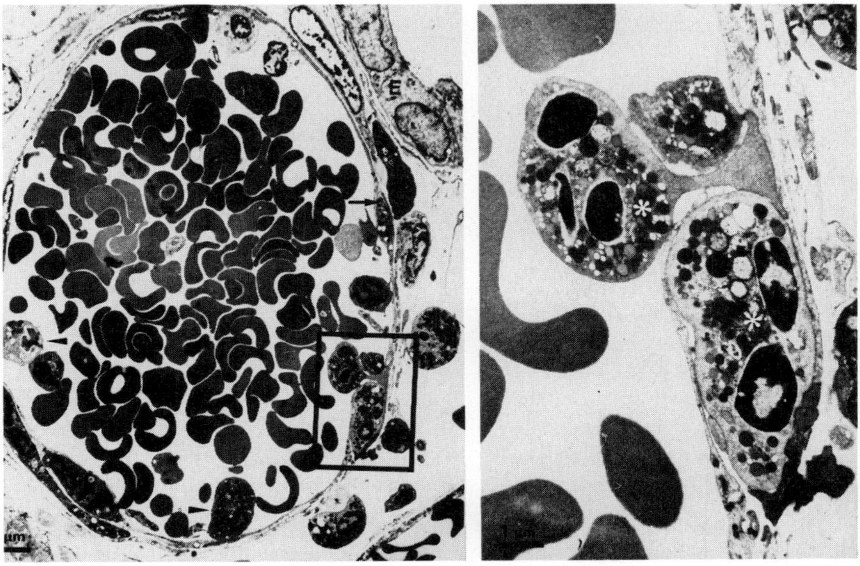

Fig. 5. Postcapillary venule of a rabbit pancreas 30 min after induction of acute pancreatitis. The vessel lumen is densely packed with erythrocytes (the boxed area in magnified on the right), suggesting hemoconcentration due to an early increase in permeability. Granulocytes are already adherent to (*arrowhead*) or even penetrating (*arrow*) the endothelium. The magnification (*right*) displays granulocytes (*white asterisk*) in the state of extravasation. These changes were significantly reduced by isovolemic hemodilution. (From [23])

animals the progressive decrease in pancreatic capillary perfusion starts at this time point [25]. Using a similar model of biliary pancreatitis, Lankisch et al. [28] demonstrated the presence of edema and pancreatic necrosis as early as 5 min after the induction. We therefore think that our experimental protocol mimics the clinical situation since in most of the cases patients present after morphologic changes of the pancreatic parenchyma have taken place.

Clinical Application

In a prospective, controlled, nonrandomized study we investigated the effect of isovolemic hemodilution with dextran 60 in 11 patients with acute alcoholic pancreatitis. Contrast-enhanced computed tomography of the abdomen was performed at admission in all patients presenting with abdominal pain and elevated serum amylase. Patients with severe clinical symptoms and initial computed tomography grading D and E [47] were included, while patients with anemia, coronary heart disease, chronic

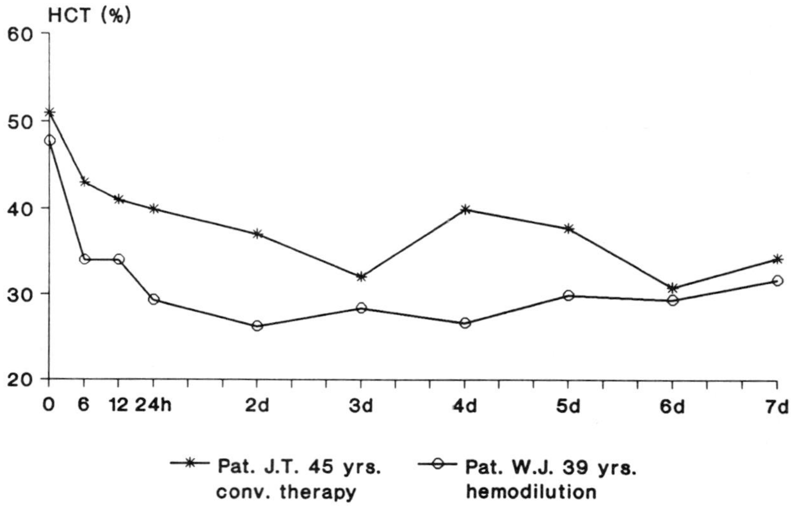

Fig. 6. Isovolemic hemodilution (*HCT*) with dextran 60 under clinical conditions. Rapid decrease in hematocrit to the optimal range concerning blood viscosity and microvessel perfusion by hemodilution. Delayed normalization of hematocrit by conventional fluid therapy alone. In both patients comparable fluid resucitation was performed based on macrohemodynamic parameters

obstructive pulmonary disease, coagulopathies, and secondary referrals were excluded from the study. The volume of blood to be exchanged for dextran 60 was calculated from a nomogram based on body surface and initial hematocrit of the patient [62]. Isovolemic hemodilution aimed at a hematocrit of 30%. Monovalent hapten dextran (Promit) was injected prior to the infusion of dextran 60 to prevent severe anaphylactic reactions. ECG, heart rate, arterial and central venous pressure were monitored throughout the study. Due to initial hemoconcentration all patients received 250 ml dextran 60 (Macrodex 6%, Schiwa, Glandorf, FRG) intravenously prior to blood exchange. Blood was withdrawn according to standard techniques of autologous blood donation. Packed red cells were prepared and stored for retransfusion when indicated. Simultaneously with blood withdrawal identical volumes of dextran 60 were administered. Following the exchange procedure Ringer's solution was given intravenously to maintain central venous pressure at 8 ± 2 mmHg. The hematocrit was maintained between 28% and 32% by dilution or retransfusion of autologous red cells.

Eight patients presented with a computed tomography grade D and three with grade E. A mean Ranson's prognostic index of 4.5 ± 1.8 was recorded, including three patients with 7 score points. The initial hematocrit of 48.4% ± 6.6% was reduced by isovolemic hemodilution to 33.9% ± 2.8% within 1 h and decreased to 31% ± 5% due to conventional fluid therapy within 24 h (Fig. 6). Abdominal pain lessened in all patients during

Table 2. Isovolemic hemodilution with dextran 60 under clinical conditions: patients' characteristics and results

Patients: $n = 11$
Time interval
Symptoms → hemodilution: 36 ± 12 h
Ranson's criteria: 4.5 ± 1.8
Hematocrit
Before hemodilution: 48.4% ± 6.6%
After hemodilution: 33.9% ± 2.8%
Exchange volume
Minimum 800 ml
Maximum 1700 ml
Necrosectomy: $n = 2$ (18%)
Mortality: $n = 1$ (9%)

or shortly after the exchange procedure; analgesics could be discontinued. In three patients the development of pancreatic necrosis was demonstrated by computed tomography on day 7; two of them underwent operative treatment, and one died on day 40 following arterial hemorrhage (Table 2).

Our first clinical experience with isovolemic hemodilution in the treatment of acute pancreatitis indicates that the promising experimental concept is feasible in patients. A beneficial effect seems likely also under clinical conditions, considering a mortality of 9% in patients with a mean Ranson's score of 4.5 and the fact that only one of three patients with 7 score points died. However, the number of patients reported is relatively low, and the described results need to be confirmed by a randomized trial.

Summary

Impairment of pancreatic microcirculation must be considered as a main mechanism in the pathogenesis of acute pancreatitis. Pancreatic capillary perfusion can be stabilized by isovolemic hemodilution with dextran 60/70 in rabbits. Improvement in pancreatic microcirculation protects pancreatic morphology in experimental pancreatitis. Isovolemic hemodilution is feasible under clinical conditions and may have a beneficial effect comparable to that in the animal studies.

References

1. Aberg M, Hedner U, Bergentz SE (1978) Effect of dextran on factor VIII (antihemophilic factor). Ann Surg 189:243–7
2. Anderson MC (1963) Venous stasis in the transition of edematous pancreatitis to pancreatic necrosis. JAMA 183:534–537
3. Anderson MC, Bergan JJ (1962) Effect of proteolytic enzymes upon pancreatic blood vessels. Surg Forum 13:304–306

4. Anderson MC, Lewis MB (1965) Low-molecular-weight dextran therapy in experimental pancreatitis. JAMA 192:138–140
5. Anderson MC, Schiller WR (1968) Microcirculatory dynamics in the normal and inflamed pancreas. Am J Surg 115:118–127
6. Anderson MC, Schoenfeldt FB, Iams WB, Suwa M (1967) Circulatory changes in acute pancreatitis. Surg Clin North Am 47:127–132
7. Arfors KE, Buckley PB (1989) Role of artificial colloids in rational fluid therapy. In: Tuma RF, White JV, Messmer K (eds) The role of hemodilution in optimal patient care. Zuckschwerdt, Munich, pp 100–123
8. Arfors K-E, Hint HC, McKenzie FN, Matheson NA, Svensjoe E (1970) Counteraction of platelet activity using laser-induced endothelial trauma. Thromb Diath Haemorrh [Suppl] 42:315–319
9. Becker H, Vinten-Johansen J, Buckberg GD, Bugyi HI (1982) Correlation of pancreatic blood flow and high-energy phosphates during experimental pancreatitis. Eur Surg Res 14:203–210
10. Binder PS, Heiskell CA, Adams JR, Cerra FB, Eilert JB, Bergan JJ (1970) Pancreatic function after normothermic ischaemia. I. In vivo ischaemia. Am J Surg 120:687–692
11. Bockman DE, Schiller WR, Anderson MC (1971) Route of retrograde flow in the exocrine pancreas during ductal hypertension. Arch Surg 103:321–329
12. Bockman DE, Schiller WR, Suriyapa C, Mutschler JHW, Anderson MC (1973) Fine structure of early experimental acute pancreatitis in dogs. Lab Invest 22:584–592
13. Crist DW, Cameron JL (1987) The current management of acute pancreatitis. Adv Surg 20:69–124
14. Donaldson LA, Schenk WG Jr (1979) Experimental acute pancreatitis: the changes in pancreatic oxygen consumption and the effect of dextran 40. Ann Surg 190:728–731
15. Donaldson LA, Williams RW, Schenk WG (1978) Experimental pancreatitis: effect of plasma and dextran on pancreatic blood flow. Surgery 84:313–321
16. Gilsdorf RB, Long D, Moberg A, Leonard AS (1965) Central nervous system influence on experimentally induced pancreatitis. JAMA 192:394–397
17. Goodhead B (1969) Vascular factors in the pathogenesis of acute hemorrhagic pancreatitis. Ann R Coll Surg Engl 45:80–97
18. Goodhead B (1969) Acute pancreatitis and pancreatic blood flow. Surg Gynecol Obstet 129:331–340
19. Gruber UF (1975) Dextran and the prevention of postoperative thromboembolic complications. Surg Clin North Am 55:679–696
20. Haas GS, Warshaw AL, Daggett WM, Aretz HT (1985) Acute pancreatitis after cardiopulmonary bypass. Am J Surg 149:508–515
21. Intaglietta M (1989) Microcirculatory effects of hemodilution: background and analysis. In: Tuma RF, White JV, Messmer K (eds) The role of hemodilution in optimal patient care. Zuckschwerdt, Munich, pp 21–40
22. Jan KM, Chien S (1977) Effect of hematocrit variations on coronary hemodynamics and oxygen utilization. Am J Physiol 233:H197
23. Klar E, Endrich B, Hammersen F, Messmer K, Herfarth C (1987) Therapeutic effect of isovolemic hemodilution with dextran 60 on the morphological integrity of the pancreas in acute biliary pancreatitis. Langenbecks Arch Chir (Suppl Chir Forum):299–302
24. Klar E, Endrich B, Messmer K (1990) Microcirculation of the pancreas. A quantitative study of physiology and changes in pancreatitis. Int J Microcirc Clin Exp 9:85–101
25. Klar E, Herfarth C, Messmer K (1990) Therapeutic effect of isovolemic hemodilution with dextran 60 on the impairment of pancreatic microcirculation in acute biliary pancreatitis. Ann Surg 211:346–353

26. Klar E, Messmer L, Warshaw AL, Herfarth CH (1990) Pancreatic ischaemia in experimental acute pancreatitis: mechanism, significance and therapy. Br J Surg 77:1205–1210
27. Knol JA, Edgcomb LP, Inman MG, Eckhauser FE (1983) Low molecular weight dextran in experimental pancreatitis: effects on pancreatic microcirculation. J Surg Res 35:73–82
28. Lankisch GP, Pohl U, Otto J, Rahlf G (1988) When should treatment of acute experimental pancreatitis be started? Res Exp Med 188:123–129
29. Lehtola A, Kivilaasko E, Puolakkainan P, Karonen S-L, Lempinen M, Schröder T (1986) Effects of dextran 70 versus crystalloids in the microcirculation of procine hemorrhagic pancreatitis. Surg Gynecol Obstet 162:556–562
30. Lindbom L, Mirhashemi S, Arfors K-E, Intaglietta M (1986) Blood flow and hematocrit distribution in response to acute normovolemic hemodilution. Int J Microcirc Clin Exp 5:278
31. Menger M, Thierjung C, Hammersen F, Messmer K (1989) Influence of isovolemic hemodilution with dextran 60 and HAES on the PMN-endothelium interaction in postischemic skeletal muscle. Eur Surg Res 21:74
32. Messmer K (1981) Compensatory mechanisms for acute dilutional anemia. Bibl Haematol 47:31–42
33. Messmer K (1987) Acceptable hematocrit levels in surgical patients. World J Surg 11:41–46
34. Messmer K (1989) Acute preoperative hemodilution: physiological basis and clinical application. In: Tuma RF, White JV, Messmer, K (eds) The role of hemodilution in optimal patient care. Zuckschwerdt, Munich, pp 54–73
35. Messmer K, Schmid-Schönbein H (eds) (1975) Intentional hemodilution. Bibl Haematol 41
36. Messmer K, Sunder-Plassmann L (1974) Hämodilution. Prog Surg 13:208–245
37. Messmer K, Lewis DH, Sunder-Plassmann L, Klövekorn WP, Mendler N, Holper K (1972) Acute normovolemic hemodilution. Changes of central hemodynamics and microcirculatory flow in skeletal muscle. Eur Surg Res 4: 55–70
38. Messmer K, Sunder-Plassmann L, Klövekorn WP, Holper K (1972) Circulatory significance of hemodilution: rheological changes and limitations. Adv Microcirc 4:1–77
39. Messmer K, Sunder-Plassmann L, Jesch F, Görnandt L, Sinagowitz E, Kessler M (1973) Oxygen supply to the tissues during limited normovolemic hemodilution. Res Exp Med 159:152–166
40. Messmer K, Sunder-Plassmann L, v. Hesler H, Endrich B (1982) Hemodilution in peripheral occlusive disease: a hemorheological approach. Clin Hemorheol 2:271
41. Mirhashemi A, Ertefai S, Messmer K, Intaglietta M (1987) Model analysis of the enhancement of tissue oxygenation by hemodilution due to increased microvascular flow velocity. Microvasc Res 34:290–301
42. Mirhashemi S, Messmer K, Arfors K-E, Intaglietta M (1987) Microcirculatory effects of normovolemic hemodilution in skeletal muscle. Int J Microcirc Clin Exp 6:359–369
43. Nordback HI, Jeffrey AC, Cameron JL (1991) The role of cholecystokinin in the pathogenesis of acute pancreatitis in the isolated pancreas preparation. Surgery 109:301–306
44. Papp M, Makara GB, Hajtman B, Csáki L (1966) A quantitative study of pancreatic blood flow in experimental pancreatitis. Gastroenterology 51: 524–528
45. Papp M, Ungvari GY, Nemeth PE, Munkacsi J, Zubeck C (1969) The effect of bile-induced pancreatitis on the intrapancreatic vascular pattern in dogs. Scand J Gastroenterol 4:681–689

46. Pissiotis CA, Condon RE, Nyhus LM (1972) Effect of vasopressin on pancreatic blood flow in acute hemorrhagic pancreatitis. Am J Surg 123: 203–208
47. Ranson JHC, Balthazar E, Caccavale R, Cooper M (1985) Computed tomography and the prediction of pancreatic abscess in acute pancreatitis. Ann Surg 201:656–665
48. Rieger H, Köhler M, Schoop W, Schmid-Schönbein H (1981) Normovolemic hemodilution in peripheral arterial disease. Ann Clin Res 13:78–83
49. Sanfey H, Cameron JL (1984) Increased capillary permeability: an early lesion in acute pancreatitis. Surgery 96:485–491
50. Schiller WR, Anderson MC (1975) Microcirculation of the normal and inflamed canine pancreas. Ann Surg 181:466–470
51. Schmid-Schönbein H, Messmer K, Rieger H (1981) Hemodilution and flow improvement. Bibl Haematol vol. 47, Karger, Basel
52. Schönberg MH, Büchler M, Schädlich H, Younes M, Bültmann B, Beger HG (1989) Involvement of oxygen radicals and phospholipase A2 in acute pancreatitis of the rat. Klin Wochenschr 67:166–170
53. Spormann H, Sokolowski A, Birkigt H-G, Letko G (1986) Contribution of pancreatic edema and short-term ischemia to experimental acute pancreatitis in the rat. I. Procedure and pathomorphological investigations. Z Exp Chir Transplant Künstliche Organe 19:323–330
54. Strand T, Asplund K, Eriksson S, Haegg E, Lithner F, Wester PO (1984) A randomized, controlled trial of hemodilution therapy in acute ischemic stroke. Stroke 15:980–989
55. Sunder-Plassmann L, Klövekorn WP, Messmer K (1976) Präoperative Hämodilution: Grundlagen, Adaptations-mechanismen und Grenzen klinischer Anwendung. Anaesthesist 25:124
56. Thal A (1954) Studies on pancreatitis. IV. The pathogenesis of bile pancreatitis. Surg Forum 5:391–393
57. Thierjung C, Menger M, Sack FU, Galla TJ, Messmer K (1988) The effect of prophylactic isovolemic hemodilution on the PMN-endothelium interaction in postischemic skeletal muscle. Int J Microcirc Clin Exp 7(Special issue):69
58. Tigno HT, Henrich H (1986): Flow characteristics of the microcirculation following intentional hemodilution. Acta Med Philipp 22:5
59. Warshaw AL, O'Hara PJ (1978) Susceptibility of the pancreas to ischemic injury in shock. Ann Surg 188:197–201
60. Wright PW, Goodhead B (1970) The value of dextrans in the treatment of experimental pancreatitis. Surgery 67:807–815
61. Zeligs JD, Janoff A, Dumont AE (1975) The course and nature of acinar cell death following pancreatic ligation in the guinea pig. Am J Pathol 80:203–226
62. Zetterström H, Wiklund L (1986) A new nomogram facilitating adequate hemodilution. Acta Anesthesiol Scand 30:300–304

Plasma Separation and Hemofiltration in Acute Necrotizing Pancreatitis

H. Zirngibl,[1] S. Mann,[1] and G. Braun[2]

Introduction

In a 1984 literature review Gebhardt [2] reported that despite the introduction of new treatment methods, the mortality of acute necrotizing pancreatitis (ANP) had not changed. It still remains between 40% and 70%.

In a retrospective study we attempted to establish a relationship between ANP-related mortality with extrapancreatic necroses and multi-organ failure (MOF) (Fig. 1). In this study, which took place between 1979 and 1987 and included 161 patients, we found that there was no correlation between the extent of the extrapancreatic necroses and hospital mortality. However, there was a correlation between hospital mortality and the number of organ failures.

In patients with no organ failure, mortality was 6%; in patients with one- to two-organ failure, mortality was between 40% and 50%; in patients with three-organ failure it was 80%; and in patients with four-organ failure it was 100%.

These data agree with those of Knaus et al. [5] who initiated a multicenter study and published results in 1985. Five-organ failure was defined as cardiovascular, respiratory, renal, hematological and neurological failure. He also observed that mortality was closely correlated with the manifesting organ failures. Mortality increased in the first 7 days from 22% on the first day to 41% on the seventh, when one organ failure had manifested itself. If a second organ failure developed, then mortality in the first week increased from 52% to 68%. In cases of three or more organ failures, nearly all patients died within 1 week.

Humoral inflammatory response and cellular immune response are out of control in septic-like syndromes and in ANP. Macromolecular enzyme inhibitors, such as $alpha_2$ macroglobulin, are rapidly consumed and are unavailable to the body in sufficient quantities. In addition, the clearance of the developing enzyme inhibitor complexes, which have vasoactive properties and sustain inflammation, is considerably reduced in the reticuloendothelial system (RES) [4, 8].

[1] Klinik u. Poliklinik für Chirurgie, W-8400 Regensburg, FRG
[2] Abteilung für Chirurgie und Anasthesiologie der Universität Erlangen-Nürnberg, Maseimiliansplatz, W-8520 Erlangen, FRG

Beger/Büchler/Malfertheiner (Eds.)
Standards in Pancreatic Surgery

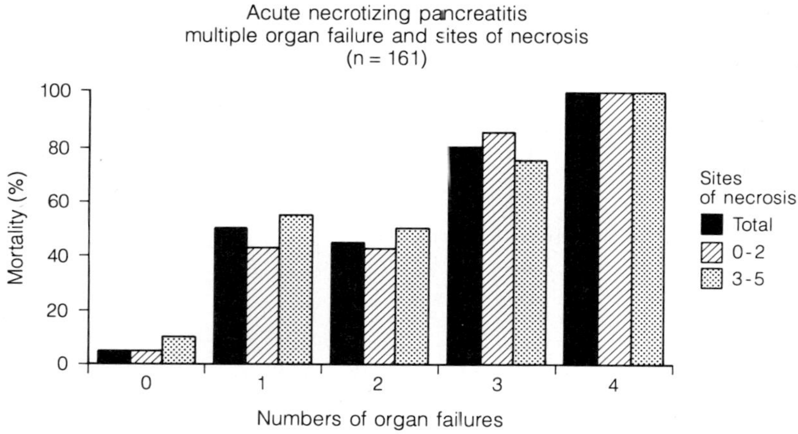

Fig. 1. Observed mortality in acute necrotizing pancreatitis in relation to the extent of extrapancreatic necroses and multiorgan failure (n = 161), 1979–1987

Table 1. Presumed cause of disease and Ranson score, age, and sex of patients (n = 11) with acute necrotizing pancreatitis who were treated with therapeutic plasma exchange

Patient	Age	Sex	Etiology	Ranson score
1	38	male	alcoholic	8
2	45	male	alcoholic	9
3	30	male	alcoholic	6
4	37	male	unknown	10
5	62	male	biliary	10
6	49	female	alcoholic	7
7	67	female	biliary?	5
8	36	male	alcoholic	7
9	34	male	alcoholic	6
10	45	male	alcoholic	5
11	41	male	alcoholic	5
Mean	44			7.1

Plasmapheresis is a blood purification technique which enables effective removal of these enzyme inhibitor complexes from the patients' plasma. Plasmapheresis controls this inflammatory cascade trigger, and with the use of fresh frozen plasma (FFP) as a substitute, the inhibitor pool is simultaneously supported.

In the literature there are reports of numerous cases in which plasmapheresis has been effectively used in severe cases of ANP [1, 6, 10, 13]. Following extensive animal studies [14] in which we were able to confirm these case reports under standardized conditions, we began a pilot study in March 1989.

Patients and Methods

In the treatment of ANP, we used therapeutic plasma exchange (TPE) in patients who, according to their Ranson score [4], were expected to have a fulminant course of disease. However, we considered five positive criteria, and not the original three, as the minimum for an expected fulminant course.

A total of two women and nine men between 30 and 67 years of age were treated. ANP was due to alcohol abuse in eight cases, biliary disease in two, and unknown in one case (Table 1).

All patients were admitted to the intensive care ward, monitored, parenterally fed and, between the second and 14th admission day, subjected to computed tomography (CT) angiography in order to assess the extent and number of extrapancreatic necroses.

As in our retrospective study, four-organ system failure was defined as cardiac/cardiovascular, lung, kidney and liver failure. Cardiac/cardiovascular failure was scored when catecholamines (dopamine, epinephrine) were administered in order to maintain a mean arterial pressure of over 50 mmHg. Lung failure was defined as a decrease in arterial PO_2 to below 50 mmHg and possible requirement of mechanical ventilation. Kidney failure was present when the volume voided was less than 500 ml/24 h, serum creatinine increased over 3.5 mg/100 ml and, in certain conditions, renal support was needed.

Because of circulatory instability, patients received continuous venovenous hemofiltration (CVVHF). Acute liver failure was defined as a decrease in cholinesterase to below 1200 U/l and a minimum of doubling of all transaminase values as well as serum bilirubin. Decreased albumin and clotting factors as well as ascites were also caused by the pancreatitis; clouding of consciousness, again due to pancreatitis, leads to the diagnosis of liver failure.

This definition, accepted in the literature, can be difficult to make because laboratory values cannot give a 100% guarantee of liver failure. They can be affected by other factors, including cell death and consumption. The time of organ failure cannot be determined because values lag behind. In the future, organ monitoring with stable isotopes may be possible. With this method, metabolic products are marked with nonradioactive substances and determined in plasma by dye-dilution methods. Grellner et al. report that on the basis of endogenous glucose production, for example, liver function can be easily quantified [3].

The disadvantages of these methods are the high costs of both the isotopes and the complicated laboratory equipment needed.

Table 2. Intensive care treatment, number of plasma separations, hemofiltrations, and extrapancreatic necroses in 11 patients with acute necrotizing pancreatitis who were treated with therapeutic plasma exchange

Patient	Days in intensive care unit	Number of hemofiltrations (CVVHF)	Number of plasma separations (TPE)	Site of necrosis
1	40	5	2	3
2	57	0	14	4
3	56	18	6	3
4	57	8	21	5
5	64	63	17	3
6	44	0	19	5
7	29	0	15	4
8	11	0	6	4
9	7	5	5	3
10	17	0	8	2
11	37	10	17	3
Mean	38.1 days	9.9	11.8	3.5

Results

The patients achieved an average of 7 points on the Ranson scale (maximum 11 points) and had an average of 3.5 (maximum five) extrapancreatic necroses as seen on CT angiography (omental bursa, paracolic bilaterally, subphrenic and mesenteric).

The patients spent an average of 38 days in the intensive care unit and received renal support for 10 days. They received 12 courses of TPE, consisting each time of 2.5–3.5 liters of plasma (Table 2). Surgical treatment consisted of on average six operations, whereby seven patients were lavaged and an additional six were necrosectomized. Patients were ventilated for an average of 28 days, cardiovascularly supported for 21 days, and were oliguric or anuric for 8 days. Patients had an average of three organ failures.

One patient, a 62-year-old man, died after 64 days of catecholamine-resistant cardiovascular failure; he had been anuric, catecholamine dependent, ventilated and had liver failure at admission. In addition to his age-related general condition, the patient also had an artificial aortic valve (Table 3).

Discussion

As already mentioned, in ANP enzymes are liberated into the bloodstream and the cellular immune response is activated. The inhibitor pool is no longer capable of resisting and controlling this attack. Shock provokes micro-

Table 3. Organ failure and outcome in patients with acute necrotizing pancreatitis who were treated with therapeutic plasma exchange

Patient	Lung	Circulatory	Renal	Liver	Outcome	Number of organ failures
1	+	+	+	+	survived	4
2	+	+	−	+	survived	3
3	+	+	+	+	survived	4
4	+	+	+	+	survived	4
5	+	+	+	+	died	4
6	+	+	−	+	survived	3
7	+	−	+	−	survived	2
8	+	−	−	−	survived	1
9	+	+	−	−	survived	2
10	+	+	−	−	survived	2
11	+	+	+	−	survived	3
Total	11	9	6	6	1/11	2.9

circulatory changes with decreased oxygen delivery to the organs and reduced energy production which in turn cause organ failure. Furthermore, a decreased clearance of the enzyme inhibitor complexes by the RES leads to an accumulation of these vasoactive mediators.

TPE is a blood purification method which has the aim of removing large molecular substances from plasma. In ANP, TPE artificially clears the vasoactive, surplus mediators which stimulate inflammation, and FFP substitution supports the inhibitor pool; both techniques give the body the opportunity to control the situation and prevent MOF.

McLelland et al. (1990) reported two cases of MOF where septic shock was successfully treated by plasmapheresis: "dramatic improvements were seen in cardiorespiratory, neurological and renal parameters, which were attributable to plasma exchange." They suspect that cytokine tumor necrosis factor (TNF) and endotoxin play a central role in the development of MOF. TNF has a molecular weight of 18 000 daltons and endotoxin-active lipid A, 2000 daltons, so these substances should be filtrable by means of a high flux membrane during hemofiltration (CVVHF). However, clinical observations have not yielded satisfactory results, which may be due to the fact that the mediators are principally protein-bound [7].

An optimal treatment could consist of TPE followed by CVVHF in order to remove the large pool of protein-bound mediators and, by means of CVVHF, to capture the newly developing unbound mediators in the body. An additional benefit of treatment with CVVHF is an unlimited volume substitution and feeding of the patient.

Schranz et al. [10] reported five cases of ANP and Larwin et al. [6] two cases where TPE was used with good results in fulminant course of disease. Bambauer et al. [1] and Tobin and Fahy [13] confirmed these observations.

Only one patient in our pilot study died. Our excellent results with TPE in the treatment of fulminant necrotizing pancreatitis have stimulated us to plan a multicenter study in order to verify the value of TPE.

References

1. Bambauer R (1988) Therapeutischer Plasmaaustausch und verwandte Plasmaseparationsverfahren. Schattauer, Stuttgart, pp 189–190
2. Gebhardt C (1984) Chirurgische Therapie der akuten Pankreatitis. In: Gebhardt C (ed) Chirurgie des exokrinen Pankreas. Thieme, Stuttgart, pp 48–68
3. Grellner F, Tschaikowsky K, Anhäupl T, Weindler J, Georgieff M (1989) Messung der hepatischen Glucoseproduktion mit Hilfe der stabilen Isotopentechnik. Lab Med 13:189
4. Hiltunen J, Kaukinen S, Pessi T, Ylitalo P (1985) The Kallikrein-Kinin system in operated and non-operated patients with acute pancreatitis. Acta Chir Scand 151:371–375
5. Knaus WA, Draper EA, Wagner DP, Zimmerman JE. (1985) Prognosis in acute organ-system failure. Ann Surg 382(6):685–693
6. Larwin M, Landsdown MRJ, McMahon MJ, Chalmers AG, Turner JH, Brownjohn AM (1988) Plasmapheresis: a rational treatment for fulminant acute pancreatitis? Br Med J 297:593
7. Mc Clelland P, Williams PS, Yaqoob M, Mostafa SM, Bone JM (1990) Multiple organ failure – a role for plasmaexchange? Intensive Care Med 16:100–103
8. McMahon MJ, Bowen M, Mayer AD, Cooper EH (1984) Relation of alpha-2-macroglobulin and other antiproteases to the clinical features of acute pancreatitis. Am J Surg 147:164–170
9. Ranson JHC, Rifkind KM, Roses DF, Fink SD, Eng K, Spencer FC (1974) Prognostic signs and the role of operative management in acute pancreatitis. Surg Gynecol Obstet 139:69
10. Schranz W, Bartels O (1986) Frühzeitiger Plasmaaustausch bei akuter Pankreatitis: Ein erfolgreiches Therapieprinzip bei extremer Hyperlipidämie. Fortschr Med 104:530–532
11. Sieberth HG (1990) Multiorganfailure – an unsolved clinical problem. 2nd international conference on continuous hemofiltration, 10–11 Sept. 1990, Baden bei Wien, Austria
12. Siegenthaler W, Kaufmann W, Hornbostel H, Waller HD (1984) Lehrbuch der inneren Medizin. Springer, Berlin Heidelberg New York, pp 13–89
13. Tobin MV, Fahy LT (1988) Plasmapheresis and fulminant acute pancreatitis. Br Med J 297:979
14. Zirngibl H (1989) Die Bedeutung der Plasmaseparation in der Behandlung der vasoaktiv-toxischen Phase der akuten hämorrhagisch nekrotisierenden Pankreatitis – eine tierexperimentelle Studie. Habilitationsschrift, University of Erlangen

Standards in Pancreas Surgery

F. KÜMMERLE[1]

Surgical Therapy of Inflammatory Diseases of the Pancreas: from Resection to Organ Preservation

For a long time surgeons exercised remarkable reserve when dealing with the pancreas. They assigned a sort of noli me tangere warning to this organ they regarded as being hostile to surgery. Consequently, the preservation of the pancreas was not in jeopardy. Due to the particular features of the pancreas it took a long time before diseases of this organ could be diagnosed. Disturbed functions were diagnosed before morphological changes were detected. X-rays, scans, and endoscopic examination of the ducts finally made the pancreas "transparent". These advances, along with the increase in inflammatory and tumor diseases of the organ, which had been treated conservatively, increased the role of surgery.

Different organ-preserving and resection methods with different therapeutic goals have become established in the surgical management of *inflammatory* diseases of the pancreas. Standards (whether actual or assumed), including those applied to clinical studies, were adopted and then abandoned – which is no wonder, given such a morphologically and functionally unique organ as the pancreas.

Acute Pancreatitis

Acute pancreatitis is divided into mildy edematous and severely necrotizing forms, according to clinical and morphological criteria. The autodigestion of the pancreas continues to represent a catastrophe in the pathology of the abdominal cavity. Its fatal course was long considered unstoppable, the patient either failing to survive the early phase of the toxic shock or dying later from septic complications. Even though intensive care medicine managed to reduce the total mortality, severe forms with extensive necrosis and local complications were still fatal. The failure of conservative medicine

[1] Am Eselsweg 31, W-6500 Mainz-Bretzenheim, FRG

Beger/Büchler/Malfertheiner (Eds.)
Standards in Pancreatic Surgery

and the new understanding of the pathogenesis of acute pancreatitis led to a return to surgical management, which had its modest beginnings in the last century. For the necessarily strict indication for surgery the disease must be clinically staged. For this purpose a staging system was developed [10, 20]. Our Mainz classification system comprising three disease stages (mild/edematous, moderate/partially necrotizing, severe/extensively necrotizing) included ultrasonography and computed tomography (CT) early on to determine changes in the pancreatic parenchyma and thus to distinguish between the two major forms of disease [12]. Hence, the influence of imaging methods was crucial to the surgical management.

The time factor governs whether or not "early" surgery should be performed after treatment has failed; that is, during the first 7–10 days after necrosis has set in, but before life-threatening organ complications occur [11]. Early operation to remove the necroses of the organ and its vicinity ranges from simple removal of the necroses (digitoclasia, "as much as necessary, as little as possible") to subtotal left resection. Many surgeons took a very aggressive approach in that they did not limit themselves to the necroses, but removed the entire organ including the duodenum, parts of the stomach, and extrahepatic bile ducts – a procedure I rejected as carrying too many risks [1]. Surgical zeal was soon curbed as it became easier to estimate the extent of the necrosis. It became evident – and was then confirmed by angio-CT – that a healthy parenchyma is preserved in the nucleus of the resection material. By removing only the necrosis this vital pancreatic tissue could be spared and thus the risk of overtreatment prevented.

Survival of the acute phase of necrotizing pancreatitis after successful intensive care, despite massive destruction of the parenchyma, depends on whether or not there is bacterial contamination of the necroses. Infected necrosis is thus an important prognostic factor in determining the course and the outcome of the disease. The diagnosis of infected necrosis by means of fine-needle aspiration is the decisive criterion for surgery, as well as for mandatory antibiotic treatment [4].

Infected necrosis in its postacute stage is characterized by demarcation, sequestration, liquefaction, and abscess formation. These findings lead to further deterioration and require "delayed" surgery [17], which consists of draining the abscesses, removing the necroses as radically as possible, and draining the abscess and necrosis cavities. Effective drainage and irrigation systems were developed to make sure of complete drainage to avoid having to perform repeat laparotomies. Necrectomy was combined with continuous bursa lavage [5], scheduled reoperation (staged reexploration) [22], or with open drainage [6]. The closed treatment seems to be superior to the open method.

The role of surgery in biliary pancreatitis to debride extrahepatic bile ducts lost importance to endoscopic therapy. This applied not only to the rare incarcerated papilla stone, but also to the severe forms of biliary necrotizing pancreatitis. In these cases the endoscopic debridement of the ducts (papillotomy and stone extraction) should precede surgery on the pancreas [7].

The better surgical results obtained in acute pancreatitis, with mortality rates of below 10% [5], can be attributed to the fact that the course of the disease can be better assessed and the operation time and procedure more reliably determined. Diverging results are due to the differences among the patient population with regard to the severity of the disease.

Chronic Pancreatitis

Principally, there are two ways of treating chronic pancreatitis: conservative therapy in uncomplicated cases of chronic pancreatitis, with the aim of allowing the excretory parenchyma to "burn out" by fibrosis and scar formation [2] and ultimately stop the pain, and surgical management in complicated cases, with the goal of alleviating the chronic pain and removing the local organ complications caused by the pancreatitis. Initially, surgery in chronic pancreatitis pursued the goal of relieving the pain by performing resections in the vegetative nervous system, such as splanchnicectomy and denervations, [15] without touching the organ per se. Such an operation – like other operations on the vegetative nervous system – could only have a limited effect. Direct operations on the gland itself were not undertaken until the 1950s.

Decompression of the ductal system, in other words, organ-preserving pain treatment, is the underlying approach behind *drainage operations* of the pancreatic duct and the jejunum, and the modifications of these procedures [8, 19, 22]. Retrograde secretion drainage end-to-end with the jejunum after resection of the pancreatic tail proved to be just as futile as the side-to-side anastomoses, which were far too narrow. I have always said that you can only drain what can be drained [13, 14]. The ductal system lacks the necessary requirements for effective drainage: a 1–1.5 cm-wide duct, which can be split to 7–10 cm. The long Roux-en-Y side anastomosis [18] can be regarded as a functionally reliable drainage procedure. Finally, the transduodenal split of the pancreatic duct by means of papillotomy was added to ensure drainage via the duodenum [21]. The advantages of the organ-sparing draining methods are the low surgical mortality and the low late morbidity caused by the operation.

Parallel to the technical development of the draining procedures, resection methods have been adopted in the last 25 years, particularly in cases with non-draining ducts. Whereas initially various degrees of left resections up to subtotal resection were the most common procedures, resections of the head (partial and total duodenopancreatectomy) later became more common, because severe lesions of the head involving the bile duct and duodenum (cholestase syndrome, duodenal stenosis) became more frequent and sometimes a suspicion of malignancy had to be clarified. The number of left resections (10%–50%) soon decreased and were only indicated when the disease was located chiefly in the region of the pancreatic tail. Subtotal left resections and total duodenopancreatectomy should be abandoned due to high risk, late morbidity, and resulting diabetes [14]. Resection to follow up suspicion of cancer has become even more rare a result of diagnostic improvement.

To counteract the effects of extensive resection in patients, most of whom are still young, and especially to limit the effect on the function of the islets, further surgical approaches were developed:

1. Islet autotransplantation after subtotal and total pancreatectomy [16]
2. Ductal occlusion in the preserved pancreatic tail during partial duodenopancreatectomy [9]
3. Duodenum-preserving pancreatic head resection as an alternative procedure to Whipple's operation, in the presence of an inflammatory pancreatic head tumor [3]

Endocrine function can be preserved to a certain degree by means of islet transplantation via the portal vein after examination of the resection material. The literature provides no information on the possibility of performing pancreatic transplantation joining the transplant to the intestine in a patient who has undergone pancreatectomy for chronic pancreatitis. Such a transplantation would be some compensation for the surgical loss of the organ.

Ductal occlusion with resorbable prolamin solution in conjunction with Whipple's operation leads to atrophy of the exocrine parenchyma while sparing the islets of Langerhans, an approach used to prevent recurrent inflammation as well as to partially preserve endocrine function.

The advantages of the organ-sparing duodenum-preserving pancreatic head resection over Whipple's procedure include the preservation of the stomach, duodenum, and bile ducts, the absence of pain, and the low rate of early and late postoperative morbidity.

Lastly, the pseudocysts in chronic pancreatitis should be mentioned, which unlike the postacute and posttraumatic cysts are not regarded as solitary cysts, but as a part of the chronic inflammation of the entire organ. Therefore, they should not be drained in isolation, but integrated in a draining or resecting procedure. Percutaneous and endoscopic internal cyst drainage can be considered.

Mortality and the late results of draining and resecting operations in the case of chronic pancreatitis are similar. This makes several surgical methods available to the surgeon that are tailored to the morphology of the particular disease.

Closing Remarks

The pancreas always presented a challenge to surgeons. Surgical measures were never attempted until conservative treatment had failed. Although a number of mechanisms in the pathogenesis of the inflammatory pancreatic disease have become known, we are still a long way from a real understanding of the various forms of inflammatory pancreatic disease.

Generally speaking, organ-preserving surgery for inflammatory pancreatic diseases is part of the modern trend to reduce surgical trauma. In looking back we must not forget what has been surgically introduced and carried out, in particular, the failures of the respective methods. In no other field has so much been learned in just one generation. In evaluating our surgical activities it is worth remembering that all of the surgical procedures were developed to treat the symptoms and not to cure the disease, with the exception of bile duct debridement in the rare case of biliary chronic pancreatitis. Whatever we do, conservatively or surgically, in the end it is the patient who determines the quality of the remainder of his or her life, which especially includes the decision whether or not to abstain from alcohol.

Strategy and tactics are terms that are derived from military terminology. In the Gulf War the term "surgical" was used to refer to a military maneuver that had been perfectly executed. I'm not sure that we can be happy with this comparison, even it does acknowledge the precision of surgical work. In the case of surgical treatment of pancreatitis with its manifold concepts we can make good use of the definition formulated by the well-known expert on war, Clausewitz: "Tactics is an unwavering procedure using a wise selection of means and methods."

References

1. Alexandre JK, Gnerrary MT (1981) Role of total pancreatectomy in the treatment of necrotizing pancreatitis. World J Surg 5:369–375
2. Ammann RW, Akovbiantz A, Largiader F, Schueler G (1984) Course and outcome of chronic pancreatitis. Gastroenterology 86:820–828
3. Beger HG, Witte C, Kraas E, Bittner R (1980) Erfahrungen mit einer das Duodenum erhaltenden Pankreaskopfresektion bei chronischer Pankreatitis. Chirurg 51:303–309
4. Beger HG, Bittner R, Block S, Büchler M (1986) Bacterial contamination of pancreatic necrosis. Gastroenterology 91:433–438
5. Beger HG, Büchler M, Bittner R, Oettinger W, Block S, Nevalainen T (1988) Necrosectomy and postoperative local lavage in patients with necrotizing pancreatitis. World J Surg 12:255–262
6. Bradley EL (1987) Management of infected necrosis by open drainage. Ann Surg 206:542–548
7. Büchler M (1990) Chirurgische Behandlung der akuten Pankreatitis. Z Gastroenterol Verh Bd 25:101–103
8. Du Val MK Jr (1954) Caudal pancreaticojejunostomy for relapsing pancreatitis. Ann Surg 140:775–785

9. Gebhardt Ch, Stolte M (1978) Pankreasgangokklusion durch Injektion einer schnell härtenden Aminosäurenlösung. Langenbecks Arch Klin Chir 346: 149–166
10. Imrie CW (1974) Observations on acute pancreatitis. Br J Surg 61:539–544
11. Kümmerle F, Neher M, Schönborn M, Mangold G (1975) Vorzeitige Operation bei akuter hämorrhagischnekrotisierender Pankreatitis. Dtsch Med Wochenschr 100:2241–2244
12. Kümmerle F (1987) Clinical staging in acute pancreatitis. In: Beger HC, Büchler M (eds) Acute pancreatitis. Springer, Berlin Heidelberg New York, pp 177–180
13. Kümmerle F, Frick S, Günther R (1982) Tendenzen in der Chirurgie der chronischen Pankreatitis. Dtsch Med Wochenschr 107:531–534
14. Kümmerle F (1987) Chronische Pankreatitis. Wandlungen in den diagnostischen und therapeutischen Konzepten. Dtsch Med Wochenschr 112:619–621
15. Mallet-Guy PA (1983) Late and very late results of resections of the nervous system in the treatment of chronic relapsing pancreatitis. Am J Surg 145: 234–238
16. Najarian JS, Sutherland DER, Baumgartner D, Burke B, Rynasiewicz JJ, Matas AJ, Goetz FC (1980) Total or near total pancreatectomy and islet autotransplantation for treatment of chronic pancreatitis. Ann Surg 192:526–542
17. Neher M, Kümmerle F, Mangold G, Schönborn H (1977) Verzögerte Operation bei akuter Pankreatitis. Chirurg 48:439–442
18. Partington PF, Rochelle REL (1960) Modified Puestow procedure for retrograde drainage of the pancreatic duct. Ann Surg 152:1037–1042
19. Puestow CB, Gillesby WJ (1958) Retrograde surgical drainage of pancreas for chronic relapsing pancreatitis. Arch Surg 76:898–907
20. Ranson JHC (1974) Prognostic signs and the role of operative management in acute pancreatitis. Surg Gynecol Obstet 139:69–78
21. Rumpf KD, Pichlmayr R (1983) Eine Methode zur chirurgischen Behandlung der chronischen Pankreatitis: die transduodenale Pancreaticoplastik. Chirurg 54:722–727
22. Teichmann W, Wittmann DH, Andreone M (1986) Scheduled reoperation (Etappenlavage). Arch Surg 121:147–152
23. Zollinger RM, Keith LM, Ellison EH (1954) Pancreatitis. New Engl J Med 251:497–501

Necrosectomy and Closed Lavage in Acute Pancreatitis

P. Pederzoli,[1] C. Bassi, S. Vesentini, F. Nifosi, R. Girelli, M. Falconi, D. Lombardi, and S. Corra[1]

Introduction

Generally, acute pancreatitis (AP) is a self-limiting disease that resolves with simple medical therapy. In a certain proportion of cases – probably higher than has been supposed up to now (15%–20%) – it is encountered in the anatomic-pathological form of necrohemorrhagic pancreatitis (NP), which is associated with elevated morbidity and mortality. Intensive medical therapy can cure many cases, but some specific situations and particular complications make surgery necessary [1].

Considering the evolutive tendency of NP, we deal here with the complications that are important for the surgeon's decision as to early or late operation. Among the indications for early surgery (within the first 2 weeks from onset), in our experience multiorgan failure nonresponsive to intensive treatment is the most frequent (this indication is still much discussed in the literature). The type of operation that we have adopted and the objectives guiding our choice correspond to the therapeutic needs of these particular patients.

Until a few years ago, biliary NP involving "fluctuating" stones or stones wedged in the papilla represented for us an absolute indication for early surgery. Today, surgical endoscopy (endoscopic sphincterotomy) is used when the patient presents within the first 2–3 days of NP [2]. There after we believe glandular damage to continue or to limit itself independently of etiology. A late complication, involving general agreement as to surgical treatment, is infection of the necrosis with clinical conditions of sepsis associated either with the infected necrosis or with pancreatic abscesses characterized by the presence of pus in the collection [3, 4]. The choice of surgery may also be dictated by less frequent complications, such as peritonitis caused by enzymatic involvement of the peritoneum or by severe bleeding due to vascular erosion.

Since 1976 in our Surgical Department we have been using a method that includes removal of necrotic areas and retroendoperitoneal draining accompanied by a post-surgical closed lavage [5, 6].

[1] Surgical Department, University of Verona, Borgo Roma Hospital, 37134 Verona, Italy

Beger/Büchler/Malfertheiner (Eds.)
Standards in Pancreatic Surgery

Table 1. Etiology

	n	%
Biliary disease	99	35.1
Alcohol abuse	96	34.0[a]
Postoperative	33	11.7
Idiopathic	20	7.1
Trauma	18	6.5
Dyslipidemia	7	2.5
Post-ERCP	6	2.1
Pancreatic cancer	2	0.7
Hypercalcemia	1	0.3

[a] Includes 31 cases associated with gall-stones or biliary sludge.

Patients and Methods

From 1976 to 1990, 282 consecutive patients underwent this type of surgical treatment for acute severe NP. The male-female ratio was 2.3:1.8; mean age was 38 years, and the mean Ranson score was 4.6. Etiology is presented in Table 1. The diagnosis was always based upon clinical, biochemical, and radiological parameters (ultrasound, computed tomography).

Surgical Procedure

An enlarged upper midline incision is made, avoiding an upper transverse approach because this incision has proven to hamper correct positioning of the drains. We proceed with the opening of the gastrocolic ligament, exposing the anterior wall of the pancreas; with a wide Kocher maneuver we explore the head of the gland posteriorly. Between the top and bottom margins of the pancreas, passing behind the splenic vessels a connection is made that is exteriorized corresponding to the body-tail passage. This maneuver – simplified by the serum necrohemorrhagic stuffing of the retropancreatic tissues – allows partial mobilization of the body and tail.

The retroperitoneal collections must be examined (also on the presurgical CT) in two distinct areas at the transverse mesocolic root level: in relation to (a) the collections from the head and corresponding to the mesenteric root at the immediate right of the upper mesenteric artery and (b) the flow from the body and tail to the left of the superior duodenal segment. Other collections can be observed in the parietocolic spaces. In our experience these features are variable, but constantly present features of the retroperitoneal types of sprues.

From these sloping areas, having cut the posterior peritoneum, we proceed to place them into communication with the connection placed behind the gland and previously prepared; in this way the more sloping parts of the collection are made to communicate with the damaged glandular sectors, creating passages for the drains. In other words, an affluxive drain is placed corresponding to the posterior wall of the head and body of the pancreas, which was mobilized previously with the Kocher maneuver, and is placed into communication with a more sloping effluxive drainage made to pass in correspondence to the mesocolon to the right of the superior mesenteric artery. The space created behind the body-tail level is used to position a new series of affluxive drains (from the top through the gastrohepatic ligament) and of defluxion (put into the connection first prepared on the mesocolon, to the left of the ligament of Treitz; Fig. 1). In the presence of collections in the parietocolic douches even these are able to be opened and drained, placing them in contact with the retroperitoneal affluxive drains [5].

Obviously the number of drains depends on the size of the injury at the retroperitoneal level. For this the two-way drain seems very useful as this reduces the number of tubes used and the risk of associated complications. We then go on to drain the retrocavity of the epiploon using two drains, one affluxive and two defluxive (Fig. 1). The sequestrectomy is always carried out simultaneously. This is done by digitoclasia when the operation is performed in a late phase to manage the infected necrosis [4]. When it is necessary in the early phases (first weeks), the necrosectomy is transferred to the mechanical action of the lavages that progressively mobilizes the necrotic tissues bordering healthy parenchyma [6].

Postsurgical Closed Lavage

The principal factor in this procedure is the postsurgical irrigation. For this reason a team of nurses is constantly being trained in our Department for correct lavages; it is important to control very carefully the patency of the drains and their correct connection.

The irrigation consists per 24 h of 8–10 l hypertonic or physiological solution containing 400 mg gabexate mesilate or 1.5×10^9 IU aprotinin per 500 ml. This was administered by continuous infusion for an average of 9 days and twice daily for an average of 12 days (range 4–96). The total daily use of liquids for the irrigation is hard to quantify; what is important is the balance between ingoing and outgoing liquids. The frequent obliteration of the drains by the surrounding necrotic tissue requires their careful management and occasionally necessitates reoperation (12 patients, 4.2%).

Serial computed tomography, enzymatic and microbiological controls of the drainage guide the decision regarding removal of the drains. In our experience they are removed at an average of 21 days (range 8–101). In cases of infected necrosis or pancreatic abscess strategies other than that of perfusion liquid include aditional medication with antibiotics chosen on the basis of the antibiogram. In the course of these lavages the defluxive drains are closed in such a way to allow the antibiotics to act locally.

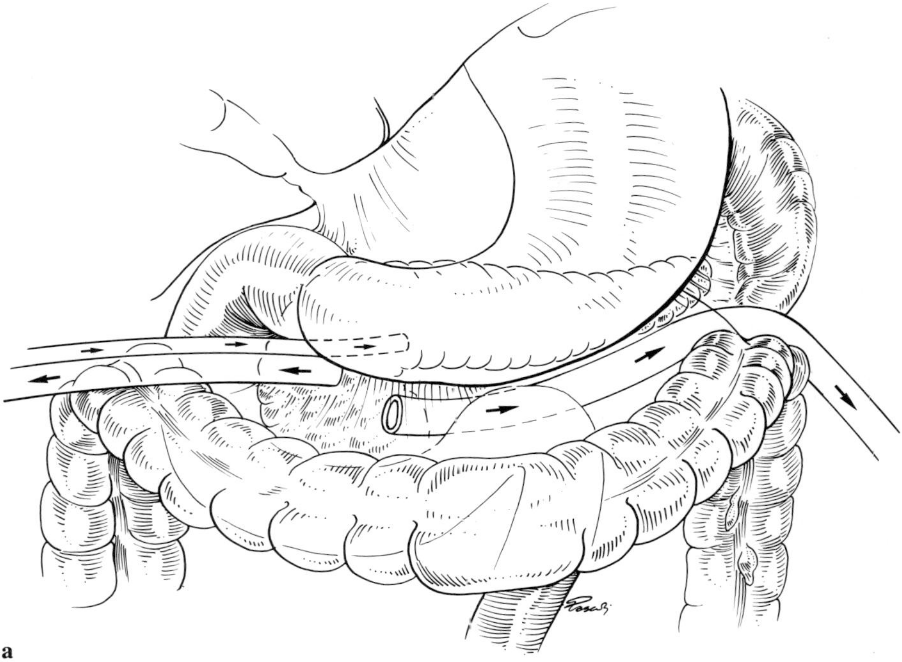

a

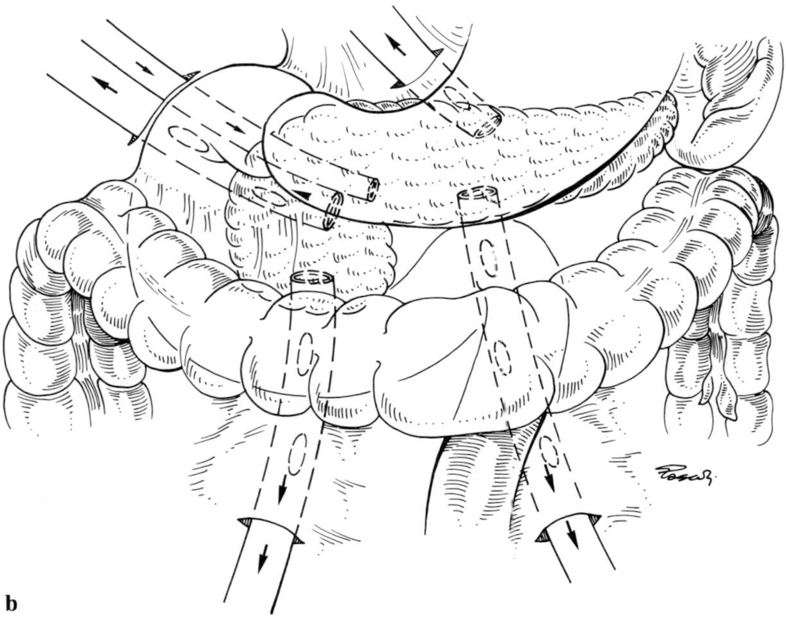

b

Fig. 1a,b. Position of the drains. **a** At the anterior wall of the pancreas. **b** At the posterior wall. *Arrows*, input and output routes of the irrigation

Table 2. Indications and timing of operation

Indications	n	%	Timing
Sepsis	181	64.2	1st week, 4 patients 2nd week, 25 patients 3rd week, 85 patients 4th week, 76 patients
Multiorgan failure	52	18.4	Within 2 days, 6 patients 2–4 days, 45 patients Over 4 days, 1 patient
Biliary pancreatitis[a]	20	7.1	Within 2 days, 4 patients (ampulla) 2–4 days, 16 patients (main BD)
Computed tomography	28	9.9	(Years from 1976 to 1980)
Bleeding	2	0.7	Over 4 days

[a] With stones into the main duct or wedged.

Table 3. Timing and results

Timing	Cases	Deaths		Findings
		n	%	
<2 days	38	3	7.9	28 patients before 1981 6 "fulminant" (3 deaths) 3 with wedged stones
2–4 days	65	8	12.3	Patients referred from other hospitals 20 surgery (2 deaths) 13 no surgery (3 deaths, 23%) Treated at the onset of NP 32 patients (3 deaths, 9.4%)
>4 days	179	37	20.6	Patients referred from other hospitals 107 surgery (35 deaths, 32.7%) 30 no surgery (1 death, 3.4%) Treated at the onset of NP 42 patients (1 death, 2.4%)
Total	282	48	17.0	

Of the 282 patients, 127 underwent surgery in other hospitals (37 deaths, 29.1%), 155 underwent surgery in our Department (11 deaths, 7.1%), and 112 were observed and operated in our Department (7 deaths, 6.2%).

Results

Table 2 presents the indications and timing of operations performed from 1976 to 1990. One sees here that 64% of patients were treated for septic complications and 18% following multiorgan failure not responsive to intensive therapy within the first 4 days of the disease. We treated 10% of patients on the basis of data regarding the presence of necrosis and retroperitoneal collections; this was revealed by CT at a time when in the

Table 4. Complications observed in 57 of 282 patients (20.2%)

Pancreatic fistulas	28	(9 surgically treated)
Enteric fistulas	24	(4 surgically treated)
Bleedings	21	(21 operations on 18 patients; 7 deaths, 38.9%)
Pseudocysts	9	(8 surgically treated)
Colonic obstruction	1	(Surgically treated)
Total	83	

Mortality rate 12.3% (7/57); all deaths due to hemorrhagic complications.

presence of necrosis a surgical procedure was preferred. Another 7% of patients were treated for NP of biliary origin. Today these cases are evaluated endoscopically and treated by sphincterotomy; in case of failure we proceeded to surgery.

Table 3 shows the results in terms of surgical timing. Examination of our case reports demonstrates remarkable differences in the death rate among those who had previously undergone surgery in other hospitals (29% death rate), those who underwent primary surgery in our department (7.1%), and those whom we observed from the beginning (6.2%).

Table 4 lists the most common postsurgical complications that we observed. The most feared of these is postsurgical hemorrhage from the drains; this was responsible for all the deaths resulting from complications. In the past 2 years we have noted that the source of such hemorrhages is generally the erosion (due to drains or "enzymatic" breakthrough) of the inferior or collateral mesenteric veins; therefore, we now electively tie such vessels. This has been associated with an important reduction in the frequency of such complications [6].

Discussion

The pathophysiological evolution of NP is considered to begin (following the action of etiological agents not always identifiable) from a parenchymal necrosis with a capsular-ductal rupture and spill of the enzymes activated in the retroperitoneum. By contact, the activated enzymes lead to retroperitoneal necrosis, creating fluid collections; this is mainly what causes the proteases (responsible for the systemic injuries) to be reabsorbed by the bloodstream (Fig. 2). The peritoneum is involved in a later phase, with an exudative type of response that seems to dilute the concentration of the active enzymes [5].

The surgical procedure that we adopt is defined in this pathophysiological context and aims at treating the glands and retroperitoneal space. The sequestrectomy (when possible) and the "slow" necrosectomy

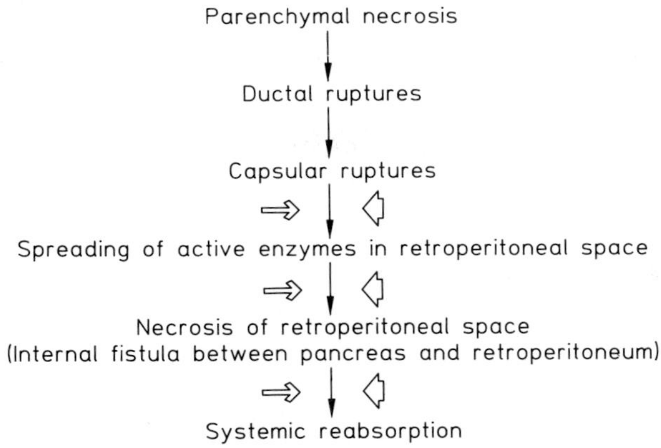

Fig. 2. Pathophysiological evolution in necrotizing pancreatitis. ►, "Attack points" of the mechanical drainage; →, "attack points" by inhibition through contact with antiproteasic substances

obtained from the mechanical action of the lavage, together with the activity of the antiproteasic substance delivered by means of the drains, seek to influence the pathophysiological evolution in various instances, such as the retroperitoneal spilling of the enzymes and their reabsorption at the level of the cycle (Fig. 2).

The closed lavage method is applicable at both the late and the early complication stages. In the latter, obtaining a "safe" sequestrectomy is extremely improbable. In fact, in the early phases the sequestrum must still be completely organized, and this is not possible by digitoclasia without complications. However, in these cases postoperative irrigation allows a spontaneous "sequestrectomy by lavage" [6] once the pathologic situation has completely matured. A recent review compares the method of simple drainage with that of drainage and lavage and of open packing [7]. Theoretically, such approaches – in particular the latter two – seem superimposable. Here one tries to remove and to drain the involved areas of NP; however, the most reliable method is that of the drainage-lavage due to the lower rate of complications associated with it.

Although important, we believe this aspect should be considered in relative terms. What we consider essential can be summarized as follows: (a) referral of severe patients to specialized centers; (b) immediate and continuous treatment to the very end; (c) close cooperation between gastroenterologists, intensive care unit operators, and surgeons; and (d) psychological suitability and material availability of long hospital stays.

References

1. Wilson L, Imrie C (1991) Current concepts in the management of pancreatitis. Drugs 41(3):358–366
2. Neoptolemos JP, London NJ, James D, Carr-Locke DL, Bailey IA, Fossard DP (1988) Controlled trial of urgent endoscopic retrograde cholangiopancreatography and endoscopic sphinterotomy versus conservative treatment for acute pancreatitis due to gallstones. Lancet ii:979–983
3. Beger HG, Bittner R, Block S, Büchler M (1986) Bacterial contamination of pancreatic necrosis: a prospective clinical study. Gastroenterology 91:433–438
4. Bassi C, Vesentini S, Nifosi F et al. (1990) Pancreatic abscess and other pus-harboring Collections related to pancreatitis: a review of 108 cases. World J Surg 14:505–512
5. Pederzoli P, Bassi C, Vesentini S, Girelli R, Cavallini G, Falconi M, Nifosi F, Riehm A, Dagradi A (1990) Retroperitoneal and peritoneal drainage and lavage in the treatment of severe necrotizing pancreatitis. Surg Gynecol Obstet 163: 428–432
6. Pederzoli P, Bassi C, Vesentini S et al. (1990) Necrosectomy by lavage in the surgical treatment of severe necrotizing pancreatitis. Acta Chir Scand 156:775–780
7. D'Egidio A, Schein M (1991) Surgical strategies in the treatment of pancreatic necrosis and infection. Br J Surg 78:133–137

Necrotizing Pancreatitis: Necrosectomy and Closed Continuous Lavage of the Lesser Sac. The Ulm Experience

M. Büchler,[1] W. Uhl, R. Isenmann, R. Bittner, and H.G. Beger

Acute pancreatitis ranges from a mild, self-limiting disease to a severe illness with sometimes fatal outcome. In about 80% of patients, acute pancreatitis takes the cause of an edematous–interstitial inflammation mainly caused by gallstones (30%) or overindulgence in alcohol (50%). A necrotizing form of acute pancreatitis develops in up to 20% of patients [1–3]. This type of acute pancreatitis, even if with slight or moderate morphologic alterations, often proceeds to local or systemic complications and may become life threatening. From a morphologic point of view, necrotizing pancreatitis shows an interstitial–edematous inflammation combined with more or less extensive necrosis of the pancreatic exocrine and endocrine parechyma, and sometimes even extensive fatty tissue necrosis in the peripancreatic and retroperitoneal tissue compartments [4]. The fluid collection around the pancreatic area in necrotizing pancreatitis contains vasoactive and toxic substances such as phospholipase A_2, endotoxin, prostacyclin, activated trypsin, complement break-down products, thromboxane, elastase, and many other undefined harmful substances [5]. The crucial risk in necrotizing pancreatitis is a bacterial infection of pancreatic necrosis [6–8].

Besides edematous–interstitial and necrotizing acute pancreatitis there are two other entities that are nowadays classified as acute pancreatitis, namely pancreatic abscess and postacute pancreatic pseudocyst [4]. The frequency of these different entities of acute pancreatitis according to the patient population in Ulm is shown in Table 1.

There is no doubt that the outcome of acute pancreatitis is closely related to the occurrence of a necrotizing type of pancreatitis. There is a significant correlation between pancreatic necrosis and the frequency of bacterial infection [3, 6]. The prognosis of acute pancreatitis is closely linked to the amount of necrosis, and to the question, whether these necrotic areas are infected or not (Table 2).

[1] Department of Surgery, University of Ulm, Steinhoevelstrasse 9, W-7900 Ulm, FRG

Beger/Büchler/Malfertheiner (Eds.)
Standards in Pancreatic Surgery

Table 1. Acute pancreatitis: frequency of the necrotizing course in 1067 patients[a]

	Patients *n*	(%)
Interstitial–edematous pancreatitis	793	(73.4)
Necrotizing pancreatitis	194	(18.2)
Pancreatic abscess	26	(2.4)
Postacute pseudocyst	54	(5.1)

[a] May 1982–December 1990 at the Departments of General Surgery and Gastroenterology, University of Ulm, FRG.

Table 2. Morphological factors in the mortality of necrotizing pancreatitis ($n = 205$)

		Patients *n*	(%)	Mortality *n*	(%)	
1. Extent of pancreatic necrosis	~30%	79	(39)	6	(8)	
	~50%	75	(37)	18	(24)	$P < 0.0001$
	Subtotal/total	51	(25)	26	(51)	
2. Extrapancreatic necrosis	Positive	96	(47)	33	(34)	$P < 0.02$
	Negative	109	(53)	17	(16)	
3. Pancreatogenic ascites	Positive	115	(56)	42	(37)	$P < 0.01$
	Negative	90	(44)	8	(9)	
4. Bacterial contamination ($n = 138$)	Positive	56	(41)	18	(32)	$P < 0.01$
	Negative	82	(59)	8	(10)	

Discrimination Between Interstitial–Edematous and Necrotizing Pancreatitis

The most important prognostic consideration in patients with acute pancreatitis is to discriminate between acute edematous–interstitial and necrotizing pancreatitis. Various clinical, radiological and single serum parameters have been analyzed in the past to stage acute pancreatitis [9–12].

In this respect, contrast-enhanced computed tomography (CT) of the inflammed pancreatic gland has been shown to have the highest rates of discrimination among imaging techniques [13–16]. Contrast-enhanced CT is better than native CT scanning, since, particularly in patients with a complicated course, this technique allows determination and the localization and measurement of the extent of the pancreatic necrosis as well as the estimation of the extent of retroperitoneal fatty tissue necrosis (Fig. 1). Besides CT scanning and with regard to biochemical parameters, the measurement of

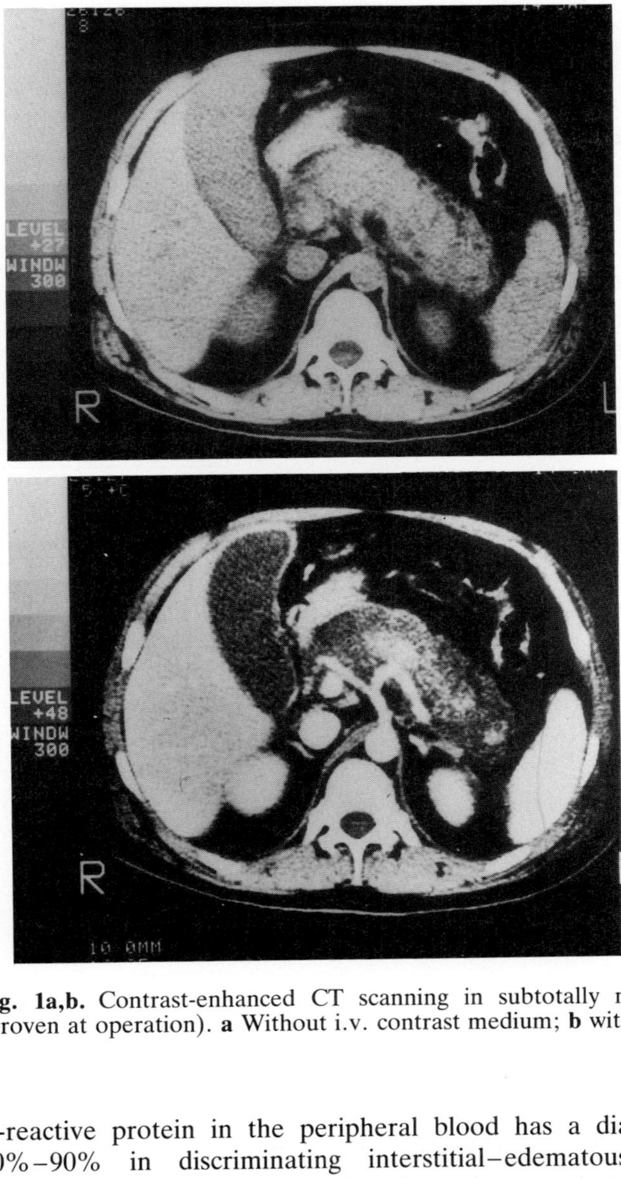

a

b

Fig. 1a,b. Contrast-enhanced CT scanning in subtotally necrotizing pancreatitis (proven at operation). **a** Without i.v. contrast medium; **b** with contrast medium

C-reactive protein in the peripheral blood has a diagnostic accuracy of 80%–90% in discriminating interstitial–edematous from necrotizing pancreatitis. The cut-off level for C-reactive protein to indicate pancreatic necrosis is above 120 mg/l [17–20]. In our Ulm concept and on the basis of series published worldwide, therefore, acute pancreatitis is staged by measuring C-reactive protein in the serum followed by contrast-enhanced CT scanning.

There are several new and possibly useful serum parameters to discriminate edematous from necrotizing pancreatitis such as the elastase

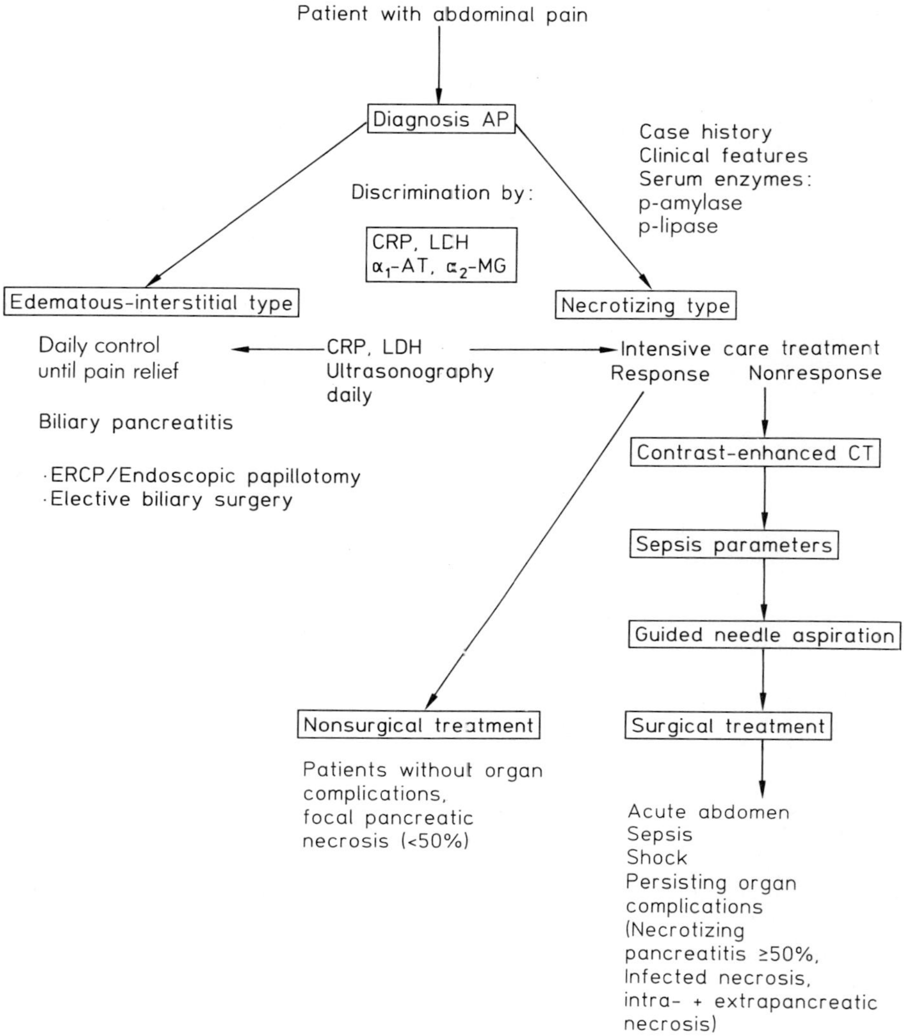

Fig. 2. Algorithm for clinical decision-making in patients with edematous–interstitial or necrotizing pancreatitis. *AP*, acute pancreatitis; *CRP*, C-reactive protein; *LDH*, lactate dehydrogenase; α_1-*At*, α_1-*antitrypsin;* α_2-*MG*, α_2-*mactoglobulin CT*; computed tomography; *ERCP*, endoscopic retrograde cholangiopancreatography

from polymorphonuclear leukocytes [20], trypsin-activating peptides [21, 22], phospholipase A_2 [23], or interleukin-6 [24] have been recently recommended, but from the point of view of clinical reliability, it still has to be proven whether these markers of necrosis will be useful in the daily clinical work-up of patients suffering from acute pancreatitis. Figure 2 shows the Ulm algorithm for the management of patients with acute pancreatitis, in-corporating the important part of staging this disease.

Necrotizing Pancreatitis: The Role of Infection

One major prognostic factor in patients suffering from necrotizing pancreatitis is bacterial infection of the necrosis. This has become a generally accepted fact [6–8]. According to the data of a prospective clinical trial, the overall contamination rate of pancreatic tissue necrosis was approximately 40%. Infected necroses were detected in 25% of the patients who had only 1-week-old disease, in 45% of the patients with 2-week-old disease, in 60% of the patients in whom the disease lasted 3 weeks, and in 58% of the patients in whom the duration of necrotizing pancreatitis was 4 weeks. Of the germ-positive samples, 75% showed gram-negative bacteria (Table 3). Most striking was the finding that the germs found in pancreatic necrosis are primarily intestinal flora derived such as *Escherichia coli*, pseudomonas and proteus [25].

A high percentage (up to 65%) of infected pancreatic necrosis was confirmed by further trials [7, 8]. These data underscore very clearly a proportionally increased risk for bacterial infection of necrosis the longer the disease lasts. Patients with infected necrosis suffer significantly more often from cardiovascular complications, pulmonary and renal insufficiency, the clinical picture of sepsis, and gastrointestinal bleeding than patients with sterile necrosis. Moreover in patients with infected necrosis, the frequency and severity of organ dysfunctions and clinical complications were increased compared with patients with sterile necrosis (Table 4). Furthermore there was a significant correlation between the quantity of pancreatic tissue necrosis and the extent of extrapancreatic fatty tissue necrosis on the one hand, and infection on the other hand (Table 5).

Conservative Treatment of Patients Suffering from Necrotizing Pancreatitis

Patients with a proven necrotizing course should receive intensive care management in accordance with generally accepted guidelines and treatment modalities in severe acute pancreatitis (Table 6). This includes nothing by mouth, electrolyte, albumin, and sometimes erythrocyte substitution, and venous-pressure-adjusted correction of hypovolemia. Placement of a gastric tube has become generally established, although controlled clinical trials have not shown subsequent improvement in morbidity. Data from controlled clinical studies with glucagon, somatostatin, aprotinin, gabexate mesylate, and H_2-blockers have not shown any effect on the course of acute pancreatitis with respect to the frequency and severity of local and systemic complications nor with regard to lowering of mortality [26–30]. Therefore,

Table 3. Frequency of bacteria in pancreatic infection

Bacteria	Frequency (%)
E. coli	25.9
Pseudomonas spp.	15.9
Staphylococcus aureus	15.3
Klebsiella spp.	10.1
Proteus spp.	10.4
Streptococcus faecalis	4.4
Enterobacter spp.	2.5
Other anaerobes	15.8
	100.0

Table 4. Preoperative morbidity in 134 patients with necrotizing pancreatitis

	Bacterial contamination			
	Positive (55 patients)		Negative (79 patients)	
	n	%	*n*	%
Pulmonary insufficiency[a]	27	49	19	24
Renal insufficiency[b]	18	33	15	19
Shock[c]	12	22	6	8
Sepsis[d]	27	49	9	11
GI-tract bleeding	5	9	1	1
None	4	7	36	46

[a] $pO_{2_a} < 60$ Torr.
[b] $Cr_s > 120\,\mu mol/l$.
[c] $RR_{sys} < 80$ mm Hg/>15 min.
[d] $T_{rec} > 38.5°C$ + WBC > 10000/mm^3 / thrombocytopenia, metabolic acidosis.

Table 5. Necrotizing pancreatitis: morbidity related to extrapancreatic fatty tissue necroses (EPN) 236 patients[a]

	Ranson points (mean)	Pancreatic necroses[b]		Bacterial infection[b] (%)	MSOF ≥2 organs[b] (%)
		Focal (%)	Extended (%)		
EPN positive (113 patients)	4.7	21	79	53	40
EPN negative (123 patients)	2.8	58	42	27	20

MSOF: multiple systemic organ failure.
[a] Surgical management November 1968–April 1986, Department of General Surgery, University of Ulm, FRG.
[b] Differences significant; χ^2 test.

Table 6. Intensive care unit treatment of acute pancreatitis (iv catheter, urine catheter, nasogastric tube)

1. Pulmonary insufficiency	paO_2 <70 mmHg	→ oxygen supply
	paO_2 <60 mmHg under oxygen	→ mechanical ventilation
2. Renal insufficiency	serum creatinine >120 μmol/l urine volume <30 ml/hr	→ dopamine (low dose) + diuretics
	BUN >30 mmol/l or serum creatinine >400 μmol/l	→ hemofiltration hemodialysis
3. Cardiocirculatory dysfunction/shock	central venous pressure ↓	→ volume replacement
	mean arterial pressure <70 mmHg	→ dopamine (high dose)
	systolic blood pressure <90 mmHg ⩾10 min	→ Swan-Ganz catheter norepinephrine
4. Metabolic disorders	hyperglycemia >11.1 mmol/l	→ insulin
	disseminated intravascular coagulation (DIC)	→ fresh frozen plasma
5. Sepsis	rectal temperature >38.5°C leukocytes <4 000/>12 000/mm^3 platelets <150 000/mm^3 metablic acidosis >−4 mmol/l	→ antibiotics surgical intervention
Fine needle aspiration	→ infected necrosis	→ surgery
Biliary pancreatitis (bilirubin ↑, ASAT ↑, alk phosphatase ↑)	endoscopic retrograde cholangiography	→ papillotomy for impacted stones

we avoid these drugs. Intensive care treatment comprises specific treatment of pulmonary, renal, and cardiocirculatory dysfunction (Table 6). Patients who develop a septic clinical picture during the course of severe acute pancreatitis should receive antibiotics that are active against mostly gram-negative bacteria. In patients with a septic course and increases in body temperature of more than 38.5°C over 48 h, a rise of leukocytes to above 12.000/m^3, thrombocytopenia, and recurrent metabolic acidosis, repeated contrast-enhanced CT scanning is performed to localize necrosis and an ultrasound- or CT-guided aspiration of the necrotic tissue is carried out to determine the presence of bacteria. If bacterial infection of necrosis is detected, surgical therapy is mandatory.

Indication for Surgical Management

From the surgeon's point of view, operative management of necrotizing pancreatitis is indicated in patients who develop signs of sepsis as determined on the basis of bacteriologically positive fine needle aspiration [31]. Besides patients with infected necrosis being suitable for operative treatment, operative treatment is mandatory if patients with necrotizing pancreatitis demonstrate persistent or increasing signs of pulmonary and renal insufficiency or cardiocirculatory failure. If these signs of major organ complications persist during maximum intensive care treatment (Table 6) for at least 3–5 days, these patients belong to the group of so-called nonresponders with a high risk of increasing morbidity and decreasingly good prognosis. Nonresponse to intensive care treatment after 3–5 days, according to our experience, is an important clinical parameter for deciding whether to change from medical to surgical treatment.

Timing of Surgery

Surgical management of necrotizing pancreatitis is based on maximum use of intensive care measures. The timing of surgical treatment is still under discussion today. According to our experience in Ulm, surgical treatment starts to become easier after the first week of the disease. Based on our data, surgery was carried out in a group of 159 patients on the ninth day (median; range 1–64 days) after the onset of acute abdominal symptoms, and on the fifth day of intensive care treatment (range 0–56 days). Early operative intervention in the first week of the disease is only indicated in the small group of patients with fulminant necrotizing pancreatitis and in patients in septic shock, after confirmation of bacterial contamination of necrosis.

Necrosectomy and Closed Continuous Lesser Sac Lavage

For surgical treatment of necrotizing pancreatitis we advocate surgical debridement – necrosectomy – supplemented by intraoperative and postoperative closed continuous local lavage of the lesser sac and the adjacent necrotic cavities. This provides an atraumatic and continuous evacuation of devitalized necrotic tissue and removes bacterially contaminated tissue in biologically active compounds. Debridement, either digital or by the careful use of instruments, permits the elimination of all demarcated, devitalized tissue, while preserving the vital pancreatic parenchyma. In our opinion, there is no place for pancreatic resection in necrotizing pancreatitis, except for a small left resection in very selected cases. After surgical debridement, thorough hemostasis is necessary with transfixation stitches using monofilament suture material. It is not mandatory to remove every gram of devitalized tissue, because any tissue that becomes necrotic is rinsed out by the lavage fluid in the early postoperative period. After necrosectomy and suturing bleeding vessels, extensive intraoperative lavage is performed using up to 12 l of normal saline in order to clear the surface of the pancreatic and peripancreatic areas. For postoperative closed continuous local lavage (Fig. 3) at least two large double-lumen silicon rubber tubes are inserted (28/34 French), so that a regionally restricted lavage within the retroperitoneal area is effective. The channels for the drainage tube are positioned at the level of

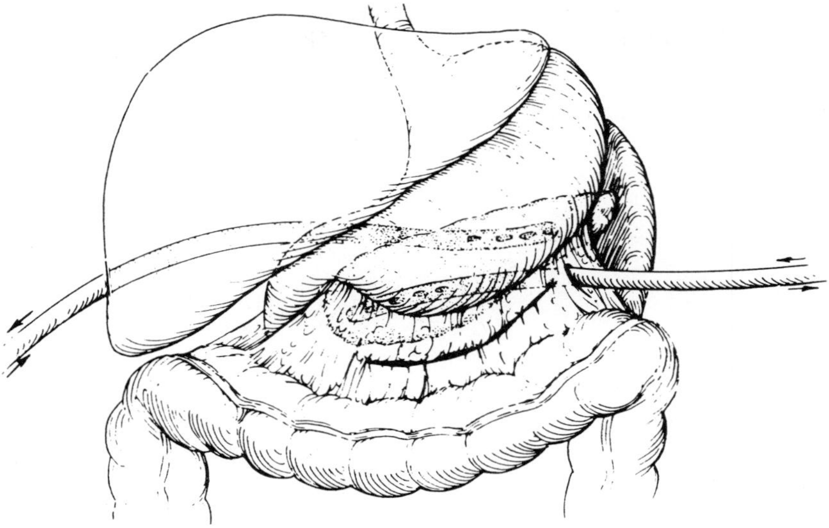

Fig. 3. Tube position for local lavage of the necrosis cavities after necrosectomy. Double-lumen lavage catheters with inflow and outflow. Suture of the gastroligament creates a closed lavage compartment

the retroperitoneal spaces in the left and right upper retroperitoneum. In cases of extended retroperitoneal necrosis cavities with fatty tissue necrosis, additional tubes are placed as required for complete elimination of devitalized tissue and exsudate. Having finished debridement, the gastrocolic and duodenocolic ligaments are sutured to create a closed retroperitoneal lesser sac compartment for postoperative continuous lavage. Meanwhile, in the first postoperative days the amount of lavage fluid ranges between 24 and 48 l. The postoperative flow of the lavage fluid through the lesser sac and the necrotic cavity cleans the inflamed area. Outflowing lavage fluid still containes enzymes, toxins, and other biologically active compounds as well as bacteria. Up to the end of the second week (mean), the lavage concept can be reduced or stopped if the signs that acute pancreatitis or clinical sepsis are vanishing and after the necrosis cavity has been completely cleansed. This is confirmed by assessing its sterility and the level of biologically active compounds such as pancreatic enzymes in the lavage fluid.

Since 1982 we have operated on 159 patients suffering from necrotizing pancreatitis (Table 7). Hospital mortality was 13.2% (21 patients). Major reasons for death were ongoing sepsis, followed by multiple organ failure (22/25; 88%) and massive local hemorrhage (3/25; 14%). The reoperation rate was 36%. This was mainly due to recurrent signs of sepsis and the need to redrain infected cavities following the primary operation. The median

Table 7. Necrotizing pancreatitis: results of necrosectomy plus continuous local lavage

Preoperatively	
Severity of necrotizing pancreatitis	4.6 Ranson points (median)
Infected necrosis	43%
Postoperatively	
Hospitalization	58 days (median among survivors)
Lavage duration	32 days (median)
Lavage fluid	8 l/24 h (median)
Reoperation	36%
Hospital mortality	13.2% (21/159)
Infected necrosis	16.4% (11/67)
Sterile necrosis	9.0% (8/89)

duration of the lavage treatment was 32 days, the median hospitalization time 58 days.

Comments

The gold standard of surgical management of necrotizing pancreatitis is the careful removal of necrotic tissue, drainage of the bacterially infected area, elimination of the pancreatogenic ascites in order to prevent systemic spread of the vasoactive and toxic substances, and interruption of the inflammatory process. For the treatment of pancreatic necrosis we strongly support surgical debridement/necrosectomy, supplemented by postoperative closed continuous lavage of the lesser sac and the adjacent necrotic cavities. In comparison with the open packing technique [32] or the multiple redressing procedures [33], our closed lavage system spares the patient several reoperations, a prolonged intensive care period, and enormous additional stress for the patient and for the several doctors generally treating these patients. However, taking into account the recent literature in the open packing technique as well as the multiple redressing approach, in experienced hands, results comparable to those achieved with the closed lavage techniques can be obtained, particularly with regard to postoperative mortality.

References

1. Warshaw AL (1980) A guide to pancreatitis. Compr Ther 6:49–55
2. Beger HG, Büchler M (1986) Decision-making in surgical treatment of acute pancreatitis: operative or conservative management of necrotizing pancreatitis? Theor Surg 1:61–68
3. Büchler M (1991) Severity staging of acute pancreatitis. Hepatogastroenterology 38:101–108

4. Beger HG, Uhl W (1990) Severe acute pancreatitis. II. The surgical approach. Clin Int Care 1:223–227
5. Beger HG, Bittner R, Büchler M, Hess M, Schmitz JE (1986) Hemodynamic data pattern in patients with acute pancreatitis. Gastroenterology 90:74–79
6. Beger HG, Krautzberger W, Bittner R, Büchler M, Block S (1986) Bacterial contamination of pancreatic necrosis. A prospective clinical study. Gastroenterology 91:433–438
7. Gerzof SG, Banks PA, Robbins AH, Johnson WC, Spechler SJ, Wetzner SM, Snider JM, Langevin RE, Jay ME (1987) Early diagnosis of pancreatic infection by computed tomography-guided aspiration. Gastroenterology 93:1315–1320
8. Bassi C, Falconi M, Girelli R, Nifosi F, Elio A, Martini N, Pederzoli P (1989) Microbiological findings in severe pancreatitis. Surg Res Commun 5:1–4
9. Ranson JHC, Rifkind KM, Roses DF, Fink SD, Eng K, Spencer FC (1974) Prognostic signs and the role of operative management in acute pancreatitis. Surg Gynecol Obstet 139:69–81
10. Bank S, Wise L, Gerstin M (1983) Risk factors in acute pancreatitis. Am J Gastroenterol 78:637–640
11. McMahon MJ, Bowen M, Mayer AD, Cooper EH (1984) Relation of a2-macroglobulin and other antiproteases to the clinical features of acute pancreatitis. Am J Surg 147:164–169
12. Warshaw A, Lee K (1979) Serum ribonuclease elevations and pancreatic necrosis in acute pancreatitis. Surgery 86:227–232
13. Block S, Maier W, Clausen C, Bittner R, Büchler, M, Malfertheiner P, Beger HG (1986) Identification of pancreas necrosis in severe acute pancreatitis. Gut 27:1035–1042
14. Kivisaari L, Somer K, Standertskjöld-Nordenstam CG, Schröder T, Kivilaakso E, Lempinen M (1984) A new method for the diagnosis of acute hemorrhagic necrotising pancreatitis using contrast-enhanced CT. Gastrointest Radiol 9: 27–30
15. Balhazar EJ (1989) CT diagnosis and staging of acute pancreatitis. Radiol Clin North Am 27:19–37
16. Bradley EL, Murphy F, Ferguson C (1989) Prediction of pancreatic necrosis by dynamic pancreatography. Ann Surg 210:495–504
17. Büchler M, Malfertheiner P, Schoetensack C, Uhl W, Beger HG (1986) Sensitivity of antiproteases, complement factors and C-reactive protein in detecting pancreatic necrosis. Results of a prospective clinical study. Int J Pancreatol 1:227–235
18. Puolakkainen P, Valtanen V, Paananen A, Schröder T (1987) C-reactive protein and serum phospholipase A2 in the assessment of severity of acute pancreatitis. Gut 28:764–771
19. Wilson C, Heads A, Shenkin A, Imrie CW (1989) C-reactive protein, antiproteases and complement factors as objective markers of severity in acute pancreatitis. Br J Surg 76:177–181
20. Uhl W, Büchler M, Malfertheiner P, Martini M, Beger HG (1991) PMN-elastase in comparison with CRP, antiproteases and LDH as indicators of necrosis in human acute pancreatitis. Pancreas 6:253–259
21. Gudgeon AM, Heath D, Hurley P, Shenkin A, Jehanli A, Patel G, Wilson C, Austen BM, Imrie CW (1988) Trypsinogen activation peptide (TAP) assay in severity assessment of acute pancreatitis. Pancreas 3:598
22. Gudgeon AM, Heath D, Jehanli A, Patel G, Hurley P, Austen B, Shenkin A, Imrie CW, Hermon-Taylor J (1989) Zymogen activation peptide (ZAP) assay in the severity prediction of acute pancreatitis. Digestion 43:145
23. Büchler M, Malfertheiner P, Schädlich H, Nevalainen TJ, Frieß H, Beger HG (1989) Role of phospholipase A2 in human acute pancreatitis. Gastroenterology 97:1521–1526
24. Leser H-G, Gross V, Scheibenbogen C, Heinisch A, Sal R, Lausen M, Rückauer K, Andreesen R, Farthmann EH, Schölmerich J (1991) Elevation of

serum interleukin-6 concentration precedes acute-phase response and reflects severity in acute pancreatitis. Gastroenterology 101:782–785
25. Büchler M, Malfertheiner P, Frieß H, Bittner R, Vanek E, Schlegel P, Beger HG (1989) The penetration of antibiotics into human pancreas. Infection 17: 20–25
26. Cox AG (1977) Death from acute pancreatitis. M.R.C. multicentre trial of glucagon and aprotini. Lancet 2(24):632–635
27. Imrie CW, Benjamin IS, Ferguson JC, Kay AJ, Mackenzie IM, O'Neill J, Blumgart LH (1978) A single-centre double-blind trial of Trasylol therapy in primary acute pancreatitis. Br J Surg 65:337–341
28. Goebell H, Ammann R, Herfarth C, Horn J, Hotz J, Knoblauch M, Schmid M, Jager J, Akovbiantz A, Linder E, Abt K, Nüesch E, Barth E (1979) A double blind trial of synthetic salmon calcitonin in the treatment of acute pancreatitis. Scand J Gastroenterol 14:881–889
29. Usadel KH, Überla KK, Leuscher U (1985) Treatment of acute pancreatitis with somatostatin: results of the multicenter double-blind trial (APTS-study) (Abstr). Dig Dis Sci 30:992
30. Büchler M, Malfertheiner P, Uhl W, Stöckmann F, Schölmerich J, Adler G, Rolle K, Ditschuneit H, Beger HG (1990) The German multicenter doubleblind randomized study of gabexate mesilate (4 g/day i.v.) in acute pancreatitis Gastroenterology 1993 (in press)
31. Gerzof SG, Banks PA, Robbins AH (1984) Role of guided percutaneous aspiration in early diagnosis of pancreatic sepsis. Dig Dis Sci 29:950
32. Bradley EL III (1984) Management of infected pancreatic necrosis by open drainage. Ann Surg 206:542–550
33. Warshaw AL, Jin G (1985) Improved survival in 45 patients with pancreatic abscess. Ann Surg 202:408–417

Programmed Reintervention in Necrotizing Pancreatitis

J. Horn[1]

Introduction

All observations on surgical procedure in the treatment of acute pancreatitis must take into consideration the requirement for continuous intensive care [6]. The question as to the "when" and, above all, "how" of the operation is still subject to controversy. The impression often arises that there are simple alternatives or methodological dogmatisms: early or late operation?; necroctomy, resection, lavage or "open packing"? [1, 4, 5, 7, 8, 17, 19, 21, 22].

Early operation seems to have been abandoned and the conviction appears to have become established that surgery should be carried out as late as possible. There is a similar situation with regard to the appraisal of the different methods of surgery. However, only a few comparative investigations have been published [3, 12], so that the selection of the method used tends to be based more on subjective conviction than on substantiated investigation results. There have been hardly any studies as to the relevance and value of the individual methods at different developmental stages of the disease. Little attention is paid to the complexity of the disease process and to the possible interaction of methodological approaches applied simultaneously. Scanty attention is also paid to the fact that a treatise concerning surgical methods is to be regarded merely as a subaspect of all therapy measures.

When comparing surgical methods, the conditions under which success or failure of the method used is to be assessed must be defined as exactly as possible.

The significance of infected necrosis was essentially established by the study group led by Beger et al. [2]. It is not the necrosis itself, but rather the associated infection which constitutes the basis for the intended surgical therapy. It is to be inferred from this that the principles of septic surgery must also be applied in the treatment of acute pancreatitis. It is crucial that appropriate principles of therapy are observed, whereas the technique may have to be adapted to the individual constellation (balanced procedure).

[1] Department of Surgery, Munich-Harlaching Municipal Hospital, Sanatoriumsplatz 2, W-8000 München 90, FRG

Beger/Büchler/Malfertheiner (Eds.)
Standards in Pancreatic Surgery

The principles of therapy in acute pancreatitis are defined in terms of the feasibility of surgical treatment. These are (a) reduction of the toxin potential, and (b) clearance of the source of infection. The principles to be observed will be defined concretely in the context of these therapy options.

Principles and Methods

Principle 1

As the first principle of therapy, the toxin potential can be reduced both by preoperative peritoneal lavage and by postoperative continuous lavage. Both methods have their own justification. As shown by several prospective investigations, the overall mortality cannot be reduced by preoperative lavage [11, 16], but this method can be regarded as exemplifying that a methodological approach must also be appraised in terms of the partial success. If it has been assumed up to now that death must be regarded as having been due to shock in about two thirds of the cases (early phase of the disease), and as due to sepsis in one third of the cases, this ratio may be reversed by peritoneal lavage [18, 20]. It is evidently possible to stabilize the circulation in a proportion of the patients using this method, whereas the septic complications increase at the same time. Notwithstanding, the latter are more readily accessible to surgical intervention than the disease characteristics of the initial phase of shock. However, preoperative peritoneal lavage is in our opinion only indicated when ascites has been detected.

Continuous lavage of the omental bursa is superior to lavage of the entire peritoneal cavity [4]. Whereas it may be regarded as a contribution to clearance of the source of infection (see below), the extent to which the toxin potential can be reduced by this method has not been investigated up to now. We perform our postoperative lavage of the pancreas space ventrodorsally (ventral inlet, dorsal outlet for the lavage fluid) in order to avoid the "pan effect" which is to be reckoned with in ventroventral application of lavage (Figs. 1 and 2).

Principle 2

By programmed reintervention with compartmentation and by postoperative continuous lavage of the pancreas space, the surgical clearance of the source of infection is to be attempted. It is very easily conceivable that a single surgical operation cannot ensure control of the infection in view of the complexity of the anatomical conditions and the often episodic nature of the necrotizing inflammation, which is underscored by the course of C-reactive protein (CRP) in some of our patients (Fig. 3).

Programmed reintervention is repeated at intervals of 2 or 3 days until necroses are no longer detectable and the wound spaces show clean, granulating conditions.

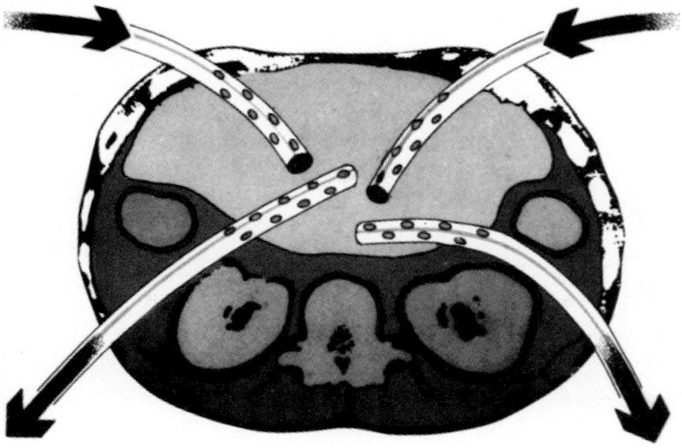

Fig. 1. Ventrodorsal positioning of drainage to carry out the continuous postoperative lavage

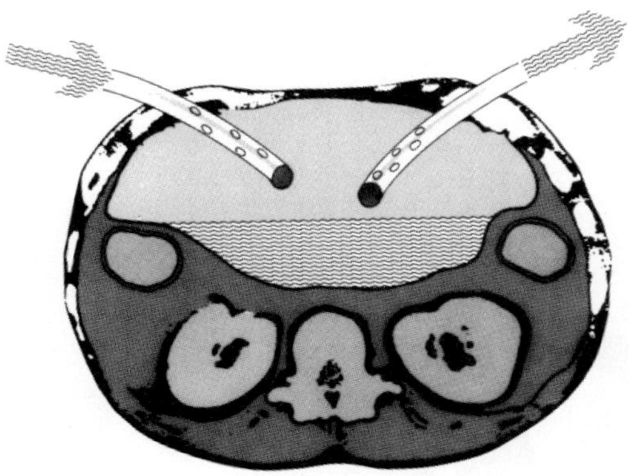

Fig. 2. Typical "pan effect" in exclusively ventral positioning of the drainages

Principle 3

One of the important principles of therapy in surgical intervention is the avoidance of peritonitis. Following inappropriate surgical procedure, it is observed far too often that the clinical picture of acute pancreatitis develops into that of suppurative fibrinous peritonitis. This must be avoided. In principle, the surgical approach is via a transverse upper abdominal incisions. The lower abdomen is flushed only in the first surgical intervention and an ileostomy is created (see below). All further operations do not impinge on the lower abdomen. We have not observed peritonitis in any of the cases treated in this way. Retroperitoneal necroses are cleared as a matter of

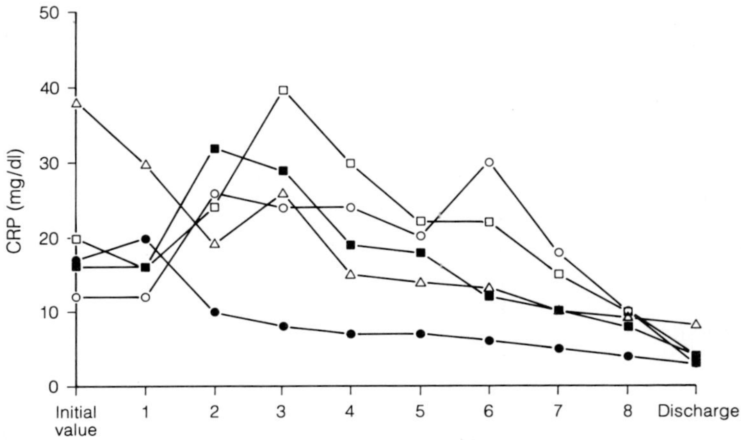

Fig. 3. Course of CRP in some patients operated on. *1–8*, first to eighth surgical interventions

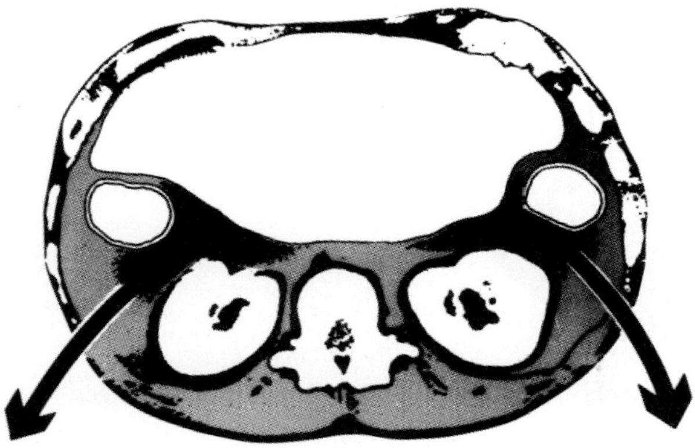

Fig. 4. Retroperitoneal necroses below the transverse colon are approached and cleared from separate flank incisions

principle via separate flank accesses, so that the integrity of the peritoneal cavity is maintained caudal to the transverse colon [10] (Fig. 4).

Principle 4

At present, it is still hypothetical to postulate that the influx of endotoxins can be reduced by orthograde lavage of the colon via the ileostomy created in the first operation [9]. There is some evidence that endotoxin plays an important role in the pathophysiology of acute pancreatitis [14]. Investiga-

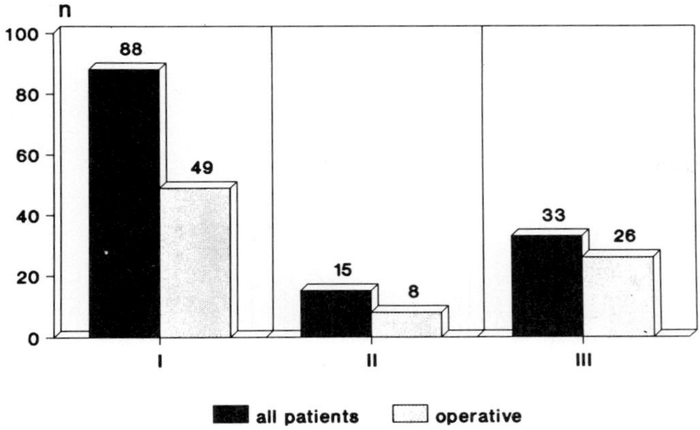

Fig. 5. Staging according to Schönborn and Kümmerle; percentage of the patients operated on in relation to the different degrees of severity

tions on individual patients show that a lowering of the endotoxin level in the portal vein is possible by orthograde lavage of the intestine. Prospective investigations are in progress to clarify these correlations. We have postulated that the course of the disease in acute pancreatitis is substantially influenced from the transverse colon. This hypothesis is yet to be documented. A substantial body of data in the literature indicates that such a correlation does indeed exist [13, 15].

Patients and Results

From July 1, 1987 to June 30, 1991, a total of 136 inpatients with acute pancreatitis were treated in our hospital (87 males, 49 females). In 58 patients a biliary genesis and in 57 patients an alcoholic genesis was assumed; six patients showed a marked hyperlipidemia, and the cause remained unclear in 15 patients.

Eighty-three patients were operated on. Whereas the operations in stage I of the disease were intended to clear the biliary tract, the surgical measures in stages II and III were designed to treat the actual pancreatitis (Fig. 5). Figure 6 shows the time of operation, and Fig. 7 the frequency of surgical interventions performed in the individual patients (stages II and III). Figure 8 shows the distribution of the Ranson criteria. Figure 9 presents the CRP values of the patients operated on in stages II and III initially and at the time of the individual surgical interventions.

Nineteen of the 34 patients operated on in stages II and III required artificial ventilation for more than 1 week (on average, 5.2 weeks). Thirteen patients underwent hemofiltration for more than 1 week (on average, 2.4 weeks). Eight patients were hemodialysed for an average of 2.8 weeks.

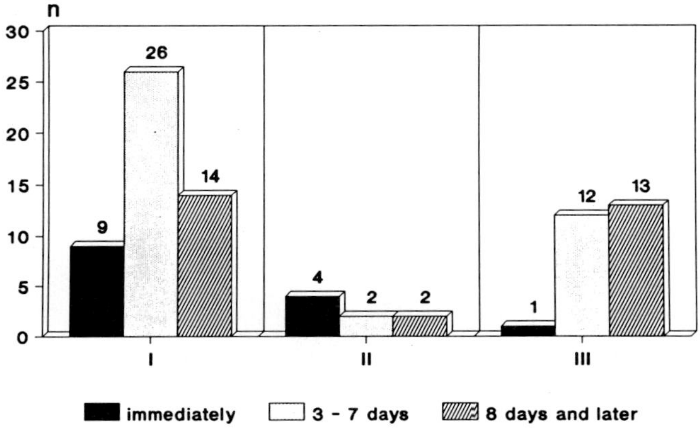

Fig. 6. Interval between inpatient admission and surgical intervention in the different stages

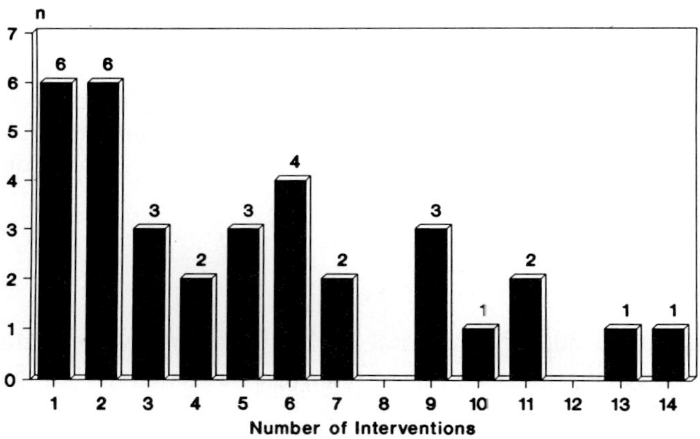

Fig. 7. Frequency of surgical revisions in the individual patients

Figure 10 shows the initial computed tomography (CT) of a 78-year-old patient (condition after three myocardial infarctions), who underwent a total of 13 surgical revisions. Figure 11 shows the final result after treatment totalling 14 weeks. Peritoneal lavage was performed preoperatively in seven patients after ascites had been detected sonographically.

Results

One patient died from an undiagnosed pneumothorax. As shown by the autopsy, the conditions were normal in the vicinity of the pancreas after a total of six surgical interventions.

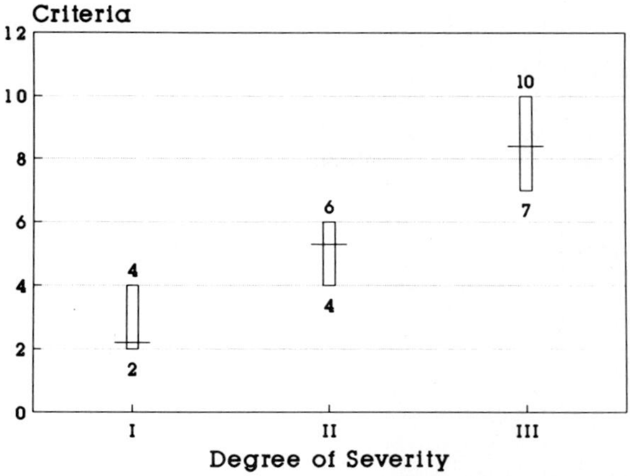

Fig. 8. Number of Ranson criteria in the different stages

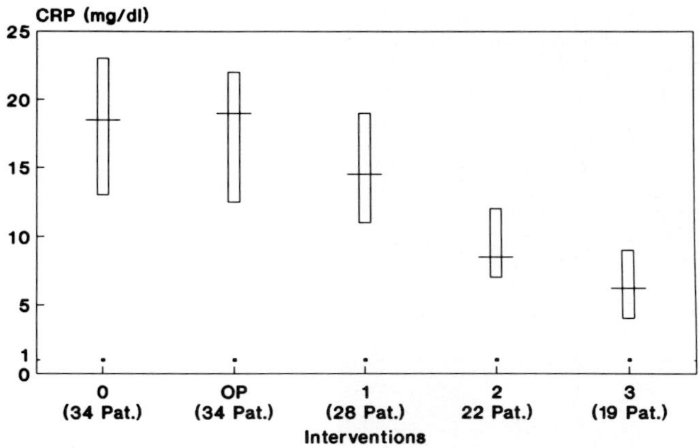

Fig. 9. CRP values of the operated patients in stages II and III initially and at the time of the sequential surgical interventions. *0*, Before operation; *OP*, at time of initial surgery; *1–3*, first to third subsequent intervention (all with number of patients)

The complications which have occurred are as follows: fistula of the duodenum ($n = 1$), fistula of the colon ($n = 3$), bile fistula after cholecystomy ($n = 1$), spontaneous splenic rupture ($n = 1$), and postoperative hernia ($n = 3$).

In relation to the overall patient population with acute pancreatitis, there was a total mortality of 0.74%. Within stages II and III, the mortality was 2.1%. In the patients operated on in stages II and III, the surgical mortality was 2.9%.

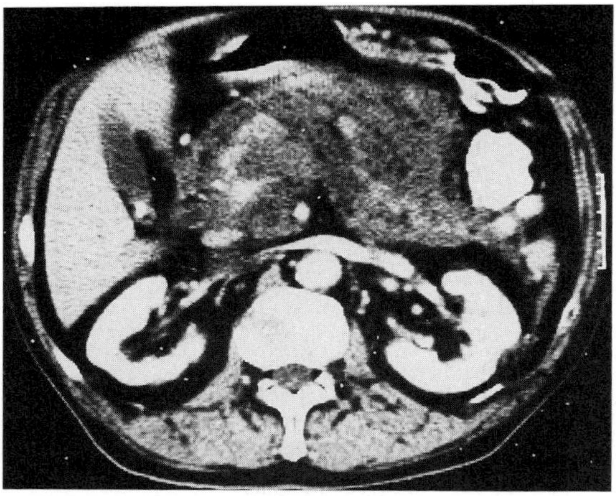

Fig. 10. The initial CT from a 78-year-old patient with severe necrotizing pancreatitis

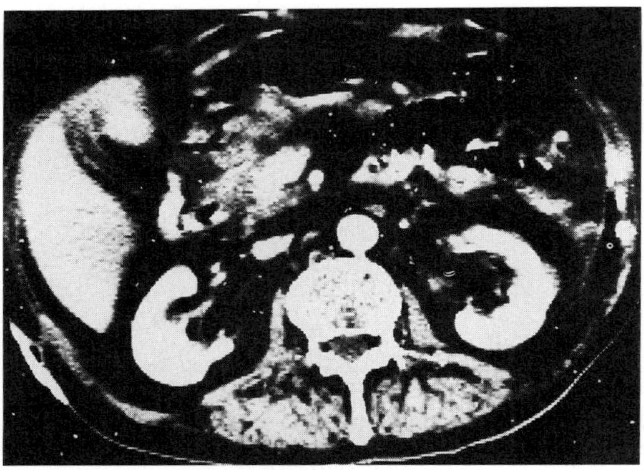

Fig. 11. CT from the same patient as in Fig. 10 after 13 surgical interventions

Summary

The results of 44 patients with severe necrotizing pancreatitis are presented (stages II and III). Thirty-four patients were operated on in accordance with the specified principles of treatment; ten patients were treated conservatively. In accordance with the possibilities of surgical therapy, four principles are defined (reduction of the toxin potential, surgical clearance of the source of infection, avoidance of peritonitis, elimination of the endotoxin), and the corresponding repertoire of methods is shown (preoperative peritoneal lavage in ascites, transverse upper abdominal laparatomy with compartmentation, programmed surgical reintervention, creation of an ileostomy, orthograde lavage of the colon). One patient died as a result of a pneumothorax after the sixth surgical intervention. The mortality of the patients in stages II and III was 2.1%, and for the patients operated on in stages II and III, 2.9%.

References

1. Aldridge MC, Ornstein M, Glazer G (1985) Pancreatic resection for severe acute pancreatitis. Br J Surg 72:796
2. Beger HG, Bittner R, Block S, Büchler M (1986) Bacterial contamination of pancreatic necrosis. Gastroenterologie 91:433
3. Beger HG, Büchler M, Bittner R, Oettinger W, Block S, Nevalainen TJ (1987) Necrosectomy and postoperative local lavage in patients with necrotizing pancreatitis. Results of a prospective clinical trial. In: Beger HG, Büchler M (eds) Acute pancreatitis. Springer, Berlin Heidelberg New York, p 335
4. Beger HG, Büchler M, Bittner R, Oettinger W, Block S, Nevalainen TJ (1988) Necrosectomy and postoperative local lavage in patients with necrotizing pancreatitis. Results of a prospective clinical trial. World J Surg 12:255
5. Bradley EL III (1987) Management of infected pancreatic necrosis by open drainage. Ann Surg 206:542
6. Creutzfeldt W, Lankisch PG (1981) Intensive medical treatment of severe acute pancreatitis. World J Surg 5:341
7. Gebhardt C, Gall FP (1981) Importance of peritoneal irrigation after surgical treatment of hemorrhagic necrotizing pancreatitis. World J Surg 5:379
8. Hölscher M, Bartels H, Siewert IR (1988) Kompartementierung des Abdomens als Behandlungsprinzip bei der akuten Pankreatitis. Chir Gastroenterol 4:113
9. Horn J (1983) Das Ileostoma als Teil der chirurgischen Therapie-konzeption bei der akuten Pankreatitis. Chirurg 54:320
10. Horn J (1989) Akute Pankreatitis: Indikationen und Erfolge der operativen Therapie. Z Gastroenterol 24:99
11. Ihse I, Evander A, Gustafson I et al. (1986) Influence of peritoneal lavage on objective prognostic signs in acute pancreatitis. Ann Surg 204:122
12. Kivilaakso E, Lempinen M, Mäkeläinen A (1984) Pancreatic resection versus peritoneal lavation for acute fulminant pancreatitis. Ann Surg 199:426
13. Kivilaakso E, Valtonen VV, Malkamäki M et al. (1984) Endotoxinaemia and acute pancreatitis: correlation between the severety of the disease and the antienterobacterial common antigen antibody titer. Gut 25:1065
14. Lange JF, van Gool J, Tytgat GNJ (1987) The protective effect of a reduction in intestinal flora on mortality of acute haemorrhagic pancreatitis in the rat. Hepatogastroenterology 34:28
15. Liehr H, Grün M, Seelig R, Seelig H-P (1980) Endotoxinämie bei akuter Pankreatitis. Leber Magen Darm 10:259
16. Mayer AD, McMahon MJ, Corfield AP, Cooper MJ, Williamson RCN, Dickson AP, Shearer MG, Imrie CW (1985) Controlled clinical trial of peritoneal lavage for the treatment of severe acute pancreatitis. N Engl J Med 312:399
17. Nordback IH, Auvinen OA (1985) Long-term results after pancreas resection for acute necrotizing pancreatitis.
18. Ranson JHC (1981) Conservative surgical treatment of acute pancreatitis. World J Surg 5:351

19. Ranson JHC (1990) The role of surgery in the management of acute pancreatitis. Ann Surg 211:382
20. Ranson JHC, Rifkind KM, Turner JW (1976) Prognostic signs and nonoperative peritoneal lavage in acute pancreatitis. Surg Gynecal Obstet 143:209
21. Stanten R, Frey CF (1990) Comprehensive management of acute necrotizing pancreatitis and pancreatic abscess. Arch Surg 125:1269
22. Teerenhovi O, Nordback I, Isolauri J (1988) Influence of pancreatic resection in systemic complications in acute necrotizing pancreatitis. Br J Surg 75:793

Management of Necrotizing Pancreatitis by Planned, Repeated Necrosectomy/Débridement with Delayed Primary Closure

M.G. SARR[1]

Introduction

The introduction of formal widespread pancreatic and peripancreatic necrosectomy, as opposed to simple peripancreatic drainage, has markedly decreased the mortality of necrotizing pancreatitis. Nevertheless, operative mortality remains about 20%. Several different techniques have been described to manage the peripancreatic space after necrosectomy to allow continued drainage and débridement. These techniques include widespread closed/open tube drainage [17], open controlled packing or so-called "marsupialization" [2–4, 11, 15], closed continuous lavage [1, 8, 16] and repeated, planned reoperative débridement [14]. This chapter discusses our technique of repeated, planned reoperative débridement following the initial operative necrosectomy. We believe that this approach maximizes débridement of pancreatic and peripancreatic necrotic tissue and thereby minimizes the incidence of recurrent intra-abdominal sepsis.

Methods

From 1986 to 1991, 31 patients with documented necrotizing pancreatitis requiring operative intervention were managed at our institution. Patients were classified carefully into those with noninfected necrosis, infected necrosis, and pancreatic abscess [14]. Patients with infected pseudocysts were excluded. Whenever possible, based on dynamic contrast-enhanced computed tomography (CT) [4] or on histopathologic review, patients were further classified into pancreatic parenchymal necrosis or primarily peripancreatic necrosis as described previously [5]. Patients were staged at the time of presentation to our institution by Ranson criteria [12], Imrie criteria [10] and APACHE II scoring [7]. Because our practice is to a great extent a tertiary referral practice, we were not able to reliably stage all patients at time of onset of pancreatitis. Morbidity and mortality until discharge were quantitated. Follow-up to date was obtained in all patients.

[1] Department of Surgery, Mayo Clinic and Mayo Foundation, 200 First Street S.W., Rochester, MN 55905, USA

Beger/Büchler/Malfertheiner (Eds.)
Standards in Pancreatic Surgery

Results

Clinical Characteristics

The 32 patients included 23 men and 9 women with a mean age of 64 years (range, 42–84 years). The etiology of the necrotizing pancreatitis was alcohol-related in one patient (3%), gallstone-induced in nine (28%), postoperative pancreatitis in four (13%), related to ERCP in four (13%), and was of indeterminate etiology in the remaining 14 (43%). Seven patients had non-infected necrosis, while infected necrosis was present in four and pancreatic abscess in 21. Significant pancreatic parenchymal necrosis occurred in 24. All but two patients were able to be staged at the time of admission to our institution but not necessarily at the time of onset of necrotizing pancreatitis. With the Ranson classification, 15 patients had 3 or less criteria, eight had 4–6 criteria, and seven had more than 6 criteria. With the Imrie staging, 13 patients had 3 or less criteria, 16 had 4–6 criteria, and no one had more than 6 criteria. Using the APACHE II scoring, 16 patients had fewer than 10 points, 11 had 11–15 points, and two had over 15 points.

Diagnosis

Necrotizing pancreatitis was diagnosed preoperatively based on a combination of clinical presentation, selected laboratory parameters, and CT scan, and confirmed at operative exploration. CT scans were obtained in all patients. All patients had variable amounts of peripancreatic fluid, and all but one had a markedly enlarged pancreas. Extraluminal gas, diagnostic of pancreatic infection, occurred in 12 of 25 patients with infected necrosis or pancreatic abscess. Intravenous contrast-enhanced scans were performed in 17 patients within 72 h of the initial necrosectomy and were diagnostic of pancreatic parenchymal necrosis [5]. CT-guided needle aspirations were performed preoperatively in 18 patients and were often repeated on a weekly basis when the clinical condition so dictated. Cultures were negative in the three patients with noninfected necrosis and were positive in two of the three patients with infected necrosis and in ten of 11 patients with pancreatic abscess. All cultures from preoperative needle aspirations corresponded with intraoperative cultures at the time of necrosectomy.

Operative Management

Operative intervention was undertaken, either because of extraluminal gas on CT (12 patients), a positive culture on percutaneous needle aspiration (12 patients), or because of a deteriorating clinical course in the absence of other treatable or likely factors (nine patients).

Celiotomy was usually performed using a bilateral subcostal incision. The necrotizing process involved significant portions of the pancreatic parenchyma in 24 of 32 patients. Two patients in whom the necrosis involved the entire gland underwent more than 95% pancreatectomy without removing the duodenum; the necrotic pancreas was removed bluntly with digital dissection. The remaining patients with parenchymal necrosis underwent localized necrosectomy of portions of the head, body and tail of the gland (nine patients) or just the body and tail (13 patients). Two patients underwent an anatomic distal pancreatectomy because the surgeon believed the body/tail region to be necrotic only to find the gland to be viable on histopathologic review. The remaining six patients underwent peripancreatic necrosectomy. Every attempt was made to excise and remove all necrotic pancreatic parenchyma and peripancreatic tissues. In addition to the immediate peripancreatic area, the necrosectomy was carried down the right and left retroperitoneal paracolic gutters, out into the base of the small bowel and transverse colon mesentery, and rostrally behind the spleen, lesser omentum, and liver whenever the necrotizing process involved these regions. The necrosectomy was performed bluntly without much sharp dissection. Care was taken to preserve any viable pancreatic parenchyma in order to avoid uncontrollable bleeding, especially from splenic, pancreatic and mesenteric vessels of the colon involved in the acute inflammatory process. One patient required transverse colectomy and proximal diversion because of colonic infarction noted at the time of the initial necrosectomy, and another was managed by diverticularization of the duodenum (pyloric stapling, tube choledochostomy, and gastrojejunostomy) because the necrosis involved a 2-cm diameter defect in the second portion of the duodenum.

After completing the necrosectomy, the peripancreatic area and all other areas involved with the necrotic process were débrided using the high pressure, Water-Pik débrider-irrigator system (Surgilav, Model 201, Stryker, Kalamazoo, Michigan, USA). Generally, 4–61 of saline irrigation were used. At this point, the surgeon decided, based on the clinical situation, whether the necrotizing process was arrested and whether all necrotic tissue had been removed. If not, the peripancreatic area was packed loosely with gauze after covering any exposed major vascular strictures (splenic artery and vein, superior mesenteric or portal vein) with a sheet of silastic. The wound was then reapproximated with the use of a zipper [9]. Patients were returned to the operating room on an every-other-day basis for repeated surgical necrosectomy and Water-Pik débridement until all devitalized tissue had been removed and the necrotizing process had ceased. Using this management approach, five patients underwent only the initial necrosectomy, five required one reoperation, 13 underwent two to four reoperations, and nine underwent five or more reoperations (range, 5–12 reoperations).

When the final necrosectomy/débridement was finished and the surgeon decided that the necrosectomy was complete, every attempt was made to close the abdominal wall fascia in a delayed primary closure fashion after leaving multiple soft, closed-suction drains or multiple Penrose drains brought out through separate lateral or inferior stab wounds. This approach was possible in 21 of 32 patients. If necessary, an artificial prosthetic mesh, either the permanent polypropylene mesh (Prolene) or the absorbable polyglycolic acid mesh (Vicryl) was employed in four patients to span the gap between the fascial edges. As the edema or abdominal distention resided, this mesh could then be removed allowing a fascia-fascia closure. In the remaining ten patients, the pancreatic bed was marsupialized completely open with gauze packing (six patients) or the lateral aspect of the wound was closed, leaving the central aspect open (four patients). This option was chosen either because of severe complication, ongoing sepsis or because severe tissue edema prevented reasonable approximation. In three patients, we elected to leave a closed irrigating system, similar to the technique of Beger and colleagues [1], because the necrotic process was limited to the lesser sac and could be contained, allowing a controlled, continuous lavage for drainage and débridement.

Mortality/Morbidity

The overall hospital mortality was 22% (seven patients). Multiple organ failure, presumably secondary to overwhelming sepsis, accounted for the majority of deaths, none of whom had evidence of recurrent intra-abdominal abscess at the time of death. One patient died the day before discharge secondary to pulmonary embolus. There were two deaths in the seven patients with noninfected necrosis, one death in four patients with infected necrosis, and four deaths in 21 patients with pancreatic abscess. Significant hospital morbidity occurred in 59% of patients manifesting as pancreatic or enteric fistulas, hemorrhage, and recurrent intra-abdominal abscess. Pancreaticocutaneous fistulas developed either from the wound (when treated with an open technique) or via the peripancreatic drains in six patients (19%), all of whom had pancreatic parenchymal necrosis. These fistulas were generally well controlled and easily managed. Three of these fistulas closed spontaneously, but three eventually required readmission and operative control by drainage into a Roux-en-Y limb. Severe hemorrhage requiring intervention occurred in eight patients (25%); seven patients underwent emergent reoperation with operative control of bleeding from splenic or pancreatic vessels in three patients, portal/superior mesenteric vein in one, and the middle colic vessels in three. One patient with hemorrhage from a pseudoaneurysm of the splenic artery was treated by angiographic embolization. Colonic fistulas developed in seven patients (25%); three patients required proximal colonic diversion, but the other four colonic fistulas caused minor if any problems and closed spontaneously. Duodenal fistulas occurred in two patients, one of whom later required operative closure. Transient gastric and small bowel fistulas occurred in three and two patients, respectively. Recurrent intra-abdominal sepsis/abscess occurred in only two patients (6%) during hospitalization. One patient was managed by percutaneous drainage of an abscess that occurred in the right paracolic gutter where a previous drain had been inadvertently removed prematurely.

This group of patients, however, were extremely ill overall. The median stay in the intensive care unit was 14 days (range, 1–90 days), while the median hospital stay was 57 days (range, 13–240 days). Nine patients (18%) required temporary tracheostomy for respiratory failure, and six patients (12%) developed acute renal failure, requiring dialysis in two.

Discussion

Recognition of the importance of necrosectomy in the management of patients with necrotizing pancreatitis requiring operative treatment revolutionalized the treatment of this severely ill group of patients. This simple change in intraoperative management decreased the mortality from over 80% to about 20%. Nevertheless, the mortality remains significant and appears to be in large part related to overwhelming sepsis.

Despite initial necrosectomy and drainage of the peripancreatic bed, recurrent intra-abdominal sepsis continues to be a major problem. The cause of recurrent sepsis is probably multifactorial, related to ongoing extension of the necrotizing process with the necrosis of pancreatic and peripancreatic tissues, development of pancreatic and enteric fistulas, but probably most commonly due to either inadequate peripancreatic drainage and incomplete necrosectomy. Just as peripancreatic drains alone were unable to evacuate the necrotic tissue of necrotizing pancreatitis, infected necrosis that is not recognized at the time of the initial necrosectomy will serve as a site of ongoing sepsis. In an attempt to provide ongoing evacuation of infected peripancreatic exudative fluids as well as to promote ongoing débridement, several techniques have been introduced to deal with the peripancreatic space after necrosectomy. Widespread peripancreatic drainage with primary wound closure has been advocated by Warshaw and colleagues [16]. Although mortality was almost unbelievably low (approximately 5%), recurrent intra-abdominal sepsis requiring reoperation was common, probably related to ongoing or overlooked necrosis that the drains were unable to evacuate. Stone, Bradley and others [3, 4, 15] have utilized controlled open packing of the peripancreatic space to maximize drainage and promote ongoing débridement by repeated open packing changes. Our previous experience with this open technique had many complications [11], which has diminished our enthusiasm. Beger and others [1, 8, 16] have utilized a system of closed, lesser sac lavage to promote drainage and débridement. While we have used this technique in selected patients, it requires a relatively localized necrotizing process limited to the lesser sac without extension down the paracolic gutters or into the small bowel mesentery.

Several years ago, our technique of managing the peripancreatic space after necrosectomy evolved to an approach consisting of planned, repeated reoperative débridements [14]. Our experience has convinced as that repeated, thorough operative exposure and reinspection of the peripancreatic area is very important. Not uncommonly, we have found significant areas of unequivocal necrosis that we judged to be viable at the time of initial necrosectomy. Some of these tissues were areas that were not operatively exposed initially or that evolved to necrosis because the necrotizing process continued due to local sepsis or ongoing leakage of pancreatic juices. It is our impression that most episodes of recurrent intra-abdominal abscess/sepsis arise in areas of peripancreatic necrosis that were overlooked inadvertently at the time of initial necrosectomy either because of failure to expose or explore the area at the time of necrosectomy or because the surgeon believed that the tissue was viable. Our approach of repeated reoperative debridement accounts for our very low incidence (6%) of recurrent intra-abdominal abscess.

The use of a zipper for reapproximation of the fascial edges between reoperations also serves several important purposes. First, it markedly speeds operative exposure and wound closure. Second, it prevents desiccation of exposed intraperitoneal tissues and repeated contact-induced tissue trauma that occurred with our previous technique of open wound management by marsupialization [11]. Third, our approach minimizes fluid losses between reexplorations and by keeping the fascial edges approximated, maintains the intra-abdominal contents within the abdominal domain, thereby facilitating an eventual delayed primary fascial closure. We continue to use this approach of repeated, planned reoperative débridement until we are convinced that the necrotizing process has been stopped and all nonviable tissue has been excised and débrided. At this point, widespread peripancreatic drainage with soft, closed-suction drains is utilized at the time of fascial closure to allow evacuation both of ongoing exudation of tissue juices and areas of pancreatic ductal disruption with leakage of pancreatic juice. This converts an undrained pancreatic ductal disruption into a controlled, external fistula. We have avoided the use of large sump-type drains for fear of erosion of these stiff drains into bowel or blood vessels. Moreover, use of a needle catheter jejunostomy [13] allows the provision of enteral nutrition, and avoids the expense and potential risks of long-term parenteral feedings.

In spite of this comprehensive and obsessive approach, mortality and major morbidity remain high (22% and 59%, respectively). Although recurrent intra-abdominal abscess has been minimized, fistula, hemorrhage and overwhelming sepsis with subsequent multiple organ failure continue to challenge all pancreatic surgeons dealing with necrotizing pancreatitis. We believe that our technique of repeated, planned reoperative necrosectomy/débridement with eventual delayed primary fascial closure over peripancreatic drains [14] minimizes recurrent intra-abdominal sepsis. Further improvements in mortality and morbidity will require earlier diagnosis and therapies designed to halt the necrotizing process and its attendant complications.

Acknowledgements. The author gratefully acknowledges the help of B.J. Poulter and D.I. Frank in the preparation of this manuscript.

References

1. Beger HG, Buchler M, Bittner R, Block S, Nevalainen T, Roscher R (1988) Necrosectomy and postoperative local lavage in necrotizing pancreatitis. Br J Surg 75:207–212
2. Bolooki H, Jaffe B, Gleidman ML (1968) Pancreatic abscesses and lesser omental sac collections. Surg Gynecol Obstet 126:1301–1308
3. Bradley EL (1987) Management of infected pancreatic necrosis by open drainage. Ann Surg 206:542–550
4. Davidson ED, Bradley EL III (1981) "Marsupialization" in the treatment of pancreatic abscess. Surgery 89:252–256
5. Johnson CD, Stephens DH, Sarr MG (1991) Necrotic pancreatitis: re-emphasis of the importance of contrast-enhanced CT. Am J Radiol 156:93–95
6. Kivisaari L, Somer K, Standertskjold-Nordenstam C-G, Schroder T, Kivilaakso E, Lempinen M (1983) Early detection of acute, fulminant pancreatitis by contrast-enhanced computed tomography. Scand J Gastroenterol 18:39–41
7. Knaus WA, Draper EA, Wagner DP, Zimmerman JE (1985) APACHE II: a severity of disease classification system. Crit Care Med 13:818–829
8. Larvin M, Chalmers AG, Robinson PJ, McMahon MJ (1989) Debridement and closed cavity irrigation for the treatment of pancreatic necrosis. Br J Surg 76:465–471
9. Leguit P Jr (1982) Zip-closure of the abdomen. Neth J Surg 34:40–41
10. Osborne DH, Imrie CW, Carter DC (1981) Biliary surgery in the same admission for gallstone-associated acute pancreatitis. Br J Surg 68:758–761
11. Pemberton JH, Becker JM, Dozois RR, Nagorney DM, Ilstrup D, ReMine WH (1986) Controlled open lesser sac drainage for pancreatic abscess. Ann Surg 203:600–604
12. Ranson JHC, Ritkind KM, Rases DF, Fink SD, Eng K, Spencer FC (1974) Prognostic signs and the role of operative management in acute pancreatitis. Surg Gynecol Obstet 139:69–81
13. Sarr MG, Mayo S (1988) Needle catheter jejunostomy: an unappreciated and misunderstood advance in the care of patients after major abdominal operations. Mayo Clin Proc 63:565–572
14. Sarr MG, Nagorney DM, Mucha P Jr, Farnell MB, Johnson CD (1991) Acute necrotizing pancreatitis: management by planned, staged pancreatic necrosectomy/debridement and delayed primary wound closure over drains. Br J Surg 78:576–581
15. Stone HH, Strom PR, Mullins RJ (1984) Pancreatic abscess management by subtotal resection and packing. World J Surg 8:340–345
16. Teerenhovi O, Nordback I, Eskola J (1989) High volume lesser sac lavage in acute necrotizing pancreatitis. Br J Surg 76:370–373
17. Warshaw AL, Gongliang J (1985) Improved survival in 45 patients with pancreatic abscess. Ann Surg 202:408–415

Open Packing for Infected Pancreatic Necrosis

E.L. Bradley[1] III

Introduction

Due to truly remarkable improvements in critical care medicine, *early* deaths from severe acute pancreatitis have become decidedly rare. Today, the majority of deaths from acute pancreatitis occur *late* in the course of the disease and are overwhelmingly dur to secondary bacterial infection of damaged pancreatic tissues [1, 2]. Not all bacterial pancreatic infections carry the same risk for affected patients, however. Of the three recognized forms of secondary bacterial infections (infected pseudocyst, pancreatic abscess, and infected pancreatic necrosis), infected necrosis is the most common, the most severe, and the most lethal [3–6]. Accordingly, accurate and consistent definitions of secondary pancreatic infections are necessary for appropriate therapy, and to provide coherent patient populations for comparison of management options [7].

Furthermore, it is becoming increasingly clear that necrotizing pancreatitis precedes the development of secondary bacterial infections of the pancreatic and peripancreatic tissues [3, 8]. Since necrotizing pancreatitis occurs in as many as 20% of patients with acute pancreatitis [3, 5, 9], and since secondary bacterial infection develops in 40%–70% of these cases [3, 9], surgeons are being be called upon with increasing frequency to manage these patients.

The current report chronicles our experience with open packing in the management of patients with infected pancreatic necrosis. The original technique of open packing, which we first applied in 1976, has undergone numerous modifications as technical advances became available and newer disease concepts replaced outmoded principles.

Patients and Methods

At the present time, 64 consecutive patients with infected pancreatic necrosis have been managed by open packing under the direct supervision of the author. Only patients with infected pancreatic necrosis documented by

[1] Emory University School of Medicine, Piedmont Hospital, Dept. of Surgery, 1958 Peachtree Road N.W., Atlanta, GA 30309, USA

Beger/Büchler/Malfertheiner (Eds.)
Standards in Pancreatic Surgery

Table 1. Patient population

Consecutive patients with operatively proved IPN	64
Sex	46 male : 18 female
Average age	44.8 years (32–84)
Average no. of Ranson signs	5.1 (2–11)
Etiology of pancreatitis	
Alcohol	31
Biliary	17
Idiopathic	5
Hyperlipidemia	4
Drug induced	3
ERCP	3
Hyperparathyroidism	1

Table 2. Bacteriology of infected pancreatic necrosis[a]

Escherichia coli	30
Aerobacter aerogenes	11
Klebsiella pneumoniae	8
Pseudomonas aeruginosa	6
Candida albicans	4
Enterococcus faecalis	2
Staphylococcus aureus	1

[a] 27 polymicrobial.

surgical exploration and bacterial culture are included in this report. Patients with pancreatic abscess or infected pseudocyst seen during this same period of time were treated by other techniques. Distinguishing between the three forms of secondary pancreatic infection (infected necrosis, pancreatic abscess, and infected pseudocyst) has occasionally been difficult, but a uniform definition of infected necrosis has facilitated this differentiation [7]. Necrotizing pancreatitis was recognized at surgery by the typical grayish-black appearance of the pancreatic and peripancreatic tissues. In most cases, a grayish fluid accompanied the necrosis ("dishwater pus"). Several of the patients also exhibited small amounts of classically purulent material.

There were 46 men and 18 women, with an average age of 44.8 years (range 32–84). The etiology of the underlying pancreatitis is shown in Table 1. The pancreatitis in these patients was particularly severe, with an average number of Ranson signs of 5.1 (range 2–11).

Bacteria were cultured from the necrotic tissue removed from each of these 64 patients (Table 2). Polymicrobial infections were demonstrated by just under half of these cases. Recently, the employment of dynamic pancreatography to detect the presence of pancreatic necrosis, combined with fine-needle percutaneous aspiration of involved areas of pancreas for bacterial smear and culture, has permitted reliable preoperative diagnosis of both the presence and extent of infected pancreatic necrosis.

The standard technique of open packing has been described in previous publications [10], and was carried out in the initial 46 cases. In brief, the abdomen was entered through a left subcostal incision, which was enlarged to bilateral subcostal when necessary. The pancreas was exposed by careful division of the gastrocolic omentum. When widespread pancreatic and peripancreatic necrosis was encountered, extensive unroofing of the superior retroperitoneum was performed. This was accomplished by taking down the splenic flexure of the colon (and the hepatic flexure if the necrosis extended to the head of the pancreas), performing a Kocher maneuver, and entering the retropancreatic space. Only necrotic tissues which could be loosened by blunt dissection were removed. Massive venous hemorrhage was uncommon when blunt dissection was used, but, when encountered, it was controlled by standard methods or by the subsequent packing technique.

No concerted attempt was made to débride all of the necrotic tissues at the first procedure, particularly those which were firmly adherent to important structures. The process of re-exploration and redébridement eventually removed all of the necrotic tissues present.

When satisfactory débridement was completed, nonadherent gauze (Adaptic, Johnson & Johnson) was placed over the surfaces of the stomach, colon, and any exposed blood vessels to prevent inadvertent débridement of these important structures by frequent dressing changes. The author considers this an important step in preventing intestinal fistulas. Laparotomy pads soaked in sodium oxychlorosene (Chlorpactin WCS 90, Guardian Chemical) were placed within the ring of Adaptic. A few sutures of no. 2 nylon were placed through all layers of the abdominal wall and loosely approximated in order to prevent evisceration and extrusion of the packs.

Re-explorations in the operating suite were planned for every 2–3 days for additional débridement. Once granulation tissue appeared in the retroperitoneum and sufficient intestinal adhesion to the abdominal wall had taken place, dressings were changed in the Intensive Care Units or on the ward. The wound was permitted to heal entirely by secondary intention.

In the most recent 18 patients the technique of open packing has been modified. Currently, when serial re-explorations have resulted in satisfactory débridement, and granulation tissue begins to appear in the retroperitoneum, two large-bore lavage catheters are placed in the débrided cavity. A constant drip of Clorpactin (0.4% at 200 cc/h) is begun through one of the catheters. Lavage is continued until all signs of infection are absent and serial fistulograms via the catheters demonstrate that the cavities have closed down around the lavage tubes (Fig. 1). The catheters are then withdrawn.

Total intravenous hyperalimentation with lipid supplements provided caloric support in the majority of these patients. More recently, feeding jejunostomies were placed for enteral alimentation. All patients were given courses of broad-spectrum antibiotics and were treated with oral Nystatin.

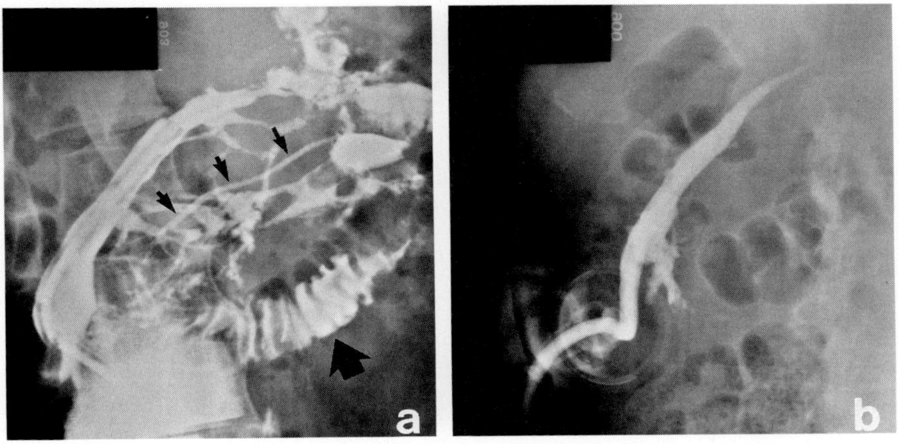

Fig. 1a,b. Fistulograms in a patient following open drainage with secondary closure and retroperitoneal lavage. Note complex of fistulas (**a**) including pancreatic duct (*small arrows*) and duodenum (*large arrow*). Following 3 weeks of continued lavage, all fistulas have closed (**b**)

Results

Of the 64 patients undergoing open packing for infected pancreatic necrosis, 55 survived during hospitalization (mortality =14%). Only two of the eight patients older than 70 years of age died. Of considerable interest is the observation that sepsis was implicated in only three of the nine deaths. The remaining causes of death are shown in Table 3.

Profound morbidity accompanied the course of these patients, however. Pancreatic fistula was seen in 31 of 64 cases (48%), no doubt attesting to the severity of the underlying necrotizing process taking place in the pancreas. Fortunately, in the vast majority of cases these fistulas closed spontaneously. Three patients required transcutaneous drainage of pancreatic juice collections prior to final closure of the pancreatic fistulas, and one required cystogastrostomy.

Twenty-three patients developed an incisional hernia through the chevron incision. In 15 of these cases the herniation was small, and the patients declined secondary repair. Six patients have undergone successful incisional herniorrhaphy.

Gastric outlet obstruction, reflecting the severity of the underlying pancreatitis, was seen in 12 patients. This obstruction persisted for varying lengths of time, resolving in all but two fatal cases. In one of these cases, massive aspiration occurred secondary to gastric retention. In the other, prolonged intravenous feeding resulted in a fatal air embolus when the patient disconnected the central feeding line. Since persistent gastric outlet

Table 3. Results of open drainage for infected pancreatic necrosis

	No. of patients
Mortality[a]	
Sepsis	3
Liver failure	2
Myocardial infarction	1
Massive aspiration	1
Air embolism	1
Adrenal hemorrhage	1
Morbidity	
Pancreatic fistula	31
Incisional hernia	23
Gastric outlet obstrucion	12
Major venous hemorrhage	5
Intestinal fistula	5

[a] Overall mortality was 14% (9/64 patients).

obstruction may be seen in patients with necrotizing pancreatitis treated without surgical intervention, this complication was not thought to be specific to open drainage.

Major venous hemorrhage was encountered in five cases; in three of these it was due to lacerations of the splenic vein and responded to splenectomy. In one case, a venous laceration occurred at the junction of the superior mesenteric and splenic veins and was corrected by a lateral venorrhaphy only with great difficulty. In another patient, diffuse venous oozing of the entire superior retroperitoneum responded well to packing.

Five cases of intestinal fistulas were encountered during the period of open packing. Two gastric fistulas were present on admission to our hospital, and represented ill-advised attempts at drainage of the infected necrosis into the stomach under the misdiagnosis of "infected pseudocyst". One patient developed a lateral duodenal fistula following an attempt at percutaneous drainage of the infected necrosis at another institution when the drainage catheter was inadvertently placed in the duodenum. One jejunal fistula arose from employment of a zipper closure early in our experience, and this was not seen again when the use of zippers was discontinued. A colonic fistula developed in the splenic flexure of the colon, which was felt to be due to the débriding action of multiple dressing changes. This was the only fistula of this type seen in this series. It is the author's contention that the untoward rate of intestinal fistulization reported in other series of open packing [11] can be minimized by careful operative technique and the use of nonadherent gauze to cover exposed intestinal surfaces. Three intestinal fistulas (one duodenal, one enteric, and one colonic) occurred after secondary abdominal closure in proximity to drainage tubes

Table 4. Weight of necrotic tissue removed at initial and subsequent re-explorations

	No. of patients[a]	Average weight (g)	Weight range (g)
Initial exploration	16	156 ± 20	54–261
First re-exploration	16	67 ± 31	33–101
Second re-exploration	16	29 ± 23	7–64
Third re-exploration	14	15 ± 12	0–38
Fourth re-exploration	13	9 ± 7	0–19

[a] Three patients had undergone secondary closure by the fourth re-exploration.

Table 5. Open packing: comparison of secondary healing vs secondary closure

	Secondary healing	Secondary closure
Patients	46	18
Re-explorations[a]	9.4 ± 3.0	5.3 ± 2.6
Mortality	15%	11%
Morbidity	31%	44%
Hospital days	48 ± 6.1	32 ± 9.2

[a] Requiring analgesia.

during prolonged lavage. Each responded to withdrawal of the offending tube.

The specific amount of necrotic tissue removed in these 64 patients was not quantitated in the initial patients. However, in a more recent group, the average weight of tissue removed at the initial exploration was 156 g (Table 4). It is the author's impression that similar amounts of necrotic tissue were removed in the initial series of patients.

In all 34 cases in which transcutaneous fine-needle aspiration was done to determine the presence of bacteria by Gram stain and culture of the aspirate, the organism cultured from the necrotic tissues removed at surgery was identical to the one obtained preoperatively by fine-needle aspiration. Two patients with an initial sterile aspirate were found (11 and 19 days later) to have positive bacterial aspirates.

A comparison of the 18 patients recently treated by secondary closure with the preceding 46 patients permitted to heal by secondary intention is shown in Table 5. Managing patients by delayed secondary closure resulted in a significant decrease in the total number of hospital days from 48 ± 6.1 to 32 ± 9.2, and this represented a considerable cost saving. However, there was an increase in morbidity associated with secondary closure, primarily due to intestinal fistulization resulting from prolonged catheter lavage and drainage.

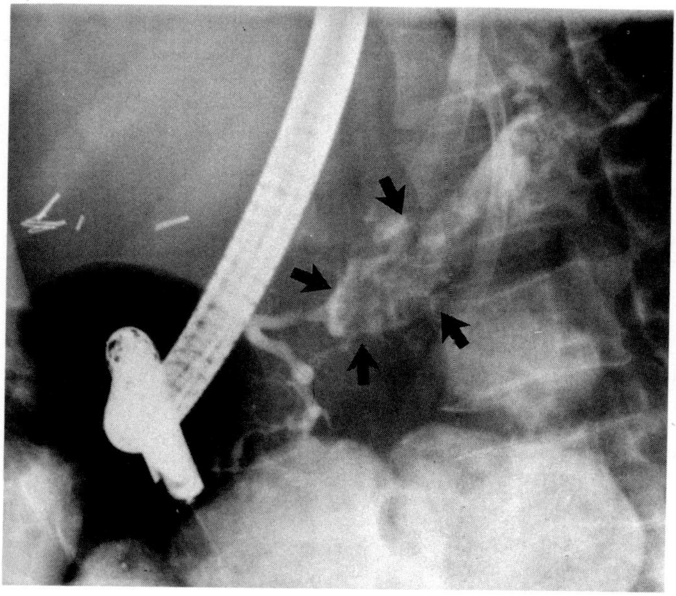

Fig. 2. Preoperative ERCP in a patient subsequently proved to have infected pancreatic necrosis. Note the loss of ductal integrity and the leak of contrast (*arrows*) into the retroperitoneum

In 12 patients, biochemical analysis of the lavage fluid following secondary closure was carried out. Constituents of the lavage effluent included markedly elevated values of immunoreactive trypsin, phospholipase A_2, and bradykinin. Preoperative endoscopic pancreatography had been carried out in three of these patients, in each case demonstrating a pancreatic duct disruption (Fig. 2).

Eleven of 13 patients consenting to postoperative endoscopic pancreatography demonstrated truncation of the pancreatic duct (Fig. 3), which emphasizes the severity of pancreatic parenchymal necrosis in these patients.

The worldwide experience with open drainage for infected pancreatic necrosis is shown in Table 6. The overall mortality in this collected series of 220 patients has been 15.5%. The diversity of investigators obtaining good results with this technique establishes that the procedure of open drainage is not operator dependent, and that good results from this approach are not geographically limited. Although minor variations in technique occurred between the technique described by the author and some of the workers in this list (such as the use of zipper abdominal closures and the direct application of laparotomy packs to unprotected intestinal surfaces), the

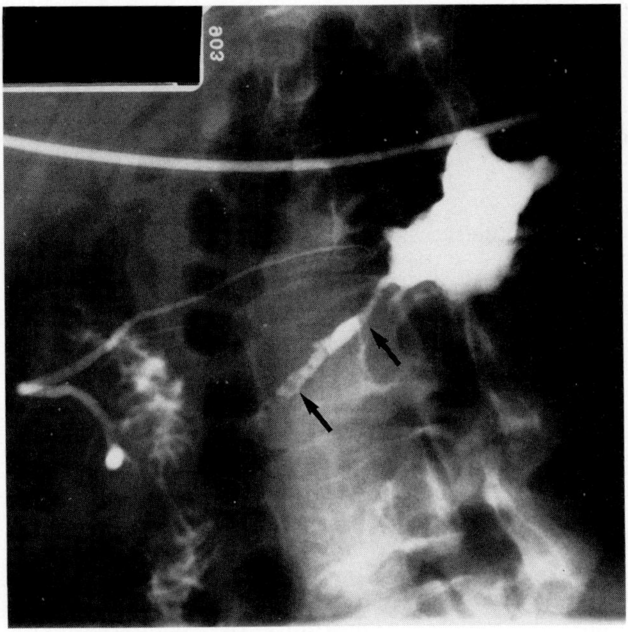

Fig. 3. Evidence of pancreatic duct disruption from an ERCP obtained 6 weeks after débridement for infected necrosis and 2 weeks after discharge (oblique view) A small sinus tract (*arrows*) arises from the pancreatic juice collection

basic principle of periodic programmed redébridement was followed throughout this collected series.

Discussion

As a result of programmed pancreatic resection for severe acute pancreatitis by several European investigators [3, 12, 13], extensive histologic studies have demonstrated that the development of necrotizing pancreatitis is the principal determinant both of the severity of the clinical course of acute pancreatitis and of ultimate survival. As a result of this clinicopathologic correlation, detection of pancreatic necrosis has become a principal focus in the modern management of acute pancreatitis.

Despite demonstrations that circulating breakdown products of pancreatic necrosis can be detected in the serum [14, 15], clinical validation of their usefulness in directing therapy is currently lacking. Dynamic contrast-enhanced CT pancreatography, introduced by Kivisaari and her associates in 1983 [16], is currently accepted as the most sensitive and

Table 6. Worldwide experience with open dreainage for infected pancreatic necrosis

Reference(s)	Year	No. of patients	Mortality (%)
Bradley et al. [9, 10] Atlanta	1981 & ff	64	14
Levy et al. [38] Paris	1984	26	23
Pemberton et al. [11] Rochester	1986	17	18
Waclawiczek et al. [39] Slazburg	1986	19	16
Wertheimer and Norris [40] Massachusetts	1986	12	17
Vogel (unpublished) Gainesville	1987	11	0
Garcia-Sabrido et al. [41] Madrid	1988	9	22
Stanten and Frey [•] Sacramento	1990	36	14
Eckhauser et al. [•] Ann Arbor	1991	18	22
Akin et al. [•] Knoxville	1991	8	0
Totals		220	15.5

reliable indicator of pancreatic necrosis, with an overall accuracy of 90% [17, 18].

Since the development of secondary bacterial infection of pancreatic necrosis results in a fourfold increase in mortality risk compared with sterile necrosis [3–6], differentiation between the clinical "toxemia" of sterile necrosis and secondary bacterial infection of necrotizing pancreatitis has assumed increasing importance. Clinical differentiation alone is not possible [19], but fortunately, transcutaneous CT-guided fine-needle aspiration for detection of bacteria has proved to be remarkably accurate in making this distinction [20].

While controversy continues regarding the role of surgery in *sterile* necrotizing pancreatitis [9], few would question the need for surgical intervention in patients with demonstrated infected pancreatic necrosis, particularly in view of the demonstrated failure of interventional radiology to benefit this group of patients [21].

Although almost all authorities agree that infected necrosis is an absolute indication for surgical exploration and débridement, a number of contentious issues have arisen. Several workers have advocated immediate exploration [12, 13], while others prefer to delay surgical intervention until demarkation between viable and nonviable tissue is better established [22, 23]. In our experience, blunt débridement of nonviable tissues is possible as early as 2 weeks following the onset of the episode of necrotizing pancreatitis. However, exploration after this time is considerably facilitated by the increasing ease with which necrotic tissues may be separated from vascularized tissues by finger dissection.

Although the majority of surgeons prefer an anterior incision, both a posterior approach [24] and a combination of anterior exploration and flank drainage [25] have also been proposed. Both of these latter approaches suffer when *extensive* infected necrosis is present, or when the necrosis presents primarily in the head of the gland.

Optimal access to the necrotizing pancreatitis is through the gastrocolic momentum [26]. Although débridement through the transverse mesocolon is possible and has been recommended [27], this approach is necessarily limited by the presence of the middle colic vessels, and extensive débridement is less easily accomplished.

While thorough débridement of all necrotic tissues is common to each of the competitive surgical approaches for infected pancreatic necrosis, it is the specific method of subsequent drainage which has characterized the various surgical options. In essence, three basic approaches to surgical drainage following débridement of infected necrosis have been proposed: closed drainage employing sump catheters [27], a semi-closed approach using continuous lesser sac lavage [28], and the open technique which employs periodic re-exploration and redébridement [29].

Choosing the conventional surgical approach of débridement and sump drainage commits the surgeon to a re-exploration rate for recurrent or persistent sepsis of 30%–50% [27, 30–32]. Moreover, the decision to reoperate is based on clinical criteria and requires considerable clinical judgment. That this judgment is not often made correctly is evidenced by the observation that 76% of the deaths in a collected series of more than 1200 cases of pancreatic infections treated by conventional drainage were due to recurrent or persistent infection [8]. Clearly, closed drainage should not be chosen by surgeons unfamiliar with these patients. Moreover, it must be noted that the favorable results with this conventional approach experienced by Warshaw and Jin [27] have not been duplicated.

It is becoming increasingly apparent that the failure of conventional surgical drainage to deal satisfactorily with patients suffering from infected pancreatic necrosis is due to continuing necrosis of retroperitoneal tissues following initial débridement. Persistence of the necrotizing process is due, at least in part, to the loss of integrity of the pancreatic ductal system demonstrated in this and other reports [33]. Continued leakage of pancreatic enzymes and cytotoxic agents from the damaged ductal systems directly into the retroperitoneal space, reported here and elsewhere [28], strongly suggests that this feature of necrotizing pancreatitis is responsible for the clinical observation that pancreatic and peripancreatic necrosis reaccumulates following initial débridement (see Table 4). Accordingly, methods for the periodic or continuous removal of the reaccumulated "toxic broth" from the retroperitoneum should provide superior clinical results to those obtained by conventional drainage.

Beger and his associates have been the principal advocates of continuous lesser sac lavage following débridement of infected pancreatic necrosis [28]. Using this technique, they were able to achieve an enviable mortality of 14% in patients with proved infected necrosis. Others, using a similar technique, have reported higher death rates, ranging from 21% to

28% [35, 36]. Furthermore, a randomized prospective comparison of lesser sac lavage and conventional sump drainage in patients with infected necrosis failed to demonstrate any superiority of lavage with respect to either morbidity or mortality [37]. Finally, we should note that surgical re-exploration for recurrent sepsis has been necessary in almost 30% of patients with infected necrosis treated by lesser sac lavage [28]. In view of these observations, contentions that the results of lesser sac lavage are equivalent to those obtained by open drainage may be premature.

How, then, should patients with infected pancreatic necrosis be managed? In the absence of a prospective trial, the available evidence favors the choice of lesser sac lavage or open drainage. The experienced pancreatic surgeon knows that each method of drainage has a place. The choice between these two approaches is best made at the time of exploration. Patients with smaller amounts of infected necrosis at initial exploration (<100 g) can often be successfully treated by débridement and lesser sac lavage and do not require the more complicated procedure of open packing. On the other hand, when infected necrosis is more extensive, or extends downward behind the colon flexures, open packing becomes the procedure of choice.

References

1. Buggy BP, Nostrant TT (1983) Lethal pancreatitis. Am J Gastroenterol 78: 810–814
2. Renner IG, Savage WT III, Pantoja JL, Renner VJ (1985) Death due to acute pancreatitis: a retrospective analysis of 405 autopsy cases. Dig Dis Sci 30: 1005–1018
3. Beger HG, Bittner R, Block S, Büchler M (1986) Bacterial contamination of pancreatic necrosis: a prospective clinical study. Gastroenterology 91:433–438
4. Bittner R, Block S, Büchler M, Beger HG (1987) Pancreatic abscess and infected pancreatic necrosis: different local septic complications in acute pancreatitis. Dig Dis Sci 32:1082–1087
5. Allardyce DB (1987) Incidence of necrotizing pancreatitis and factors related to mortality. Am J Surg 154:295–299
6. Pederzoli P, Bassi C, Elio A, Corra S, Nifosi F, Benetti G (1989) The infected necrosis is a prognostic factor in necrotizing pancreatitis. Gastroenterology 96:1389
7. Frey CF, Bradley EL III, Beger HG (1988) Progress in acute pancreatitis. Surg Gynecol Obstet 167:282–286
8. Lumsden A, Bradley EL III (1990) Secondary pancreatic infections: abscess, infected pseudocyst, and infected necrosis. Surg Gynecol Obstet 170:459–468
9. Bradley, EL III, Allen KA (1991) Management of necrotizing pancreatitis: results of prospective longitudinal trial. Am J Surg 161:19–25
10. Bradley EL III, Fulenwider JT (1984) Open treatment of pancreatic abscess. Surg Gynecol Obstet 159:509–513
11. Pemberton JH, Becker JM, Dozois RR, Nagorney DM, Ilstrup D, Remine WH (1986) Controlled open lesser sac drainage for pancreatic abscess. Ann Surg 203:600–604
12. Alexandre JH, Guerrieri MT (1981) Role of total pancreatectomy in the treatment of necrotizing pancreatitis. World J Surg 5:369–377

13. Kivilaakso E, Fraki O, Nikki P, Lempinen M (1981) Resection of the pancreas for acute fulminant pancreatitis. Surg Gynecol Obstet 152:493–498
14. Gudgeon AM, Heath D, Hurley P, Sheikin A, Iehanli A, Patel G, Wilson C, Austen B, Imrie C, Hermon-Taylor J (1988) Trypsinogen activation peptide (TAP) assay in severity assessment of acute pancreatitis. Pancreas 3:598–600
15. Büchler M, Malfertheiner P, Schoetensack C, Uhl W, Beger HG (1986) Sensitivity of antiproteases, complement factors and C-reactive protein in detecting pancreatic necrosis. Int J Pancreatol 1:227–235
16. Kivisaari L, Somer K, Standertskjold-Nordenstam C-G, Schroder T, Kivilaakso E, Lempinen M (1983) Early detection of acute fulminant pancreatitis by contrast-enhanced computed tomography. Scand J Gastroenterol 18:39–41
17. Bradley EL III, Murphy F, Ferguson C (1989) Prediction of pancreatic necrosis by dynamic pancreatography. Ann Surg 210:495–501
18. Nuutinen P, Kivisaari L, Schroder T (1988) Contrast-enhanced computed tomography and microangiography of the pancreas in acute human hemorrhagic/necrotizing pancreatitis. Pancreas 3:53–60
19. Nordback I, Pessi T, Auvinen O, Autio V (1985) Determination of necrosis in nectrotizing pancreatitis. Br J Surg 72:225–227
20. Banks PA, Gerzof SG, Rovvins AH, Johnson WC, Spechler SJ, Wetzner SM, Snider JM, Langevin RE, Jay ME (1988) Diagnosis of pancreatic infection by CT-guided aspiration: an update. Pancreas 3:590
21. Steiner E, Mueller PR, Hahn PF, Saini S (1988) Complicated pancreatic abscesses: problems in interventional management. Radiology 167:443–446
22. Machado MCC, Bacchella T, da Cunha JEM, Faintuch J, Penteado S, Giovanoli ACV, Pinotti HW (1986) Surgical treatment of pancreatic necrosis. Dig Dis Sci 31:25S
23. White TT, Heimback DM (1976) Sequestrectomy and hyperalimentation in the treatment of hemorrhagic pancreatitis. Am J Surg 132:270–274
24. Fagniez P-L, Rotman N, Kracht M (1989) Direct retroperitoneal approach to necrosis in severe acute pancreatitis. Br J Surg 76:264–267
25. Berne TV, Donovan A (1981) Synchronous anterior and posterior drainage of pancreatic abscess. Arch Surg 116:252–256
26. Davidson ED, Bradley EL III (1981) "Marsupialization" in the treatment of pancreatic abscess. Surgery 89:252–256
27. Warshaw AL, Jin G (1985) Improved survival in 45 patients with pancreatic abscess. Ann Surg 202:408–415
28. Beger HG, Büchler M, Bittner R, Oettinger W, Block S, Nevalainen T (1988) Necrosectomy and postoperative local lavage in patients with necrotizing pancreatitis: results of a prospective clinical trial. World J Surg 12:255–262
29. Bradley EL III (1987) Management of infected necrosis by open drainage. Ann Surg 206:542–550
30. Aranha GV, Prinz RA, Greenlee HB (1982) Pancreatic abscess: an unresolved surgical problem. Am J Surg 144:534–538
31. Holden JL, Berne TV, Rosoff L (1982) Pancreatic abscess following acute pancreatitis. Arch Surg 111:858–861
32. Watters JM, Mullens JE (1982) Pancreatic abscess. Can J Surg 25:460–462
33. Gebhardt C (1987) Indications for surgical intervention in necrotizing pancreatitis. In: Beger HG, Büchler M (eds) Acute pancreatitis. Springer, Berlin Heidelberg New York, pp 310–313
34. Nicholson ML, Mortensen NJ McC, Espiner HJ (1988) Pancreatic abscess: results of prolonged irrigation of the pancreatic bed after surgery. Br J Surg 75:88–91
35. Larvin M, Chalmers AG, Robinson PJ, McMahon MJ (1989) Débridement and closed cavity irrigation for the treatment of pancreatic necrosis. Br J Surg 76: 465–471

36. Pederzoli P, Bassi C, Vesentini S (1990) Retroperitoneal and peritoneal drainage and lavage in the treatment of severe necrotizing pancreatitis. Surg Gynecol Obstet 170:197–203
37. Teerenhovi O, Nordback I, Eskola J (1989) High-volume lesser sac lavage in acute necrotizing pancreatitis. Br J Surg 76:370–373
38. Levy E, Hannoun L, Parc R, Honiger J, Herguet C, Loyguc J (1984) Le drainage activ prolongé des pancreatites aiguës necrotico-hémorrhagiques: indications, techniques, resultuts preliminaires a propos de vingt-six cas. Ann Chir 38:351–356
39. Waclawiczek HW, Pimpl W, Chmelizek F (1986) Perioperative interdisciplinary management in acute necrotizing pancreatitis. Dig Dis Sci 31:359
40. Wertheimer MD, Norris CS (1986) Surgical management of necrotizing pancreatitis Arch Surg 121:152–156
41. Garcia-Sabrido JL, Tallado JU, Christion NV, Polo JR, Valdecantos E (1988) Treatment of severe intraabdominal sepsis and/or necrotic foci by an open-abdomen approach. Arch Surg 123:152–156

Laparostomy – Open Packing – for Infected Pancreatic Necroses

H.W. WACLAWICZEK,[1] F. CHMELIZEK, and O. BOECKL

Acute necrotizing pancreatitis still poses a central problem for general surgery, mainly when infected pancreatic necroses have to be treated. In spite of all the progress – especially in intensive care medicine – and despite better findings in the field of pathogenesis, mortality is still up to 50% in literature reports. Only a few centers can report a mortality rate below 20% [2–4, 7, 8].

The aim surgical treatment of acute pancreatitis with infected pancreatic necroses is clearly defined and includes removal of the septic sources and the peripancreatic and paracolic necroses, as well as continuous lavage and drainage of the pancreatic bed and the affected retroperitoneal spaces respectively. Yet, due to the "disadvantageous" topography of the pancreas and because of the rapidly spreading retroperitoneal inflammation processes these goals can rarely be achieved with only one surgical intervention.

Laparostomy (open packing) represents only one of several surgical treatment methods for necrotizing pancreatitis, but excellent results can be achieved when good teamwork, sufficient experience of the surgeons and nursing staff and well organized intensive care medicine are present.

Patients

Because of unsatisfactory results with closed methods (necrosectomy and/or peritoneal lavage) for infected pancreatic necroses (mortality up to 70%) our approach to this serious disease since 1985 has been exclusively the open packing method. Out of 284 patients with acute pancreatitis a necrotizing course of disease occurred in 73 cases (28%). All these patients underwent dynamic computed tomography (CT) within a few hours of admission. If the clinical symptoms gave reason to suspect infected pancreatic necroses they were carefully aspirated under CT or sonographic guidance.

In the case of negative bacteriologic findings (n = 30) the patients with these sterile pancreatic necroses were conservatively treated using all intensive care measures, hemofiltration included. Only six patients had to be

[1] Ist Surg. Dept., LKA Salzburg, Müllner Hauptstraße 48, A-5020 Salzburg, Austria

Beger/Büchler/Malfertheiner (Eds.)
Standards in Pancreatic Surgery

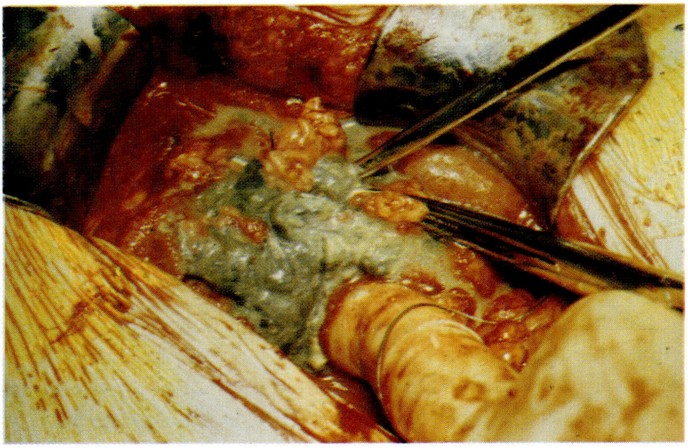

Fig. 1. Infected peripancreatic necroses after dissection of the gastrocolic ligament

treated surgically or endoscopically for pseudocysts in the following period of 4 months.

In the case of positive bacteriologic findings and thus proof of infected pancreatic necroses ($n = 43$) the patients were operated on: 33 men, 10 women, average age 37.2 years (range 23–78 years). According to CT criteria and the classification of stages by Kümmerle the extent of necrosis amounted to below 30% in 10 patients and to 40%–90% in 33 patients.

Basically we tried to bring these patients into a "postacute" phase from day 12 after onset of the disease by means of all intensive care measures. The aim of delaying operation in this way was clear demarcation of the pancreatic necroses from the remaining healthy tissue, making necrosectomy easier and less risky. Therefore a sonographic check was performed daily and a CT control on average every 3 days was performed during this time. These delayed operation tactics succeeded in 32 out of 43 patients. For this reason preoperative renal failures amounted to the very high rate of 74%. An absolute indication for immediate laparotomy was the existence or early occurrence of lung failure in the sense of acute respiratory distress syndrome (ARDS) ($n = 11$).

Surgical Technique

The abdomen was always opened by an extended bilateral subcostal laparotomy. After dissection of the gastrocolic ligament the bursa omentalis was entered and first of all the purulent peripancreatic necroses were removed (Fig. 1). Only then the exact extent of pancreatic necroses and of peripancreatic necrotic abscesses could be verified. Subsequently, if

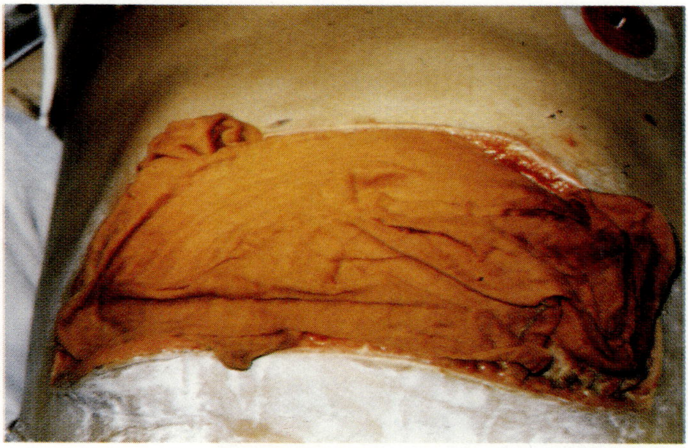

Fig. 2. Tamponade of the laparostomy with laparotomy pads (soaked in povidone solution)

possible, a digitoclastic necrosectomy was performed. In 17 of the 43 patients a left pancreatectomy and splenectomy were carried out during the first intervention, whereas in eight further cases these procedures were necessary within the first postoperative week. After mobilization of both colon bends the paracolic and retroperitoneal and retrogastric spaces were debrided. Ample lavage with up to 20 l physiological saline followed. Large-bore sump drains were placed in both subphrenic spaces and the pancreatic bed. In order to protect the peritoneal cavity from (further) infection the partly resected greater omentum was always sutured to the lower fascia of the laparotomy wound, thus creating an omental compartment (laparostomy). Finally, this laparostomy was packed with up to 10 pads, soaked in povidone (Betadine) solution (Fig. 2). In a few cases only ($n = 5$), the laparostomy was temporarily closed by means of a zipper technique (Ethizip).

Further daily interventions were carried out under sterile conditions at the patient's bedside in the intensive care unit. After removal of the laparotomy pads further digitoclastic necrosectomies and lavages with up to 10 l saline were performed (Fig. 3). Then the laparostomy was repacked with laparotomy pads and a continuous lavage of the pancreatic bed followed wtih 10–15 l saline via the sump tubes for 24 h. These daily procedures demanded an average operation time of 40 min.

At the first signs of clinical deterioration or increasing sepsis the procedure was carried out in the operating theater with complete exploration of all intra- and extraperitoneal spaces.

If no source of sepsis could be located, an immediate CT scan was obtained; this proved very helpful in ten cases as further necroses or

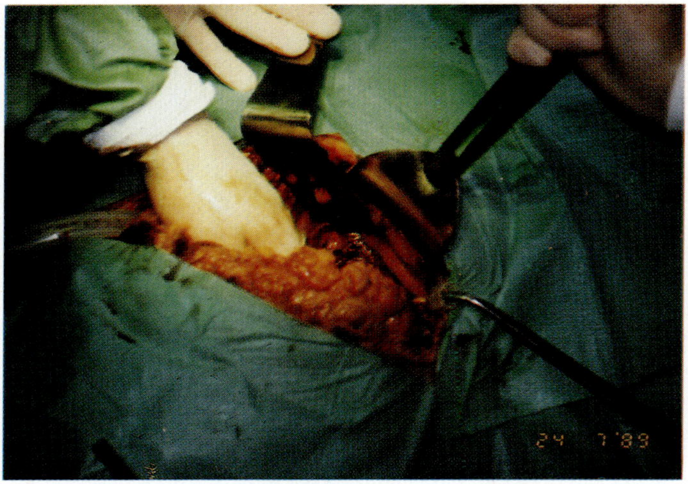

Fig. 3. Digitoclastic necrosectomy via the laparostomy at the bedside in the intensive care unit

abscesses, mainly located in the mesenterium, could be detected, thus permitting an exact necrosectomy.

In order to be able to perform all these daily surgical interventions via the laparostomy, intubation and respiration were required for an average of 15 days (range 4–168 days). Despite this long-term respiration no tracheotomy was necessary. Due to renal failures, mostly combined with ARDS, 18 patients required hemofiltration for 12 days on the average. Parenteral, high-caloric nutrition was obligatory; in addition, in 13 patients enteral feeding was started via a jejunostomy catheter, placed transcutaneously, after the first postoperative week. Antibiotic therapy was changed constantly according to the latest bacteriological state.

With these daily, exact, and careful necrosectomies the preservation of as much healthy pancreatic tissue as possible was achieved in many cases. After an average of 7 days progressive closing of the laparostomy with fresh granulation tissue started. Therefore the laparostomy could be closed surgically between days 10 and 27 and no plastic operation of the abdominal wall was required (Fig. 4). In the initial 13 patients though, we allowed the abdomen to close solely by granulation; this happened after 45 days on average.

The mean stay in the intensive care unit amounted to 22 days (range 6–190 days), the overall hospital stay to 42 days (range 25–245 days).

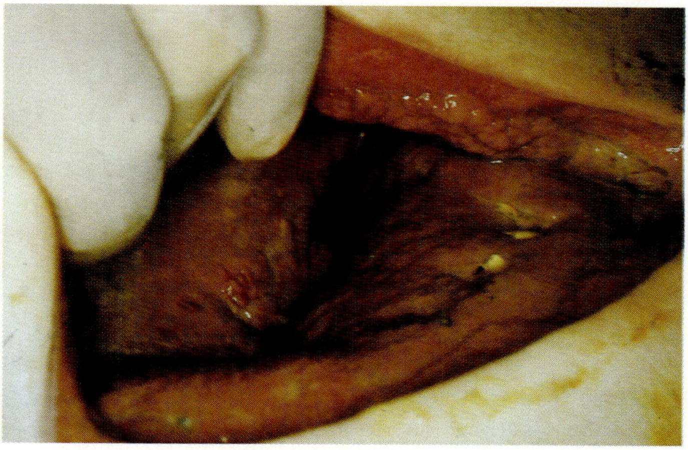

Fig. 4. Pancreatic bed, cleaned by granulation tissue (post-operative day 15)

Results

In 25 patients (58%) the postoperative course was without serious complications, although 17 had renal and four had lung failures. These patients underwent respiration for 13 ± 4 days; the laparostomy could be closed after 16 ± 5 days.

The rate of major surgical complications amounted to 28% (n = 12), mostly caused by incisional hernias and fistulae. In five patients duodenal or colo-cutaneous fistulae were observed. Three more developed pancreatic fistulae; one of these patients expired 14 months postoperatively (see mortality). The fistulae of the other seven patients were treated conservatively (partly with somatostatin) or by oversewing. Only in one case postoperative insulin-dependent diabetes occurred after extended pancreas resection.

Six of the 43 patients died (mortality rate 14%). The causes of death were multiple organ failures due to acute sepsis (n = 4) and one myocardial infarction. A 45-year-old male patient developed multiple gastro-entero-cutaneous fistulae. After the failure of conservative therapy, the patient was subjected to 23 surgical interventions (gastrectomy, colon resections etc.); he died due to *Candida* sepsis 14 months postoperatively.

Thirty-three of the 43 patients (74%) developed organ failures either preoperatively or very soon after operation. When only one organ (lung, liver, kidney) failed (n = 23), the mortality rate was only 4.3% (n = 1), but this rate escalated significantly to 30% (n = 3) when two or more organ failures occurred (n = 10).

In keeping with the extent of necrosis the mortality in stage III (more than 30% necrosis; n = 33) amounted to 18% (n = 6). With an extent of

Table 1. Mortality in acute pancreatitis (n = 284)

Disease stages	Patients (n)	Therapy		Mortality	
		Surgical	Conservative/endoscopic	(n)	(%)
I (no necroses)	211	0	211	1	0.4
II (necroses <30%)	40	10	30	0	
III (necroses >30%)	33	33	0	6	18
Stages I and II	73	43	30	6	8.2
Total (all stages)	284	43	241	7	2.4

necrosis below 30% (stage II; n = 40), non patient died. A laparostomy was necessary in only ten of these patients due to infected necroses; in the other 30 patients conservative treatment, using all intensive care measures, was successful. For this reason the overall mortality rate in necrotizing pancreatitis including the conservatively treated sterile necroses (n = 73) amounted to only 8.2% (Table 1).

Discussion

Alongside resection procedures and necrosectomy with continuous closed peritoneal lavage [2, 3, 7], laparostomy (open packing) represents only one of the operative methods for the treatment of infected pancreatic necroses. While subtotal pancreas resection can not be recommended because of the high surgical risk and the resultant high mortality, Büchler reports excellent results, with a mortality rate of around 11%, achieved with necrosectomy, drainage and continuous peritoneal lavage; yet contrary to our patients, in almost 40% of his cases noninfected necroses were treated. Furthermore, in those cases with a severe course of the disease several relaparotomies had to be performed [3].

Surgical treatment with laparostomy (open packing method) is not new, as Körte had already described it in 1894 [6]. Over recent years several centers have taken up this method because of the progress in intensive care medicine [2, 4, 8]. Especially Bradley demonstrated that the open packing method for infected pancreatic necroses could significantly help to reduce mortality [1, 2].

Essential advantages of laparostomy over the other methods are in our opinion the possibilities of daily exploration and careful necrosectomy, performed under sterile conditions mostly at the patient's bedside in the intensive care unit. Additional continuous peritoneal lavages serve to remove endotoxins and necrotic material. Complications such as arrosion bleedings, fistulae etc. are quickly managed via the laparostomy. Also, the often difficult decision on relaparotomy is thus avoided [8]. A disadvantage of this method is that it is labor-intensive and time-consuming especially in the intensive care unit. With an average daily operation time of 40 min, and a mean duration of 15 days, the surgical interventions amounted to 12–14 h per patient. In our opinion a further, very important point is that the same surgeon who performed the laparostomy must carry out the daily dressing changes and necrosectomies, as he is the only one who is familiar with the individual and the varying course of the disease. This surgeon needs to have sufficient experience in pancreatic and abdominal surgery to be able to manage any complications. In the case of deterioration of the patient's state, mainly in the case of reappearance of sepsis, an immediate CT scan proved helpful; the source of sepsis could always be found in the retroperitoneum [1, 5].

These surgical measures for necrotizing pancreatitis combined with sepsis and organ failure naturally require good teamwork from the intensive care physicians. Due to good intensive care nursing and exact hygienic measures tracheotomies could be avoided despite long-term respiration. Therefore we attribute our good results with the open packing method for infected pancreatic necroses exclusively to the success of this interdisciplinary cooperation.

References

1. Bradley EL III, Murphy F, Ferguson C (1989) Prediction of pancreatic necrosis by dynamic pancreatography. Ann Surg 210:495–504
2. Bradley EL III (1990) The role of open packing in the management of infected pancreatic necrosis. In: Waclawiczek HW, Boeckl O, Pauser G (eds) The open packing – laparostomy – in pancreatitis and peritonitis. Springer, Berlin Heidelberg New York, pp 105–112
3. Büchler H, Beger HG (1990) Necrosectomy and continuous closed bursa lavage in necrotizing pancreatitis. In: Waclawiczek HW, Boeckl O, Pauser G (eds) The open packing – laparostomy – in pancreatitis and peritonitis. Springer, Berlin Heidelberg New York, pp 175–183
4. Chmelizek F, Waclawiczek HW (1985) Perioperatives interdisziplinäres Management bei der akut nekrotisierenden Pankreatitis. Anaesthesia 34:607–611
5. Crass RA, Meyer AA, Jeffrey RB et al. (1985) Pancreatic abscess: impact of computerized tomography on early diagnosis and surgery. Am J Surg 150:127–131
6. Körte W (1894) Zur chirurgischen Behandlung der Pankreas-Eiterung und Pankreas-Nekrose. Arch Klin Chir 48:720–724
7. Levy E, Frileux P, Fontaine E et al. (1988) Management of acute necrotizing pancreatitis with marsupialization, prolonged active drainage, and continuous enteral nutrition through the jejunostomy. A study of 80 cases. Neth J Surg 74:75
8. Waclawiczek HW, Boeckl O, Chmelizek F (1990) Interdisciplinary management in necrotizing pancreatitis. In: Waclawiczek HW, Boeckl O, Pauser G (eds) The open packing – laparostomy – in pancreatitis and peritonitis. Springer, Berlin Heidelberg New York, pp 113–123

Management of Pancreatic Necrosis and Abscess

D.W. Rattner[1] and A.L. Warshaw

Introduction

The treatment of acute pancreatitis is primarily supportive. Management of severe pancreatitis entails evaluation of multiple clinical, radiologic, and biochemical parameters to determine the timing and type of intervention when it becomes necessary to alter the natural course of the disease. Recent work by Beger and others [1–4] has emphasized that when pancreatitis is complicated by the development of necrosis, infection is the primary determinant of outcome. Others have therefore extrapolated that the presence or absence of infection should determine whether or not surgical intervention is undertaken [3, 4]. Minimally invasive therapy (such as diagnostic needle aspiration) or observation alone have been advocated for sterile necrosis [3, 4]. Furthermore, the successful experience with percutaneous radiologically guided drainage of abdominal abscesses [5, 6] has brought enthusiasm for this technique to the treatment of pancreatic sepsis [7, 8]. Amid these trends we chose to examine the experience at our institution with cases of severe necrotizing pancreatitis during the past 5 years.

Materials and Methods

Hospital charts and office records were retrospectively reviewed for all patients (n = 253) admitted to the Massachusetts General Hospital between 1 January 1985 and 31 December 1989 with a primary or secondary diagnosis of acute pancreatitis. Patients with simple fluid collections, sterile and infected pseudocysts, and trivial amounts of necrosis which did not preoduce symptoms were excluded. Among 253 records reviewed, 73 patients with significant pancreatic necrosis or abscess were identified. All underwent an invasive radiologic or surgical procedure. We did not identify any patient with extensive necrosis who was treated with observation alone.

[1] Department of Surgery, Massachusetts General Hospital and Harvard Medical School, Boston, MA 02114, USA

Beger/Büchler/Malfertheiner (Eds.)
Standards in Pancreatic Surgery

Table 1. Etiology of pancreatitis

	Gallstone		Ethanol		Other	
	n	%	*n*	%	*n*	%
Transferred ($n = 59$)	21	36	13	22	25	42
Primary admission ($n = 14$)	4	29	1	7	9	64
Total	25	34	14	19	34	47

Computed tomographic (CT) scans were reviewed concurrently by a radiologist who was unaware of the clinical details of each case and graded according to Balthazar's criteria (grade A, normal pancreatic morphology; B, pancreatic enlargement only; C, peripancreatic inflammation only; D, one fluid collection; E, two or more fluid collections) [9]. Further analysis and categorization of the collection morphology was performed by reviewing the operative and pathology reports. Bacteriologic studies were performed by the Massachusetts General Hospital microbiology laboratory according to standard clinical practice.

Statistical analysis was performed using Primer of Biostatistics software (McGraw-Hill, New York). Comparison between groups was made using Student's unpaired t test with Bonferonni correction for interval variables, χ^2 analysis of proportions, and Mann-Whitney rank sum test for ordinal variables. Values of p less than 0.05 were considered significant.

Results

General Characteristics of Patients with Pancreatic Necrosis and Abscess

The median age was 60 years (range 20–90). There were 20 women (27%) and 53 men (73%). Most patients were referred from outside hospitals (61/73) after an average pretransfer hospital stay of 13 days. The etiology of pancreatitis was gallstone related in 25 patients, ethanol abuse in 14 patients, and a variety of other causes in 34 patients (Table 1). Particularly notable among the patients whose pancreatitis was related to neither gallstones nor ethanol were 15 cases of postoperative pancreatitis (Table 2). In 62 patients the initial collection was primarily semisolid necrotic material whereas in 11 it was primarily fluid. Of the preoperative CT scans available for analytic review ($n = 42$) 70% were grade E ($n = 29$), 26% grade D ($n = 11$), and 5% grade C ($n = 2$).

Nearly all patients were symptomatic. The indications for intervention were: infection proven by needle aspiration (or indwelling percutaneous drainage catheter) in 24 patients, persisting pancreatitis manifested by pain, inability to eat, or failure to thrive in 16 patients, clinical picture consistent

Table 2. Etiology of pancreatitis due to "other" causes

Etiology	Number of cases
Idiopathic	13
After cardiac surgery	9
After aortic surgery	3
After gastrointestinal surgery	3
After ERCP	2
Carcinoma	1
Trauma	1
Hyperlipidemia	1
Steroids	1

with intraabdominal sepsis in 15 patients, radiographic evidence of pancreatic abscess in 10 patients, severe acute abdominal pain in 6 patients, and large asymptomatic collections in 2 patients. The overall mortality of the series was 24.6% (18/73). Of the 73 patients 59 experienced a complication following surgical or radiologic intervention (80%).

Factors Correlated with Mortality

Because most patients were referred from outside hospitals well after the onset of pancreatitis, Ranson's criteria [10] at the time of first admission could not be assessed. However, the APACHE II score [11] was determined at our institution 24 h prior to the first intervention and proved to be an excellent predictor of outcome. Patients with an APACHE II score of 15 or higher had a 50% mortality rate whereas those whose APACHE II score was under 15 had a mortality rate of 14% ($p < 0.02$). The mean APACHE II score in survivors was 9.7 ± 5.6 versus 14.8 ± 6.0 in nonsurvivors ($p = 0.005$). Preintervention respiratory failure requiring mechanical ventilation (12/19 died), hypotension (6/9 died), and multisystem failure (11/20 died) were grave prognostic indicators. Furthermore, preoperative acute renal failure had an adverse effect on survival but in this series did not quite reach statistical significance ($p = 0.06$). Preoperative blood transfusion to replace blood lost in the retroperitoneum or gastrointestinal tract was also significantly different between survivors (1.8 ± 3.4 U packed red blood cells) and nonsurvivors (6.8 ± 4.5 U; $p < 0.01$).

No patient with alcohol-induced pancreatitis died in this series. The mortality rate in patients with "other" etiologies of pancreatitis (14/34, 41%) was significantly higher than those with either gallstone-induced or alcoholic pancreatitis (4/39, 10%; $p = 0.018$). Seven of 14 patients with postoperative pancreatitis, including three of four patients with pancreatitis following abdominal surgery, died.

The most important postintervention predictor of death was development of recurrent pancreatic sepsis. Among 39 patients who required only

Table 3. Factors not correlated with mortality

	Survivors	Nonsurvivors
Age (years)	55 ± 16	61 ± 14
Days between onset and first intervention	23 ± 17	22 ± 14
Previous episodes of pancreatitis	10/45 (22%)	6/15 (40%)
Lowest serum calcium (mg/dl)	7.1 ± 1.1	6.3 ± 1.2
Highest WBC	24 300 ± 6200	23 100 ± 7400
Highest amylase (IU/l)	1961 ± 2422	2542 ± 3688
Lowest albumin (g/dl)	2.4 ± 0.7	2.1 ± 0.6
Intraoperative blood loss (units)	1.64 ± 2.4	1.60 ± 1.5
Total hospital days	78 ± 39	62 ± 41
Total TPN days	36 ± 31	50 ± 39
Infected collection	35/55 (64%)	15/18 (83%)

Table 4. Effect of duration of pancreatitis from onset of symptoms until first intervention on outcome

Interval from onset to first intervention (days)	*n*	Infected		Recurrence		Deaths	
		n	%	*n*	%	*n*	%
0–7	3	2	66	1	50	0	
8–14	16	10	63	6	38	3	19
15–21	14	9	64	8	57	7	50
22–28	11	8	73	5	46	2	18
29–35	6	4	66	3	50	1	16
36–42	3	3	100	1	33	1	33
>43	9	8	89	4	44	1	11

one intervention (surgical in all cases) there was one death. In contrast, 17/34 who required reintervention died. Those factors which were important in the development of recurrent sepsis are discussed below.

Factors which did not correlate with mortality are listed in Table 3. Of particular interest is the lack of significant correlation between bacteriologic status of necrosis and death. Furthermore, the time from the onset of pancreatitis until the first intervention did not correlate with death, recurrent abscess, or the presence of infection (Table 4).

The Role of Infection

Bacterial cultures obtained during the first intervention were available in 72 patients. Of these, 29 had a monomicrobial infection, 17 had a polymicrobial infection, and in 26 the initial culture was sterile. *Escherichia coli* was the most common pathogen in monomicrobial collections whereas enterococcus was the most common pathogen in polymicrobial collections. There were a

Table 5. Comparison of sterile and infected collections

	Sterile collection	Infected collection
Number of patients	23	50
Deaths	3 (13%)	13 (26%)
Days between onset and first intervention	25	23
APACHE II score (mean)	11.2	10.8
Lowest albumin (g/dl)	2.42	2.25
Lowest calcium (mg/dl)	6.46	6.86
Preoperative blood transfusion (units)	1.7	3.6
Total blood transfused (units)	11.9	15.9
ICU days	17	16
TPN days	37	40
Hospital days	62	56
Recurrent abscess	7 (39%)	21 (49%)

There was no significant difference between groups in any category.

median of three types of organisms per polymicrobial collection (from two to five).

To discern whether infection was the primary determinant of outcome we analyzed the effect of infection on multiple parameters as well as mortality. The mortality rate in patients with infected collections (26%) was higher than in patients with sterile collections (13%), but this difference was not statistically significant ($p = 0.2$). APACHE II score, which was the most reliable index of severity of illness in these patients, was similar in patients with infected and non-infected collections. The time interval between the onset of pancreatitis and intervention was comparable in patients with sterile (20 ± 10 days) and infected collections (26 ± 18 days). Likewise, the mean interval from onset of pancreatitis to intervention was similar in patients whose collections were primarily fluid (25 days) and in patients whose collections were a heterogeneous mix of liquid and solid debris, i.e., necrosis (23 days). Furthermore, the original bacteriologic status of the collection did not correlate with either the development of post-operative complications or recurrent pancreatic sepsis (Table 5).

Causes of Recurrent Pancreatic Sepsis

Since the development of recurrent pancreatic sepsis following the initial intervention at Massachusetts General Hospital seemed critically important in determining outcome, we sought a correlation between recurrent pancreatic sepsis and other variables. The rate of recurrent sepsis varied widely among individual surgeons. One surgeon had eight recurrent collections among nine patients whereas another surgeon had seven recurrences among 24 cases. The mortality rate of different surgeons paralleled the recurrence

Table 6. Variation in recurrent pancreatic sepsis following surgical débridement

Surgeon	*n*	Recurrences		Deaths	
		n	%	*n*	%
A	24	7	29	3	12.5
B	19	8	42	5	26
C	21	11	52	4	21
D	9	8	88	6	66

Table 7. Comparison of patients treated with surgery versus surgery plus PD

	PD + surgery	Surgery alone	*p*
Number of patients	31	42	
APACHE II score	12.3 ± 5.7	9.9 ± 6.2	NS
Deaths	10 (32%)	8 (19%)	NS
Preoperative transfusion	4.4 ± 5.1	1.6 ± 2.6	<0.05
Lowest calcium (mg/dl)	6.33 ± 1.03	7.42 ± 1.0	0.002
Lowest albumin (g/dl)	2.0 ± 0.5	2.6 ± 0.7	0.01
Number of CT scans	7 (2–18)	3 (0–6)	
TPN days	57 ± 39	27 ± 24	<0.001
ICU days	31 ± 31	6 ± 9.6	<0.001
Hospital days	82 ± 40	42 ± 25	<0.001

rate but the numbers were too small to achieve statistical significance (Table 6).

Three other factors (determined prior to the first intervention) correlated with the development of recurrent sepsis: respiratory failure, APACHE II score, and lowest serum calcium. These factors reflect both the debilitated general condition of the patient and the severity of the underlying pancreatitis. No other factor including age, etiology, highest amylase, highest WBC, lowest albumin, number and type of drains, extent of necrosis [12], and monomicrobial versus polymicrobial infection, predicted recurrent sepsis.

Percutaneous Radiologic Intervention

Twenty surgically treated patients had diagnostic radiologic aspiration performed preoperatively to determine the presence or absence of infection. In two patients the gram stain of the aspirate showed no organisms but the culture was positive (*E. coli* and *Staphylococcus aureus*). In two other patients the culture from the aspirate was sterile, but the operative culture was positive (*Aspergillus flavus* and *Staphylococcus epidermidis*). Therefore

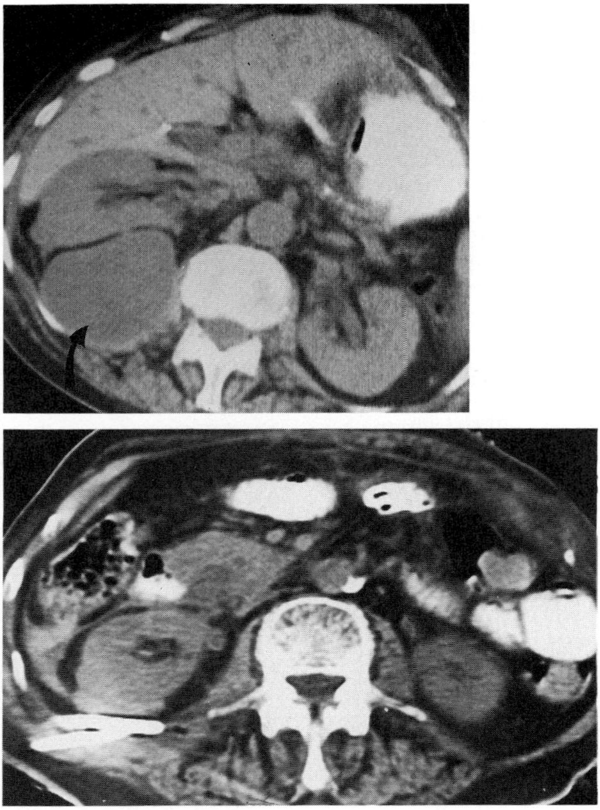

a

b

Fig. 1. **a** CT scan showing a homogeneous low attenuation fluid collection in the right posterior pararenal space (*arrow*) prior to percutaneous drainage. **b** CT scan following percutaneous drainage of fluid collection seen in **a** showing complete resolution of the collection

the initial diagnostic aspirate gave a temporarily false sense of security in 4/20 patients. There were no false positive aspirates.

Thirty-one patients had percutaneous radiologically guided drainage procedures (PD; Table 7). In six patients, PD was the initial intervention. In the majority of patients (25/31) PD was employed to drain collections which developed following an initial surgical debridement. All six patients in whom PD was the initial procedure subsequently required surgical débridement and drainage. No patient was successfully treated by percutaneous drainage alone.

A total of 81 catheters were inserted in 59 collections with an average of 2.7 catheters inserted per patient (from one to ten). These patients required an average of seven CT scans (range 2–18) and three catheter manipulations

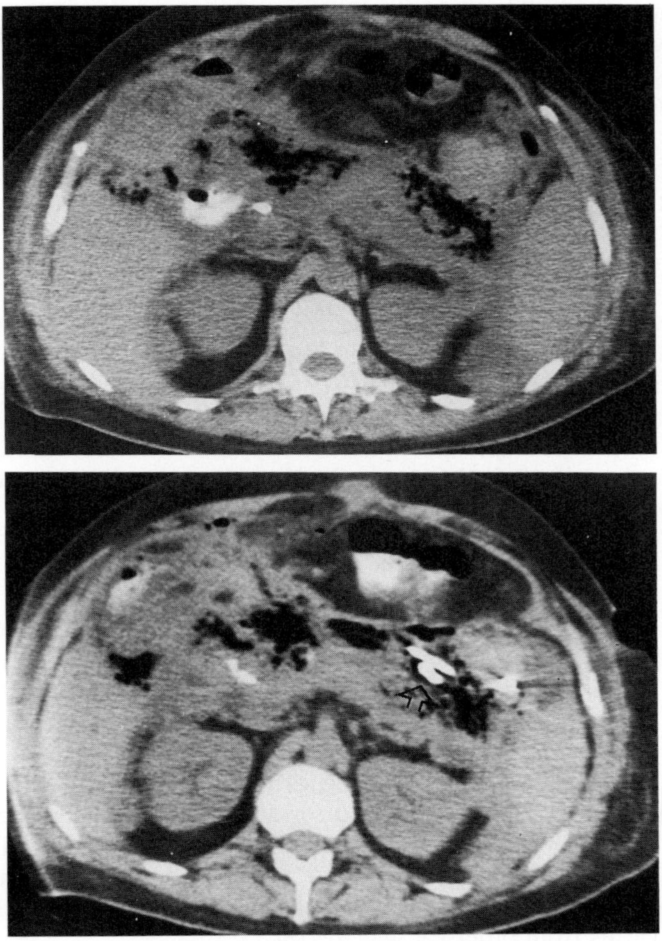

a

b

Fig. 2. a CT scan showing a complex collection containing fluid, solid material, and gas in the lesser sac prior to attempted percutaneous drainage. **b** CT scan of the collection shown in **a** after attempted percutaneous drainage. Drainage catheters (*arrow*) lie in the middle of the collection. There was little change in the radiographic appearance and the patient was unimproved and subsequently required surgical débridement

(range 1–9). PD was considered successful in 14 patients (45%; all of whom had undergone a prior surgical debridement) whose collections were completely drained, obviating the need for further surgery. In nine patients (29%) PD ameliorated sepsis temporarily and allowed a less urgent definitive surgical drainage, or successfully drained one of multiple collections and changed the surgical approach. In eight other patients (26%) PD failed to drain a collection, did not temporarily relieve sepsis, and may have delayed necessary surgery.

Percutaneous drainage was most effective for homogeneous, low attenuation (on CT scan) collections. Successful drainage was achieved less often for heterogeneous collections or collections containing gas. Of 15 simple collections 14 (93%) were completely drained by percutaneous intervention (Fig. 1) whereas only 21/44 complex collections were successfully drained (Fig. 2).

Patients treated with PD required significantly more days of total parenteral nutrition (TPN), intensive care, and hospitalization (Table 7). In at least eight patients, failed PD clearly delayed ultimate surgical débridement and contributed to a prolonged hospital stay. Prior to the first intervention, patients treated with PD had APACHE II scores which were similar to those treated by solely surgical methods. However, this group of patients had more preoperative blood transfusion, lower serum calcium, and lower serum albumin than the surgically treated group and thus may represent the most severe cases of pancreatitis.

Discussion

The patients who comprise this series represent the severe end of the spectrum of necrotizing pancreatitis. The median age was 60 years, and 81% of patients were referred after it was apparent at an outside hospital that complications of the initial bout of pancreatitis were developing. Furthermore, 92% had either major or extended necrosis and 95% of the patients had grade D or E changes on their CT scans. The etiology of pancreatitis was also different than most other reported series [1, 13–15] in that nongallstone, nonalcoholic causes were most frequent (47%). It is interesting that no patient with alcoholic pancreatitis died. Several other authors have found that alcoholic pancreatitis may have a better prognosis than acute necrotizing pancreatitis from other causes [16–18].

Since most patients were not seen at our institution at the onset of their illness, it was not possible to assess Ranson's criteria [10] as outcome predictors. Likewise all patients included had markedly abnormal CT scans so that CT grade could not be used as a predictor of mortality [9]. Serum markers which may relate to severity of the necrotizing process, such as C-reactive protein [19], polymorphonuclear leukocyte elastase [20], and trypsinogen activation peptide [21], were not routinely measured. We therefore evaluated the APACHE II scoring system [11] and found it to be a good predictor of both mortality and recurrent sepsis. This confirms previous work that APACHE II may be the best clinical scoring system for stratifying patients with severe pancreatitis [22, 23]. We, like most other authors, found the presence of major organ system failure prior to intervention to be a harbinger of poor outcome [10, 17, 18, 24]. This is partially reflected in the APACHE II score.

A great deal of emphasis has recently been placed on the differentiation of infected and sterile necrosis. Since Beger reported that bacterial infection of pancreatic necrosis was associated with significantly higher morbidity and mortality [1] there has been enthusiasm for basing decisions about the need for surgical débridement upon the bacteriologic status of the tissue in question. In Beger's series [1] the incidence of infection was maximal (71.1%) in patients operated upon 15–21 days after the onset of symptoms. This is the same as the incidence of infected necrosis in the current series (44/62, 70.9%). Those patients in Beger's series who underwent exploration early in the course of pancreatitis (days 1–21) did poorly if the tissue was infected. However, in patients operated upon 3 weeks or more after the onset of illness, the presence of infection did not affect outcome. Since the need for operation was determined by clinical criteria in Beger's series and not necessarily by the known preoperative presence of infection, it is possible that early operation was performed on patients with more severe pancreatitis than those operated upon later in the course of their illness. Beger's observation that bacterial infection is an important determinant of outcome appears to apply only to patients undergoing *early* operation for necrotizing pancreatitis. Because no clinical, biochemical, or hemodynamic parameters have been shown to correlate with the presence of pancreatic infection [25], the severity of the underlying pancreatitis may be as important a determinant of outcome as infection.

In this series, the presence of infection had very little impact on the clinical course of the patients. It is important to note, however, that the first intervention in our institution occurred at an average of 3 weeks following the onset of symptoms. Although patients whose collections were infected had a somewhat higher mortality rate than those with sterile collections, the difference was not statistically significant. Likewise, recurrent collections (all infected) occurred with nearly equal frequency among the two groups (46% in patients with infected collections versus 43% in those with initially sterile collections). Patients with infected necrosis were no more ill than those with sterile collections as determined by the criteria shown in Table 5. Beger also noted that the systemic complications of sterile and infected necrosis were similar [26].

These data should not be interpreted to belittle the importance of infection. No case of infected pancreatic necrosis or pancreatic abscess has ever been cured by antibiotic treatment alone. Since there is no clinical or biochemical test which reliably detects the presence of infection, radiologically guided aspiration of pancreatic collections plays an important role in determining a need for intervention. The finding of infection is an absolute indication for débridement and drainage. The converse, however, is not true. Although it has been reported that sterile necrosis in some asymptomatic patients may be safely observed [4], patients who are symptomatic (systemically ill, cannot eat, anorexic, febrile, in pain or have other effects secondary to a necrotic collection) should not be denied a laparotomy simply because a necrotic collection is sterile. We have seen patients who suffered low grade, but significant symptoms for up to a year because their physicians were committed to avoiding an operation. Symptoms due to mass effect and local inflammation can only be relieved by debridement and drainage. Although some authors claim to be able to exclude infection on the basis of a diagnostic needle aspiration [27], we and others [13] have observed a 10% false negative rate with this technique. Also some sterile collections will surely become infected subsequently resulting in urgent operations in more seriously ill patients. Therefore, because infection is not the sole or even the primary determinant of outcome, we conclude that symptomatic collections should be drained irrespective of their bacteriologic status.

Just as it has become fashionable to utilize the presence of infection as the sole determinant of need for intervention, it has also been stated that pancreatic abscess (a circumscribed liquid collection of pus) is a different entity than infected pancreatic necrosis (a predominantly solid, somewhat ill-defined collection of dead tissue) [2]. While these terms are useful morphologic descriptions, most patients have elements of both abscess and necrosis. The protean manifestations of necrotizing pancreatitis span the entire morphologic spectrum from infected, solid unperfused tissue to saclike collections of liquid with virtually no solid component. Most often the clinician is dealing with the middle of this spectum with a mixture of solid and liquid components. Thus we feel that differentiating abscess from infected necrosis is somewhat artificial.

The most important factor determining mortality in this series was the development of recurrent pancreatic sepsis after the initial drainage. This effect has been previously noted [13, 17, 24]. It was not related to the bacteriologic status of the initial collection. It appears to be related to the severity of the antecedent pancreatitis as evidenced by the association with hypocalcemia, preoperative respiratory failure, and APACHE II score. These patients either had further progression of the local injury caused by pancreatitis or were debilitated enough to have impaired ability to clear the debris of pancreatitis.

Because recurrent sepsis is such a serious development, it is imperative that the initial débridement be aggressive and thorough. The importance of the initial surgical debridement may be reflected in the outcomes by different surgeons within this institution (Table 6). Since the severity of illness, the ICU care, the surgical residents and ancillary services, and the timing of operation were similar for all of our patients, the importance of the primary surgeon is highlighted. The timing of the initial operation appears to be less important than the adequacy of the initial débridement. At the time of laparotomy, the entire pancreas from head to tail should be explored. Often the capsule of the pancreas must be incised to identify a necrotic sequestrum (Fig. 3). Necrotic tissue should be removed as completely as possible within the limits of safety. Simply placing drains adjacent to dead tissue is not

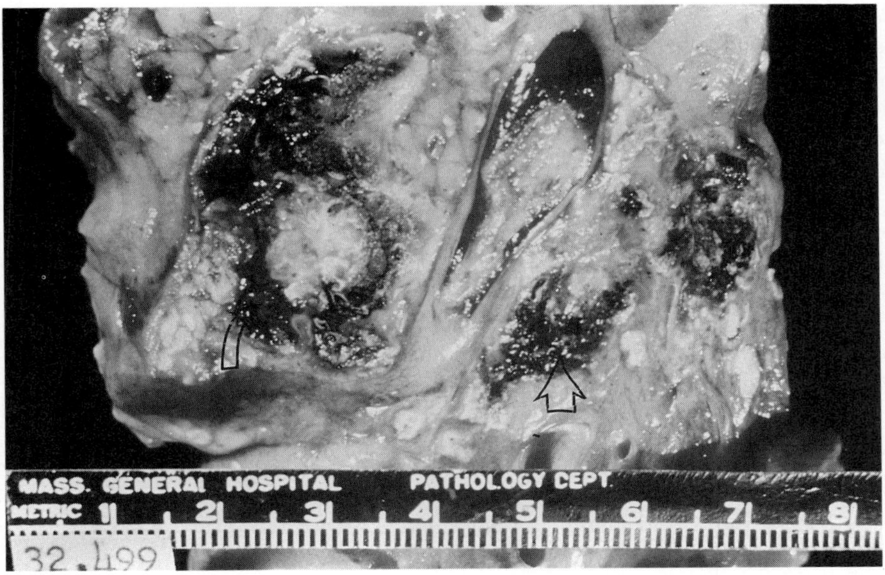

Fig. 3. Cross-section of resected pancreas showing areas of necrosis (*arrows*) beneath the pancreatic capsule

adequate therapy. We prefer to use a combination of soft silicone suction drains and large gauze-filled penrose drains to ensure easy egress of fluid, debris, and pus [28]. Others have championed the use of continuous irrigation of the lesser sac [26] or employed open packing techniques to prevent recurrent sepsis and allow further débridement [29, 30]. Open packing was employed in two patients in this series, both of whom died of sepsis. Open packing may be particularly useful when the limits of the necrotizing process are indeterminate and when it seems likely that further slough will occur. Continuous irrigation of the lesser sac has only been employed in a few cases during the past year, and we cannot comment upon its efficacy.

Percutaneous radiologically guided drainage of intraabdominal collections has been a great advance in the management of intraabdominal sepsis due to a variety of causes. It can obviate the need for laparotomy and reduce both morbidity and cost when properly employed. Enthusiasm for percutaneous drainage has prompted widespread use in complicated pancreatitis. Gerzof and others [7, 27, 31, 32] have recognized that the efficacy of PD in complicated pancreatitis depends on the precise indication for its use. While some fluid collections and even infected pseudocysts can be treated with PD, infected solid material cannot be evacuated through a catheter! Several caveats are apparent in reviewing the experience with PD in this series. PD can be life saving and cost-effective when used to drain simple fluid collections, especially those which develop following surgical débridement. On the other hand, failure is likely if there is a significant solid component in the collection. In this series of severe pancreatitis, PD was not effective for pancreatic necrosis when employed prior to surgical débridement probably because there was almost invariably a significant solid component to the collection. Thus PD should not be the primary mode of therapy in acute necrotizing pancreatitis.

In this era of cost-consciousness it is important to recognize that appropriate use of PD may be cost-effective, but attempts to treat collections containing a significant amount of necrotic tissue are not. Inappropriate use of PD increases cost and delays necessary surgical intervention. This point is apparent in comparing the TPN days, ICU days, and hospital days in patients treated with PD and surgery (Table 7). In a previous series from this institution, prior to the extensive use of PD, the length of stay was 49 days, similar to the 42 days in the surgery alone group in the current series [28], both being significantly less than the 82 days required for those treated by catheter drainage.

References

1. Beger HG, Bittner R, Block S, Büchler M (1986) Bacterial Contamination of pancreatic necrosis: a prospective clinical study. Gastroenterology 91:433–438
2. Bittner R, Block S, Büchler M, Beger HG (1987) Pancreatic abscess and infected pancreatic necrosis – different local septic complications in acute pancreatitis. Dig Dis Sci 32:1082–1087
3. Reber HA (1986) Surgical intervention in necrotizing pancreatitis. Gastroenterology 91:479–482
4. Bradley EL (1991) A prospective longitudinal study of observation verses surgical intervention in the management of necrotizing pancreatitis. Am J Surg 161:19–24
5. Johnson WC, Gerzof SG, Robbins AH et al. (1981) Treatment of abdominal abscesses: comparative evaluation of operative drainage vs percutaneous catheter drainage under computed tomography or ultrasound. Ann Surg 194:510–520
6. Gerzof SG, Johnson WC, Robbins AH, Nabseth DC (1985) Expanded criteria for percutaneous abscess drainage. Arch Surg 120:227–232
7. Gerzof SG, Johnson WC, Robbins AH, Spechler SJ, Nabseth DC (1984) Percutaneous drainage of infected pancreatic pseudocysts. Arch Surg 19: 888–893
8. Adams DB, Harvey TS, Anderson MC (1990) Percutaneous catheter drainage of infected pancreatic and peripancreatic fluid collections. Arch Surg 125: 1554–1557
9. Ranson JHL, Balthazar E, Caccavale R, Cooper M (1985) Computed tomography and the prediction of pancreatic abscess in acute pancreatitis. Ann Surg 201:656–663
10. Ranson JHL, Rifkind KM, Roses DF et al. (1974) Prognostic signs and the role of operative management in acute pancreatitis. Surg Gynecol Obstet 139:69–81
11. Knaus WA, Draper EA, Wagner DP, Zimmerman JE (1985) APACHE II: a severity of disease classification. Crit Care Med 13:818–829
12. Beger HG, Krautzberger W, Bittner R, Block S, Büchler M (1985) Results of surgical treatment of necrotizing pancreatitis. World J Surg 9:972–979

13. Fink AS, Hiatt JR, Pitt HA, Bennion RS, Souza JR, McCoy RD, Meyer JP, Thompson J et al. (1988) Indolent presentation of pancreatic abscess: experience with 100 cases. Arch Surg 123:1067–1072
14. Mainwaring R, Kern J, Schenk WG, Rudolf LE (1989) Differentiating pancreatic pseudocysts and pancreatic necrosis using computed tomography. Ann Surg 209:562–566
15. Lumsden A, Bradley EL (1990) Secondary pancreatic infections. Surg Gynecol Obstet 170:459–467
16. Aranha GV, Prinz RA (1982) Pancreatic abscess: an unresolved surgical problem. Am J Surg 144:534–538
17. Becker JM, Pemberton JH, DiMagno EP (1984) Prognostic factors in pancreatic abscess. Surgery 96:455–461
18. McClare SA, McAllister EW, Karl RC, Nord HJ (1986) Pancreatic abscess: 10 year experience at the University of South Florida. Am J Gastroenterol 81: 180–184
19. Büchler M, Malfertheiner P, Schoetenstack C, Uhl W, Beger HG (1988) Sensitivity of antiproteases, complement factors, and C-reactive protein in detecting pancreatic necrosis. Int J Pancreatol 1:227–235
20. Uhl W, Büchler M, Malfertheiner P, Martini M, Beger HG (1990) Serum necrosis factors and imaging procedures: competitive or complementary factors in severe acute pancreatitis. Gastroenterology 98:A238
21. Gudgeon AM, Heath DI, Hurley P, Jehanl A, Patel G, Wilson L, Slenkin A, Ausen BM, Imrie CW, Hermon-Taylor J (1990) Trypsinogen activation peptides assay in the early prediction of severity of acute pancreatitis. Lancet 335:4–8
22. Larvin M, McMahon MJ (1989) APACHE II. Score for assessment and monitoring of acute pancreatitis. Lancet ii(8656):201–205
23. Stanten R, Frey CF (1990) Comprehensive management of acute necrotizing pancreatitis and pancreatic abscess. Arch Surg 125:1269–1274
24. Malangoni M, Richardson D, Shallcross JC, Seiler JG, Polk HC (1986) Factors contributing to fatal outcome after the treatment of pancreatic abscess. Ann Surg 203:605–613
25. Beger HG, Bittner R, Büchler M, Hess W, Schmitz JE (1986) Hemodynamic data pattern in patients with acute pancreatitis. Gastroenterology 90:74–79
26. Beger HG, Büchler M, Bittner R, Oettinger W, Block S, Nevalainen T (1988) Necrosectomy and postoperative local lavage in patients with necrotizing pancreatitis: results of a prospective clinical trial. World J Surg 12:255–262
27. Banks PA, Gerzof SG, Chong FK, Worthington MG, Doos W, Sullivan JG, Johnson WC (1990) Bacteriologic status of necrotic tissue in necrotizing pancreatitis. Pancreas 5:330–333
28. Warshaw AL, Jin G (1985) Improved survival in 45 patients with pancreatic abscess. Ann Surg 202:408–415
29. Bradley El, Fulenwider JH (1984) Open treatment of pancreatic abscess. Surg Gynecol Obstet 159:509–513
30. Pemberton JH, Becker JM, Dozois RR, Nagorrez DM, Ilstrup D, Remire WH (1986) Controlled open lesser sac drainage for pancreatic abscess. Ann Surg 203:600–604
31. Adams DB, Harvey TS, Anderson MC (1990) Percutaneous catheter drainage of infected pancreatic and peripancreatic fluid collections. Arch Surg 125: 1554–1557
32. White ME, Wittenberg J, Mueller PR, Simeone JF, Butch RJ, Warshaw AL, Neff CC, Nardi GL, Ferucci JT (1986) Pancreatic necrosis: CT manifestations. Radiology 158:343–346

Pancreatic Abscess in Biliary Acute Pancreatitis

J. KLINGER-ROITMAN[1], M.S. GALVEZ, G.L. CAIMI, T.P. OLIVARES, M. DIAZ, and M. SAAVEDRA

Introduction

The incidence of pancreatic abscess (PA) in acute pancreatitis (AP) is between 2% and 9% [2, 6, 11, 13, 21, 23]. PA is a severe complication with a mortality rate of 30%–50%, which has remained constant over recent decades [11, 14, 21]. Before the advent of imaging techniques, diagnosis was difficult and usually not achieved until late in the evolution. Now, however, using computed tomography (CT), diagnosis is made earlier, when there is a pancreatic fluid collection.

In Chile, biliary origin is the main etiologic factor of AP (60%–75%), and PA is the most frequent complication [1, 12, 22, 23] (Table 1). This chapter examines the incidence, diagnosis, surgical treatment, morbidity, and mortality of PA in biliary AP (BAP).

Material and Methods

In a retrospective study we analyzed 56 cases of PA in patients admitted to the intensive care unit of the G.C. Fricke Hospital, Vina del Mar, Chile during the years 1988–1990. In 38 cases, the etiology was BAP. Of these, 17 (45%: eight men, nine women) developed PA: 2/4 (50%) in 1988, 10/18 (56%) in 1989, and 5/16 (31%) in 1990. All cases of infected pseudocysts were excluded, as were five cases in which biliary etiology could not be established with certainty. Cases were classified in terms of Ranson's criteria of severity, acute physiology score (APS-2 scale), and trauma index and severity score (TISS). There were eight cases with a Ranson score of less than 3, seven with a score of 3 or 4, one with a score of 5 or 6, and one with a score of more than 6. On the APS-2 scale there were ten with a score under 9, three with a score of 10–14, three with a score of 15–19 and one with a score over 20 (average 9.3); 41% thus presented with an APS-2 score above 10, which predicted a mortality at admission of 20%. Diagnosis was made in seven cases by CT and in three by ultrasound. The diagnosis was

[1] Surgical Service and Intensive Care Unit G.C. Fricke Hospital, Vina del Mar, Chile and Department of Surgery, School of Medicine, University of Valparaiso, Chile

Beger/Büchler/Malfertheiner (Eds.)
Standards in Pancreatic Surgery

Table 1. Pancreatic abscess in patients with acute pancreatitis

Etiology	Number of patients	Pancreatic abscesses *n*	%
Gallstones	38	17	45
Alcoholic	7	0	0
Traumatic	2	0	0
Metabolic[a]	2	0	0
Postoperative	2	1	50
Idiopathic	5	0	0
Total	56	18	32

[a] One hyperlipidemia, one chronic failure.

confirmed in 15 cases at operation and in two by percutaneous guided puncture (PGP).

Bacteriological study was carried out on the pancreatic tissue and pus obtained in 12 cases during operation and in two cases by PGP. Analysis for anaerobic bacteria was not possible for technical reasons.

All patients were treated in the intensive care unit with medication, antibiotics, and decontamination of the gastrointestinal (GI) tract; 15 were submitted to total parenteral nutrition and 11 required mechanical respiratory assistance.

We examined the effect of age, sex, diagnosis, operation, timing of initial operation, complications and the factors probably involved in cases of death.

Results

In about 59% of cases the diagnosis of PA was confirmed at operation. The indications for surgery were based on clinical and laboratory aspects that showed a persistent septic status before other septic foci were eliminated. In 1989 we incorporated the use of repeated CT (every 7–10 days) in AP, and this allowed us an earlier diagnosis of pancreatic fluid collections and better planning of surgical treatment. In the 12 cases, bacteriological study showed infection due to Enterobacteriacea in nine, to coagulase-positive staphylococci in five, and to *Candida albicans* in one.

Of our cases 75% were operated on during the first 4 weeks of the disease, almost 30% in the first 2 weeks. No relationship to the Ranson criteria was found (Table 2). Fifteen patients had been operated on previously (on the biliary tract); the average period was 26 days before the diagnosis of PA. The indication for this type of surgery was a very acute attack in 11, and AP was a surgical finding. The remaining four patients were operated on because there was evidence of acute cholecystitis in

Table 2. Ranson score and the timing of operation

Ranson score	Timing of operation (weeks)			
	<2	2–4	>4	Unknown
<3	2	4	1	1
⩾3	3	4	2	0
Total	5 (29.4%)	8 (47%)	3 (17.6%)	1 (6%)

Table 3. Reoperations

Number of reoperations	Number of patients	Type of surgery
One	7	– SEQ + TPB
Two	3	– SEQ + TPB/choledochorraphy + SEQ – SEQ + TPB (twice) – SEQ + TPB/subtotal pancreatectomy + splenectomy
Four	1	– SEQ + TPB (twice)/subtotal pancreatectomy + splenectomy/suture incision due to hemorrhage

SEQ, sequestrectomy; TPB, toilet of pancreatic bed.

combination with AP. There were three instances of cholecystostomy, three of cholecystectomy, eight of combined cholecystostomy and cholecystectomy, and one of choledochostomy.

Once the diagnosis of PA was established, surgical treatment was performed within 24 h. Two cases were treated by PGP; operation was due to failure of adequate drainage in one and to a subphrenic abscess in the other. In ten of the 17 cases a sequestrectomy was performed at the first intervention (five with drainage, five with content laparostomy).

A pancreatic resection was performed in only one case, drainage alone in four, and percutaneous drainage in two. Of the 17 cases 11 required reoperation (Table 3). Sequestrectomy and toilet of the pancreatic bed was carried out, and four patients needed between two and four reoperations for persistent infected pancreatic parenchyma or for complications of previous surgery.

The average period of total hospitalization was 45 days (18–77 days), and the average period in the intensive care unit was 35 days (3–68 days). The most severe complications in the postoperative period were sepsis and multiple organ failure (11 cases). Each case presented more than one complication. Other complications included: intraabdominal abscess (four),

Table 4. Factors in mortality

Factor	Patient number						
	1	2	3	4	5	6	7
Age (years)	41	58	26	26	28	67	58
Sex	w	w	w	w	m	m	w
Ranson score	4	3	3	2	7	2	3
APS-2 score	28	–	12	11	15	12	–
TISS score	42	–	24	26	44	27	–
No. of reoperations	2	–	1	0	2	–	4
Cause of death	MH	MOF	MOF	MH	MOF	TR	MOF

MH, massive hemorrhage; MOF, multiple organ failure; TR, tracheal rupture.

pneumonia (four), pancreatic fistula (three), hemodynamic hemorrhage (three), massive hemorrhage (two), small intestinal fistula (one), and biliary peritonitis (one).

Overall mortality was 41% (seven cases); in four there was multiple organ failure, in two, severe massive hemorrhage of the pancreatic bed, and in one, tracheal rupture during respiratory assistance. Table 4 presents the factors implicated in each patient's mortality. There was a tendency to decreased mortality during the last year of the study. Death occurred in 2/2 cases of PA in 1988, 4/10 in 1989, and 1/5 in 1990.

Discussion

In Chile the main etiology of PA is clearly biliary lithiasis, with an incidence of 60%–75% [1, 6, 7, 12, 22, 23]. In the present series this etiology was responsible for 68% of cases of PA. Some authors, though, have reported lower figures [2, 4, 18, 20]. The incidence of PA due to BAP is 40%–86%, although Saxon et al. [20] found only 19%; in our study the figure was 45%. Bittner et al. [4] found alcohol abuse to be the most frequent etiology in primary PA.

At the present time it is accepted that PA is related to the severity of AP. Ranson et al. [17] report 40.7% of patients with a score ⩾3.

In the Chilean literature it is emphasized that PA is more frequent in the 4th and 5th decades, with a male predominance. However, 47% of our patients were aged under 30 years, and 76% were younger than 40 years of age, without predominance of one sex.

Due to the fact that PA symptoms are not pathognomonic and X-ray studies and laboratory findings are not specific (except with high and persistent levels of pancreatic ribonuclease, which is not available to us), the diagnosis was based exclusively on imaging techniques. Bittner et al. [4]

reported that abdominal pain and sepsis are the most important symptoms in 50% of cases.

CT scan is the most sensitive and specific diagnostic method. Ranson et al. [16, 17] stated that the finding of two or more fluid collections in patients with two or more positive criteria is a sign of high risk for developing PA. CT does not differentiate between infected collections and others, and for this reason clinical evaluation is mandatory [3, 5, 19].

PGP is the only method that guarantees a preoperative diagnosis of PA. As a therapeutic means in our hands, results were not good, and the two patients needed reoperation. Bittner's findings are in accord with this.

The bacteria involved were gram negative, mostly from the GI tract. The mechanism for this is not clear, and the dissemination channels are not defined, but direct hematogenous or lymphatic paths have been suggested [9, 12], and there was a predominance of Enterobacteriacea. Bittner et al. [4] found two mixed flora in 43.8% of their cases.

It is well known that there is a higher incidence of PA after biliary surgery, but the role of the operation in the development of PA is still under study [8, 10].

Our tendency is to treat the biliary pathology when operation is decided, and in all cases exploration of the common bile duct is performed. The treatment for PA is surgical drainage. There is controversy in relation to laparotomy or access, but the important thing is to obtain sufficient exposure of the pancreas, install the drainage tubes, and perform aggressive débridement of necrotic pancreatic tissue. In all cases the access was transperitoneal, and in all aggressive digital débridement was performed. In six cases a laparostomy was used to facilitate the toilet of the pancreatic zone at the patient's bedside as needed.

In eight of 11 cases reoperations were related to the necessity of removing remaining necrotic tissue, and only two patients were operated on due to complications from the previous surgery. In 90% of cases complications derived from sepsis, pancreatic or abdominal. Mortality in the seven cases was secondary to multiple organ failure. Overall mortality was 41%, and 5/7 patients (75%) had three or more positive Ranson criteria, and 57% were older than 40 years. The average APS-2 score in those who died was 15.6, which is a 40% mortality index [7]. Mortality in PA is decreasing, and is reported in the literature to range between 20% and 25% [1, 8, 25]. Malagnoni et al. [12] and Warshaw and Gongliang [23], however, reported 18% and 5% mortality respectively. On the basis of our limited experience we feel that this is due to the effectiveness of medical treatment in the intensive care unit, the CT scan of all cases of acute pancreatitis, GI decontamination, the semiaggressive surgery performed upon the pancreas and peripancreatic area, and the use of laparostomy in selected cases.

Summary and Conclusions

In Chile the etiology of PA is mainly biliary lithiasis, with an incidence in the literature of 60%–75% and in our experience of 68%. The incidence of PA due to BAP ranges between 40% and 85% and in this series was 45%. Half of the patients with PA had severe AP (Ranson score ⩾3), which is not in accordance with other Chilean publications, where two thirds of patients are reported as having a score ⩾3. The most useful diagnostic technique is CT, and PGP is very important for establishing the differential diagnosis with any type of fluid collections. From the therapeutic point of view we were not satisfied with PGP, and the two patients submitted to the procedure needed to be operated on. In all, 88% of the PA patients had been operated on previously, at an average of 96 days before the diagnosis of PA was established. Basically, surgical drainage is the treatment for PA, and the removal of all the necrotic tissue is mandatory in the control of sepsis. Mortality remains high, (41%) but showed a tendency to decrease during the last year of this study.

References

1. Agar R, Bastias J, Yarmuch J, Silva J, y Vergas R (1988) Absceso pancreatico. Rev Chil Chir 40:224–226
2. Aranha G, Prinz R, y Greenlee H (1982) Pancreatic abscess, unresolved surgical problem. Am J Surg 144:534–538
3. Beger HG, Block S, Bittner R (1987) The significance of bacterial infection in acute pancreatitis. In: Beger HG, Büchler M (eds) Acute pancreatitis. Springer, Berlin Heidelberg New York, pp 79–86
4. Bittner R, Block S, Büchler M, Beger HG (1987) Pancreatic abscess and infected pancreatic necrosis: different local septic complications in acute pancreatitis. In: Beger HG, Büchler M (eds) Acute pancreatitis. Springer, Berlin Heidelberg New York, pp 216–223
5. Freise J (1987) Evaluation of sonography in the diagnosis of acute pancreatitis. In: Beger HG, Büchler M (eds) Acute pancreatitis. Springer, Berlin Heidelberg New York, pp 118–131
6. Galvez S (1990) Documentos estadisticos UCI Hospital Gustavo Fricke, 1988–1990
7. Galves S, Engels R, Vega J, Torres H, Merino C, Jerez R, Clavero R (1989) Manejo del paciente quirúrgico critico. Monografía ACS, pp 108–110
8. Guzmán S, Zamorano L, León P, Rahmer A, Zúniga Y, y Llanos O (1983) Absceso pancreático; experiencia clinica. Rev Chil Cir 35:432–436
9. Hancke E, Marklein G (1987) Bacterial contamination of the pancreas with intestinal germs: a cause of suppurative pancreatitis. In: Beger HG, Büchler M (eds) Acute pancreatitis. Springer, Berlin Heidelberg New York, pp 87–89
10. Imrie CW (1987) Gallstone-associated acute pancreatitis. In: Beger HG, Büchler M (eds) Acute pancreatitis. Springer, Berlin Heidelberg New York, pp 227–232
11. Jara L, Flores MP, Fernández E, Arredondo G, Garay M (1990) Rol de la cirugia en pancreatitis aguda necrohemorrágica. Rev Chil Cir 42:75–77
12. Malanogi M, Richarson D, Cotton J, Seiler J, Polck H (1986) Factors contributing to fatal outcome after treatment of pancreatic abscess. Ann Surg 203:605–610

13. Palacios R (1990) Pancreatitis aguda. Rev Chil Cir 42:297–313
14. Pemberton J, Becker J, Dozois R, Nagorney D, Ilstrup D, Remine W (1986) Controlled open lesser sac drainage for pancreatic abscess. Ann Surg 203: 600–604
15. Potts J (1988) Acute pancreatitis. Surg Clin North Am 68:281–297
16. Ranson J, Berman R (1990) Long peritoneal lavage decreases pancreatis sepsis in acute pancreatitis. Ann Surg 211:708–711
17. Ranson J, Balthazar E, Caccavale R, Cooper M (1985) Computed tomography and the prediction of pancreatic abscess in acute pancreatitis. Ann Surg 656–663
18. Rattner D, Warshaw A (1988) Surgical intervention in acute pancreatitis. Critical Care Med 16:93–94
19. Roscher R, Beger HG (1987) Bacterial infection of pancreatic necrosis. In: Beger HG, Büchler M (eds) Acute pancreatitis. Springer, Berlin Heidelberg New York, pp 314–317
20. Saxon A, Reynolds J, Doolas A (1981) Management of pancreatic abscess. Ann Surg 194:545–552
21. Videla C, Boria H, Bastias E (1983) Protocolo y manejo de la pancreatitis aguda. Bol Hosp Vina del Mar 39:27–36
22. Videla C, Cenitagoya G, Bergn C, Caimi L (1989) Sobrevida a corto plazo en la pancreatitis aguda grave. Rol del lavado peritoneal y cirugia conservadora. Rev Med Chil 117:258–265
23. Warshaw A, Gongliang J (1985) Improved survival in 45 patients with pancreatic abscess. Ann Surg 202:408–415
24. Welch J, White C (1982) Acute pancreatic of biliary origin: is urgent operation necessary? Am J Surg 143:120–125
25. Yarmuch J, Burdiles P, Schutte H, Csendes A, Meza P, Chiong H (1990) Absceso pancratico. Rev Chil Cir 42:234–237

II. Chronic Pancreatitis

Epidemiology of Chronic Pancreatitis

J. Mössner[1]

The epidemiology of chronic pancreatitis (CP) can be seen in terms of various aspects. A prerequisite is a clear definition of the disease, which enables us to compare reports in the literature on epidemiology of CP in various parts of the world [25]. In the following we discuss aspects of the various etiologic factors of CP, such as alcohol, diet, and genetics. Knowledge about etiology may help to explain data on incidence and prevalence of CP with regards to sex, age, and demography. Special emphasis is placed on the discussion of tropical pancreatitis. Prognosis of CP is another epidemiological aspect. Thus, we must discuss special aspects of the clinical course of the disease and the association with other diseases.

Etiology of Chronic Pancreatitis

An etiologic classification of pancreatic insufficiency comprises alcohol abuse, dietary factors (tropical CP), hypercalcemia, and in very rare cases trauma [16]. True hereditary pancreatitis is also very rare. Chronic obstructive pancreatitis is a separate entity [25]. Pancreatic insufficiency may exist without underlying CP. These diseases can be divided into primary pancreatic insufficiency (cystic fibrosis, Shwachman syndrome, lipase deficiency, pancreatic resections) or secondary insufficiency (mucosal small – bowel disease with lack of release of cholecystokinin and secretin, gastric resections, gastrinoma, and enterokinase deficiency) [16].

Alcohol consumption is associated with a wide variety of effects on the exocrine pancreas [63, 64]. These divergent effects are dependent on the amount and duration of alcohol consumption, whether humans or animals are studied, on the route of alcohol application, etc. Furthermore, the effects of ethanol on the exocrine pancreas may be indirect, mediated by neurotransmitters, hormones, or direct.

Chronic ethanol abuse is the most common cause of acute and chronic pancreatitis in industrialized nations [64]. There is still controversy whether

[1] Medizinische Poliklinik, University of Würzburg, Klinikstraße 8, W-8700 Würzburg, FRG

Beger/Büchler/Malfertheiner (Eds.)
Standards in Pancreatic Surgery

alcohol-induced pancreatitis always leads to chronic disease, or whether a nonprogressive alcohol-induced pancreatitis exists [54, 60]. In industrialized countries probably about 85% of all cases of CP are caused by alcohol abuse [1, 2, 17, 53–55]. There is no doubt about a strong correlation between the amount of alcohol consumption and the risk of developing CP [14, 27, 59]. The Marseille group reported a linear relationship between the logarithm of the risk of developing CP and the daily consumption of ethanol (Durbec 1978). Thus, there is no threshold for alcohol toxicity as compared to liver cirrhosis [59]. However, the female pancreas seems to be more sensitive to alcohol. In countries with a higher mean alcohol consumption the duration of alcohol consumption before the onset of symptoms is shorter [59]. Quantity and duration of alcohol consumption is the major risk factor, while neither the type of alcoholic beverage (wine, beer, sugar-cane based, rice alcohol, whisky) nor the rhythm of alcohol consumption (regularly or weekends) seem to have any influence [57].

Patients with alcohol-induced CP are very often in the fourth decade of age at onset of the first symptoms, as compared to patients with liver cirrhosis who are about 10 years older in most cases. In France the average duration of alcohol abuse before the onset of the first attack of pancreatitis is 18 ± 11 years in men and 11 ± 8 years in women [18]. This may explain the age difference between CP and liver cirrhosis because it obviously needs a longer duration of alcohol abuse to cause cirrhosis.

The incidence and prevalence of CP is therefore related to the general alcohol consumption of a population. In Europe CP is especially frequent in France and Italy; in Germany there seems to be an increase as well as in Sweden, Denmark, and the United Kingdom [7, 14, 20, 43, 56]. In Germany consumption of beer increased continuously after World War II and reached a plateau around 1973 with about 150 l beer per year per capita [27]. Alcoholism is also the major cause of CP in South Africa except among the black Africans in Durban where protein deficiency seems to play the major role [32, 37]. Probably due to the lower alcohol consumption in Japan, the incidence of CP is relatively low in this country [28]. Because alcohol consumption is higher in men than in women, CP is mostly seen in men [49]. Thus, alcohol abuse is the main cause of CP in Europe, the United States, South America [15, 39], Mexico, South Africa, and Japan [57]. In some countries of Africa alcohol consumption also seems to be the major etiologic factor, such as in Senegal [11], Madagascar [33], and Uganda [62].

It has been hypothesized that a diet high in fat and protein predisposes alcoholics to pancreatitis [18, 56, 57]. The amount of total proteins consumed is said to be related to the logarithm of the relative risk of developing CP in a linear fashion. Fat intake, however, is related quadratically to the risk of developing CP [18]. Both high (above 100 g/day) and very low (below 85 g/day) fat consumption are reported to be risk factors. This hypothesis, however, has not been confirmed by studies on nutritional intake in the United States and Australia [34, 48, 69].

Many alcoholics smoke. This may explain the strong association between CP and smoking cigarettes. This association, however, was seen only in men [70].

There are some reports that heredity may be a risk factor for alcoholic pancreatitis [29]. There seem to be more patients with blood group 0 [32]. The phenotype P_1MZ of α_1-antitrypsin was more prevalent and P_1MM less prevalent in CP in South Africa. The authors suggest that a heterozygous deficiency of this protease inhibitor may be responsible for the pancreas being more vulnerable to ethanol [45]. Other studies found an increased frequency of HLA Cw5, B40 in Europe, HLA B13 in Japan, HLA-w23 and w24 in Brasil, and HLA Bw39 in Australia [59, 63, 64]. True hereditary CP is very rare [13, 23, 65]. Recently, eight cases of hereditary CP were reported in a 35-member three-generation kindred [44]. No linkage was found between CP and either ABO/Rh blood groups or HLA haplotypes in this family.

A variable proportion of up to 30% of patients are labeled as having idiopathic CP [16].

Association of Pancreatitis with Acute Alcohol Consumption

Blood samples of 300 subjects suspected of drunken driving were analyzed for concentrations of pancreatic and hepatic enzymes. Serum amylase and trypsin levels were higher than twice the upper normal limit in only three subjects. The authors conclude that other factors in addition to alcohol are necessary to initiate pancreatitis [42].

Incidence and Prevalence of Chronic Pancreatitis

There are no exact data with regards to the true incidence and prevalence of the disease in various countries. This lack of knowledge may be explained by many factors. (a) Diagnosis of CP is still not easy, especially at the beginning of the disease, with no signs of maldigestion and no endocrine insufficiency. (b) Despite the revised definition of CP given by the second symposium at Marseilles [25], CP may be misdiagnosed as acute pancreatitis. (c) Very often a diagnosis of CP may be simply wrong in those patients who actually have functional abdominal problems. (d) Statistics derived from postmortem examinations [27] cannot be extrapolated to the general population because in most countries the rate of autopsies has decreased dramatically. (e) The diagnosis on death certificates does not help for exact statistical analysis [27]. This diagnosis may be wrong, or the diagnosis may be mentioned regarding only the cause of death but excluding other relevant diseases such as CP; this may be particularly true in those cases in which CP was not directly related to the cause of death.

In two studies, one from the Mayo Clinic and one from Copenhagen, the incidence of CP was remarkably similar; 3.5 and 4 per 100 000 population [14, 47]. In Copenhagen the prevalence of documented and possible CP per 100 000 citizens aged 20 years or more was 27.4.

Tropical-Type Chronic Pancreatitis

In many Third World countries, such as India, Indonesia, Sri Lanka, Tunisia, Uganda, and Nigeria, most cases of chronic calcifying pancreatitis are clearly not related to alcohol abuse [12]. Patients are younger at the onset of the disease and malnutrition seems to play a major pathogenetic factor [9, 21, 40, 46, 61, 71]. This typical tropical form is especially found in the southern Indian state of Kerala [21]. The mean age at onset is 12.5 years. There is no sex difference. Pain is less common, and first symptoms are very often a consequence of insulin insufficiency. The diet in Kerala is very low in fat and protein. However, the demographic distribution of tropical CP and kwashiorkor is not identical [59]. Cyanogenetic glycosides present in cassava have been suggested as a potential pathogenetic factor. However, cassava is also ingested in large amounts in the Ivory Coast, where CP is rare [58]. There is one case report of a 40-year-old woman who was taking a cassava-based diet and developed calcific pancreatitis and goiter [41].

In Mexico there are two groups of patients with CP: one with typical alcohol-induced CP, consisting mainly of men with a mean age at clinical onset of 41 years and a high dietary intake of fat and protein, and the other a nonalcoholic group with female preponderance and a mean age at onset of 23 years. This group does not exactly ressemble tropical pancreatitis because patients are not malnourished [51, 67].

Some Aspects on Clinical Course and Outcome of Chronic Pancreatitis

In a prospective long-term observation of 205 cases of alcoholic and 82 cases of nonalcoholic pancreatitis from Switzerland, a typical continuous alteration in the clinical picture, pancreatic function, and morphology is reported [6]. According to the Swiss experience there are three typical models of the disease: (a) early and (b) late stage of uncomplicated CP, and (c) complicated CP with mostly pseudocysts or duct obstruction. Persistent freedom of pain occurs in parallel with the decrease in pancreatic functional capacity. In patients with alcoholic relapsing calcific pancreatitis 85% were pain free within a median time of 4.5 years from the clinical onset of the disease [3]. Of these patients 47% underwent surgery, mostly due to complications such as pseudocysts. The rate of progression of exocrine function and the incidence of diabetes are higher in alcoholic CP as compared to nonalcoholic idiopathic CP [4, 16]. Up to 90% of patients develop calcifications. However, interestingly, one-third of patients in the Swiss study showed a decrease in calcifications in late phases of the disease [5]. Our own experience on 100 patients with documented CP from northern Bavaria confirms the Swiss experience in many aspects, such as frequency of operations and development of a painless stage [38]. However, in most cases we do not see a decrease in calcifications.

Prognosis

According to the reports from Zurich, the 50% survival time in chronic alcoholic pancreatitis is 20–24 years after the clinical onset of disease, thus being shorter as compared to nonalcoholic CP. Only 20% of deaths were related to pancreatitis; the extrapancreatic causes were malignancies, cardiovascular diseases, severe infections, and nonpancreatic surgery [3]. Abstinence from alcohol clearly has a beneficial effect on the further outcome of the disease [10, 26, 31, 59]. However, despite cessation of alcohol abuse the pancreatic functional impairment progresses [24]. According to a French study on 240 patients with CP followed for a mean time of 8.7 years the "overmortality" after 20 years was 35.8%. During the observation period 57 patients (23.7%) died. CP was the direct cause of death for only 19.3% of patients. Main other causes of death were alcoholic hepatopathy (n = 10), cancer (n = 9), and postoperative mortality (n = 8) [30]. In a Japanese study a low rate of deaths directly related to CP was also found. Frequent causes of death were cancer- and diabetes-associated conditions such as renal failure, hypoglycemia, and pneumonia [35].

Mortality of CP is highest in Hungary (0.9 per 100000) and lowest in Japan (0.06) [43]. In 1986 in the Federal Republic of Germany CP was the cause of death in 1.8 cases per 1000 deaths in the age group between 31 and 40. This rate decreased with further increase in age [43]. However, with regard to the size of population the death rate due to CP increased continuously with age (24 deaths per 1000000 living citizens in the age group above 80 years; about ten cases were reported in the age group between 61 and 70 [43]. These results, however, may conceal a considerable bias due to the problem of accuracy of diagnosis on death certificates.

Association of Chronic Pancreatitis with Other Diseases

In an Italian study on 40 patients with alcoholic CP, 29 had abnormal liver histology with 5 documented cases of liver cirrhosis. Five out of 32 liver cirrhosis patients hat CP according to typical duct abnormalities on endoscopic retrograde cholangiopancreatography (ERCP) [8]. Since the simultaneous occurrence of liver cirrhosis and CP was low, the authors conclude that besides alcohol other important factors may play a role in the pathogenesis of both diseases. There is no prospective study published in the literature investigating the coexistance of CP and liver cirrhosis in a non-selected group of alcoholics [66]. However, the coexistence of these two diseases is probably higher than believed, according to earlier studies by Ammann and Sarles [66], and may be in the range of about 20%–30% ([19, 22, 50] for further literature see Teschke 1983 [66]). In a study from Germany on 107 patients with radiologically confirmed pancreatic calcifications, liver cirrhosis or advanced alcoholic hepatitis was found in 28%. The authors suggest that the time factor may explain the lack of a greater association [36]. In a retrospective study on 112 chronic alcoholics ERCP and liver biopsy was performed; 65 patients had CP according to typical signs on ERCP, and 20/65 (30.7%) suffered from additional liver cirrhosis [22].

According to 26221 sections performed at the Institute for Pathology at the University of Heidelberg beween 1950 and 1982, there was a significant coexsistence of several other diseases such as duodenal ulcer, bile stones, cholecystitis, thrombosis of the portal vein, general arteriosclerosis, colonic polyps, and diverticula together with CP [27]. According to studies on 132 patients with proven CP in Northern Italy, the disease characteristics were similar to those described in France by Sarles and coworkers [56]. However, a higher frequency of gallstones was found [68].

It has been suggested that CP is an independent risk factor of pancreatic as well as extrapancreatic cancers [52]. However, the epidemiolgical data discerning the risks related to alcohol, smoking, and malnutrition from CP per se are scarce.

References

1. Ammann RW, Hammer B, Fumagalli I (1973) Chronic pancreatitis in Zürich, 1963–1972. Clinical findings and follow-up studies of 102 cases. Digestion 9: 404–415
2. Ammann RW, Knoblauch M, Möhr P et al. (1980) High incidence of extra-pancreatic carcinoma in chronic pancreatitis. Scand J Gastroenterol 15:395–399
3. Ammann RW, Akovbiantz A, Largiader F, Schüler G (1984) Course and outcome of chronic pancreatitis. Longitudinal study of a mixed medical-surgical series of 245 patients. Gastroenterology 86:820–828
4. Ammann RW, Bühler H, Münch R, Freiburghaus AW, Siegenthaler W (1987) Differences in the natural history of idiopathic (nonalcoholic) and alcoholic chronic pancreatitis. A comparative long-term study of 287 patients. Pancreas 2:368–377
5. Ammann RW, Münch R, Otto R, Bühler H, Freiburghaus AU, Siegenthaler W (1988) Evolution and regression of pancreatic calcification in chronic pancreatitis. A prospective long-term study of 107 patients. Gastroenterology 95:1018–1028
6. Ammann R (1989) Klinik, Spontanverlauf und Therapie der chronischen Pankreatitis. Unter spezieller Berücksichtigung der Nomenklaturprobleme. Schweiz Med Wochenschr 119:696–706

7. Andersen BN, Pedersen NT, Scheel J, Worning H (1982) Incidence of alcoholic chronic pancreatitis in Copenhagen. Scand J Gastroenterol 17:247–252
8. Angelini G, Merigo F, Degani G, Camplani N, Bovo P, Fratta Pasini A, Cavallini G, Brocco G, Scuro LA (1985) Association of chronic alcoholic liver and pancreatic disease: a prospective study. Am J Gastroenterol 80:998–1003
9. Banwell JG, Hutt MRS, Leonard PJ, Blackman V, Connor DW, Marsden PD, Campbell J (1967) Exocrine pancreatic disease and the malabsorption syndrome in tropical Africa. Gut 8:388–401
10. Capitaine Y, Roche B, Wiesner L, Hahnloser P (1988) Pancreátite chronique: histoire naturelle et évolution en relation avec l'alcoolisme. Schweiz Med Wochenschr 118:817–820
11. Carayon A, Onde M, Rousselet M (1967) Evolution de la pathologie pancreatique de l'Africain (a propos de 26 observations). Bull Soc Med Afr Noire Lang Fr 12:287–293
12. Chatti N, Chaieb L, Jemni L, Letaief R, Tlili-Graies K, Hochlef S, Zinelabidine Y, Allegue M, Hamida RB (1990) Juvenile idiopathic chronic calcifying pancreatitis: report of 10 cases from central Tunisia. Pancreas 5:354–357
13. Comfort MW, Steinberg AG (1952) Pedigree of a family with hereditary chronic relapsing pancreatitis. Gastroenterology 21:54–63
14. Copenhagen Pancreatitis Study Group (1981) An interim report from a prospective epidemiological multicenter study. Scand J Gastroenterol 16: 305–312
15. Dani R, Noguera CED, Furtado M, Leal S (1974) Epidemiology and aetiology of chronic calcifying pancreatitis in Belo Horizonte, Brazil, and chronic calcifying pancreatitis in Brazil. Morphological study. Rendic Gastroenterol 6:153–164
16. DiMagno EP, Clain JE (1986) Chronic pancreatitis. In: Go VLW, Gardner JD, Brooks FP, Lebenthal E, DiMagno EP, Scheele GA (eds) The exocrine pancreas. Raven, New York, pp 541–575
17. Dürr HK (1978) Alkoholschädigung des Pankreas. Internist 19:123–130
18. Durbec JP, Sarles H (1978) Multicenter survey on the etiology of pancreatic diseases. Relationship between the relative risk of developing chronic pancreatitis and alcohol, protein, and lipid consumption. Digestion 18:337–350
19. Dutta SK, Mobrahan S, Iber FL (1978) Associated liver disease in alcoholic pancreatitis. Dig Dis 23:618–622
20. Gastard J, Joubaud F, Farbos T, Loussouarn J, Marion J, Pannier M, Renaudet F, Valdazo R, Gosselin M (1973) Etiology and course of primary chronic pancreatitis in western France. Digestion 9:416–428
21. Gevarghese PJ, Pillai VK, Joseph MP, Pitchumoni CS (1962) The diagnosis of pancreatogenous diabetes mellitus. J Assoc Physicians India 10:173–180
22. Greiner L, Schubert E, Franken FH (1983) Koinzidenz von chronischer Pankreatitis und Leberzirrhose bei Alkoholabusus. Eine röntgen- und histomorphologische Studie. Z Gastroenterol 21:526–532
23. Gross J, Gambill EE, Ulrich JA (1962) Hereditary pancreatitis. Description of fifth kindred and summary of clinical features. Am J Med 33:358–362
24. Gullo L, Barbara L, Labò G (1988) Effect of cessation of alcohol use on the course of pancreatic dysfunction in alcoholic pancreatitis. Gastroenterology 95:1063–1068
25. Gyr K, Singer M, Sarles H (1984) Proceedings of the 2nd International Symposium of Pancreatitis. Elsevier, Amsterdam
26. Hayakawa T, Kondo T, Shibata T, Sugimoto Y, Kitagawa M (1989) Chronic alcoholism and evolution of pain and prognosis in chronic pancreatitis. Dig Dis Sci 34:33–38
27. Höpker WW (1987) Epidemiology of pancreatic diseases. Verh Dtsch Ges Pathol 71:144–160

28. Ishii K, Nakamura K, Takeuchi T, Hirayama T (1973) Chronic calcifying pancreatitis and pancreatic carcinoma in Japan. Digestion 9:429–437
29. Lankisch PG, Hierholzer E, Koop H, Kaboth U, Koch HF (1980) HLA-antigens in acute and chronic pancreatitis. Z Gastroenterol 18:524–526
30. Levy P, Milan C, Pignon JP, Baetz A, Bernades P (1989) Mortality factors associated with chronic pancreatitis. Gastroenterology 96:1165–1172
31. Little JM (1987) Alcohol abuse and chronic pancreatitis. Surgery 101:357–360
32. Marks IN, Bank S, Louw JH (1973) Chronic pancreatitis in the western Cape. Digestion 9:447–453
33. Merlihot J (1963) Quelques observations de pancreatites chroniques a Madagascar. Med Trop (Mars) 23:52–62
34. Mezey E, Kolman CJ, Diehl AM, Mitchell MC, Herlong HF (1988) Alcohol and dietary intake in the development of chronic pancreatitis and liver disease in alcoholism. Am J Clin Nutr 48:148–151
35. Miyake H, Harada H, Ochi K, Kunichika K, Tanaka J, Kimura I (1989) Prognosis and prognostic factors in chronic pancreatitis. Dig Dis Sci 34:449–455
36. Mörl M, Piechulek H (1987) Leberschaden bei chronisch-kalzifizierter, alkoholinduzierter Pankreatitis. Z Gastroenterol 25:325–330
37. Moshal MG (1973) A study of chronic pancreatitis in Natal. Digestion 9:438–446
38. Mössner J, Weth G (1981) Verlaufsbeobachtung bei der chronischen Pankreatitis. Therapiewoche 31:8167–8176
39. Mott C de R, Ohki Y, Barros MIB, Conte VP, Machado MCC, Bove P, Bettarello A (1975) Aspectos etic patogenicos das pancreatitas cronicas. Observacao de 80 casos. Rev Assoc Med Minas Gerais 21:281–284
40. Nagaratnam N, Gunawardene KRW (1972) Aetiological factors in pancreatic calcification in Ceylon. Digestion 5:9–16
41. Narendranathan M (1988) Calcific pancreatitis and goitre in cassava toxicity. Indian J Gastroenterol 7:169–170
42. Niederau C, Niederau M, Strohmeyer G, Bertling L, Sonnenberg A (1990) Does acute consumption of large alcohol amounts lead to pancreatic injury? A prospective study of serum pancreatic enzymes in 300 drunken drivers. Digestion 45:115–120
43. Niederau M, Niederau C (1991) Epidemiologie der Pankreaserkrankungen. In: Niederau C (ed) Neue Aspekte in der Diagnostik und Therapie von Pankreaserkrankungen. TM Verlag, Hameln (in press)
44. Nordback I, Saarenpaeae-Heikkilae O, Koskimies S (1990) Screening a family for hereditary chronic pancreatitis. Panminerva Med 32:19–24
45. Novis BH, Young GO, Bank S, Marks IN (1975) Chronic pancreatitis and alpha$_1$-antitrypsin. Lancet ii:748–749
46. Olurin EO, Olurin O (1969) Pancreatic calcification: a report of 45 cases. Br Med J 4:534–539
47. O'Sullivan JN, Nobrega FT, Morlock CG, Brown AL, Bartholomew LG (1972) Acute and chronic pancreatitis in Rochester, Minnesota, 1940 to 1969. Gastroenterology 62:373–379
48. Pitchumoni CS, Sonnenshein M, Candido FM, Panchacharam P, Cooperman JM (1980) Nutrition in the pathogenesis of alcoholic pancreatitis. Am J Clin Nutr 33:631–636
49. Read G, Braganza JM, Howat HT (1976) Pancreatitis – a retrospective study. Gut 17:945–952
50. Renner IG, Savage WT 3d, Stace NH, Pantoja JL, Schultheis WM, Peters RL (1984) Pancreatitis associated with alcoholic liver disease. A review of 1022 autopsy cases. Dig Dis Sci 29:593–599
51. Robles-Diaz G, Vargas F, Uscanga L, Fernandez-del Castillo C (1990) Chronic pancreatitis in Mexico City. Pancreas 5:479–483
52. Rocca G, Gaia E, Iuliano R, Caselle MT, Rocca N, Calcamuggi G, Emanuelli G (1987) Increased incidence of cancer in chronic pancreatitis. J Clin Gastroenterol 9:175–179

53. Sarles H, Sarles JC (1964) Chronische alkoholische Pankreatitis. Chronische calcifizierende Pankreatitis. Verh Dtsch Ges Inn Med 70:773–780
54. Sarles H, Sarles J-C, Camatte R, Muratore R, Gaini M, Guien C, Pastor J, LeRoy F (1965) Observations on 205 confirmed cases of acute pancreatitis, recurring pancreatitis, and chronic pancreatitis. Gut 6:545–559
55. Sarles H (1971) Alcoholism and pancreatitis. Scand J Gastroenterol 6:193–198
56. Sarles H (1973) An international survey on nutrition and pancreatitis. Digestion 9:389–403
57. Sarles H, Cros RC, Bidart JM and International Group for the Study of Pancreatic Diseases (1979) A multicenter inquiry into the etiology of pancreatic diseases. Digestion 19:110–125
58. Sarles H, Sauniere JF, Attia Y, Lombardo A, D'ri Yoman T, Manlan K, Laugier R, Sahel J (1984) Pancreatic function in children and chronic calcified pancreatitis in Ivory Coast. The tropical form of CCP is not due to kwashiorkor or cassava. In: Gyr KE, Singer MV, Sarles H (eds) Pancreatitis. Concepts and classification. Elsevier, Amsterdam, pp 365–366
59. Sarles H (1986) Chronic pancreatitis: etiology and pathophysiology. In: Go VLW, Gardner JD, Brooks FP, Lebenthal E, DiMagno EP, Scheele GA (eds) The exocrine pancreas. Raven, New York, pp 527–540
60. Seligson U, Cho JW, Ihre T, Lundh G (1982) Clinical course and autopsy findings in acute and chronic pancreatitis. Acta Chir Scand 148:269–274
61. Shaper AG (1960) Chronic pancreatic disease and protein malnutrition. Lancet i:1223–1224
62. Shaper AG (1964) Aetiology of chronic pancreatic fibrosis with calcification seen in Uganda. Br Med J 1:1607–1609
63. Singer MV (1985) Pankreas und Alkohol. Schweiz Med Wochenschr 115: 973–987
64. Singh M, Simsek H (1990) Ethanol and the pancreas. Current status. Gastroenterology 98:1051–1062
65. Stafford RJ, Grand RJ (1982) Hereditary disease of the exocrine pancreas. Clin Gastroenterol 11:141–170
66. Teschke R (1983) Hohe Inzidenzrate von chronischer Pankreatitis und Leberzirrhose bei chronischem Alkoholabusus? Z Gastroenterol 21:533–535
67. Uscanga L, Robles-Diaz G, Sarles H (1985) Nutritional data and etiology of chronic pancreatitis in Mexico. Dig Dis Sci 30:110–113
68. Vantini I, Piubello W, Cavallini G, Enderle A, Benini L, Scuro LA (1978) Chronic pancreatitis in north-east Italy: a clinical and pathological study. Acta Hepato-Gastroenterol 25:130–135
69. Wilson JS, Bernstein L, McDonald C, Tait A, McNeil D, Pirola RC (1985) Diet and drinking habits in relation to the development of alcoholic pancreatitis. Gut 26:882–887
70. Yen S, Hsieh CC, MacMahon B (1982) Consumption of alcohol and tobacco and other risk factors for pancreatitis. Am J Epidemiol 116:407–414
71. Zuidema PJ (1959) Cirrhosis and disseminated calcification of the pancreas in patients with malnutrition. Trop Geogr Med 11:70–74

Some Etiological and Pathogenetic Aspects of Chronic Alcoholic Pancreatitis

M.K. MÜLLER[1] and M.V. SINGER[1]

This short overview concentrates on some relevant new data on the etiology and pathogenesis of chronic alcoholic pancreatitis. For further information the reader is referred to more extensive reviews on alcohol and chronic alcoholic pancreatitis which have been published recently [25, 28, 31, 36].

In the majority of patients chronic pancreatitis is caused by nutritive factors (Table 1). Chronic alcohol consumption often in connection with a diet rich in fat and protein in industrialized countries or a macro- and micronutrient deficient diet in childhood in areas with endemic protein deficiency are most often associated with chronic pancreatitis. Other forms of chronic pancreatitis are caused by or associated with metabolic disorders, ductal obstruction, or hereditary factors, or they are idiopathic:

Nutritive causes
- Alcohol
- Deficiency in protein and trace elements; toxins

Metabolic causes
- Hypercalcemia

Pancreatic duct obstruction
- Pancreas divisum
- Scarring, strictures
- Tumors

Unknown causes
- Hereditary
- Idiopathic

Alcoholic Chronic Pancreatitis

Alcohol is the dominant etiological factor in chronic pancreatitis, and the significant increase in the incidence rate in the industrialized countries is paralleled by a marked increase in alcohol consumption. This connection has been clearly demonstrated by a linear relationship between alcohol

[1] Department of Medicine IV, (Gastroenterology), University Hospital of Heidelberg at Mannheim, Theodor Kutzer Ufer, W-6800 Mannheim, FRG

Beger/Büchler/Malfertheiner (Eds.)
Standards in Pancreatic Surgery

Table 1. Etiology of chronic pancreatitis in western Europe

Etiology	Frequency (%)
Nutritive causes, alcohol, deficiency in protein and trace elements; toxins	50–70
Metabolic causes, hypercalcemia	0–5
Pancreatic duct obstruction, scarring, strictures, tumors, pancreas divisum	2–20
Unknown causes, idiopathic, hereditary	10–30

consumption and the logarithmic risk for chronic pancreatitis [9]. Depending on regional variation in alcohol consumption, the form of chronic alcoholic pancreatitis ranges from 40%–50% in northern Europe to 90% in southern Europe [27].

Alcoholic chronic pancreatitis normally becomes clinically manifest about the middle or end of the 4th decade of life [4, 9, 28]. The interval between the beginning of regular alcohol consumption in substantial quantities and the first clinical manifestation averages 17–18 years in men and 10–12 years in women [9]. Numerous studies have shown that the appearance of calcifications increases with the duration of the disease. After about 15 years pancreatic calcifications are evident in more than 90% of patients [2, 5].

Although only a minority of alcoholics develop clinically apparent disease, distinct morphological alterations in the pancreas can be found at a much higher rate at autopsy, ranging from 19% to 58% [23, 26, 32].

In contrast to studies on the liver, no threshold toxic dose of daily alcohol consumption has been observed for the development of chronic pancreatitis. However, the average daily quantity of pure alcohol usually exceeds 60–80 g. Thus the quantity of pure alcohol but not the quality of the alcoholic beverage plays the decisive role.

Individuals who develop chronic pancreatitis early or even while consuming low amounts of alcohol or individuals who do not develop pancreatitis in spite of consuming higher amounts are possibly genetically more or less sensitive to the noxious effect of alcohol. In general, women – who represent 15% of patients with chronic alcoholic pancreatitis – seem to have both a lower threshold for developing the disease and are affected earlier than men [30].

Nutritional Factors Associated with Chronic Alcoholic Pancreatitis

Epidemiological data have shown that the risk for alcoholic pancreatitis increases with a diet high in protein and fat [9]. However, this relationship was not found in other studies in which patients did not have an increased consumption of calories [34] or had even a significantly lower intake of calories, fat, and protein as compared with a matched group of controls [23]. These findings can be reconciled by the notion that nutritional factors are additive, and that the absence of one factor can be compensated by the increase of one or several other factors. However, the relationship between chronic pancreatitis and protein and fat consumption is much weaker than that for alcohol. There are further indications that an insufficient supply of zinc or other trace elements such as copper or selenium [10, 12] plays a role.

Pathogenensis of Chronic Alcoholic Pancreatitis

The mechanism by which alcohol induces chronic pancreatitis is still a matter of dispute. Four theories are under discussion. The first step in the development of chronic pancreatitis is the effect of alcohol primarily on pancreatic exocrine secretion with resulting formation of protein plaques, leading to obstruction of intrapancreatic ductules; chronic pancreatic ischemia in addition to incomplete pancreatic duct obstruction causes chronic pancreatic lesions; the intracellular effect of alcohol on tissue integrity causes secondary alteration of pancreatic secretion; or an alcohol-induced dysfunction of the hepatic mixed-function oxidases releases emerging products which are toxic for the pancreas. In detail, the hypotheses are:

1. Primary intraductal obstruction (due to protein precipitates and calcifications)
   - Decrease in secretion of lithostathine S
   - Increase in viscosity of pancreatic juice
   - Increase in secretion of calcium
   - Decrease in secretion of citrate
2. Combined chronic ischemic and incomplete duct obstruction
   - Inflammatory, embolic, arterosclerotic lesions in combination with precipitates
3. Primary toxic-metabolic actions of alcohol
   - Toxic metabolites of the lipid metabolism
4. Primary disordered hepatic "detoxification"
   - Regurgitation of free radicals and lipid peroxidation products

Theory of Primary Intraductal Obstruction

Clinical and experimental findings indicate that chronic alcohol uptake decreases bicarbonate and water secretion followed by an increase in protein secretion [24, 26]. Both actions increase the concentration of intraductal proteins and juice viscosity. Several factors, such as oversaturation, activation of enzymes, or reduction of substances which keep proteins soluble, may further contribute to the formation of protein plugs and calcifications in the pancreatic ductules. Recent data support the concept that chronic calcific pancreatitis results from precipitation of calcium salts with a specific pancreatic protein, lithostathine, a new family of secretory calcium stabilizers. These precipitations may cause focal obstructions.

Role of Lithostathine

Intraductal protein precipitates have been observed before ultrastructural or pathological damage to acinar and ductal cells. It was concluded from these observations that the initial lesion of chronic calcific pancreatitis is intraductal stone formation, i.e. chronic pancreatitis is a lithiasis. Precipitations would thus be the prime mover of the pathological process which finally leads to damage of the ductal basal membranes, atrophy of epithelia, and formation of other pathologic lesions [29].

Within the past few years Sarles and coworkers have described a protein which is involved in the process of protein calcification. Eosinophilic precipitates of protein have been found in the pancreatic juice and within the acini of patients with early chronic calcific pancreatitis [13, 19]. Protein plugs were also found in the pancreatic juice in 10% of normal controls, 21% of asymptomatic alcoholics, but in 65% of patients with chronic calcific pancreatitis. They are uncommon in the juice of patients with the obstructive form of chronic pancreatitis.

Biochemical studies revealed that the protein plugs are partly consistent of fibrillar protein. This protein was named lithostathine H2. It contains 133 amino acids, and is insoluble at neutral pH where it precipitates as fibrils [29]. Lithostathine H2 is derived from lithostathine S by hydrolytic cleavage. Lithostathine S is known as a secretory calcium salt stabilizer in pancreatic juice. Calcium stabilizers are secreted by the pancreas to prevent calcium nucleation and growth by blocking the growth sites of crystals. Such stabilizers are also present in other fluids such as saliva and urine.

Lithostathine is the major calcium stabilizer in pancreatic juice. It comprises a group of glycoproteins with a molecular mass of 15 000–19 000. The finding of a messenger RNA in acini, which is specific for lithostathine has confirmed its immunological entity [13, 14]. Lithostathine S is synthesized as a 144 amino acid precursor form. After cleavage from its initiation peptide, it is concentrated in zymogen granules and secreted into the pancreatic juice. Lithostathine S can be actively hydrolyzed by tryptic digestion, resulting in two forms: the N-terminal undecapeptide (lithostathine H1), which is glycosylated and soluble at physiological pH, and the non-glycosylated 133 C-terminal amino acid residue which is insoluble at neutral pH. Lithostathine S1 and H1, but not H2, inhibit nucleation and growth of calcium crystals (Fig. 1).

According to Sarles' group, the formation of calcium crystals in patients with chronic calcific pancreatitis is due to decreased synthesis of lithostathine. This theory is based on the observation that the specific messenger RNA encoding for lithostathine is decreased within the acini and in the pancreatic juice of patients with chronic calcific pancreatitis compared. This

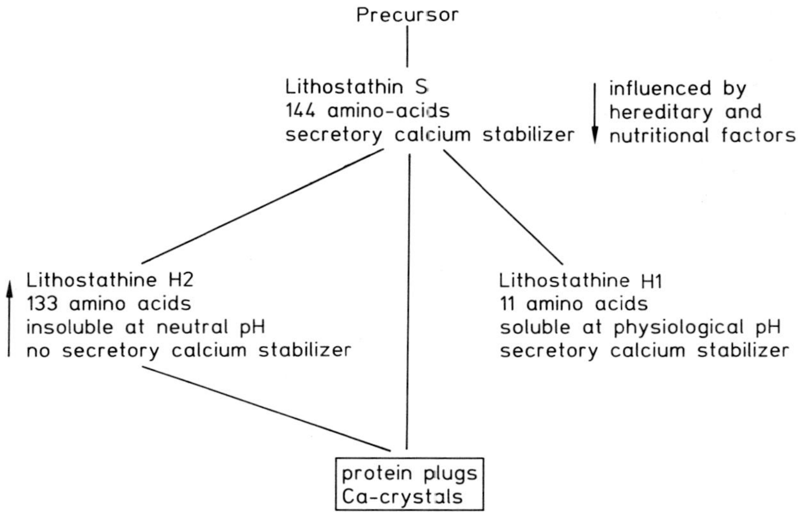

Fig. 1. Theory of primary intraductal obstruction as proposed by Sarles et al. 1989 [29]

occurs whether the disease is of alcoholic, hereditary, tropical, or idiopathic origin [8].

It seems clear from the available epidemiological data that decreased lithostathine secretion is probably due to hereditary and nutritional factors. These data may indicate that an endogenous disposition together with noxious factors which somehow interfere somewhere with acinar cell integrity might play an important role in the development of chronic calcific pancreatitis. Although this concept of the pathogenensis of chronic pancreatitis and the role of lithostathine S and H2 is not yet confirmed and not generally accepted, it seems at present to be the most plausible working hypothesis to explain the process of protein plugs and calcification in pancreatic ductules.

However, several questions need to be answered. It is still unknown what mechanisms cause enzymatic hydrolysis of lithostathine S to yield insoluble lithostathine H2, which is proposed to be a major part of protein-precipitates. Trypsin, lysosomal, or bacterial and coagulation enzymes and spontaneous cleavage of the unstable protein have been discussed without showing clear evidence for anyone of the mechanisms. It is also unclear, why diminished secretion of lithostathine S, a calcium stabilizer increases the formation of protein precipitations by its hydrolysis product lithostathine H2, which is thought to become the nucleus of pancreatic stones.

Other Factors Associated with Calcium-Protein Precipitations

Besides lithostathine there are other factors which are possibly of importance in alcoholics for the calcification of protein in the pancreatic

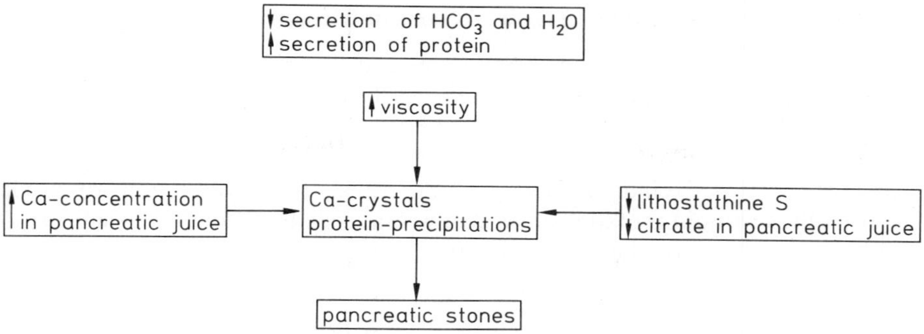

Fig. 2. Factors contributing to pancreatic calcifications

ductules: increase in viscosity of the pancreatic juice due to increased protein secretion, increase in secretion of calcium by acinus cells [17], and decrease in the concentration of citrate in the pancreatic juice [16] (Fig. 2).

Theory of Combined Chronic Ischemia and Incomplete Pancreatic Duct Obstruction

Investigations on the pathogenesis of chronic pancreatitis have recently stressed the importance of intrapancreatic blood perfusion in addition to ductal obstruction.

Investigations in experimental models have shown that complete obstruction of the pancreatic duct results in atrophy of the pancreatic parenchyma but incomplete or intermittent obstruction in histologic changes [11, 15, 33] which resemble those seen in human chronic pancreatitis. The role of pancreatic perfusion has been well established for acute pancreatitis, and studies with microspheres have clearly shown that acute pancreatitis can be produced with mechanical vascular blockage of small intapancreatic vessels [22]. Postmortem studies on patients with infarcts of the pancreas [18], celiac axis compression [35], thromboembolic occlusion of small pancreatic arteries [1], and a distinct form of chronic pancreatitis in elderly patients, which was termed senile pancreatitis [3], have also stressed the role of impaired blood perfusion for chronic pancreatitis due to inflammatory, embolic, or arterosclerotic lesions.

Recent investigations have now shown in an experimental model that chronic ischemia in combination with incomplete pancreatic duct obstruction results in histologic changes which were considered to resemble closely human chronic pancreatitis [33]. Pancreatic duct obstruction is here seen as a strong aggravating factor for the cellular damage which is primarily caused by chronic ischemia. The authors believe that these pathogenetic events are involved in the pathogenesis of chronic alcoholic pancreatitis.

Theory of Primary Toxic-Metabolic Actions of Alcohol

In contrast to Sarles' hypothesis which considers acinar cell damage primarily as a consequence of ductular obstruction by protein precipitates, Bordalo and coworkers have suggested that these alterations are secondary to fatty degeneration of pancreatic cells associated with loss of zymogen content and periacinar fibrosis [6, 20, 21]. The production of toxic metabolites of lipid metabolism in pancreatic cells by alcohol was suggested to be responsible for the development of chronic pancreatitis.

Theory of Primary Disordered Hepatic "Detoxification"

Another concept postulates disordered hepatic detoxification as the principal cause of chronic pancreatitis [7]. This concept is based on the findings that alcohol can induce hepatic mixed function oxidases. This process may be facilitated by an abundant nutritional intake of unsaturated fatty acids and is thought to be dependent on the individual genetic disposition. Products of hepatic "detoxification" (free radicals, lipid peroxidation products) are excreted into the bile and thus may cause damage to the pancreas after regurgitation into the duct system.

These hypotheses on the development of chronic alcoholic pancreatitis are still speculative. The hypothesis put forward by Sarles and coworkers is more substantiated than the others although many open questions remain. Most likely, however, the cause of alcoholic pancreatitis is multifactorial, comprising an interaction of vascular and metabolic-toxic as well as secretory changes in the acini on the basis of a genetically determined sensitivity to alcohol.

References

1. Aach R, Kissane I (1972) Chronic relapsing pancreatitis with cardiac and renal disease. Am J Med 53:335–343
2. Ammann R (1989) Klinik, Spontanverlauf und Therapie der chronischen Pankreatitis, unter spezieller Berücksichtigung der Nomenklaturprobleme. Schweiz Med Wochenschr 119:696–706
3. Ammann R, Sulser H (1976) Die "senile" chronische Pankreatitis – eine nosologische Einheit? Schweiz Med Wochenschr 106:429–437
4. Andersen BN, Thorsgaard Pedersen N, Scheel J, Worning H (1982) Incidence of alcoholic chronic pancreatitis in Copenhagen. Scand J Gastroenterol 17:247–252
5. Bernardes P et al. (1983) Histoire naturelle de la pancreatique chronique. Etude de 120 cas. Gastroenterol Clin Biol 7:8–13
6. Bordalo O, Bapista A, Dreiling D, Noronha M (1984) Early pathomorphological pancreatic changes in chronic alcoholism. In: Gyr KE, Singer MV, Sarles H (eds) Pancreatitis – concepts and classification. Elsevier, Amsterdam (Exerpta Medica, International Congress series no 642)
7. Braganza JM (1983) Pancreatic disease: a casualty of hepatic "detoxification"? Lancet ii(8357):1000–1003

8. De Caro A, Lohse J, Sarles H (1979) Characterization of a protein isolated from pancreatic calculi of men suffering from chronic calcifying pancreatitis. Biochem Biophys Res Commun 87:1176–1182
9. Durbec JP, Sarles H (1978) Multicenter survey of the etiology of pancreatic diseases. Relationship between the relative risk of developing chronic pancreatitis and alcohol, protein, and lipid consumption. Digestion 18:337–350
10. Dutta SK, Miller PA, Greenberg LB, Lavander OA (1983) Selenium and acute alcoholism. Am J Clin Nutr 38:713–718
11. Engel S, ReMine WH, Dockerty M, Grindlay J, Bartholomew LG (1962) Effect of ligation of pancreatic ducts on chronic pancreatitis. Arch Surg 85:1031–1035
12. Fell BF, King TP, Davies NT (1982) Pancreatic atrophy in copper-deficient rats: histochemical and ultrastructural evidence of a selective effect on acinar cells. Histochem J 14:665–680
13. Giorgi D, Bernhard JP, De Caro A, Multigner L, Lapointe R, Sarles H, Dagoren JC (1985) Pancreatic stone protein. I. Evidence that it is encoded by a pancreatic messenger ribonucleic acid. Gastroenterology 89:381–386
14. Giorgi D, Bernhard JP, Ranquier S, Iovanna J. Sarles H, Dagoren JC (1989) Secretary pancreatic stone protein messenger RNA. Nucleotide sequence and expression in chronic calcifying pancreatitis. J Clin Invest 84:100–106
15. Hermann RE, Davis JH (1960) The role of incomplete pancreatic duct obstruction in the etiology of pancreatitis. Surgery 48:318–329
16. Lohse J, Schmid D, Sarles H (1983) Pancreatic citrate and protein secretion of alcoholic dogs in response to graded doses of caerulein. Pflugers Arch 397:141–143
17. Lohse J, Pfeiffer A (1984) Duodenal total and ionised calcium secretion in normal subjects, chronic alcoholics, and patients with various stages of chronic alcoholic pancreatitis. Gut 25:874–880
18. McKay JW, Baggenstoss AH, Wollaeger EE (1958) Infarcts of the pancreas. Gastroenterology 35:256–264
19. Multigner I, Sarles H, Lombardo D, De Caro A (1985) Pancreatic stone protein II. Implication in stone formation during the course of chronic calcifying pancreatitis. Gastroenterology 89:387–391
20. Noronha M, Bordalo O, Dreiling DA (1981) Alcohol and the pancreas. II. Pancreatic morphology of advanced alcoholic pancreatitis. Am J Gastroenterol 76:120–124
21. Noronha M, Bapista A, Bordalo O (1984) Sequential aspects of pathology in chronic alcoholic disease of the pancreas. In: Gyr KE, Singer MV, Sarles H (eds) Pancreatitis – concepts and classification. Elsevier, Amsterdam (Excerpta Medica, International Congress series no 642)
22. Pfeffer RB, Lazzarini-Robertson A, Safadi D, Mixter G Jr, Secoy CF, Hinton JW (1962) Gradations of pancreatitis, edematous, through hemorrhagic, experimentally produced by controlled injection of microspheres into blood vessels in dogs. Surgery 51:764–769
23. Pitchumoni CS, Sonneshein M, Candido FM, Panchacharam P, Cooperman JM (1980) Nutrition in the pathogenesis of alcoholic pancreatitis. Am J Clin Nutr 33:631–636
24. Planche NE, Palasciano G, Meullenet J, Laughier R, Sarles H (1982) Effects of intravenous alcohol on pancreatic and biliary secretion in man. Dig Dis Sci 27:449–453
25. Reber HA (1987) Etiology, pathology and diagnosis. In: Howa IM, Jorda GL, Reber HA (eds) Surgical diseases of the pancreas. Lea and Febiger, Philadelphia
26. Renner IG, Savage WT, Pantoja JL, Renner VJ (1985) Death due to acute pancreatitis: a retrospective analysis of 405 autopsy cases. Dig Dis Sci 30:1005–1018
27. Sarles H (1985) Chronic calcyifing pancreatitis. Scand J Gastroenterol 20:651

28. Sarles H (1986) Chronic pancreatitis: ethiology and pathophysiology. In: Go VLW et al. (eds) The exocrine pancreas; chap 37. Raven, New York, pp 527–540
29. Sarles H, Bernhard JP, Johnson CD (1989) Pathogenesis and epidemiology of chronic pancreatitis. Ann Rev Med 40:453–468
30. Sarles H, Cros RC, Bidart JM (1979) A multicenter inquiry into the etiology of pancreatic disease. Digestion 19:110–125
31. Singer MV, Goebel H (1985) Acute and chonic actions of alcohol pancreatic exocrine secretion in humans and animals. In: Seitz HK, Kommerell B (eds) Alcohol diseases in gastroenterology. Springer, Berlin Heidelberg New York
32. Stigendal L, Olsson R (1984) Alcohol consumption pattern and serum lipids in alcoholic cirrhosis and pancreatitis. A comparative study. Scand J Gastroenterol 19:582–587
33. Tanaka T, Ichiba Y, Fujii Y, Itoh H, Kodama O, Dohi K (1988) New canine model of chronic pancreatitis due to chronic ischemia with incomplete pancreatic duct obstruction. Digestion 41:149–155
34. Voirol M, Infante F, Brahime-Reteneo O, Raymond L, Hollenweger V, Loizeau E (1980) Consommation d'alcool de tabac et de nutriments dans les affecitons pancréatiques. Schweiz Med Wochenschr 110:854–855
35. Watson WC, Sadikali F (1977) Experience with 20 patients and a critical appraisal of the syndrome. Ann Intern Med 86:278–284
36. Worning H (1989) Etiologic aspects of chronic pancreatitis. Int J Pancreatol 5:1–9
37. Worning H (1990) Incidence and prevalence of chronic pancreatitis. In: Beger HG, Büchler M, Ditschuneit H, Malfertheiner P (eds) Chronic pancreatitis. Springer, Berlin Heidelberg New York, pp 8–14

PSP, PTP, or REG Protein? The Role of Pancreatic Stone Protein*

W. Schmiegel[1]

Introduction

The occurrence of pancreatic calcifications in chronic pancreatitis (CP) has long been recognized [1–3] and accepted as a diagnostic criterion [3]. Among different pancreatic secretory proteins identified in the last decade, like pancreatic stone protein (PSP [4]), protein X [5], human pancreatic thread protein (PTP [6]), it has been argued that PSP plays a crucial role in the development of pancreatic calcifications, i.e., pancreatic stone formation.

PSP, a pancreatic acinar cell product [7], was initially characterized as a glycosylated acidic phosphoprotein of 14 kDa found as the major constituent of human pancreatic stones by H. Sarles and associates [4, 8]. Furthermore, by immunoprecipitating cell-free translation products of human pancreatic messenger RNA, the same group reported that PSP was a molecular entity [9] and not a degradation product of trypsinogen 1 or other pancreatic proteins as has been suggested by others [10].

PSP – referring to the acidic glycosylated phosphoprotein cited above – had been reported to suppress in vitro calcium carbonate precipitation [11]. Recent clinical investigations showed that PSP concentrations quantitated by radial immunodiffusion with a polyclonal antiserum were decreased in most pancreatic secretions derived from patients with chronic pancreatitis compared to controls. Decreased levels were especially prominent when pancreatic calcifications were present [12]. These findings continuously supported speculations about the etiopathogenic role of PSP in stone development during the course of chronic pancreatitis/chronic calcifying pancreatitis (CCP) ("lithiasis before being a pancreatitis") [12, 13].

In a preliminary investigation [14] we failed to confirm reduced PSP levels in pancreatic secretions of CP/CCP patients. This discrepancy has been related by others to the different assays applied [13, 15]. In an extended study [16] we report on PSP quantitations in pancreatic secretions and for

* This work was supported in part by grants No. 01 GA 8805, DFVLR-Bundes ministerium für Forschung und Technologie, and DFG-Schm/603-2, Deutsche Forschungsgemeinschaft

[1] Medizinische Kernklinik und Poliklinik, Universitätskrankenhaus Eppendorf, Martinistraße 52, W-2000 Hamburg 20, FRG

Beger/Büchler/Malfertheiner (Eds.)
Standards in Pancreatic Surgery

the first time in sera of patients suffering from chronic pancreatitis and other pancreatic diseases. These data confirmed our initial findings. They will be discussed in the light of recent reports by others [17] showing that PSP is actually highly homologous to protein X [5] and to bovine PTP [18] and most probably identical with the human PTP [6] described earlier.

Immunoassays

To quantitate PSP an antigen inhibition assay was developed. In this fluorochromogenic [19] assay the binding of PSP-specific monoclonal antibody (mAb) D4 [20, 21] to a solid phase bound target antigen (pure PSP or pancreatic secretion rich in PSP) is proportionately inhibited by prior incubation with soluble PSP (purified PSP for calibration, or PSP-containing samples). This incubation results in immunocomplex formation (PSP: mAb D4) which are removed before mAb D4 still free to react with solid phase bound target antigen is detected by a second antibody (antimouse immunoglobin) enzyme complex and subsequent substrate reaction. The extent of substrate turnover is inversely related to PSP concentrations analyzed.

The detection limits of the assay for PSP were 0.002 μg/ml–1.0 μg/ml, the optimal working range was reproducibly found to be linear in the range of 0.015–0.5 μg/ml.

Inter- and intra-assay variabilities rontinely estimated were at mean 0.013 μg/ml $\pm$ 0.015 μg/ml.

For better comparison with previous findings [22] PSP concentrations of pancreatic secretions were related to protein content and expressed in μg PSP per total pancreatic secretion protein minus albumin.

Patients

Pancreatic juice samples were obtained from a total of 70 patients by direct transduodenal cannulation of the pancreatic duct and aspiration under stimulation (secretin, 50 units i.v.; Boots, Nottingham, UK) [23]. Samples were transferred immediately to tubes and cleared by centrifugation for 5 min at 3000 g, 4°C. The supernatants were stored at −80°C until further analysis. Protease activity was routinely estimated by azocoll-substrate reaction (Calbiochem, Frankfurt, FRG) and not found to exceed 6×10^{-6} Anson units (range 0–5 units).

Group 1 comprised 31 patients suffering from chronic pancreatitis, with calcifications disclosed by abdominal X-ray, ultrasound or computed tomography (CT) in ten patients. Group 2 contained 22 patients with pancreatic cancer, group 3 consisted of 17 patients in whom a disorder of the pancreas had been excluded: sclerosing cholangitis (n = 1), cholelithiasis (n = 5), gastritis (n = 4), no disease (n = 7). Diagnostic pancreatograms were performed in all these patients prior to pancreatic juice aspiration which was done separately.

Serum samples were obtained from 20 patients with acute pancreatitis. In eight patients (three females, five males, age 33–75 years, mean 49 years) pancreatitis was ethanol related, in seven patients (three females, four males, age 65–83 years, mean 75 years) with acute pancreatitis bile stones were present, in one patient (female, age 29 years) apolipoprotein C-II deficiency associated hypertriglyceridemia (triglyceride: 6000 mg/100 ml) was found, while the etiology of the acute pancreatitis remained obscure in four patients. All patients had increased serum amylase (>34 U/l) and lipase (>190 U/l) enzyme activities.

Sixty-six serum samples were collected from patients suffering from chronic pancreatitis. This group comprised 26 females and 40 males, age 26–74 years, mean 48 years, who were admitted to hospital because of continuous or intermittent abdominal pain. All patients had a history of recurrent attacks of pancreatitis. Elevated serum amylase activities were noted in 26, and elevated lipase activities in 38 of these patients upon admission. ERCP was performed in 31 patients disclosing typical findings for chronic pancreatitis [24]. Pancreatic calculi were detected in 21 patients. In 38 patients chronic pancreatitis was clearly ethanol related, as was suspected but could not be proven in a further 11 patients, abuse of analgetics was

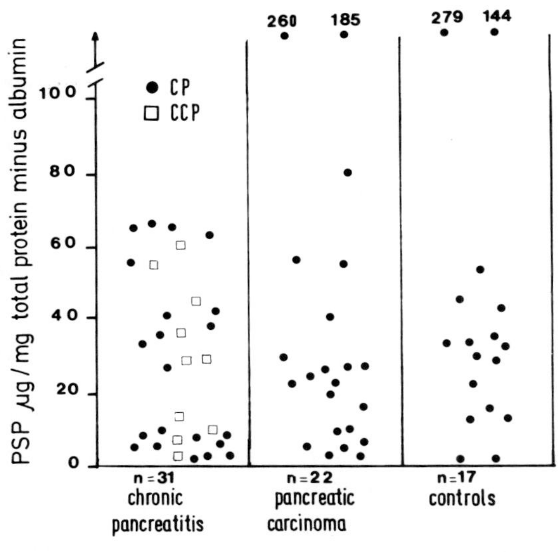

Fig. 1. Concentration of pancreatic stone protein (µg PSP per mg pancreatic secretion protein minus albumin) determined out of pancreatic secretions from patients with chronic pancreatitis (n = 31) with (□, n = 10) or without (●, n = 21) calcifications, pancreatic cancer (n = 22), nonpancreatic diseases (n = 17) as controls

discussed in three patients, and in 14 patients the etiology of chronic pancreatitis remained obscure.

Serum samples from normal blood donors ($n = 68$) served as controls.

PSP Quantitation in Pancreatic Juice Samples

PSP concentrations assessed from pancreatic secretions were related to protein content and expressed in μg PSP per total pancreatic secretion protein minus albumin. Three groups were analyzed:

Group 1. Chronic pancreatitis ($n = 31$): $\bar{x} = 27.5 \pm 23.4$ (0.4–67.0 μg PSP per mg protein).
Group 2. Pancreatic cancer ($n = 22$): $\bar{x} = 41.1 \pm 62.9$ (0.4–260 μg PSP per mg protein).
Group 3. Nonpancreatic diseases ($n = 17$): $\bar{x} = 47.1 \pm 67.9$ (0.6–279 μg PSP per mg protein).

The distribution of single PSP values of pancreatic secretions showed a considerable overlap between the three diagnostic groups (Fig. 1). Statistical analyses revealed no significant changes in PSP concentrations in chronic pancreatitis compared with pancreatic cancer ($p = 0.91$) or with normals ($p = 0.59$; Kruskal-Wallis test).

PSP Quantitation in Sera

Serum concentrations (μg/ml) were determined for four diagnostic groups:

Group 1. Chronic pancreatitis ($n = 66$): $\bar{x} = 2.101 \pm 3.112$ (0.15–20.0 PSP μg/ml). Patients suffering from chronic pancreatitis but normal serum pancreatic enzyme activities ($n = 31$) were separately evaluated for PSP concentrations: $\bar{x} = 3.32 \pm 5.01$ (0.15–20.0 PSP μg/ml).
Group 2. Acute pancreatitis ($n = 20$): $\bar{x} = 2.824 \pm 2.885$ (0.26–11.0 PSP μg/ml).
Group 3. Pancreatic cancer ($n = 25$): $\bar{x} = 1.052 \pm 1.171$ (0.16–4.0 PSP μg/ml).
Group 4. Serum of normal blood donors ($n = 68$): $\bar{x} = 0.326 \pm 0.158$ (0.16 – 0.9 PSP μg/ml).

A cut-off line for normal PSP values giving the 95% percentile of the control group (4) was made at ≤0.7 μg/ml (Fig. 2). In chronic pancreatitis approximately 60% (39/66) of the patients were found to have PSP values of >0.7 μg/ml, compared to 80% in acute pancreatitis, and 36% of the pancreatic cancer patients. The PSP levels of every pancreatic disease group differed highly significantly from serum PSP levels of normal blood donors ($p < 0.001$; Kruskal-Wallis test), and was not strictly correlated to the serum pancreatic enzyme activities in CP.

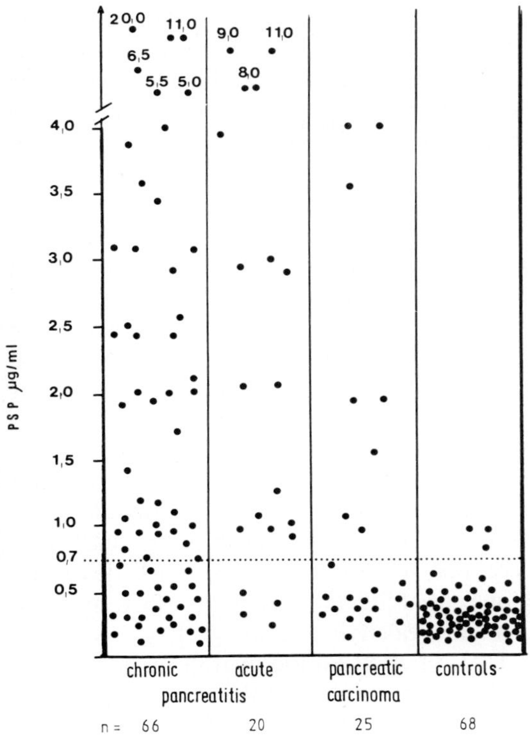

Fig. 2. Concentration of pancreatic stone protein in serum samples from patients with chronic pancreatitis ($n = 66$), acute pancreatitis ($n = 20$), pancreatic cancer ($n = 25$), and controls ($n = 68$)

Discussion

After PSP – extracted as an acidic glycosylated phosphoprotein [8] out of pancreatic stones – had been shown to be a potent inhibitor of calcium carbonate precipitation [11] both the Cambridge [25] and the subsequent second Marseille Classification of Pancreatitis [26] recommended PSP and its role in the pathogenesis of chronic pancreatitis as an important area for further investigations.

In accompanying papers it was demonstrated that PSP was not a degradation or release product but synthesized de novo (pre-PSP: M_r 16000), and was significantly lower within the pancreatic secretions of patients with chronic calcifying pancreatitis than in other diseases or controls [9, 12]. Until very recently the paradigmatic role attributed to PSP in the etiopathogenesis of chronic pancreatitis [27] has been largely based on these studies.

In a preliminary study we had failed to confirm reduced PSP concentrations within the pancreatic secretions of patients with chronic pancreatitis (CP/CCP) [14], thus the aim was to reinvestigate the pathological importance of pancreatic stone protein in chronic pancreatitis in an extended study. To survey the distribution of PSP in pancreatic secretions and in sera derived from patients suffering from chronic pancreatitis a sensitive quantitative immunoassay was established.

By means of this assay, PSP concentrations from pure pancreatic secretions were determined and expressed as micrograms of PSP per milligram of total pancreatic secretion protein minus albumin, as suggested recently [12]. The lowest PSP values were recorded in chronic pancreatitis patients ($\bar{x} = 27.5 \pm 23.4$). The values in pancreatic carcinoma were $\bar{x} = 41.1 \pm 62.9$, and in controls with nonpancreatic diseases, $\bar{x} = 47.1 \pm 67.9$. However, as outlined (Fig. 1), there was a considerable overlap in PSP values, and no statistical differences between groups could be found (CP/CCP vs controls $p = 0.59$; CP/CCP vs pancreatic cancer $p = 0.91$; Kruskal-Wallis test). Even in patients with chronic calcifying pancreatitis no obvious distinctions were observed compared with the noncalcifying form and/or other diagnostic groups, respectively. This is in contrast to recent findings which described generally decreased concentrations of PSP in pancreatic secretions in chronic pancreatitis, particularly in the calcifying forms [12], yet confirms our first preliminary experiments [14]. In addition the overall ranges of PSP values obtained in our study were lower, regardless of the diagnostic group, than those initially reported, which were assessed by polyclonal antiserum using the radial immunodiffusion technique [12]. To explain these continuing discrepancies, the different assays applied to quantitate PSP and new data evolved recently on the structure of PSP need further consideration.

Our preliminary results [14] have been confirmed very recently using mAb D4 [13, 15]. In contrast, radial immunodiffusion or radioimmunoassay applying polyclonal antiserum directed to PSP have been reported to show decreased concentrations of PSP within pancreatic secretions in chronic pancreatitis, and particularly in the calcifying forms [15] again. It was claimed that the polyclonal antiserum to PSP, in contrast to mAb D4, would specifically measure the PSP-S_{2-5} forms. These have been assumed to be particularly active in the inhibition of calcium carbonate precipitation [13] and reduced in CCP. This might be conceivable, yet no immunobinding studies (immunoprecipitation, western blotting) substantiating the postulated sub-specificities of the polyclonal antisera used in these assays have been made available so far. Likewise, mAb D4 used in preparative immunoadsorption to purify so-called secretory PSP-S_1 and the "active" higher molecular weight forms PSP-S_{2-5} [17, 20, 21] has not been cross-checked in analytical immunobinding studies (immunoprecipitation, western blotting) actually to provide specificities for the higher molecular weight forms (PSP-S_{2-5}). In our previous studies [16] studies these bands were not detected by western blotting, thus PSP quantitations referred to the 14 kDa molecule.

As already outlined, PSP was initially characterized as a glycosylated acidic phosphoprotein of 14 kDa [8]. The phosphoserine/phosphothreonine residues were considered essential for its function as a suppressor of in vitro calcium carbonate precipitation [11]. Recently, an amino acid composition rich in aromatic amino acids was reported by the same group [17], indicating that PSP is highly homologous to protein X [5] and to bovine PTP [18] and most probably identical with the human PTP [6] described earlier by Gross and colleagues. As for PTP, no phosphate residues were reported. The carbohydrate content was cited to be 5% (w/w) for PSP-S_{2-5} [28] in contrast to PTP, which lacks carbohydrate residues [6], yet estimated on the basis of detection by the Schiff reagent only [17]. In contrast to previous findings showing that PSP was de novo synthesized [9], recently, the PSP-S_{1-5} forms – all homologous in their C-terminal portions [29] – were related to tryptic release products of an unknown precursor molecule [29].

In contrast to pancreatic secretions serum analyses of the mAb D4-defined 14-kDa protein showed marked differences between the diagnostic groups. Highly significant ($p < 0.0001$; Kruskal-Wallis test) PSP elevations were noted in the majority of acute (80%) and chronic (60%) pancreatitis patients and pancreatic cancer patients when compared to controls. No comparable data on PSP or PTP serum concentrations in acute or chronic pancreatitis have been reported to date. PTP was not detected in a recent large series of normal sera [6], while in this study no PSP or low levels ($\leqslant 0.7\,\mu g/ml$) were found in the majority (95%) of the controls. It is noteworthy that PSP in chronic pancreatitis was also found significantly ($p < 0.0001$; Kruskal-Wallis test) elevated in patients with normal serum pancreatic enzyme activities. This may point to a release mechanism for PSP different from that employed by pancreatic enzymes. Whether this implies that serum PSP provides a suitable new indicator for pancreatic inflammation requires further exploration. Likewise further investigations will show whether the elevated PSP serum levels observed in 36% of the pancreatic cancer patients in this study are related to pancreatic duct obstruction by the underlying disease or to chronic pancreatitis occasionally found to coincide with pancreatic cancer (for review see [30]).

In summary, many questions addressed are waiting for a scientific resolution: What is the relationship of the PSP [4], originally described as a glycosylated acidic phosphoprotein [8], an inhibitor of calcium carbonate precipitation [11], synthesized de novo [9], and reduced in pancreatic secretions in CCP [12] to the PSP described later [17], rich in aromatic amino acids and identical to the PTP described by Gross before [6]? Without these data the renaming of PSP as "Lithostathine" as proposed recently [31] may be premature and confusing.

Moreover, our attention has been focused on the recent findings of Terazono and colleagues. They have identified [32] and meantimes sequenced [33] the entire reg gene encoding for the REG protein, which seems to be identical to PTP/PSP. Besides its expression in regenerating islets (for review see [34]), the REG protein has been found to be synthesized by distinct tumors like colorectal cancer [33]. Keeping this in mind as well as its reported homologies to pancreatic secretory trypsin inhibitor (PSTI) and to endothelial cell growth factor 2a [34] functions of PSP/PTP/REG other than that of a stone formation inhibitor may be found.

References

1. Friedreich N (1878) In: van Ziemssen H (ed) Cyclopaedia of the practice of medicine. Wood, New York, pp 600–603
2. Klob J (1860) Zur pathologischen Anatomie des Pankreas. Oesterr Z Prakt Heilkde (Wien) 6:629–634
3. Ring EJ, Eaton SB, Ferrucci JT, Short WF (1973) Differential diagnosis of pancreatic calcification. Am J Roentgenol 117:446–452
4. De Caro A, Lohse J, Sarles H (1979) Characterization of a protein isolated from pancreatic calculi of men suffering from chronic calcifying pancreatitis. Biochem Biophys Res Commun 87:1176–1182
5. Guy-Crotte O, Amouric M, Figarella C (1984) Characterisation and N-terminal sequence of a degradation product of 14000 molecular weight isolated from human pancreatic juice. Biochem Biophys Res Commun 125:516–523
6. Gross J, Carlson RI, Brauer AW, Margolies MN, Warshaw AL, Wands JR (1985) Isolation, characterization, and distribution of an unusual pancreatic human secretory protein. J Clin Invest 76:2115–2126
7. Lechene de la Porte P, De Caro A, Amouric M, Sarles H (1981) Localisation imunocytochimique de la protéine majoritaire de calculs pancréatiques humaines. Nouv Presse Med 10:3851
8. De Caro A, Multigner L, Lafont H, Lombardo D, Sarles H (1984) The molecular characteristics of a human pancreatic acidic phosphoprotein that inhibits calcium carbonate crystal growth. Biochem J 222:669–677
9. Giorgi D, Bernard JP, De Caro A, Multigner L, Lapointe R, Sarles H, Dagorn JC (1985) Pancreatic stone protein: I. Evidence that it is encoded by a pancreatic messenger ribonucleic acid. Gastroenterology 89:381–386
10. Figarella C, Amouric M, Guy-Grotte O (1984) Proteolysis of human trypsinogen 1. Pathogenic implication in chronic pancreatitis. Biochem Biophys Res Commun 118:154–161
11. Multigner L, De Caro A, Lombardo D, Campese O, Sarles H (1983) Pancreatic stone protein, a phosphoprotein which inhibits calcium carbonate precipitation from human pancreatic juice. Biochem Biophys Res Commun 110:69–74
12. Multigner L, Sarles H, Lombardo D, De Caro A (1985) Pancreatic stone protein: II. Implication in stone formation during the course of chronic calcifying pancreatitis. Gastroenterology 89:387–391
13. Sarles H (1986) Etiopathogenesis and definition of chronic pancreatitis. Dig Dis Sci 31:91S–107S
14. Schmiegel W-H, Burchert M, Kalthoff H, Thiele HG, Bützow GH, Klose G, Greten H (1986) Pancreatic stone protein in serum of patients with pancreatitis. Lancet ii:686
15. Bernard JP, Provansal-Cheylan M, Mariani A, Dupuy P, Sarles H (1989) Pancreatic stone protein: quantification in pancreatic juice by enzyme-linked immunosorbent assay and comparison with other methods. Gastroenterology 96:A955
16. Schmiegel W, Burchert M, Kalthoff H, Roeder C, Bützow G, Grimm H, Kremer B, Soehendra N, Schreiber H-W, Thiele H-G, Greten H (1990) Immunochemical characterization and quantitative distribution of pancreatic

stone protein in sera and pancreatic secretions in pancreatic disorders. Gastroenterology 1421–1430
17. Montalto G, Bonicel J, Multigner L, Rovery M, Sarles H, De Caro A (1986) Partial amino acid sequence of human pancreatic stone protein, a novel pancreatic secretory protein. Biochem J 238:227–232
18. Gross J, Brauer AW, Bringhurst RF, Corbett C, Margolies MN (1985) An unusual bovine pancreatic protein exhibiting pH-dependent globule-fibril transformation and unique amino acid sequence. Proc Natl Acad Sci USA 82:5627–5631
19. Neurath AR, Strick N (1981) Enyzme-linked fluorescence immunoassays using β-galactosidase and antibodies covalently bound to polystyrene plates. J Virol Methods 3:155–165
20. Montalto G, Lusher M, De Caro A, Multigner L, Sarles H, Delaage M (1985) Analysis of human pancreatic juice constituents related to the pancreatic stone protein using monoclonal antibody. CR Acad Sci (Paris) 300:199–202
21. Provansal-Cheylan M, Lusher M, De Caro A, Multigner L, Montalto G, Sarles H, Delaage M (1986) Monoclonal antibodies to pancreatic stone protein. Radioimmunoassay and immunological comparison with trypsin 1. Biochimie 68:1109–1113
23. Schmiegel WH, Kreiker C, Eberl W, Arndt R, Classen M, Greten H, Jessen K, Kalthoff H, Soehendra N, Thiele HG (1985) Monoclonal antibody defines CA 19–9 in pancreatic juice and sera. Gut 26:456–460
24. Axon ATR, Classen M, Cotton PB, Cremer M, Freeny PC, Lees WR (1984) Pancreatography in chronic pancreatitis: international definitions. Gut 25: 1107–1112
25. Sarner M, Cotton PB (1984) Classification of pancreatitis. Gut 25:756–759
26. Sarles H, Gyr K, Singer MV (1984) Revised classification of pancreatitis-Marseille 1984. Presented at the American Pancreatic Association Meeting, 8 November, 1984, Chicago
27. De Caro A, Multigner L, Dagorn JC, Sarles H (1988) The human pancreatic stone protein. Biochimie 70:1209–1214
28. De Caro AM, Bonicel JJ, Rouimi P, De Caro JD, Sarles H, Rovery M (1987) Complete amino acid sequence of an immuno-reactive form of human pancreatic stone protein isolated from pancreatic juice. Eur J Biochem 168:201–207
29. Rouimi P, Bonicel J, Rovery M, De Caro A (1987) Cleavage of the Arg-Ile bond in the native polypeptide chain of human pancreatic stone protein. FEBS Lett 216:195–199
30. Klöppel G (1984) Pancreatic, non-endocrine tumours. In: Klöppel G, Heitz UP (eds) Pancreatic pathology. Edinburgh, pp 79–113
31. Sarles H, Dagorn JC, Giorgi D, Bernard JP (1990) Renaming pancreatic stone protein as "Lithostathine". Gastroenterology 99:900–901
32. Terazono K, Yamamoto H, Takasawa S, Shiga K, Yonemura Y, Tochino Y, Okamoto H (1988) A novel gene activated in regenerating islets. J Biol Chem 263:2111–2114
33. Watanabe T, Yonekura H, Terazono K, Yamamoto H, Okamoto H (1990) Complete nucleotide sequence of human reg gene and its expression in normal and tumoral tissues. J Biol Chem 265:7432–7439
34. Terazono K, Watanabe T, Yonemura Y (1990) A novel gene, reg, expressed in regenerating islets. In: Okamoto H (ed) Molecular biology of the islets of Langerhans. Cambridge University Press, Cambridge, pp 301–315

The Morphologic Basis for the Evolution of Acute Pancreatitis into Chronic Pancreatitis

G. KLÖPPEL[1] and B. MAILLET

Introduction

The pathogenesis of chronic pancreatitis is still unsettled. The most commonly cited theory postulates that the deposition of protein plugs which later calcify leads to duct obstruction with subsequent fibrotic replacement of the acinar tissue upstream of the occlusion [13]. Alternatively, we have proposed a working hypothesis that relates the pathogenesis of chronic pancreatitis with that of acute pancreatitis [8, 9]. The sequence of events that we believe may connect acute with chronic pancreatitis starts with interstitial fat necrosis and hemorrhage that induces perilobular fibrosis. Perilobular fibrosis, in turn, may also distort the interlobular ducts, creating stenoses and dilatations. The ducts, once altered, hamper the normal flow of pancreatic secretions, thereby enabling the precipitation of proteins (protein plugs) and eventually their calcification (calculi). If duct obstruction becomes more extensive, the acinar cells upstream of such a stenosis disappear, leaving dense intralobular fibrosis.

This chain of events has been provisionally termed the necrosis-fibrosis sequence (Fig. 1). If this necrosis-fibrosis sequence is indeed the basic pathogenetic principle underlying chronic pancreatitis, it must also be consistent with a number of observations that seemingly contradict it. In this contribution special emphasis is therefore placed on answering the following questions: (a) Why has pancreatic fibrosis characterizing chronic pancreatitis typically a patchy pattern, although acute pancreatitis is thought to be a diffuse disease; (b) why does biliary pancreatitis virtually never progresses to chronic pancreatitis [5, 6]; and (c) why does not every relapsing alcoholic pancreatitis progress to chronic pancreatitis, and when does chronic pancreatitis progress?

[1] Department of Pathology, Academic Hospital Jette, Free University of Brussels, Laarbeeklaan 101, B-1090 Brussels, Belgium

Beger/Büchler/Malfertheiner (Eds.)
Standards in Pancreatic Surgery

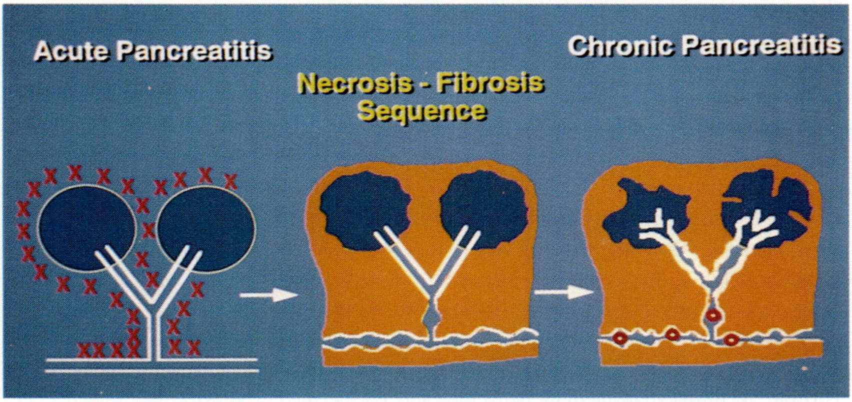

Fig. 1. The "necrosis-fibrosis sequence" schematically summarizes the main events and findings that connect acute with chronic pancreatitis. *Left*, pancreatic lobule and duct surrounded by interstitial fat necroses (*red crosses*); *center*, pancreatic lobule encased by fibrosis (*orange areas*) that also involves the draining interlobular duct; *right*, pancreatic lobule partly replaced by intralobular fibrosis and encased by advanced perilobular fibrosis. The distorted draining duct is obstructed by calculi (*red circles*)

Why Is Chronic Pancreatitis a Focal Disease?

There is general agreement that the fibrotic process characterizing chronic pancreatitis affects the pancreas unevenly [7, 9, 15]. In a typical case, areas with some perilobular fibrosis, or even normal acinar parenchyma, alternate with severe perilobular and intralobular fibrosis. If such a patchy pattern of fibrosis is to be due to a necrotic process, this process must be focal as well. Yet, acute pancreatitis is thought to be a diffuse disease, implying that all parts of the pancreas are evenly affected. This conception, however, is not consistent with the distribution pattern of necrosis that one usually finds in severe acute pancreatitis. Although the surface of pancreatic specimens with severe acute pancreatitis show confluent fat necrosis and hemorrhage suggesting diffuse involvement of the organ, analysis of the parenchyma of the gland reveals, as a rule, that it is for large parts well preserved and displays only foci of hemorrhage and interstitial fat necrosis [11, 14]. These focal changes may be confined to only one area of the pancreas, for instance, the head or tail, leaving the other parts of the gland completely unaffected. It is totally unclear which mechanisms govern the distribution of the necrotic lesions within the pancreas because the damage patterns differ from patient to patient and do not follow any recognizable rule.

From these findings it is evident that acute pancreatitis is, morphologically speaking, not a diffuse disease, but a focal process, the pattern of which compares well with the irregularity of fibrosis seen in chronic pancreatitis. We therefore believe that the primarily focal nature of chronic pancreatitis reflects the intrapancreatic damage pattern observed in severe acute pancreatitis.

Why Does Biliary Pancreatitis Seldom Progress to Chronic Pancreatitis?

According to clinical studies it appears that gallstone pancreatitis, even if relapsing, rarely (or virtually never) progresses to chronic pancreatitis [5, 6]. This observation seems to contradict our necrosis-fibrosis hypothesis for the pathogenesis of chronic pancreatitis, since it implies that there is a large group of patients whose acute pancreatitis is obviously never followed by pancreatic fibrosis. To explain this finding, it must be taken into account that biliary pancreatitis is usually a mild (also called interstitial-edematous) acute pancreatitis. The morphology of mild acute pancreatitis is characterized by some spotty peripancreatic fat necroses that barely involve the gland [7, 10]. Accordingly, these peripancreatic lesions resolve without any influence on the architecture of the pancreatic parenchyma, and even if the same lesions recur, the glandular tissue remains intact (Fig. 2). It can thus be concluded that mild acute pancreatitis never produces intrapancreatic

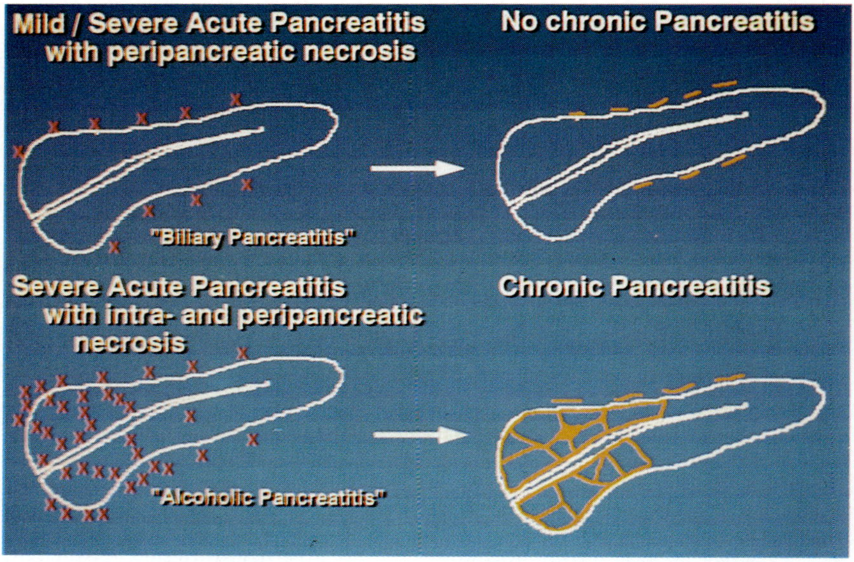

Fig. 2. Natural history of acute pancreatitis *Upper panel*, acute pancreatitis that is characterized by peripancreatic fatty tissue necrosis (mild or severe) and clinically often corresponds to biliary pancreatitis, does not proceed to chronic pancreatitis. *Lower panel*, acute pancreatitis that is characterized by peripancreatic and intrapancreatic necroses and clinically often corresponds to alcoholic pancreatitis, may go on to chronic pancreatitis

changes such as perilobular or periductal fibrosis. Biliary pancreatitis is therefore not likely to evolve into chronic pancreatitis.

Why Does Not Every Relapsing Alcoholic Pancreatitis Progress to Chronic Pancreatitis, and When Does Chronic Pancreatitis Progress?

It has been shown that, apart from biliary pancreatitis, also some patients with relapsing alcoholic pancreatitis do not clinically progress to chronic pancreatitis [2]. Conversely, it is also well known that the morphologic substrate of relapsing alcoholic pancreatitis is usually chronic pancreatitis with the tendency for self-perpetuation [1, 4, 12]. To explain these observations and to get an idea about a patient's risk to develop a progressive chronic pancreatitis, the possible extent of damage in severe acute pancreatitis, its localization in and around the pancreas, and its consequences to the pancreatic duct system must be considered (Fig. 2).

In a great number of patients, severe acute pancreatitis leads predominantly to massive peripancreatic fat necrosis over the surface of the pancreas, while the intrapancreatic regions are virtually unaffected. The massive peripancreatic necrosis is transformed into extrapancreatic

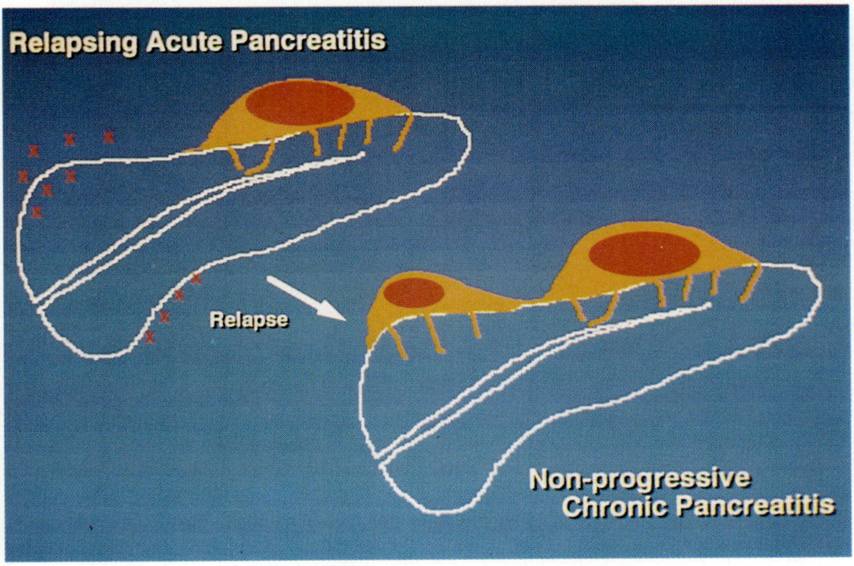

Fig. 3. Natural history of relapsing severe acute pancreatitis with necroses restricted mainly to the peripancreatic fatty tissue and the peripheral pancreatic parenchyma. The postnecrotic sequelae, i.e., pseudocyst and peripheral scarring, do not go on to progressive chronic pancreatitis

pseudocysts that may cause complications but do not lead to significant intrapancreatic fibrosis with duct alterations (Fig. 3). Consequently, this type of severe acute pancreatitis does not progress to chronic pancreatitis.

In other patients with severe acute pancreatitis, peripancreatic necrosis is associated with some small foci of intrapancreatic necrosis. The sequelae of these lesions are extrapancreatic pseudocysts and small foci of scarring within the pancreas. If the intrapancreatic fibrotic foci do not involve the main pancreatic duct and its direct branches, progression of the disease is unlikely to occur. It will, however, progress, when the patient continues to abuse alcohol so that further pancreatitis attacks can occur which now affect regions adjacent to the main pancreatic duct resulting in alterations of the branches and eventually of the main duct (Fig. 4).

The third group of patients shows severe acute pancreatitis with marked extrapancreatic fat necrosis as well as large foci of intrapancreatic necrosis (Fig. 4). This pancreatitis, particularly if relapsing, causes not only pseudocysts but also pancreatic fibrosis that already initially involves the main duct in the affected areas and leads to its distortion. In these patients, progression to chronic pancreatitis is most likely, even after alcohol abstinence. The clinical severity of the resulting chronic pancreatitis then

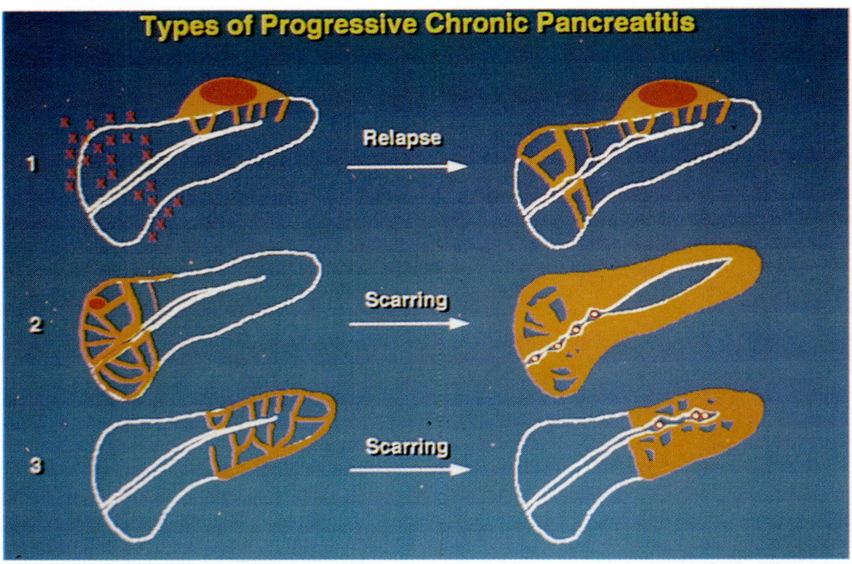

Fig. 4. Natural history of progressive chronic pancreatitis. The first type is characterized by acute relapses that involve the peripancreatic tissue as well as the pancreatic parenchyma including the duct system. The second type is characterized by chronic damage to the pancreatic head which subsequently induces progressive obstructive changes in the body and tail of the pancreas. The third type is characterized by damage to the body/tail that in time will locally progress but remain restricted to this area

depends on whether the damage was mainly to the head of the pancreas or to the body and/or tail. When the head was the main target, the resulting duct obstruction causes dilatation of the main duct and its branches in the body and tail of the pancreas, and subsequently also fibrosis (Fig. 4). After months or some years this patient will, apart from pain, suffer from severe exocrine and endocrine pancreatic insufficiency. When the damage was limited to the body and/or tail, the patient, even with abstinence from alcohol, may suffer from pain but will not develop pancreatic insufficiency, because of normal tissue remaining in the head of the pancreas (Fig. 4).

Conclusions

There are many reasons to believe that the necrosis-fibrosis sequence is the basic pathogenetic event in the evolution of chronic pancreatitis. This sequence implies that acute pancreatitis, probably in its severe relapsing form, may be the cause of chronic pancreatitis. To make this concept relevant to the individual patient and the natural course of his disease, the extent and distribution pattern of necrosis in acute pancreatitis must be carefully evaluated with regard to the restitutional processes (i.e., restitutio ad integrum, pseudocyst, intrapancreatic fibrosis) that may follow. Such an analysis reveals that only after severe acute pancreatitis and only under certain conditions, i.e., occurrence of intrapancreatic necrosis involving the main duct, can development of chronic pancreatitis be anticipated. The individuality of each patient's pancreatitis demands a thorough clinical and morphologic assessment of the pancreas in order to asign the appropriate therapy to this disease and to halt its progression [16].

References

1. Ammann RW, Akovbiantz A, Largiader F, Schueler G (1984) Course and outcome of chronic pancreatitis. Longitudinal study of a mixed medical-surgical series of 245 patients. Gastroenterology 86:820–828
2. Ammann RW, Buehler H, Bruehlmann W, Kehl O, Muench R, Stamm B (1986) Acute (nonprogressive) alcoholic pancreatitis: prospective longitudinal study of 144 patients with recurrent alcoholic pancreatitis. Pancreas 1:195–203
3. Angelini G, Pederzoli P, Caliari S, Fratton S, Zrocco G, Mavzoli G, Bovo P, Cavallini G, Scuro LA (1984) Long-term outcome of acute necrohemorrhagic pancreatitis. Digestion 30:131–137
4. Comfort MW, Gambill EE, Baggenstoss AH (1946) Chronic relapsing pancreatitis. A study of 29 cases without associated disease of the biliary or gastrointestinal tract. Gastroenterology 6:239–285
5. Dürr GHK (1979) Acute pancreatitis. In: Howat HT, Sarles H (eds) The exocrine pancreas. Saunders, London, pp 352–401
6. Gullo L, Priori P, Labo G (1984) Natural history of acute pancreatitis and its relationship to chronic pancreatitis. In: Banks PA, Porro GB (eds) Acute pancreatitis. Masson, Milan, pp 87–93

7. Gyr K, Singer MV, Sarles H (eds) (1984) Pancreatitis. Concepts and classification. In: Proceedings of the second international symposium on the classification of pancreatitis. Excerpta Medica, Amsterdam
8. Klöppel G (1990) Pathology of chronic pancreatitis and pancreatic pain. Acta Chir Scand 156:261–265
9. Klöppel G, Maillet B (1991) Pseudocysts in chronic pancreatitis: a morphological analysis of 57 resection specimens and 9 autopsy pancreata. Pancreas 6:266–274
10. Klöppel G, von Gerkan R, Dreyer T (1984) Pathomorphology of acute pancreatitis. Analysis of 367 autopsy cases and 3 surgical specimens. In: Gyr KE, Singer MV, Sarles H (eds) Pancreatitis. Concepts and classification. Excerpta Medica, Amsterdam, pp 29–35
11. Klöppel G, Dreyer T, Willemer S, Kern HF, Adler G (1986) Human acute pancreatitis: its pathogenesis in the light of immunocytochemical and ultrastructural findings in acinar cells. Virchows Arch [A] 409:791–803
12. Nagata A, Homma T, Tamai K et al. (1981) A study of chronic pancreatitis by serial endoscopic pancreatography. Gastroenterology 81:884–891
13. Sarles H (1986) Chronic pancreatitis: etiology and pathophysiology. In: Go VLW, Gardner JD, Brooks FP, Lebenthal E, DiMagno EP, Scheele GA (eds) The exocrine pancreas. Biology, pathobiology, and diseases. Raven, New York, pp 527–575
14. Schmitz-Moormann P (1981) Comparative radiological and morphological study of the human pancreas. IV. Acute necrotizing pancreatitis in man. Pathol Res Pract 171:325–335
15. Uys CJ, Bank S, Marks IN (1973) The pathology of chronic pancreatitis in Cape Town. Digestion 9:454–468
16. Warshaw AL (1990) Indications for surgical treatment in chronic pancreatitis. In: Beger HG, Büchler M, Ditschuneit H, Malfertheiner P (eds) Chronic pancreatitis. Springer, Berlin Heidelberg New York, pp 395–399

Diagnosis and Staging of Chronic Pancreatitis

P. Malfertheiner,[1] J.E. Domínguez-Muñoz, and M. Büchler

Improvement of imaging techniques to visualize the pancreas, and the development of non-invasive pancreatic function tests have facilitated and greatly improved the diagnostic approach to chronic pancreatitis (CP) in clinical routine. However, the limited sensitivity of diagnostic procedures and difficulty in obtaining pancreatic tissue specimens hinder detection in early stages of CP. Diagnosis of CP is based on clinical history, pathognomonic changes of pancreatic structure assessed by ultrasonography (US), computed tomography (CT) and/or endoscopic retrograde pancreatography (ERP), and impaired exocrine and/or endocrine pancreatic function. Staging of CP is based on the degree of morphological and functional changes. This article updates the current knowledge of clinical, morphological, and functional aspects of CP that allow diagnosis and staging.

Clinical Manifestations

Pain is the major and usually the first clinical manifestation in CP. The typical clinical picture of the disease is characterized by recurrent attacks of upper abdominal pain occurring at intervals of months or years. These attacks tend to be progressively more frequent until the pain becomes persistent or, contrarily, diminishes in frequency and severity as pancreatic fibrosis progresses. In about 50% of patients the disease starts with an episode of acute pancreatitis, and in 40% the onset of pain is insidious.

The painless form of CP is rather infrequent (around 10% of patients), and occurs preferentially in the elderly. The first clinical manifestations in these patients with no pain are related to impairment of pancreatic exocrine and/or endocrine function. Symptoms of diabetes mellitus, malabsorption, jaundice, or upper gastrointestinal bleeding lead usually to the diagnosis of CP in these cases.

Intensity, site, character, and duration of pain vary considerably, but in acute attacks pain is generally severe, diffused over the upper abdomen,

[1] Abteilung Innere Medizin II, Universitätsklinik Ulm, Robert-Koch-Straße 8, W-7900-Ulm, FRG

Beger/Büchler/Malfertheiner (Eds.)
Standards in Pancreatic Surgery

radiating to the back, and persistent for several days. Nausea, vomiting and mild jaundice are often present.

Despite the fact that there are various causes of CP, chronic alcohol abuse is the predominant etiology and accounts for more than 90% of adult patients in industralized countries. Typically CP patients present initially with an attack of pancreatitis in early adulthood after several years of excessive drinking and recover, but continue to drink, thereby setting the stage for recurring episodes. Most of these patients have CP at the time of the first attack. Weight loss, diabetes, and steatorrhea appear usually in the advanced stage of the disease. The most frequent local complications during evolution of CP are:

- Pseudocysts
- Obstruction of common bile duct
- Bowel obstruction
- Splenic vein thrombosis
- Hemorrhage
- Ascitis
- Pancreatic fistula

Morphological Diagnosis of Chronic Pancreatitis

Imaging procedures are the mainstay in the diagnosis of CP based on the development and improvement of imaging techniques to visualize the pancreas (US, CT, ERP and magnetic resonance imaging). The recognition and further definition of pathognomonic morphological signs of CP relegated the use of function tests in the diagnosis of this disease. Conventional

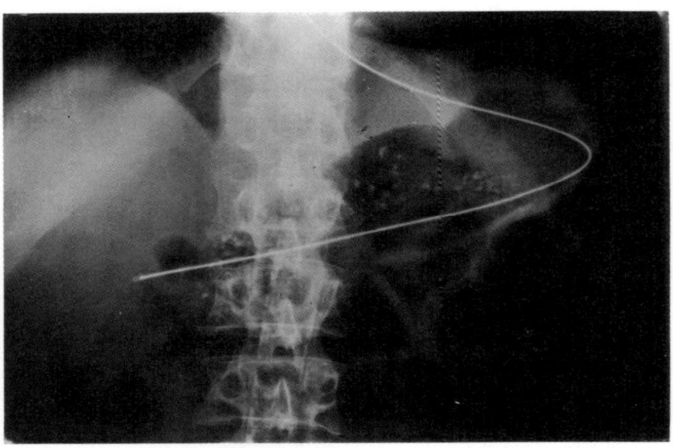

Fig. 1. Plain film of the upper abdomen showing pancreatic calcifications in a patient with chronic pancreatitis

radiography may also indicate CP if pancreatic calcifications are present (Fig. 1).

Ultrasonography in Chronic Pancreatitis

Ultrasonography is the imaging technique of choice as a first diagnostic approach to a patient with abdominal symptoms. US is inexpensive, noninvasive, available everywhere, and well tolerated by patients. In the diagnosis of CP, the modern real-time US systems have a higher sensitivity, allowing high-quality visualization of the pancreas and the main pancreatic duct. The pancreatic head, anatomically close to the liver, is the easiest part to explore with US, while the tail of the gland is not so easily accessible. Meteorism and increased regional deposition of abdominal fat are the two major obstacles to adequate US pancreatic exploration.

Size, shape and echo-texture of the pancreas, the main pancreatic duct, and the presence of complications (i.e., cysts, dilatation of the common bile duct, vascular involvement) can be assessed in great detail by US (Table 1). However US findings in CP can be extremely variable, depending on the nature and severity of pancreatic damage.

The size of the pancreas in CP is related to the activity and stage of the disease [1]. The pancreas is more enlarged during an acute relapse, while it becomes normal sized or even smaller as atrophy progresses [2, 3]. Focal enlargement of the gland can also be detected, generally secondary to localized inflammation during an acute relapse [4]. However, the usefulness of size alterations in the diagnosis of CP is limited, because changes of pancreatic size may be found in physiologic and pathological conditions other than CP and, furthermore, because they are only present in 38%–55% of patients with CP [2, 5]. Due to the enlargement and irregular delineation of the gland, an altered shape of the pancreas may be observed in advanced CP [2]. This finding is not specific for CP, and it is frequently observed in other pathological conditions and even in anatomic variations (pancreatic tumors, pancreas divisum) [6].

Increased echogenicity of the pancreatic parenchyma is the most frequently described abnormal US finding in CP. Nevertheless, this finding

Table 1. Pathological features of chronic pancreatitis detected by imaging procedures

Ultrasonography	Computed tomography	Endoscopic retrograde pancreatography
Changes in size of the gland	Changes in size of the gland	Changes in the main duct
Changes in caliber of the main duct	Changes in caliber of the main duct	Changes in the side branches
Changes in echo pattern	Changes in parenchyma	Presence of cavities
Calcifications	Calcifications	
Fluid collections	Fluid collections	

secondary to an increment in fat and fibrous content of the pancreas [7] is relatively sensitive but nonspecific for CP. An abnormal parenchymal echotexture can be demonstrated in only 53%–74% of patients with CP [2, 8]. On the other hand, pancreatic echogenicity in healthy people tends to increase with age and in the presence of increased subcutaneous fat [9].

The detection of a dilated main pancreatic duct is the most specific US sign of CP. The normal main pancreatic duct has a diameter of up to 2 mm on US, bounded by echogenic walls. In early stages of CP an increase in echogenicity of the walls of the main duct can be observed, the main duct becoming irregularly dilated with advancing disease [10]. This feature is important in differentiating dilatation of the main pancreatic duct due to CP from that in pancreatic cancer. Using US, a dilated duct has been found in 11%–54% of patients with CP according to published reports [2, 5]. However, sensitivity does improve with simultaneous secretin stimulation [11, 12]. US is similarly useful to detect the existence of complications of CP, such as fluid collections, dilatation of the common bile duct, and lienal and portal vein thrombosis.

The accuracy of US in diagnosing CP varies between 60% and 80%, depending on the diagnostic US criteria used (Table 1) and the stage of CP to be evaluated [5, 8, 13–15]. In early stages of the disease, a large number of false-negative results can occur. On the other hand, the risk of false-positive results is also considerably high if too much confidence is placed in nonspecific signs. In these cases, the combination of functional tests and US can be of great use in the primary diagnostic approach to CP [16].

Computed Tomography in Chronic Pancreatitis

The introduction of high-resolution CT scans entailed an important advance in the diagnosis of pancreatic disease by displaying the parenchyma. In patients with CP the pathological features in CT are similar to those in US (Table 1): changes in size of the gland and main pancreatic duct, together with the presence of calcifications and fluid collections are the basic alterations to be considered.

The above considerations for US regarding size alterations of the gland and dilatation of the main pancreatic duct can also be applied to CT. So, enlargement of the pancreas is a frequent but nonspecific CT feature of CP. Dilatation of the pancreatic duct system is easily detected with CT. However, mild duct dilatation (less than 4 mm), even associated with gland enlargement and contour changes, may not be sufficient to establish the diagnosis of CP. In this case, the evidence of pancreatic dysfunction may be of help [16]. An irregular duct dilatation greater than 4 mm is a pathognomonic CT finding of advanced CP.

CT has a high sensitivity in detecting even small pancreatic calcifications [16] (Fig. 2). This sign is considered as unequivocal of the advanced stage of CP [17].

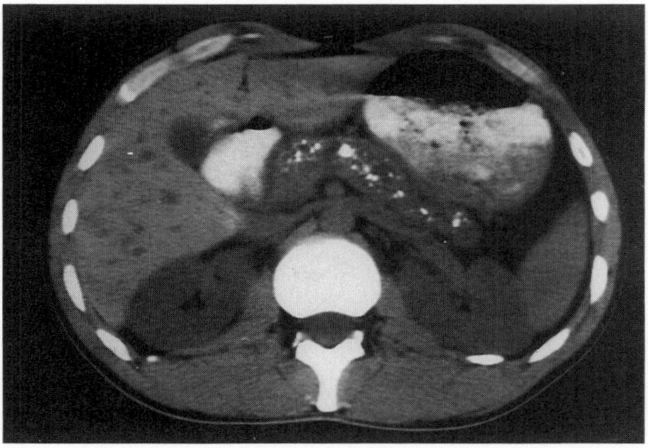

Fig. 2. Pancreatic calcifications in chronic pancreatitis detected by computed tomography

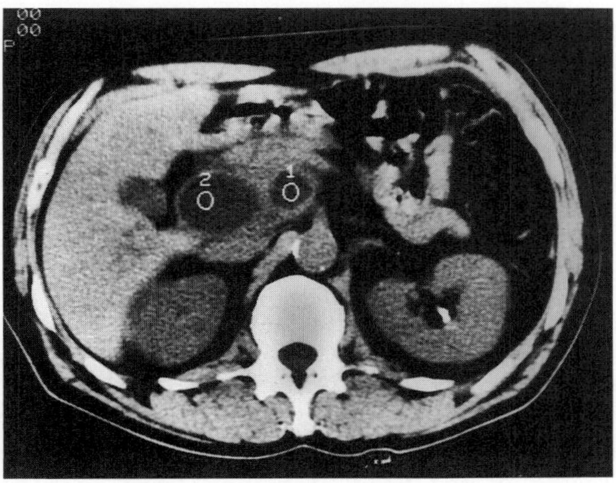

Fig. 3. Pancreatic psudocysts in chronic pancreatitis detected by computed tomography

Pseudocysts are the most frequent complication in CP. CT has a great reliability in detecting these pseudocysts, even if they are as small as 1.5 mm [16] (Fig. 3). Furthermore, CT is useful in detecting cyst complications such as infection (presence of gas within the cyst) or rupture within the gastrointestinal tract.

As with US, the accuracy of CT in diagnosing CP depends basically on the stage of the disease and on the diagnostic CT criteria applied. In this way, the sensitivity of CT in diagnosing CP has been reported to vary between 56% and 95%, with a specificity of 85%–90% [15, 18–20]. In early

Table 2. Cambridge classification of pancreatograms in chronic pancreatitis (CP)[a]

Terminology	Main duct	Abnormal side branches	Additional features
Normal	Normal	None	
Equivocal	Normal	Fewer than 3	
Mild changes of CP	Normal	3 or more	
Moderate changes of CP	Abnormal	More than 3	
Marked changes of CP	Abnormal	More than 3	One or more of: large cavity, obstruction, filling defects, severe dilatation or irregularity

[a] Pathological changes are defined as local or diffuse, based on the involvement of less or more than one third of the gland, respectively.

stages of CP, the diagnostic accuracy of CT is about 50% [20, 21]. CT appears to be an useful method for the diagnosis of CP, being essential for planning the strategy of surgical intervention.

Endoscopic Retrograde Pancreatography in Chronic Pancreatitis

Since experience was gained in the mid-1970s with this procedure, ERP has allowed a marked improvement in the diagnosis of CP, as the pancreatic duct system can be displayed in high detail. Abnormalities of the main pancreatic duct and its side branches are highly specific findings for CP, in such a way that ERP appears to be the most adequate morphological method for diagnosing this disease (Table 1).

During a meeting of experts in Cambridge in 1983, the current international definitions of pancreatographic findings in CP were established [22, 23]. The Cambridge criteria are shown in Table 2. The caliber and contour of the main pancreatic duct and side branches, the number and length of side branches, parenchymal opacification, presence of cavities, and the common bile duct in the region of the head of the pancreas must be analyzed in detail. Local or diffuse irregular dilatation of the main duct or side branches is specific for CP. Diameters of the main pancreatic duct are considered normal up to 6.5, 5.0, and 3.0 mm for head, body, and tail, respectively [23]. If alterations are limited to the side branches, they indicate mild CP (Fig. 4). Abnormalities of the main pancreatic duct are present in moderate CP (Fig. 5). Severe CP is characterized by abnormal main duct in the ERP (Fig. 6) with at least one of the following features: large cavity, obstruction, filling defects, severe dilatation or irregularity.

The accuracy of ERP in diagnosing CP is superior to that of US and CT (21), but ERP operators need more and special training and the technique is more invasive than US and CT. ERP has a sensitivity higher than 80%, with a specificity of about 90% [13, 20, 24–28] (Table 3). However, in early stages of CP the sensitivity of ERP in the diagnosis of this disease is limited,

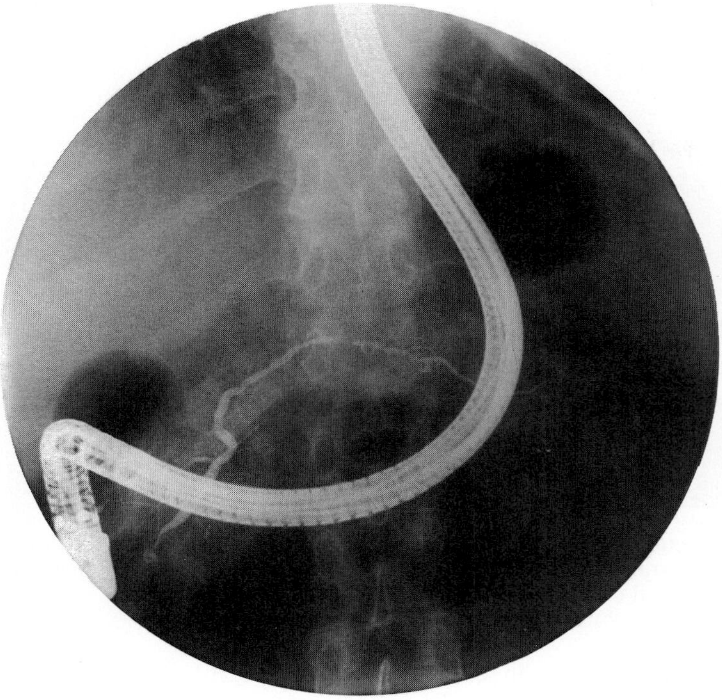

Fig. 4. Mild ductular changes in chronic pancreatitis assessed by endoscopic retrograde pancreatography. Alterations are limited to the side branches

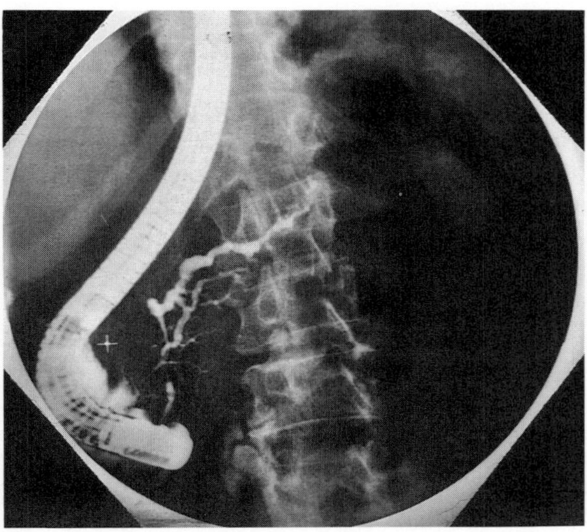

Fig. 5. Moderate ductular changes in chronic pancreatitis assessed by endoscopic retrograde pancreatography. Moderate alterations of the main pancreatic duct and side branches

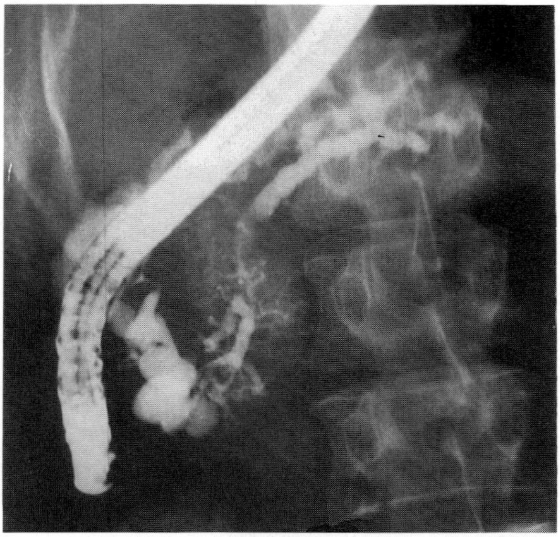

Fig. 6. Marked ductular changes in chronic pancreatitis assessed by endoscopic retrograde pancreatography. Marked irregularities of the main pancreatic duct and side branches intraductal caecue

while its specificity decreases in elderly patients [16, 36]. In both cases pancreatic function tests may be useful in interpreting ERP findings [20]. Problems in the differential diagnosis with pancreatic cancer by ERP findings arise in less than 10% of patients presenting with duct abnormalities.

Function Tests in Diagnosis of Chronic Pancreatitis

A series of new and modified pancreatic function tests have been introduced in the clinical practice which greatly enhance the diagnosis of pancreatic insufficiency. Nevertheless, the detection of mild and moderate forms of CP remains a problem for these tests too. The spectrum of function tests comprises intubation tests with direct or indirect stimulation of the pancreas, oral tests, determination of serum and fecal pancreatic enzyme concentrations, and tests that evaluate the endocrine function of the gland. These tests have to be evaluated in the basis of several criteria which include accuracy, precision, difficulty in performance, and cost.

Direct Function Tests

The most valuable pancreatic function test is still the duodenal intubation test based on the analysis of duodenal aspirates following exogenous hormonal stimulation of the pancreas [37–39]. The exocrine pancreas is usually stimulated with a combination of secretin and cholecystokinin

Table 3. Accuracy of endoscopic retrograde pancreatography in the diagnosis of chronic pancreatitis

Author	Reference	Patients (*n*)	True positive		False negative		Unsuccessful (%)
			n	%	*n*	%	
Classen et al.	[29]	25	17	68	8	32	0
Kasugai	[30]	69	58	84	2	3	14
Liguory and Caletti	[31]	77	52	68	1	2	30
Löffler et al.	[32]	66	53	80	0	0	20
Belohlavek	[33]	193	178	92	15	8	15
Rolny et al.	[34]	30	21	70	9	30	0
Anacker et al.	[35]	269	224	83	8	3	14
Valentini et al.	[25]	65	52	80	9	14	6
Braganza et al.	[26]	45	37	82	8	18	0
Malfertheiner et al.	[20]	74	69	89	5	11	13

(CCK) or cerulein (SC test). Amylase, trypsin, chymotrypsin, lipase and bicarbonate are determined in the sampling fractions of duodenal aspirate [16]. In advanced stages of CP, all these parameters are significantly decreased. However, in early stages of CP, only one or two parameters may be found to be reduced, and it has been suggested that lipase is the first to be impaired [37]. The accuracy of this test in the diagnosis of CP is very high, with a sensitivity and specificity usually higher than 90% [37–39]. However, it is invasive, time-consuming, expensive, and its performance is restricted to specialized centers.

The same disadvantages arise with the Lundh test. This function test is based on the induction of an endogenous stimulation of the pancreas by a test meal. The parameter usually determined in duodenal aspirates is mean tryptic activity [38, 40, 41]. The accuracy of the Lundh test in the diagnosis of CP appears to be lower than that of the SC test, since it is less sensitive in cases of mild pancreatic damage [38, 41].

Indirect Function Tests

Exocrine pancreatic function is indirectly reflected by measuring pancreatic enzymes in serum and feces, or by determining the enzyme effect on a test meal.

Serum and Fecal Pancreatic Enzymes

Serum concentration of individual pancreatic enzymes in patients with CP may either be abnormally low, increased, or normal [42–44]. In our experience, low values appear in 20%–32% of CP patients, increased values in 22%–39%, and normal values in 49%–71% of patients [45]. An abnormally low serum concentration of any individual pancreatic enzyme is highly specific but not very sensitive for the diagnosis of CP [45], since it is a typical finding in patients with pancreatic steatorrhea [42, 44, 46].

Analyzing the ratios between different serum pancreatic enzymes, we have found that low values of the P-isoamylase/lipase ratio are highly specific for CP and, in addition, this ratio shows high accuracy in the differentiation between mild to moderate and advanced CP as classified by ERP [45].

Determination of trypsin and, basically, chymotrypsin activities in feces has been used in the diagnosis of CP because of its simplicity and noninvasivity. However, the probability of false-positive results is high, as well as the probability of false-negative results in patients without pancreatic steatorrhea [47]. This limits the use of this test.

Oral Function Tests

The most widely accepted indirect pancreatic function tests are those based on the urinary recovery of *para*-aminobenzoic acid (nitro blue tetrazolium-

para-aminobenzoic acid, NBT-PABA, test) or fluorescein (pancreolauryl test), which are liberated from complex substrates into the intestinal lumen by specific pancreatic enzymes [48–50]. Both tests have a high reliability in the detection of severe exocrine pancreatic insufficiency, but not in cases of mild to moderate disease [48–50]. The limitations of these tests related to urine sampling have been overcome with the development of serum determination methods of PABA and fluorescein [51, 52]. Furthermore, the duration of the serum pancreolauryl test (PLT) has been shortened, and its sensitivity in detecting mild to moderate forms of CP improved by means of the intravenous administration of metoclopramide and secretin to stimulate pancreatic secretion [53]. In our experience, this modified serum PLT shows sensitivity and specificity near to 90% in the diagnosis of CP, considering patients in the different evolutive stages of the disease. A pathological result of this test in postgastrectomy patients, in patients with extensive intestinal inflammatory disease, or in presence of hepatobiliary diseases and marked jaundice must be carefully analyzed because of interferences with the gastrointestinal transit and absorptive capacity of free fluorescein [54].

Other Indirect Pancreatic Function Tests

A new exocrine pancreatic function test has been developed, based on the consumption of plasma amino acids by the pancreas following stimulation with secretin and/or cerulein. In patients with severe pancreatic insufficiency, a significantly lower decrease in plasma amino acid concentration is produced than in controls [55, 56]. However, the accuracy shown by this test in the diagnosis of CP varies widely according to different authors [56, 57].

Quantitative fecal fat analysis is only able to detect exocrine pancreatic insufficiency at the end stage. The use of this test is only indicated to find out the need to control the effect of enzyme replacement therapy. Other methods, like breath analysis tests using stable isotopes (i.e., C_{13}-octanoate), have the potential to be useful in the future.

Endocrine Function Tests

Abnormalities in the endocrine pancreatic function are frequently present in patients with advanced stage of CP. Investigation of the endocrine pancreatic function may reflect the severity of CP. Nevertheless, the role of blood glucose levels, the glucose tolerance test, insulin and C peptide blood levels is unimportant as diagnostic tool. The determination of pancreatic plasma glucagon after arginine infusion seems to be useful in differentiating primary diabetes from diabetes secondary to CP [58]. The pancreatic glucagon response to arginine is impaired in patients with CP but not in those with primary diabetes.

Table 4. Accuracy of imaging and functional procedures in the diagnosis of chronic pancreatitis[a]

	Sensitivity (%)	Specificity (%)
Imaging procedures		
Ultrasonography	74	84
Computed tomography	81	87
Endoscopic retrograde pancreatography	89	92
Exocrine function		
Direct funtion tests		
Secretin/cerulein test	90	94
Lundh test	80	85
Indirect function tests		
Serum enzymes	30	95
Fecal chymotrypsin	75	84
NBT-PABA test	87	89
Pancreolauryl test	82	87
Amino acid consumption test	69–96	54–100
Endocrine function		
Pancreatic polypeptide	76	90
Arginine test	75	

NBT-PABA, nitro blue tetrazolium-*para*-aminobenzoic acid.
[a] Mean values estimated on the basis of studies quoted in this article.

The integrated plasma pancreatic polypeptide (PP) response to food, secretin infusion, or cerulein infusion seems to be a reliable test in the diagnosis of CP, and in differentiating between moderate and severe stages of the disease [59, 60]. The PP response is related to pancreatic exocrine function in advanced stages of CP [61]. However, the sensitivity of this test in the diagnosis of early stages of CP is limited.

Values of sensitivity and specificity of the different procedures in the diagnosis of chronic pancreatitis are shown in Table 4. Variability among studies is high, basically due to the different stage of CP in the studied patients, to the different control group selected, and to the different diagnostic criteria applied for each one of the tests to define CP.

Correlation of Imaging and Function in Chronic Pancreatitis

A significant correlation between ductal abnormalities (ERP) and parenchymal lesions (CT, US) with pancreatic function impairment has been found only in advanced stages of CP; the correlation is frequently weak in earlier stages [16]. Studies comparing the degree of ductal abnormalities in ERP with the degree of functional impairment in the SC test have demonstrated a significant correlation [20, 26, 62]. However, a high discrepancy exists between these two tests in early stages of CP [20, 26, 62]. A high correlation has been also observed between the SC test and morphological changes in CT [20], while the discrepancy between authors regarding the correlation between the SC test and US findings is greater [5, 21, 63]. When individual secretory parameters in the SC test with morphological findings are compared, amylase secretion appears to be more closely correlated with CT parenchymal abnormalities than with ERP ductal changes, while bicarbonate secretion is more closely correlated with the degree of ERP ductal abnormalities [20]. In spite of the significant correlation between imaging procedures and function tests in CP, prediction of exocrine function based on morphological alterations, or vice versa, is not possible [26].

Conclusions

Because of its low cost, and noninvasiveness, high-resolution US is firmly placed as the first step in the diagnostic approach to CP. Because of its high accuracy in detecting small cysts and calcifications, CT is a valid method if US findings are inconclusive. The most accurate imaging procedure in diagnosing and staging CP is ERP, with which ductal changes can be detected at a relatively early stage. ERP provides the most valuable information about morphological alterations since strictures and stones, within the pancreatic duct system can be exactly located; it is, therefore, essential for the planning of surgical therapy in CP. The sensitivity and specificity

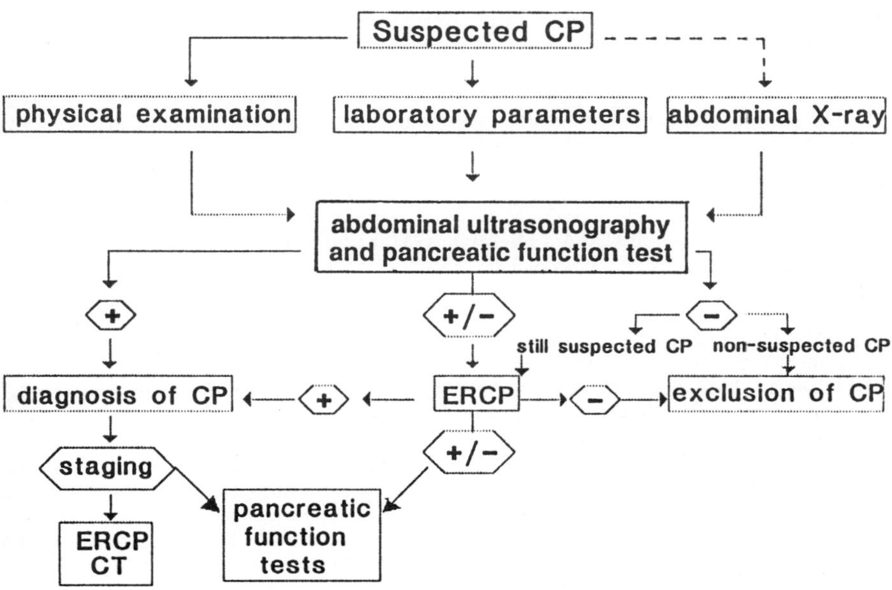

Fig. 7. Diagnostic algorithm of chronic pancreatitis (*CP*)

of the imaging procedures decrease markedly in the detection of early pancreatic damage. Pancreatic function tests may be of value in the interpretation of mild to moderate morphological abnormalities. Moreover, therapeutic management of patients with CP requires the knowledge of the functional status of the pancreas. The most efficient and reliable pancreatic function test is still the analysis of duodenal aspirates following exogenous stimulation with secretin and CCK or cerulein. However, indirect tests, basically the modified serum PLT, is a valid alternative because of its high accuracy, noninvasiveness, practicability, and simplicity. The steps to be in the diagnosis of CP are summarized in the algorithm in Fig. 7.

Acknowledgements. J.E. Domínguez-Muñoz is the recipient of a grant from the Alexander von Humboldt Foundation.

References

1. Niederau C, Grendell JH (1985) Diagnosis of chronic pancreatitis. Gastroenterology 88:1973–1995
2. Otte M (1986) Ultrasound in chronic pancreatitis. In: Malfertheiner P, Ditschuneit H (eds) Diagnostic procedures in pancreatic disease. Springer, Berlin Heidelberg New York, pp 143–148
3. Swobodnik W, Meyer W, Brecht-Kraus D et al. (1983) Ultrasound, computed tomography and endoscopic retrograde cholangiopancreatography in the morphologic diagnosis of pancreatic disease. Klin Wochenschr 61:291–296
4. McCain AH, Berkman WA, Bernardino ME (1984) Pancreatic sonography: past and present. JCU 12:325–332
5. Bolondi L, Priori P, Gullo L et al. (1987) Relationship between morphological changes detected by ultrasonography and pancreatic exocrine function in chronic pancreatitis. Pancreas 2:222–229
6. Bolondi L (1984) The pancreas. In: Bolondi L, Gandolfi L, Labo G (eds) Diagnostic ultrasound in gastroenterology: instrumentations, clinical problems and atlas. Butterworths, Padua, pp 261
7. Marks WM, Filly RA, Callen PW (1980) Ultrasonic evaluation of normal pancreatic echogenicity and its relationship to fat deposition. Radiology 137:475–479
8. Alpern MB, Sandler MA, Heilman GM et al. (1985) Chronic pancreatitis: ultrasonic features. Radiology 155:215–219
9. Worthen NJ, Beaben O (1982) Normal pancreatic echogenicity: relation to age and body fat. AJR 139:1095–1098
10. Bolondi L, Bassi S, Gaiani S, Barbara L (1989) Sonography of chronic pancreatitis. Radiol Clin N Am 27:815–833
11. Glaser J, Hogemann B, Krummenerl T et al. (1987) Sonographic imaging of the pancreatic duct. New diagnostic possibilities using secretin stimulation Dig Dis Sci 32:1075–1081
12. Bolondi L, Bassi S, Gaiani S, Santi V, Gullo L, Barbara L (1989) Impaired response of main pancreatic duct to secretin stimulation in early chronic pancreatitis. Dig Dis Sci 34:834–840
13. Gowland M, Kalantzis N, Warwick F, Braganza J (1981) Relative efficiency and predictive value of ultrasonography and endoscopic retrograde pancreatography in diagnosis of pancreatic disease. Lancet 2:190–193

14. Foster PN, Mitchell CJ, Robertson DRC et al. (1984) Prospective comparison of three non-invasive tests for pancreatic disease. Br Med J 289:13–16
15. Hessel SJ, Siegelman SS, McNeil BJ et al. (1982) A prospective evaluation of computed tomography and ultrasound of the pancreas. Radiology 143:129–133
16. Malfertheiner P, Büchler M (1989) Correlation of imaging and function in chronic pancreatitis. Radiol Clin N Am 27:51–64
17. Ammann RW, Akovbiantz A, Largiader F et al. (1984) Course and outcome of chronic pancreatitis. Longitudinal study of a mixed medical-surgical series of 245 patients. Gastroenterology 86:820–828
18. Ferruci JT, Wittenberg J, Black EB, Kirkpatrick RH, Hall DA (1979) Computed body tomography in chronic pancreatitis. Radiology 130:175–182
19. Freeny PC, Marks WM (1984) Computed tomography of chronic pancreatitis. In: Sarles H, Singer M, Gyr K (eds) Pancreatitis – concepts and classification. Elsevier, Amsterdam, pp 219–223
20. Malfertheiner P, Büchler M, Stanescu A, Ditschuneit H (1986) Exocrine pancreatic function in correlation with ductal and parenchymal morphology in chronic pancreatitis. Hepatogastroenterology 33:110–114
21. Malfertheiner P, Büchler M, Beger HG, Ditschuneit H (1984) Exocrine pancreatic function in correlation to morphological findings (assessed by different imaging procedures) in chronic pancreatitis. In: Sarles H, Singer M, Gyr K (eds) Pancreatitis – concepts and classification. Elsevier, Amsterdam, pp 291–299
22. Axon ATR, Classen M, Cotton PB, Cremer M, Freeny PC, Less WR (1984) Pancreatography in chronic pancreatitis: international definitions. Gut 25:1107–1112
23. Axon ATR (1989) Endoscopic retrograde cholangiopancreatography in chronic pancreatitis. Cambridge classification. Radiol Clin N Am 27:39–50
24. Cotton PB, Less WR, Vallon AG, Cottone M, Croker JR, Chapman M (1980) Gray-scale ultrasonography and endoscopic pancreatography in pancreatic diagnosis. Radiology 143:453–459
25. Valentini M, Cavallini G, Vantini I et al. (1981) A comparative evaluation of endoscopic retrograde cholangiopancreatography and the secretin-cholecystokinin test in the diagnosis of chronic pancreatitis: a multicentre study in 124 patients. Endoscopy 13:64–67
26. Braganza JM, Hunt LP, Warwick R (1982) Relationship between pancreatic exocrine function and ductal morphology in chronic pancreatitis. Gastroenterology 82:1341–1347
27. Girwood AH, Hatfield ARW, Bornman PC et al. (1984) Structure and function in noncalcific pancreatitis. Dig Dis Sci 29:721–726
28. Heij HA, Obertop H, Van Blankenstein M, Nix GAJJ, Westbroek DL (1987) Comparison of endoscopic retrograde pancreatography with functional and histologic changes in chronic pancreatitis. Acta Radiol 28:289–293
29. Classen M, Koch H, Demling L (1972) Diagnostische Bedeutung der endoskopischen Kontrastdarstellung des Pankreasgangsystem. Leber Magen Darm 2:79–81
30. Kasugai T (1975) Recent advances in the endoscopic retrograde cholangiography. Digestion 13:79–99
31. Liguory Cl, Caletti G (1976) An evaluation of endoscopic retrograde pancreatography (ERP) in chronic and relapsing acute pancreatitis. Endoscopy 8:59–64
32. Löffler A, Miederer SE, Glänzer K (1976) Endoskopische retrograde Pankreatikographie (ERP) und exokrine Funktion bei verschiedenen Pankreatitisformen und Papillenstenose. Leber Magen Darm 6:235
33. Belohlavek D (1977) Diagnostische Möglichkeiten der endoskopisch retrograden Cholangiopankreatikographie. Postdoctoral thesis, University of Ulm, FRG

34. Rolny P, Lukes PJ, Gamklou R (1978) A comparative evaluation of endoscopic retrograde pancreatography and secretin-CCK test in the diagnosis of pancreatic disease. Scand J Gastroenterol 13:777–781
35. Anacker H, Weiss HD, Kramann B, Gmelin E (1981) Die Treffsicherheit der endoscopisch retrograden Pankreatiko-Cholangiographie in der Diagnostik der Pankreaskrankheiten. DMW 106:230–233
36. Schmitz-Moormann P, Malchow H, Himmelmann GW et al. (1983) Pancreatitis-like changes in ERCP and their morphological patterns: the validity of ERCP. Digestion 28:60
37. Gullo L (1990) Value and clinical role of intubation tests in chronic pancreatitis. In: Beger HG, Büchler M, Ditschuneit H, Malfertheiner P (eds) Chronic pancreatitis. Springer, Berlin Heidelberg New York, pp 287–290
38. Gyr H, Agrawal NM, Felsenfeld O et al. (1975) Comparative study of secretin and Lundh tests. Am J Dig Dis 20:506–512
39. Wormsley KG (1978) Test of pancreatic secretion. Clin Gastroenterol 7:529–544
40. Ashton MG, Axon ATR, Lintott DJ (1978) Lundh test and ERCP in pancreatic disease. Gut 19:910–915
41. Arvanitakis C, Cooke AR (1978) Diagnostic tests of exocrine pancreatic function and disease. Gastroenterology 74:932–948
42. Johnson SG, Levitt MD (1978) Relation between serum pancreatic isoamylase concentration and pancreatic exocrine function. Dig Dis Sci 23:914–918
43. Ventrucci M, Pezzilli R, Gullo L, Plate L, Sprovieri G, Barbara L (1989) Role of serum pancreatic enzyme assays in diagnosis of pancreatic disease. Dig Dis Sci 34:39–45
44. Fahrenkrug J, Magid E (1980) Concentration of immunoreactive trypsin and activity of pancreatic isoamylase in serum compared in pancreatic diseases. Clin Chem 26:1573–1576
45. Domínguez-Munoz JE, Pieramico O, Büchler M, Malfertheiner P (1992) Ratios of different serum pancreatic enzymes in the diagnosis of chronic pancreatitis and in the evaluation of the morphological stage. Digestion (submitted)
46. Lankisch PG, Koop H, Otto J (1986) Estimation of serum pancreatic isoamylase: its role in the diagnosis of exocrine pancreatic insufficiency. Am J Gastroenterol 81:365–368
47. Dürr HK, Otte M, Forell MM, Bode JC (1978) Fecal chymotrypsin: a study on its diagnostic value by comparison with the secretin-cholecystokinin test. Digestion 17:404–409
48. Toskes PP (1983) Bentiromide as a test of exocrine pancreatic function in adult patients with pancreatic exocrine insufficiency. Determination of appropriate dose and urinary collection interval. Gastroenterology 85:565–569
49. Malfertheiner P, Peter M, Junge U, Ditschuneit H (1983) Indirect pancreatic function test pancreolauryl- its value in diagnosis of chronic pancreatitis. Klin Wochenschr 61:193–198
50. Lankisch PG, Schreiber A, Otto J (1983) Pancreolauryl test. Evaluation of a tubeless pancreatic function test in comparison with other indirect and direct tests for exocrine pancreatic function. Dig Dis Sci 28:490–493
51. Lang C, Gyr K, Tonko I, Conen D, Stalder GA (1984) The value of serum PABA as a pancreatic function test. Gut 25:508–512
52. Lagger A, Bastian L, Prager J, Pointner H, Deutsch E (1981) Pankreas-Funktionsdiagnostik. Vereinfachtes Screening mit Fluorescein-Dilaurat durch Serumkonzentrations-bestimmungen. Fortschr Med 589–591
53. Malfertheiner P, Büchler M, Müller A, Ditschuneit H (1987) Fluorescein dilaurate serum test: a rapid tubeless pancreatic function test. Pancreas 2:53–60
54. Malfertheiner P, Büchler M, Müller A, Ditschuneit H (1985) Influence of extrapancreatic digestive disorders on the indirect pancreatic function test with fluorescein dilaurate. Clin Physiol Biochem 3:166–173

55. Domschke S, Heptner G, Kolb S, Sailer D, Schneider MU, Domschke W (1986) Decrease in plasma amino acids level after secretin and pancreozymin as an indicator of exocrine pancreatic function. Gastroenterology 90:1031–1038
56. Gullo L, Pezzilli R, Ventrucci M, Barbara L (1990) Caerulein induced plasma amino acid decrease: a simple, sensitive, and specific test of pancreatic function. Gut 31:926–929
57. Kemmer TP, Häberle H, Friess H, Büchler M, Malfertheiner P (1991) Is the amino acid consumption test valuable for the diagnosis of pancreatic insufficiency? Digestion 49:30
58. Keller U, Szollosy E, Varga L, Gyr K (1984) Pancreatic glucagon, secretin and exocrine function (BT-PABA test) in chronic pancreatitis. Dig Dis Sci 29:853–857
59. Campbell D, Slaff J, McGuigan J, DesJardin L, Toskes P (1985) Integrated pancreatic polypeptide response in pancreatic diseases. Gastroenterology 88:1341
60. Adrian TE, Besterman HS, Mallinson CM, Garalotis C, Bloom SR (1979) Impaired pancreatic polypeptide release in chronic pancreatitis with steatorrhoea. Gut 20:98–101
61. Imrie CW, Devine B, McKenzie J (1989) The assessment of chronic pancreatitis. Int J Pancreatol 5:11–15
62. Oguri T (1979) Statistical evaluation on the correlation between endoscopic retrograde cholangiopancreatography and pancreozymin-secretin test – structure and function in chronic pancreatitis. In: Takemoto T, Kasugai AT (eds) Endoscopic retrograde cholangiopancreatography. Igaku-Shoin, Tokyo, pp 48–57
63. Malfertheiner P, Büchler M, Stanescu A et al. (1984) Ultrasound findings in correlation to the exocrine function in chronic pancreatitis. Digestion 30:113–114

Hemorrhagic Complications of Pancreatitis

G. Flati,[1] P. Negro, B. Porowska, D. Flati, and M. Carboni

Introduction

Bleeding in pancreatitis may be due either to gastroduodenal causes (e.g., acute gastric erosions, mucosal congestions, peptic ulceration, Mallory-Weiss syndrome, and alcoholic gastritis), which are usually managed with conservative treatment [1], or to direct involvement of vascular structures by pancreatitic local sequelae. The latter, although uncommon, is usually characterized by massive hemorrhage, which is considered the most severe and rapidly lethal complication of pancreatitis [2, 3]. It may be associated with either acute or chronic pancreatitis and is caused by major vessels' erosion, followed in most cases by vessel disruption or pseudoaneurysm formation. Pseudocysts, severe inflammation, regional necrosis, and infection are the most important pathogenetic factors [4, 5]. Although the incidence of major bleeding in pancreatitis is relatively low (1.7%–2.5%), it is associated with a prohibitively high mortality rate reaching 40%–80% [6, 7, 8].

Stimulated by our experience with three cases of massive postpancreatitic hemorrhage, we carried out a literature review covering the past ten decade.

Patients and Review of the Literature

Case 1

A 30-year-old alcoholic man was transferred to our unit in January 1977 with a diagnosis of severe acute pancreatitis. The patient was in a state of shock, and the abdomen was tender. After 24 h of intensive care the cardiocirculatory and local conditions dramatically worsened. Blood pressure was persistently under 80 mmHg; hematocrit was 20% and hemoglobin 7.5 mmol/l. Exploratory laparotomy was performed, and a massive hemorrhagic pancreatitis was found. Two large drains were placed in the pancreatic region after partial débridement. The early postoperative course was troublesome,

[1] II Department of Surgery, University of Rome "La Sapienza", Via Raimondo D'Aronco 18, 00164 Roma, Italia

Beger/Büchler/Malfertheiner (Eds.)
Standards in Pancreatic Surgery

and the patient died 20 h later of massive hemorrhage. At postmortem examination the peritoneal cavity and the bursa omentalis were full of blood, and the whole pancreas was necrotic. A diffuse necrotic destruction of minor blood vessels appeared to be responsible for the fatal postoperative bleeding.

Case 2

This case has been discussed in detail elsewhere [9]. On August 24, 1983, a 50-year-old single man with an unknown clinical history was admitted to our hospital with signs of peritonitis and severe shock (SBP = 60 mmHg, HR = 160/min). The man was a heavy drinker. Shortly before admission, he had complained of acute diffuse abdominal pain. During the ambulance transport, he suddenly worsened and lost consciousness. Shock treatment was immediately instituted and a nasogastric tube was applied. The aspirate did not reveal any blood, and rectal exploration was negative. Clinical evidence of intra-abdominal hemorrhage and a suspected aortic aneurysm rupture prompted us to perform an emergency laparotomy. On the way to the operating theater, however, the patient died (about 20 min after admission). At autopsy a massive amount of blood (4 l) was found within the peritoneal cavity. Pancreatic body and tail along with the surrounding organs were devastated by the necrotico-hemorrhagic process. The liver was diffusely atrophic and presented clear macroscopic features of Laennec cirrhosis. Splenomegaly and indirect signs of portal hypertension were also observed. The head of the pancreas was slightly increased in size and moderately indurated. The body and tail were almost completely destroyed. A wide erosive rupture of the splenic vein could be seen at a more detailed evaluation. The retroperitoneum was full of clots and blood which extravasated into the peritoneal cavity in extensive amounts (4 l). The histologic diagnosis was acute necrotico-hemorrhagic pancreatitis with signs of chronic lesions in the remaining pancreas and erosive destruction of the proximal splenic vein.

Case 3

A 38-year-old nonalcoholic man was admitted in May 1990 with severe melena. One month previously he had undergone a jejunal drainage of a postacute pancreatic tail pseudocyst. On admission the patient was afebrile and had a normal serum amylase level. The white blood cell count was 4600/μl, hematocrit 24%, and hemoglobin 8.6 mmol/l. An upper GI tract endoscopy was negative. Five hours later the patient experienced a new severe bleeding episode. Hematocrit dropped to 17.2%, and hemoglobin was 6 mmol/l. An emergency celiac angiogram disclosed a pseudoaneurysm of the splenic artery communicating with the pseudocystojejunostomy (Fig. 1). Coil embolization was performed (Fig. 2), and bleeding was temporarily controlled, allowing hemodynamic and metabolic resuscitation of the patient.

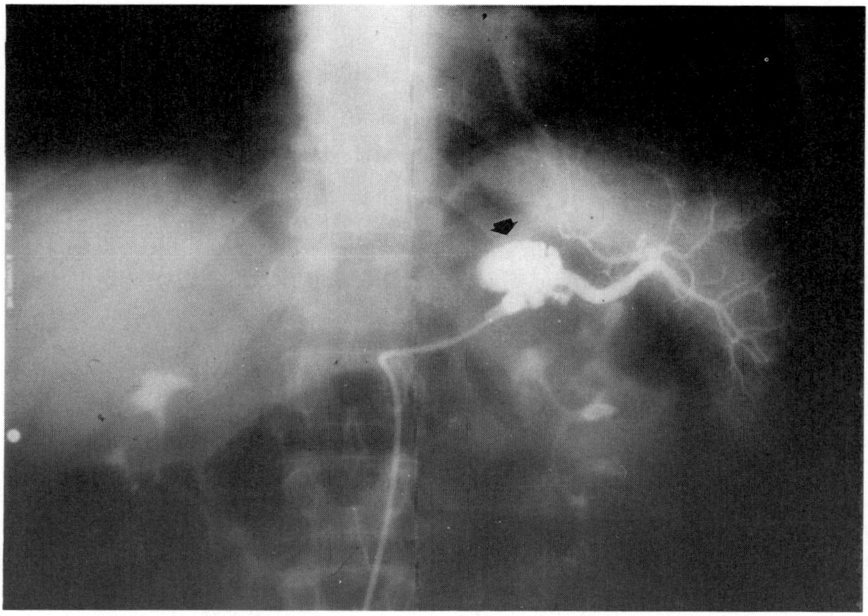

Fig. 1. Case 3. Splenic arteriogram showing extravasation of contrast (*arrow*) into the pseudoaneurysm communicating with the pseudocystojejunostomy

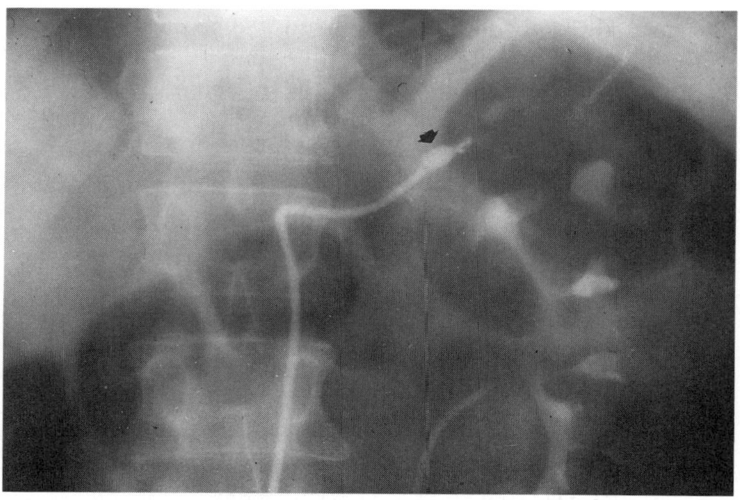

Fig. 2. Case 3. Splenic arteriogram after successful steel coil embolization (*arrow*)

Forty hours later he experienced a new massive bleeding episode. An emergency celiotomy with splenectomy and proximal splenic artery ligation was performed. Perioperatively 11 U blood was transfused; the postoperative course was uneventful, and the patient was discharged in good health 14 days later.

Literature Review

In 1985 the present authors reported a literature review on 159 cases of major hemorrhage in pancreatitis. We present here a more comprehensive review covering almost ten decades. A total of 277 cases reported by 101 authors have been collected and analyzed. The mean age of patients was 47.4 years and male/female ratio was 7 to 1. Mean bood transfusion per patient was 20.3 U. Although this value is related to 41 cases in which the quantity of blood transfused was clearly stated, in the remaining cases the level of bleeding was usually referred to as massive, major, or severe. According to the definition of Shankar and Russel [10], major bleeding should be considered that in which the patient presents with a drop in hemoglobin concentration over 4 g/dl, has a transfusion requirement of over 4 U, and has a peripheral circulatory impairment. The present review was aimed at defining the most important clinical features of what is considered to be the most lethal complication of acute and chronic pancreatitis, but in many aspects it is still a scarcely defined entity. In particular we focused on the following points: (a) etiopathogenetic factors and mechanisms involved in the bleeding process; (b) etiology-related mortality; (c) mortality related to the bleeding sources, to the sites of bleeding, and to the particular anatomo-pathologic sequelae of pancreatitis (e.g., infected necrosis, abscess); (d) diagnostic detection of the bleeding sources; and (e) therapeutic possibilities and treatment-related mortality.

Results and Discussion

Massive hemorrhage is a rare and fatal complication of acute pancreatitis, but, as is shown in Table 1, it has been observed more frequently in chronic pancreatitis. The grade of activity of the chronic form is probably an important factor. Therefore we considered a particular subgroup of patients, those who presented a chronic pancreatitis associated with clinical and morphologic evidence of acute pancreatitis. In all, 107 patients out of 277 reported died, for an overall mortality of 38.6%, which is similar to the rate reported by Stabile et al. [11] in his review of 131 cases. The highest mortality rate (69.2%) was observed among patients who had undergone drainage procedures for the treatment of pancreatic pseudocysts. Similarly high mortality rates were observed when bleeding occurred in patients with acute pancreatitis or in patients with chronic pancreatitis presenting severe

Table 1. Etiology of bleeding and related mortality in different types of pancreatic diseases

	n	%	Deaths	Mortality (%)
Chronic pancreatitis	175	63.1	48	27.4
Acute necrotizing pancreatitis	44	15.8	27	61.4
Chronic + acute pancreatitis	7	2.5	4	57.1
Postdrainage	26	9.4	18	69.2
Traumatic pancreatitis	1	0.4	–	–
Not specified	24	8.6	10	41.6
Total	277	–	107	38.6

acute morphologic and clinical alterations (Table 1). For a better understanding of these data we believe it important to consider the pathogenesis of massive bleeding. With regard to acute pancreatitis it seems likely that uncontrolled severe inflammation and activated lytic enzymes (elastase) might cause lysis of the elastic component of the vessel wall with consequent erosion and disruption. Regional necrosis, particularly when it is infected, may destroy the microcirculation, leading to diffuse uncontrollable bleeding or may cause major vessel disruption.

A second pathogenetic mechanism involves the presence of pseudocysts. In the majority of patients these were associated with a long-standing chronic pancreatitis. Pseudocysts may produce erosions of vessels as a consequence of persistent compression, ischemia, and elastolytic action of its enzymatic content [2, 3]. Frequently this chronic mechanism results in pseudoaneurysm formation. When a pseudoaneurysm ruptures within the pseudocyst cavity, the latter becomes pseudoaneurysmatic or the so-called "pulsatile pseudocyst," which may eventually rupture in the retroperitoneum or peritoneal cavity or may communicate with adjacent hollow structures such as stomach, duodenum, jejunum, and colon. Occasionally, rupture of the pseudoaneurysm or the pseudoaneurysmatic pseudocyst takes place directly into the pancreatic duct, producing hemosuccus pancreaticus. Wirsungrrhagia and pancreatic duct hemorrhage are synonyms. The same meaning is sometimes erroneously attributed to hemoductal pancreatitis. This refers to a pancreatitis caused by pancreatic duct obstruction as a result of bleeding within the pancreatic duct. This may originate from true splenic aneurysms or from pancreatic cancer.

A third important pathogenetic mechanism may explain our second case report and a few other similar cases reported in the literature. Inflammatory process and pseudocyst may result in portal or splenic vein erosion or may cause their thrombosis or simply their compression, leading to localized portal hypertension. When erosion takes place, it usually produces massive fulminant bleeding. In some cases secondary gastroesophageal varices are the bleeding source.

Table 2. Bleeding sources and associated mortality

	n	Deaths	Mortality (%)
Splenic a.	65	14	21.5
Gastroduodenal a.	26	10	38.4
Superior pancreaticoduodenal	18	11	61.1
Inferior pancreaticoduodenal	10	5	50
Diffuse bleeding	10	7	70
Hepatic a.	8	2	25
Drainage edges	6	5	83.3
Splenic vein	5	3	60
Superior mesenteric a.	5	3	60
Cyst wall	5	4	80
Left gastric a.	4	–	–
Dorsal pancreatic a.	3	–	–
Pancreatic veins	1	1	100
Portal vein	2	2	100
Splenic parenchima	1	1	100
Left gastroesophageal a.	1	1	100
Aorta	2	1	50
Right gastric a.	2	–	–
Transverse pancreatic a.	2	–	–
Renal a.	1	–	–
Right colic a.	1	–	–
Left inferior phrenic a.	1	–	–
Right gastroesophageal a.	1	–	–
Not descrided	72	29	40.3
Total	252	99	39.3

Table 3. Mortality related to the site of bleeding

	n	%	Deaths	Mortality (%)
External drainages	4	3	4	100
Gastrointestinal	28	21	15	53.6
Colon	26	19.5	13	50
Peritoneal cavity	17	12.8	9	52.9
Retroperitoneum + duodenum	2	1.5	1	50
Duodenum	12	9	6	50
Stomach	20	15	6	30
Pancreatic ducts	15	11.3	4	26.6
Pseudocyst	5	3.7	–	–
Peritoneal cavity + duodenum	2	1.5	–	–
Retroperitoneum	2	1.5	–	–
Total	133	100	58	42.5

Tables 2 and 3 show the mortality rates related to the source and the site of bleeding, respectively. Splenic artery, gastroduodenal artery, and superior pancreaticoduodenal artery are the vessels most frequently involved. The highest associated mortality rates have been observed among vessels of the pancreatic head region. Portal vein and splenopancreatic veins have occasionally been involved, and the related mortality has been extremely high, varying between 60% and 100%. Analyzing the mortality rates associated with the site of bleeding, it appears that when the colon, peritoneal cavity, or duodenum are involved, the number of fatal cases is higher as compared to the stomach and pancreatic ducts. Stomach bleeding is as promptly diagnosed as Wirsung duct bleeding usually is. The anatomic characteristic of the latter may also limit blood loss. Colonic bleeding due to acute pancreatitis was associated with a mortality rate of 85.7%, while in the presence of chronic pancreatitis 38.8% of patients died. Higher mortality was observed among patients with colon bleeding due to pancreatic abscess compared to patients with bleeding pseudocysts (Table 4). It is clear that in necrotizing pancreatitis the tissue and vessel wall dissolution is much more devastating in the presence of septic contamination. As a consequence, bleeding may assume a rapidly lethal course, and its surgical treatment becomes extremely hazardous. In fact, bleeding due to infected necrosis and abscess has been found associated with a worse prognosis compared to bleeding due to pseudocyst or pseudoaneurism (Table 5). The over-

Table 4. Mortality (%) due to colon bleeding ($n = 26$) in relation to the etiology and the presence of abscess and pseudocyst

Etiology	Overall ($n = 26$)	Abscess ($n = 10$)	Pseudocyst ($n = 13$)
Acute pancreatitis ($n = 7$)	85.7	66.6	100
Chronic pancreatitis ($n = 13$)	38.8	50	44.4
Not reported ($n = 6$)	33.3	66.6	0
Total	50	60	38.8

Table 5. Massive bleeding in pancreatitis: anatomo-pathologic findings and related mortality (%)

	Acute pancreatitis ($n = 24$)	Chronic pancreatis ($n = 34$)	Not reported ($n = 138$)	Total ($n = 196$)
Infected necrosis ($n = 13$)	53.8	–	–	53.8
Abscess ($n = 12$)	75	25	50	50
Pseudocyst and pseudoaneurysm ($n = 140$)	–	0	38.8	37.1
Pseudocyst ($n = 26$)	42.8	21	–	26.9
Pseudo-aneurism ($n = 5$)	–	20	–	20

all mortality of postoperative postdrainage bleeding is higher than that of spontaneous bleeding (48.6% versus 33%). In patients undergoing pseudocyst drainage procedures underlying vessel injuries might result in massive bleeding episodes, which are facilitated by a sudden fall in intracystic pressure and by bacterial contamination of the residual cavity.

Diagnosis and Treatment

Spontaneous bleeding due to pancreatitis can represent a diagnostic challenge since it is often attributed to more common causes of bleeding in the alcoholic population such as gastroduodenitis, ulcer diseases, or gastroesophageal varices [1, 11]. This may delay a correct diagnosis. In the majority of cases upper and lower endoscopic examinations are useful only to exclude primary gastrointestinal bleeding. In patients with pancreatic pseudocysts or long-standing pancreatitis or in patients who had undergone internal pseudocyst drainage, clinical suspicion of severe hemorrhagic complication is mandatory. The triad of protracted pancreatitis, abdominal mass, and hematochezia [12, 13] is highly suggestive of bleeding coming from a fistula between a pseudoaneurysmatic pseudocyst and the colon. Even in such circumstances colonoscopy might be inconclusive although it should be routinely performed for differential diagnosis. Barium enema may show the presence of a fistulous tract. It is generally accepted that celiac angiography is the most useful investigation when massive bleeding due to pancreatitis is strongly suspected. It allows the visualization of the bleeding site and possibly the embolization of the involved vessel. Balloon occlusion, bucrylate embolization, and coil occlusive devices have occasionally been successfully employed to achieve temporary or definitive bleeding control.

Although several authors have reported enthusiastic results with either diagnostic or therapeutic angiographic approaches to bleeding in pancreatitis [7, 14, 15, 16], some limitations of the procedure have been reported as well [17]. The failures to demonstrate bleeding with angiography may be related to venous bleeding, to intermittent arterial bleeding, or to bleeding from a large surface area. In these circumstances, angiographic control is impossible and may be disappointing when major arteries are involved. In our case 3, although recurrence of bleeding occurred 40 h after embolization of the splenic artery, we had enough time to resuscitate the patient before surgery. Also in Waltman's experience [6] angiographic control of bleeding reduced the rate of bleeding, saved blood, added time for surgical decision making, and reduced the wasting of patient's physical reserves. Duplex ultrasound (real-time and pulsed Doppler ultrasound) and contrast-enhanced computed tomography have occasionally been useful in establishing a correct diagnosis [18]. Table 6 shows the prevalence of various diagnostic means used to identify the bleeding sources in 245 patients. It is evident that diagnosis of this severe complication of pancreatitis is far from established. Exploratory

Table 6. Diagnostic determination of the source of bleeding (n = 245)

	n	%
Surgery	70	28.6
Angiographic		
Preoperative	57	23.3
Postoperative	4	1.6
Clinical	7	2.8
Combined (clinical, surgery, angiography)	18	7.3
CT, duplex US, angiography	5	2
Enhanced CT	3	1.2
Duplex US	1	0.4
Endoscopy	3	1.2
Autopsy	22	8.9
Not specified	55	22.4

CT, Computed tomography; US, ultrasound.

Table 7. Massive bleeding in pancreatitis: mortality associated with treatment

	Acute pancreatitis (n = 19)	Chronic pancreatitis + pseudocyst (n = 106)	Abcess (n = 4)	Postdrainage (n = 15)	Total (n = 144)
Resection					
Proximal (n = 15)	0/1	5/11	1/1	0/2	40%
Distal (n = 39)	0/2	9/37	–	–	23%
Ligature (n = 25)	1/1	5/15	–	5/9	44%
Ligature + drainage (n = 13)	–	2/11	1/1	1/1	30.7%
Ligature + splenectomy (n = 4)	0/1	0/3	–	–	0%
Embolization (n = 28)	6/11	2/17	–	–	28.6%
Embolization + surgery (n = 4)		0/2	0/2	–	0%
Nonope-rative (n = 16)	3/3	9/10	–	2/3	87.5%

laparotomy was diagnostic in a consistent number of patients (28.6%), and in 9% of the cases exact diagnosis could be achieved only at postmortem examination.

Angiographic control of bleeding plays a key role among the therapeutic possibilities and is certainly a valuable complement to surgery. Several surgical options have been proposed to control bleeding. Intracystic suture ligation (possibly followed by a drainage procedure), bipolar arterial ligation, splenectomy, distal resection, and pancreatico-duodenectomy are the most popular ones. Suture ligation of the bleeding point and drainage of the pseudocyst should be abandoned as they are inappropriate in the presence of inflammatory, friable, necrotic, bacterially contaminated tissue. Recurrent severe bleeding is likely to follow. On the other hand, bipolar arterial ligation possibly associated with splenectomy or with internal drainage is a rational and safe conservative procedure in patients with underlying chronic pancreatitis. When bleeding occurs in the presence of friable inflammatory tissues, contaminated necrosis, abscess, or fistula with adjacent organs (e.g., colon, duodenum), distal or proximal resection should be the treatment of choice [10]. Mortality rates associated with this type of treatment are reported in Table 7. It is almost impossible to draw conclusions from these data due to the heterogeneity of the collected experience. We feel the association of embolization and surgery to be the way toward reducing the high mortality observed among severely ill pancreatitic patients.

Finally, we would like to stress the importance of prophylaxis to massive bleeding. Particular care should be dedicated to the surgical treatment of pancreatic pseudocysts contiguous with major blood vessels or when they present a brownish content. Their drainage could result in fatal postoperative bleeding. In such circumstances resective treatment should be strongly considered. Surgical management of severe necrotizing pancreatitis is another crucial point for massive bleeding prevention. As strongly claimed by Beger et al. [19] as well as by Waltman et al. [6], a more aggressive attitude is necessary to identify and treat regional liquefaction necrosis, infected necrosis, and abscesses. Delays and inadequate débridement or insufficient postoperative local lavage may increase the risk of vessel injuries and consequently of severe bleeding complications.

In conclusion, although severe bleeding still represents the most rapid lethal complication of pancreatitis, leading to the death of almost 40% of patients, we believe that this figure might be considerably reduced. The following guidelines are suggested (a) awareness of high-risk predisposing conditions (infected necrosis, abscesses, insufficient necrotic tissue débridement, long-standing pancreatic pseudocysts) and their inadequate treatment; (b) activism in diagnosis for an early identification of the bleeding sources; (c) angiographic attempt to achieve bleeding control; and (d) accurate and definitive surgical procedures.

References

1. Marks NI, Banks S, Louw JH, Farman J (1967) Peptic ulceration and gastrointestinal bleeding in pancreatitis. Gut 8:253–259
2. Stroud WH, Cullom JW, Anderson MC (1981) Hemorrhagic complications of severe pancreatitis. Surgery 90/4:657–665
3. Brown RA, Immelman EJ, Harries-Jones EP (1985) Pancreatic duct haemorrhage. Br J Surg 72/3:223–224
4. Breitenecker R (1960) Fatal gastrointestinal hemorrhage due to chronic relapsing pancreatitis. Report of two cases, one with abscess and one with pseudocyst formation. New Engl J Med 260:1167–1169
5. Eckhauser EF, Stanley JC, Zelenock GB, Borlaza GS, Freier TD, Lindenauer MS (1980) Gastroduodenal and pancreaticoduodenal artery aneurysms: a complication of pancreatitis causing spontaneous gastrointestinal hemorrhage. Surgery 88:335–344
6. Waltman AC, Luers PR, Athanasoulis CA, Warshaw AL (1986) Massive arterial hemorrhage in patients with pancreatitis. Arch Surg 121:439–443
7. Bretagne JF, Heresbach D, Darnault P, Raoul JL, Gosselin M, Carsin M, Gastard J (1990) Pseudoaneurysms and bleeding pseudocysts in chronic

pancreatitis: radiological findings and contribution to diagnosis in 8 cases. Gastrointest Radiol 15:9–16
8. Henne-Bruns D, Froschle G, Grimm H, Kremer B (1991) Acute gastrointestinal bleeding as a complication of pancreatic pseudocysts. Hepatogastroenterology 38:75–77
9. Negro P, Flati G, Flati D, Porowska B, Tuscano D, Bianchini A, Carboni M (1985) Massive fulminant hemorrhage due to splenic rupture in pancreatitis. Dig Surg 2:231–234
10. Shankar S, Russel RCG (1989) Haemorrhage in pancreatic disease. Br J Surg 76:863–866
11. Stabile BE, Wilson SE, Debas HT (1983) Reduced mortality from bleeding pseudocysts and pseudoaneurysms caused by pancreatitis. Arch Surg 118:45–51
12. Berne TV, Edmondson HA (1966) Colonic fistulization due to pancreatitis. Am J Surg 111:359–363
13. Poole GV, Wallenhaupt SL (1984) Massive rectal bleeding from colonic fistula in pancreatitis. Arch Surg 119:732–735
14. Walter JF, Chuang VP, Bookstein JJ, Reuter SR, Cho KJ, Pulmano CM (1977) Angiography of massive hemorrhage secondary to pancreatic disease. Diagn Radiol 124:337–342
15. Huizinga WKJ, Kalideen JM, Bryer JV, Bell PSH, Baker LW (1984) Control of major haemorrhage associated with pancreatic pseudocysts by transcatheter arterial enbolization. Br J Surg 71:133–136
16. Triller VJ, Seiler C, Blumgart LH (1989) Akute intestinale Blutung bei pankreatikopseudozysto-kolischer Fistel. Fortschr Geb Rontgenstr 151/5: 527–531
17. Vujic I, Andersen BL, Stanley JH, Gobien RP (1984) Pancreatic and peripancreatic vessels: embolization for control of bleeding pancreatitis. Radiology 150:51–55
18. Falkoff GE, Taylor KJW, Morse S (1986) Hepatic artery pseudoaneurysms: diagnosis with real-time and pulsed Doppler US. Radiology 158:55–56
19. Beger HG, Buchler M, Bittner R, Block S, Nevalainen T, Roscher R (1988) Necrosectomy and postoperative local lavage in necrotizing pancreatitis. Br J Surg 75:207–212

Conservative Management of Chronic Pancreatitis

E.P. DiMagno[1]

Introduction

Pain and the symptoms of malabsorption are the cardinal manifestations of chronic pancreatitis that require treatment. Complications such as bile duct obstruction secondary to fibrosis or intrapancreatic retention cysts and pseudocysts may also arise and require treatment.

To appropriately manage patients with pain or malabsorption, it is necessary to understand that the natural history and the association and tempo of pain, calcification, and exocrine and endocrine pancreatic insufficiency differ in the alcoholic and nonalcoholic forms of the disease.

Natural History

Patients with alcoholic chronic pancreatitis typically begin having pain in the third to fourth decade (median age 44 years) and rapidly progress to developing pancreatic calcifications and insufficiency within 10 years [1, 2]. Of patients with alcoholic pancreatitis, 10%–20% never have pain and instead present with calcifications, diabetes, or malabsorption. By contrast, in patients with idiopathic chronic pancreatitis, the presence of painful or pain-free pancreatitis, the severity of pain, and the time to calcification and pancreatic insufficiency are related to the age at onset of pancreatitis [1–3].

In our studies [1, 3] we found that idiopathic pancreatitis is comprised of two populations. One group all had the onset of pain before the age of 35 (median age 19 years) and developed calcification and pancreatic insufficiency after 20–25 years (two times slower than patients with chronic alcoholic pancreatitis). By contrast, patients with idiopathic pancreatitis beginning after the age of 35 developed calcification and pancreatic insufficiency much more rapidly (at the same rate as patients with chronic alcoholic pancreatitis).

The severity of pain also is related to the type of pancreatitis. Forty percent of patients with early onset idiopathic pancreatitis have severe pain, whereas 10%–20% of patients with late-onset idiopathic pancreatitis or alcoholic pancreatitis have severe pain. Approximately 50% of the patients

[1] GI Unit, Mayo Clinic, Rochester, MN 55905, USA

Beger/Büchler/Malfertheiner (Eds.)
Standards in Pancreatic Surgery

with late-onset idiopathic pancreatitis may have no pain and present with calcification or pancreatic insufficiency.

With both early- and late-onset idiopathic pancreatitis and alcoholic pancreatitis calcifications and exocrine and endocrine insufficiency eventually developed in similar numbers of patients. Calcifications occurred in 56%, 37%, and 59% of patients with early- and late-onset idiopathic pancreatitis and alcoholic pancreatitis, respectively. Exocrine and endocrine insufficiencies occurred in 40%–50% and 30%–40% of patients, respectively, in all three groups. However, the complications of pseudocyst (27% vs. 15%) and bile duct obstruction (11% vs. 5%) arise more frequently in alcoholics than in patients with the idiopathic forms of chronic pancreatitis.

Medical Management of Pain

The underlying mechanisms of pain in chronic pancreatitis are not well understood. The currently most popular hypothesis is that pain occurs because the low amount of proteases fails to fully activate the normal pancreatic enzyme-dependent negative-feedback regulation of pancreatic secretion [4, 5]. As a result, hypercholecystokinemia occurs, and the subsequent stimulation of the pancreas causes pain. Thus, the major medical strategies for pain relief are to increase intraluminal enzyme content, reduce pancreatic secretion by dietary and pharmacologic means, and provide analgesia by simple oral analgesics or by celiac ganglion plexus blockade.

When a patient with chronic pancreatitis first presents with pain or develops a different pain pattern, appropriate tests are done to determine if there is an anatomic reason for the pain (pseudocyst, phlegmon, or even a peptic ulcer). If no anatomic explanation is found, we advise cessation of *all* ethanol ingestion, ingestion of 8 tablets of a nonenteric coated pancreatic enzyme preparation, e.g., Viokase, with meals consisiting of high amounts of carbohydrate and low amounts of fat and protein (provides sufficient calories, but minimally stimulates pancreatic enzyme secretion) [6], and use of aspirin or acetaminophen for pain. If this program is unsuccessful, a percutaneous celiac ganglion block often is followed by several months of pain-free life [7]. Because repeated treatments are also effective, the necessity of surgery for pain relief is often forestalled or even eliminated. In the past, approximately 30% of patients have failed medical treatment for pain and undergone surgical treatment for pain. Currently, Sandostatin, a somatostatin analogue, is under evaluation as a potential treatment for patients with painful chronic pancreatitis, and cholecystokinin (CCK) antagonists theoretically might provide pain relief, but none are clinically available.

The effectiveness of celiac ganglion blocks and enzymes is controversial. Contrary to our view, the prevailing opinion is that pain of chronic pancreatitis rarely should be treated with nerve block [8]. Multiple studies on the effect of enzyme therapy on pancreatic pain have been done and variable results reported [9]. The lack of uniform pain relief in the studies has usually been ascribed to inadequate release of microencapsulated enzymes in the duodenum. Alternative or additional explanations have not been investigated. None of the trials of enzyme therapy to treat painful chronic pancreatitis have accounted for the possible effect of diet on enzyme secretion [6]. Also, it is possible that the amount of protein in diets might variably bind the ingested proteolytic enzymes and affect their ability to hydrolyze CCK-releasing factor and reduce the pain-relieving effect of ingested enzymes.

Increasingly, on the basis of anecdotal reports, endoscopic placement of stents into the pancreatic duct is gaining popularity as a treatment for pain relief. For example, McCarthy et al. [10] reported symptomatic relief after endoscopic stent placement in 17% of 22 patients with pancreas divisum (an unlikely cause of pancreatitis!) and in 8% of 15 patients with chronic pancreatitis. Even proponents of stenting, however, concluded that prospective clinical trials are needed to determine if stent occlusion is associated with recurrent symptoms [10], and that success depends heavily on the anatomic situation and on the skill of the endoscopist [11].

In my opinion, further application of endoscopic stenting of the pancreatic duct should be stopped until controlled studies are done to determine the long-term effects of this procedure. This extreme position is warranted by the significant mortality and complication rate associated with the procedure. Of 32 patients, Huibregtse et al. [10] reported that seven (22%) had complications. One of these died (3%). Three patients had surgery as a result of the procedure (9%), two developed acute pancreatitis, and two developed pancreatic abscess (6%).

Even more disquieting is the recent report by Kozarek [12] that duct abnormalities occurred in 36% of patients who had stents placed for a variety of problems, including disrupted ducts, isolated strictures, pancreas divisum, and hypertensive duct sphincters. Stent occlusion was associated with development of pseudocyst or diffuse duct enlargement, which resolved after stent removal or exchange. More ominous was the development of irregular stenosis and side-branch ectasia, indistinguishable from the findings of chronic pancreatitis in patients with patent stents. Of major concern, however, was the failure of these abnormalities to resolve with stent removal. Similarly, Derfus et al. [13] reported that 76% (n = 22) of patients with previously normal ducts (n = 28) had abnormal ducts at the time of stent removal. Six months post stent, 15 patients underwent an ERCP and two (13%) continued to have abnormal pancreatic ducts. It is possible that stent placement produces chronic pancreatitis in a significant number of patients.

Medical Management of Malabsorption

Treatment of steatorrhea is the major problem in managing malabsorption of chronic pancreatitis, as protein malabsorption is almost always abolished with standard pancreatin therapy. However, we showed almost two decades ago in carefully done studies that steatorrhea can be abolished if enough lipase is given (30 000 IU per meal) and gastric acid secretion is inhibited [14]. We also showed that other factors may be involved in the maldigestion and malabsorption of fat, such as precipitation of bile acid by low intraduodenal pH [15] and proteolytic inactivation of ingested lipase. These findings recently have again been largely confirmed [17, 18].

In patients with severe pancreatic insufficiency secondary to alcoholic pancreatitis, azotorrhea will be abolished and steatorrhea satisfactorily reduced by ingesting 8 tablets of Viokase or the equivalent of at least 30 000 IU of lipase and 10 000 units of trypsin with meals that consist of 25 g of fat. To prevent immediate inactivation of lipolytic activity by gastric acid and to increase mixing of the enzymes with meals, we recommend ingesting one fourth of the enzyme dose after a few bites of the meal, one half of the dose during the meal, and one fourth of the dose at the end of the meal. Most patients on this regimen achieve satisfactory nutritional status and become relatively asymptomatic.

As to the remaining symptomatic patients, in the past it has been accepted that simple reduction in the amount of dietary fat usually will alleviate symptoms. However, the proper diet for patients with severe pancreatic insufficiency is under current study. In recent in vitro studies [19] we have found that lipolytic activity is maximized by nutrient mixtures that contain high amounts of fat and protein and are low in carbohydrates, and that low concentrations of lipolytic activity undergo proportionally greater inactivation than high concentrations. These data suggest that to maximize survival of lipolytic activity in patients with pancreatic insufficiency, a diet should be recommended that is high in protein (24%), moderate in fat (30%), and low in carbohydrates (40%).

For the occasional patient who remains symptomatic, the addition of cimetidine to standard pancreatin treatment will usually totally eliminate steatorrhea and will alleviate troublesome diarrhea [14]. Similar results have been achieved with bicarbonate [20]. Ranitidine and other H_2 blockers should be as effective as cimetidine, and omeprazole may be more effective. In certain circumstances in which gastric pH is greater than 4 for approximately 2 h postprandially, altering the dose schedule from 8 tablets with meals to 2 tablets hourly may alleviate steatorrhea. In the opposite situation, in which gastric pH does not exceed 5 and duodenal pH is maintained relatively acidic (less than 4) for long periods of time postprandially, enteric coated preparations may be effective.

Difficult patients who continue to have symptoms and steatorrhea may require intubation studies to determine whether intraluminal conditions are present for certain dosage schedules to be effective or whether intraluminal conditions have been altered by adjunctive therapy. For example, if administration of 300 mg of cimetidine does not keep the gastric pH greater than 4, gastric secretion has not been reduced enough. Either more cimetidine should be given, omeprazole substituted for cimetidine, or, if intraluminal conditions are constantly acidic, an enteric coated formulation may be the best preparation to use.

The treatment of steatorrhea remains controversial because practically all studies are uninterpretable due to invalid experimental designs. At the very least, the amount of lipase administered should be the same across treatment groups and the investigators need to independently test the amount of lipolytic activity of the treatment. In five recent trials [16, 21–24] the investigators gave variable amounts of lipase with the treatments and accepted the manufacturer's claims of lipolytic activity and adequacy of the enteric coating if these types of preparations were used. The latter two points are extremely important; it is a well-known fact that lipolytic activity may vary greatly among many enzyme preparations and may not contain the amount of lipolytic activity or bioeffective enteric coating claimed [25].

The major need is for enzyme preparations containing a lipase that can withstand both acid denaturation and proteolytic inactivation. Thus far, fungal lipases, which are acid stable, have not proven to be better than standard pancreatitis preparations [21], but well-done studies have not been performed. Lipase from other organisms or synthetic lipases may fulfill this need. Also, dietary alterations may improve survival of lipase during gastrointestinal transit [19].

Management of Pancreatic Diabetes

The principles of managing pancreatic diabetes are no different from those for diabetes mellitus. However, hypoglycemia may complicate pancreatic diabetes. Inappropriate release of insulin from damaged islet cells, trapped or unavailable hepatic glycogen, or impaired release of glucagon in patients with chronic pancreatitis may contribute to hypoglycemia in patients with late chronic pancreatitis and overt diabetes. The most common causes of hypoglycemia, however, in chronic pancreatitis are continuing abuse of alcohol and irregular caloric intake due to alcohol or variable absorption due to malabsorption. Thus, diabetes was usually undertreated, particularly in the unreliable patient. This approach was taken because it was believed that there was a low incidence of vascular complications and ketoacidosis. However, data from Gullo et al. [26] indicate that the risk and characteristics of retinopathy are similar in patients with diabetes secondary to chronic pancreatitis and patients with idiopathic diabetes mellitus. These findings emphasize the need for appropriate treatment of endocrine insufficiency. If insulin is required, 20–40 units/day usually suffice.

References

1. DiMagno EP, Clain JE (1986) Chronic pancreatitis. In: Go VLW, Gardner JD, Brooks FP, Lebenthal E, DiMagno EP, Scheele GA (eds) The exocrine pancreas: biology, pathobiology and diseases. Raven, New York, pp 541–575
2. Ammann RW, Buehler H, Muench R, Freiburghaus AW, Siegenthaler W (1987) Differences in the natural history of idiopathic (nonalcoholic) and alcoholic chronic pancreatitis. A comparative long-term study of 287 patients. Pancreas 2:368–377
3. Layer P, Kalthoff L, Clain JE, DiMagno EP (1985) Nonalcoholic chronic pancreatitis – two diseases? Dig Dis Sci 30:980
4. Owyang C (1989) Control of exocrine pancreatic secretion. Regul Pept 1:1–7
5. Rowell WG, Toskes PP (1989) Pain in chronic pancreatitis. In: Barkin J, Rogers A (eds) Difficult decisions in digestive diseases. Yearbook Medical, Chicago, pp 192–197
6. Boivin M, Lanspa SJ, Zinsmeister AR, Go VLW, DiMagno EP (1990) Are diets associated with different rates of human interdigestive and postprandial pancreatic enzyme secretion? Gastroenterology 99:1763–1771
7. Pap A, Nauss LA, DiMagno EP (1990) Is percutaneous celiac plexus block (PCPB) associated with pain relief in chronic pancreatitis? A comparison among analgesic, alcohol and steroid PCPB. Pancreas 5:725
8. Bengtsson M, Lofstrom JB (1990) Nerve block in pancreatic pain. Acta Chir Scand 156:285–291
9. Ihse I, Permerth J (1990) Enzyme therapy and pancreatic pain. Acta Chir Scand 156:281–283
10. Huibregtse K, Schneider B, Vrij AA, Tytgat (1988) Endoscopic pancreatic drainage in chronic pancreatitis. Gastrointest Endosc 34:9–15
11. McCarthy J, Geenen JE, Hogan WJ (1988) Preliminary experience with endoscopic stent placement in benign pancreatic diseases. Gastrointest Endosc 34:16–18
12. Kozarek RE (1989) Pancreatic stents can induce ductal changes consistent with chronic pancreatitis. Gastrointest Endosc 35:A170
13. Derfus GA, Geenen JE, Hogan WJ (1989) Alterations in pancreatic duct morphology associated with endoscopic stent placement. Pancreas 4:613
14. Regan PT, Malagelada J-R, DiMagno EP, Glanzman SL, and Go VLW (1977) Comparative effects of antacids, cimetidine, and enteric coating on the therapeutic response to oral enzymes in severe pancreatic insufficiency. N Engl J Med 297:854–858
15. Regan PT, Malagelada J-R, DiMagno EP, Go VLW (1979) Reduced intraluminal bile acid concentrations and fat maldigestion in pancreatic insufficiency: correction by treatment. Gastroenterology 77:285–289
16. Thiruvengadam R, DiMagno EP (1988) Inactivation of human lipase by proteases. Am J Physiol 255:G476–G481
17. Mundlos S, Kühnelt P, Adler G (1990) Monitoring enzyme replacement treatment in exocrine pancreatic insufficiency using the cholesteryl octanoate breath test. Gut 31:1324–1328
18. Andersen JR, Bendtsen F, Ovesen L, Pedersen NT, Rune SJ, Tage-Jensen U (1990) Pancreatic insufficiency. Duodenal and jejunal pH, bile acid activity, and micellar lipid solubilization. Int J Pancreatol 6:263–270
19. Kelly DG, Sternby B, DiMagno EP (1991) How to protect human pancreatic enzyme activities in frozen duodenal juice. Gastroenterology 100:189–195
20. Graham DY (1982) Pancreatic enzyme replacement: the effect of antacids or cimetidine. Dig Dis Sci 27:485–490
21. Schneider MU, Knoll-Ruzicka ML, Domschke S, Heptner G, Domschke W (1985) Pancreatic enzyme replacement therapy: comparative effects of conventional and enteric-coated microspheric pancreatin and acid-stable fungal

enzyme preparations on steatorrhoea in chronic pancreatitis. Hepatogastroenterology 32:97–102
22. Robinson PJ, Sly PD (1990) High-dose pancreatic enzymes in cystic fibrosis. Arch Dis Child 65:311–312
23. Williams J, MacDonald A, Weller PH, Fields J, Pandov H (1990) Two enteric coated microspheres in cystic fibrosis. Arch Dis Child 65:594–597
24. Jorgensen BB, Thorsgaard Pedersen N, Worning H (1991) Monitoring the effect of substitution therapy in patients with exocrine pancreatic insufficiency. Scand J Gastroenterol 26:321–326
25. Hendeles L, Dorf A, Stecenko A, Weinberger M (1990) Treatment failure after substitution of generic pancrelipase capsules. JAMA 263:2459–2461
26. Gullo L, Parenti M, Monti L, Pezzilli R, Barbara L (1990) Diabetic retinopathy in chronic pancreatitis. Gastroenterology 98:1577–1581

Endoscopic Therapy in Chronic Pancreatitis

R.A. KOZAREK[1]

Chronic pancreatitis, usually presenting with recurrent attacks of clinical pancreatitis or chronic pain, is usually the consequence of alcoholism [1]. Less commonly, childhood malnutrition, familial and idiopathic forms, and hyperparathyroidism are felt to be etiologic [2]. Less common still are causes such as papillary stenosis, pancreas divisum, and other obstructive etiologies. Finally, the latter occasionally occurs when chronic pancreatic duct structural damage follows a severe insult, e.g., blunt abdominal trauma or biliary pancreatitis with associated pancreatic duct (PD) disruption. Traditionally, endoscopy has been primarily utilized in conjunction with noninvasive imaging modalities for diagnosis and to direct subsequent surgical intervention [3]. More recently, a number of interventional techniques have been applied at endoscopic retrograde cholangiopancreatography (ERCP) in such patients [4]. Including PD sphincterotomy, stent or drain placement, stone extraction, and pseudocyst drainage, data are accumulating which suggest that endoscopic management is effective in a subset of patients with chronic pancreatitis (Table 1).

Chronic Pain/Relapsing Pancreatitis

Although it is uncertain why patients develop recurrent attacks of clinical pancreatitis or suffer chronic pain in chronic pancreatitis, ductal obstruction may play a role. This is supported by evidence of ductular dilation distal to stones or local stenoses in many patients, an elevation of main PD pressures when compared to controls, and symptomatic relief following longitudinal pancreaticojejunostomy [5–8].

Despite the question of ductal obstruction, however, endoscopic sphincterotomy of the PD has had few adherents. This is related both to fear of eliciting severe pancreatitis and to previous suboptimal results when such patients were treated with surgical septoplasty [9]. More recently, a number of endoscopic series have evolved that suggest an acceptable complication rate, particularly if undertaken in conjunction with stent placement or stone extraction.

---

[1] Virginia Mason Clinic, Dept. of Gastroenterology, University of Washington, P.O. BOX 900, Seattle, WA 98111, USA

Beger/Büchler/Malfertheiner (Eds.)
Standards in Pancreatic Surgery

Table 1. Endoscopic therapies in chronic pancreatitis

Pain, recurrent pancreatitis
Sphincterotomy, biliary/pancreatic
Stricture dilation
Stent/drain placement
Stone extraction
Duct obliteration/occlusion (?)
Complications
Biliary (jaundice, cholangitis, cirrhosis)
Drain and stent placement
Pancreatic Leak
Ascites: stent
Pseudocyst: cystgastrostomy, cystduodenostomy, transpapillary endoprosthesis

a 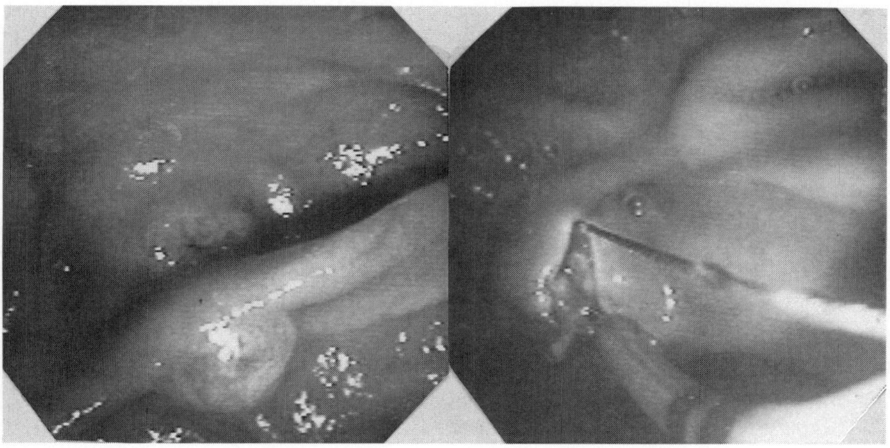 b

Fig. 1a,b. Pancreatic duct sphincterotomy. Note separate biliary and pancreatic ductal orifices (**a**), completed sphincterotomy (**b**)

Sphincterotomy (Fig. 1)

Although evidence of primary sphincter of Oddi dysfunction is lacking in most patients with chronic pancreatitis, pancreaticobiliary manometry suggests that up to one-sixth of patients with idiopathic relapsing pancreatitis have sphincter dysfunction, most commonly an elevated basal pressure [10]. Venu et al. reported 17 such patients, 12 of whom had endoscopic sphincterotomy, 4 pancreatic septoplasty, and one who refused treatment [10]. Ninety-four percent (16/17) remained asymptomatic for periods up to 3 years. While encouraging, data such as these are gleaned from patients

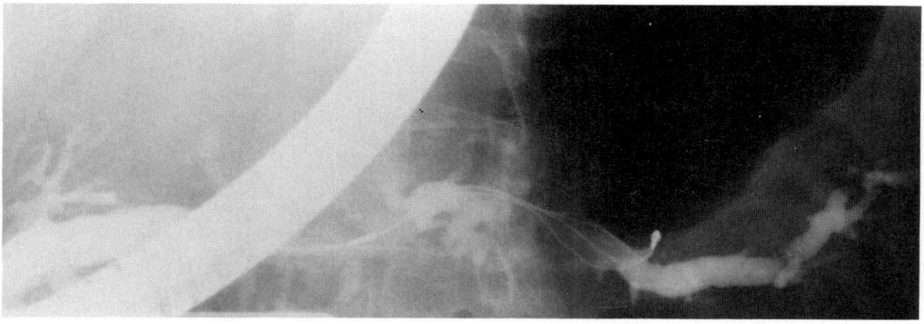

Fig. 2. Stone retrieval in patient with idiopathic chronic pancreatitis. Obstructing calculus has been pushed to midbody during retrieval attempts

with recurrent acute pancreatitis, some of whom may be passing gravel through the biliary tree, and should not be generalized to chronic pancreatitis patients. Further manometric studies are required prior to widespread sphincter section in this patient group.

Stone Extraction (Fig. 2)

Pancreatic calculi are usually felt to be the consequence as opposed to the cause of chronic pancreatitis [11, 12]. Occasionally, however, such stones themselves cause obstruction, particularly when located in the head of the gland. Fuji et al. successfully performed PD sphincterotomy in 10 of 13 patients with chronic pancreatitis, removing calculi in two and placing stents in three [13]. Three patients developed mild clinical pancreatitis and nine of the ten successful procedures were associated with relief of chronic pain.

Sherman et al., in turn, attempted endoscopic PD stone removal in 32 patients with ERCP evidence of chronic pancreatitis [14]. Although 72% of the patients had complete or partial stone removal and two-thirds improved after endoscopic therapy, most patients underwent a significant number of ancillary procedures making the stone extraction significance uncertain. In this series, eight patients had simultaneous biliary, ten pancreatic, four combined, and six minor sphincterotomy. Five patients had stents placed in the dorsal and five in the main pancreatic duct, four had stricture dilation, and five underwent nasopancreatic drain placement. Mild pancreatitis was noted in 8% of patients, 42% had a decrease in the main PD diameter, and one-quarter had regression of chronic pancreatitis changes noted at ERCP. Additional case reports or series have been reported by Ponsky and Duppler [15], Huibregtse et al. [16], Cremer et al. [17] and Schneider and Lux [18] with similar results. Moreover, six of eight patients with chronic pancreatitis (relapsing pancreatitis six, chronic pain two) in a personal series of chronic pancreatitis patients undergoing stone extraction have had no recurrence of symptoms at a mean follow-up of 18 months. Neither patient with chronic pain improved.

In addition to pancreaticobiliary sphincterotomy and direct stone extraction, several authors have recently combined ERCP plus extracorporeal shock wave lithotripsy (ESWL) for PD calculi. Sauerbruch et al. utilized a Dornier renal lithotriptor in 8 patients with chronic pancreatitis and 5–20 mm^2 calculi [19]. After baseline PD sphincterotomy, patients received a mean of 1356 shock waves allowing clearance of the larger stones in seven of eight patients and improvement in pain intensity in half. One patient developed mild pancreatitis. Delhaye et al., in turn, treated 104 patients with endoscopic pancreatic sphincterotomy and nasopancreatic drain followed by lithotripsy (Lithostar, Erlangen, FRG) [20]. Stone fragmentation occurred in 99%, decrease in PD diameter in 82%, and ultimate complete stone clearance from the main PD following additional endoscopic manipulation in 54%. Although all patients were purported to have relief of chronic pain, 41% developed recurrence related to stone migration, relapsing stricture, or stent occlusion (placed in 1/2 of the patients). Complications occurred in one-quarter of cases, usually pancreatitis or pancreaticobiliary sepsis, and there was no mortality. Finally, Grimm et al. treated 15 patients with ESWL following PD sphincterotomy [4]. Thirteen patients had successful stone retrieval and no complications were noted. Long-term follow-up is pending.

Stent Placement (Figs. 3, 4)

Pancreatic stents have been primarily used to bypass obstructing strictures or stones or to protect a sphincterotomized site from acute obstruction.

Major Papilla

Huibregtse et al. endoscopically treated 32 patients with chronic pancreatitis with a variety of therapeutic maneuvers to include sphincterotomy, PD stone extraction, and biliary or PD stent placement [16]. Five patients had transpapillary endoprostheses placed into communicating pseudocysts, one patient had an endoprosthesis placed following sphincterotomy for papillary stenosis, and an additional six endoprostheses were placed beyond obstructing calculi with subsequent stone clearance in two of these patients. Clinical outcomes were better in patients with relapsing pancreatitis and total complication rate was 22%, including one death from perforation at time of sphincterotomy. Specific stent-related complications consisted of occlusion of two of the prostheses, including one placed for pseudocyst drainage with subsequent abscess development. The latter patient ultimately required distal pancreatectomy. McCarthy et al. in turn, treated 35 patients with PD stent placement, including 15 through the major papilla [21]. Successful in 14 patients, 4 of 5 patients with alcoholic pancreatitis and stricture, 3 of 7 with papillary stenosis and recurrent pancreatitis, and 1 of 2

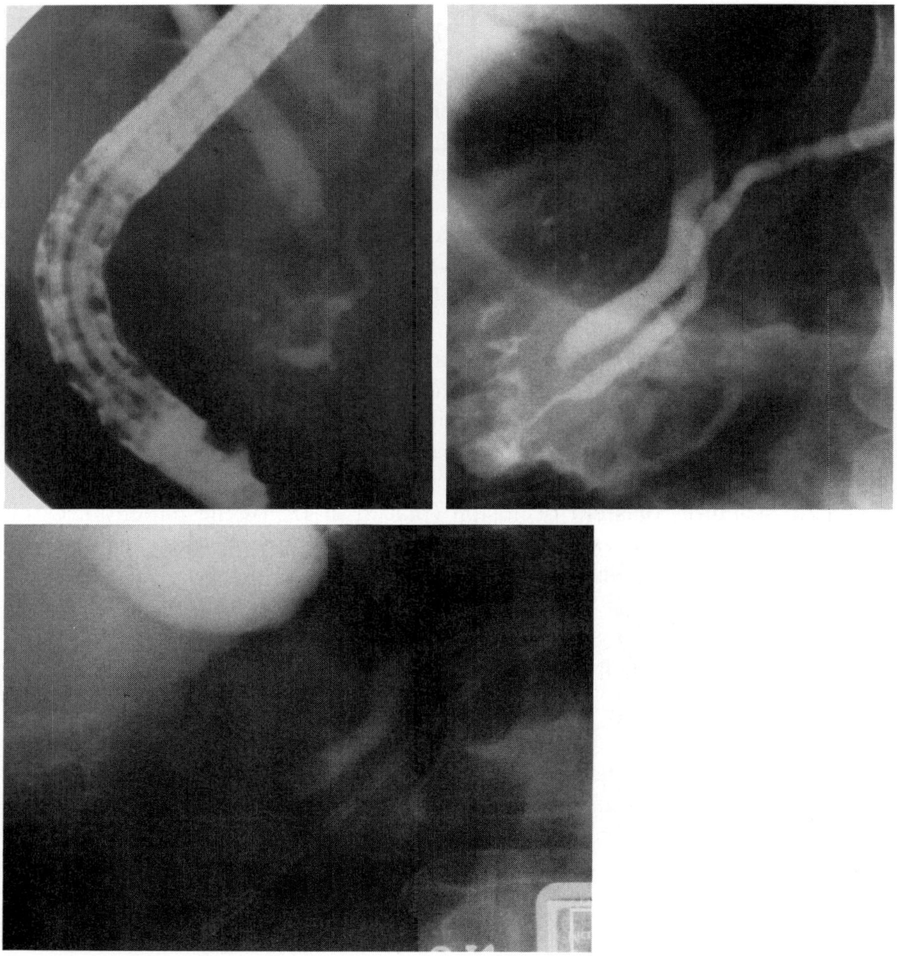
a c b

Fig. 3. **a** Small pseudocyst in patient with relapsing pancreatitis. **b** Stent placement in same patient. **c** Pancreatogram in same patient after 6 weeks of stent. Pancreatitis has not recurred at 6-month follow-up

patients with idiopathic pancreatitis were purported to have symptomatic improvement. In the entire 35 patients, five stents occluded early, four stents migrated spontaneously including two within the body of the PD, and two required removal because of early pain. Five patients developed mild pancreatitis with stent placement.

Additional studies by our group [22] as well as those by Cremer et al. [23] also suggest that placement of pancreatic endoprostheses may be useful

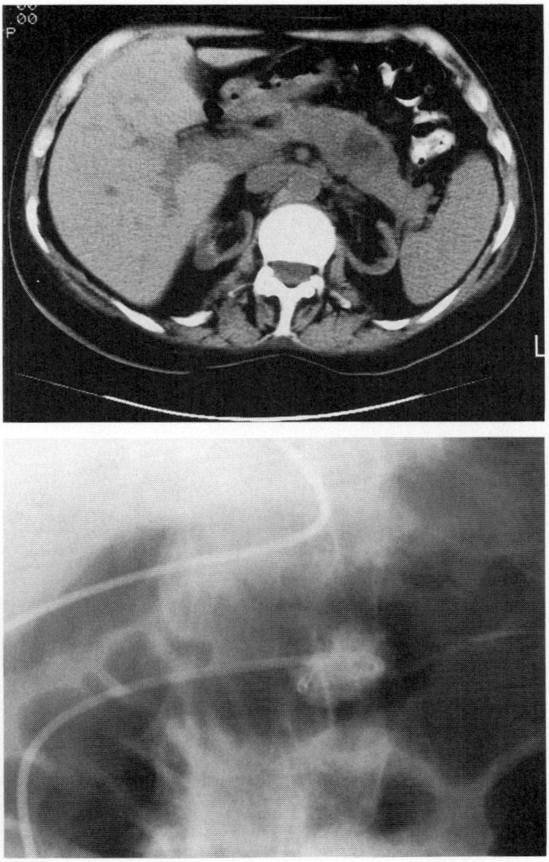

a

b

Fig. 4. a CAT scan showing pseudocyst at junction of body and tail in renal transplant patient. **b** Transnasal pancreatic drain in pseudocyst. Distal pancreatectomy ultimately required

in a subset of chronic pancreatitis patients with papillary stenosis or obstructing strictures or stones. In the latter series, 50 patients with strictures of the main PD and distal dilation were stented using a 10-F endoprosthesis after PD sphincterotomy. At a mean follow-up of 2 years, 55% of the patients were purported to be symptom free, and half of these patients retain an endoprosthesis. In addition to use of conventional polyethylene, prostheses in chronic pancreatitis, Cremer et al. have also placed expandable metal prostheses in a subset of patients [24]. Early reports claim pain relief and reduction in distal duct diameter in all patients. No complications were reported. Whether such prostheses will ultimately be associated with occlusion, as has been noted when used in the biliary tree [25], remains speculative but ultimately likely.

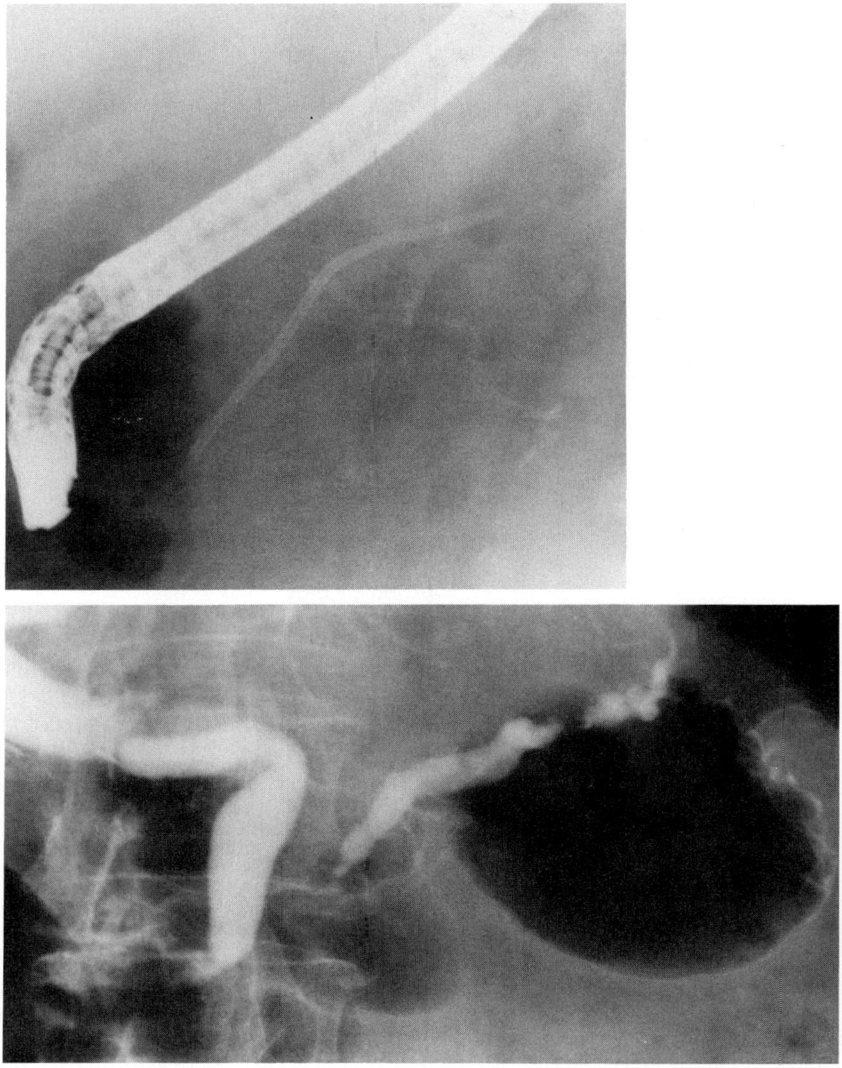

a

b

Fig. 5. a Stent in minor papilla in patient with relapsing pancreatitis. **b** Note moderate ductal dilation, localized stenoses. Subsequent cytology brushings of PD showed dysplasia and pancreatic resection, low-grade carcinoma

Stents: Minor Papilla (Fig. 5)

Occurring in 5%–10% of autopsy and ERCP series, pancreas divisum is thought to predispose to recurrent attacks of pancreatitis by offering a relative obstruction to dorsal pancreatic duct (DPD) [26–30] flow. Its relationship to chronic abdominal pain and localized chronic pancreatitis of the DPD has been more contentious, and reported series approaching the minor papilla endoscopically usually admix all three clinical groups (acute relapsing pancreatitis, chronic abdominal pain, and chronic pancreatitis). McCarthy et al. successfully placed stents in 19 of 22 divisum patients reporting symptomatic improvement in 17 [21]. Sherman et al. undertook sphincterotomy of the minor ampulla, using a needle-knife over an endoscopically placed stent in 33 patients [31]. Twenty of these patients had relapsing pancreatitis and 13 chronic abdominal pain. There was an acute reduction in pancreatitis attacks in 19 of 20 patients initially, although this fell to 15 patients (75%) after a 6- to 54-month follow-up. Patients with chronic pain had a 38% symptomatic improvement after a 2- to 36-month follow-up, a figure that approximates the improvement in such patients following minor sphincteroplasty done surgically. Overall, at a mean follow-up of 19 months, 73% of patients were clinically improved, one-third of whom were asymptomatic. This improvement came at the expense of mild clinical pancreatitis at time of stent placement in most patients. In contrast to the series by McCarthy in which prostheses were traded out every 3–4 months for 1 year, the latter series utilized prostheses for only days or weeks in an attempt to prevent post sphincterotomy edema and occlusion of DPD flow. Other series by Siegel et al. [32], Liguory et al. [33] and Soehendra et al. [34] report similar results as does an unreported personal experience. There is some concern with placement of stents within the PD, however, regardless of whether that stent has been placed through the major or minor papilla. In a retrospective review of 34 patients in whom 38 PD stents were placed, 36% of all patients and 72% of patients with normal initial pancreatograms were found to have subsequent ductal changes [35]. These changes were felt to be related either to stent occlusion (diffuse duct enlargement, pseudocyst) or direct stent trauma and side branch occlusion (irregular stenoses and side branch ectasia possibly related to local pancreatitis). Although most of these changes resolved, and there may be less reason for concern in chronic pancreatitis, PD endoprostheses are obviously not innocuous and demand further study.

Endoscopic Approach to Chronic Pancreatitis Complications

Pseudocyst Drainage (Fig. 6)

Pseudocysts can be endoscopically managed whether by direct fistulization between the bowel wall and the cyst cavity or by transpapillary drain or stent placement through a ductal disruption. Using the former methodology with a diathermic knife, Sahel et al. were successful in creating a cystduodenostomy in 17 of 19 patients with chronic calcific pancreatitis and 20 total pseudocysts [36]. Two patients, one of whom died, experienced bleeding, two patients had local perforations that responded to conservative therapy,

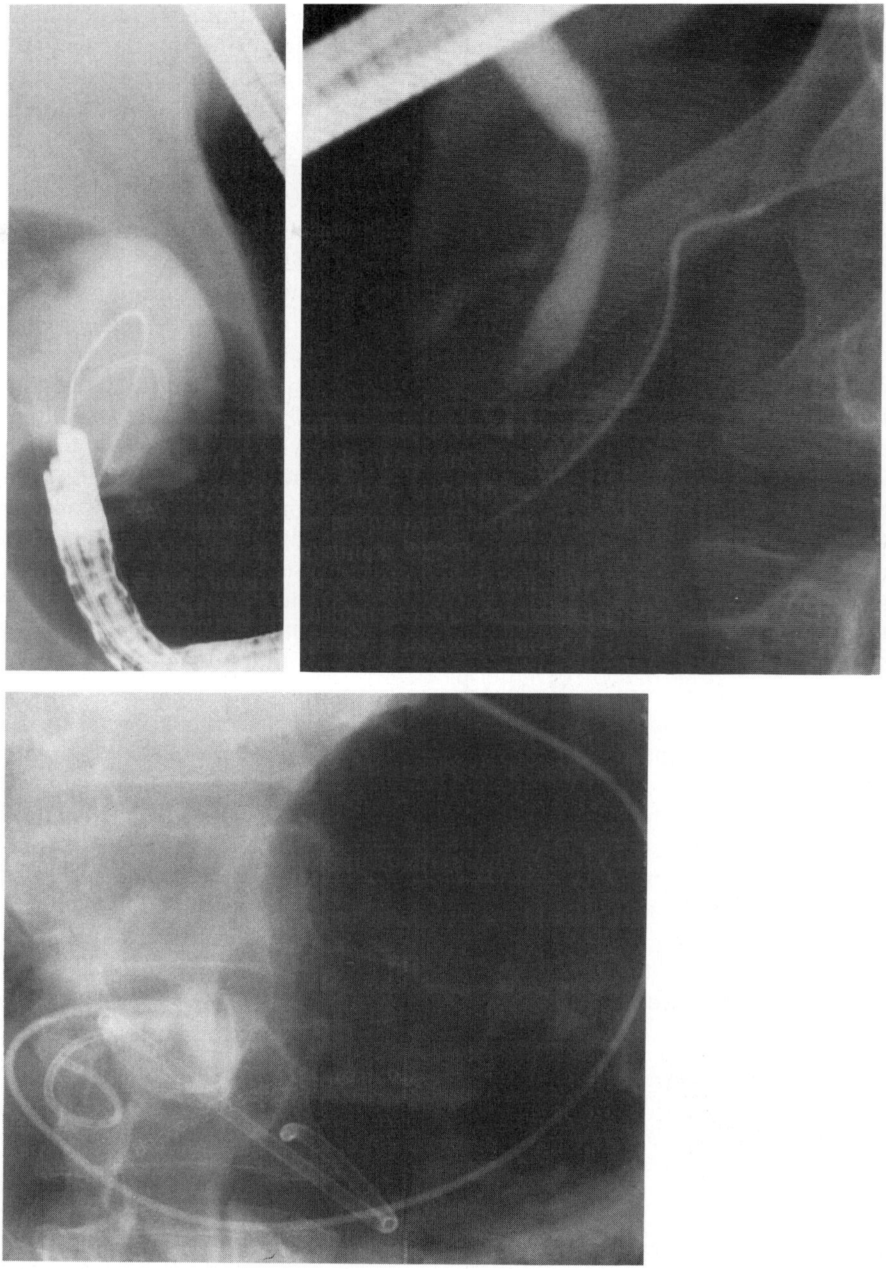

a c b

Fig. 6. **a** Transgastric pseudocyst puncture. Note double pigtail stent and guide wire being placed into cyst cavity. **b** Transcyst nasal drain and 10-F double-pigtail stent in pseudocyst cavity. Note staple line from previous cystgastrostomy. Resolution of cyst with endoscopic drainage. NP drain removal 2 days. Stent retrieval 6 weeks. No recurrence 2 years. **c** ERCP in same patient. Note occluded PD (guide wire to level of obstruction)

and one had transient cholangitis. Overall, 18 of the pseudocysts (90%) could be endoscopically drained and long-term efficacy (>6 months) was ultimately noted in 64% of patients.

In the largest series to date, Cremer et al. reported their results in 33 patients including 22 in whom they performed a cystduodenostomy and 11 in whom a cystgastrostomy was performed [37]. Technical success rates were 96% and 100%, respectively. Side effects included one case of retroperitonitis following duodenal pseudocyst puncture, and one case each of gastric hemorrhage and iatrogenic pseudocyst infection at time of transgastric pseudocyst drainage. Endoscopic drainage, utilizing diathermic puncture, fistula extension with cautery, and nasocyst tube placement was definitive therapy in 19 of 22 patients undergoing cystduodenostomy and 8 of 11 cases in whom cystostomy was performed. Additional case reports or smaller series have been reported by Hershfield [38], Huibregtse et al. [16], Kozarek et al. [39], Henkenbrant and Davaux [40], Delmott et al. [41], Rogers et al. [42], Spinelli et al. [43] and Knecht and Kozarek [44].

All of these series stress the necessity for visualization of the pseudocyst bulge against gastric or duodenal wall, a small amount of intervening tissue as evidenced by abdominal computed tomography or ultrasound, and control of the fistula after it has been created. I no longer extend fistula size with diathermy after entrance into the cyst proper, but instead place a nasocyst tube and double pigtail stent between the pseudocyst and gut lumen. The former allows access to the cyst fluid contents for bacteriologic and chemical analysis as well as to assure progressive reduction in size over a several-day period. The latter is left in place for several weeks to months to assure complete cyst collapse and formation of a chronic fistulous tract prior to its endoscopic retrieval. Moreover, I now suggest applying this technique at the time of endoscopic ultrasonography, a technology not available when the procedure was originally described. Finally, the application of this procedure must be placed into the perspective of other radiologic and surgical drainage techniques as well as local medical expertise within a practice setting.

In addition to direct puncture of the gut wall into a pseudocyst cavity, acute and chronic pseudocysts, peripancreatic fluid collections without a definable wall, pancreatic ascites, and pancreaticopleural/mediastinal fistulae can all be treated with a transpapillary endoprosthesis. Such treatment is predicated on demonstrating the site of ductal disruption and either passing a stent directly into the pseudocyst/fluid collection proper or bridging the site of ductal disruption. The latter probably allows duct healing less by a mechanical sealing mechanism than by bypassing a relative obstruction at the sphincter mechanism. Similar results have been noted in the treatment of biliary fistulae with sphincterotomy, nasobiliary drains, or endoprosthesis placement. Huibregtse et al. reported transpapillary pseudocyst drainage in six patients, five of whom had excellent results and one of whom developed infection following stent occlusion [16].

In the largest series reported to date, Kozarek et al. placed transpapillary drains in 17 patients with PD disruption, nine with acute and eight with chronic pancreatitis. An attempt to avoid acute but not necessarily elective surgical intervention [45], 14 patients had successful treatment of duct disruption. Complications included mild flare of pancreatitis in two and subsequent stent occlusion with recurrent pseudocyst (one) and infection of pseudocyst (one). Surgical intervention was ultimately required in one-third of patients but was primarily undertaken for chronic pain as opposed to complications of ongoing ductal disruption. Since the publication of this initial experience, we have successfully treated other forms of ductal disruption with endoprostheses to include massive pancreatic ascites and pancreaticomediastinal fistulae.

Treatment of Biliary Obstruction

Occurring in 10%–63% of patients with chronic calcific pancreatitis [46], distal biliary stenoses are usually asymptomatic and found incidentally at ERCP, surgery, or autopsy. Due to edema or cicatrization of the mid or distal bile duct within the pancreatic head, these strictures are occasionally symptomatic. Complications include jaundice, cholangitis, liver abscess, and occasionally, biliary cirrhosis, the former three usually considered indications for surgical biliary bypass (choledochoduodenostomy/choledochojejunostomy) [47–49]. Although there have been incidental reports utilizing biliary endoprostheses in the treatment of such stenoses, the largest series to date has been compiled by Deviere et al. [50]. In 25 chronic pancreatitis patients with significant cholestasis (mean bilirubin 4.7 mg/100 ml; mean alkaline phosphatase 5 × normal; 7 evidence of cholangitis), endoscopic stent placement was successful in 23 and in an additional 2 following placement of a percutaneous biliary drainage catheter. Migration of the stent occurred in ten patients and occlusion in eight, four of these patients developing cholangitis. Two patients died of sepsis, including one after surgical cholecystectomy. Only 3 of 21 patients with complete follow-up were asymptomatic without a stent in place. The authors concluded that biliary drainage was satisfactory for the acute complications of pancreatitis-induced biliary stricture (cholangitis, cholestasis), but were not a satisfactory long-term therapy.

Waxman and Huibregtse, in turn, have followed 26 patients with chronic pancreatitis stented for persistent cholestasis plus biliary stenosis [51]. Six patients (23%) remain well after stent retrieval, and 15 retain their stents and have undergone multiple exchanges. Eight patients developed stent occlusion, three patients cholangitis, and one patient died in septic shock. The Amsterdam group also concluded that endoprosthesis placement affords temporary relief of cholestasis related problems and results in stricture resolution in only a minority of chronically treated patients. To this end it should be reserved for the extremely high surgical risk patient or as a temporizing measure prior to definitive biliary-enteric bypass. More recently, a small number of self-expanding metal stents have been placed in patients having biliary stenoses related to chronic pancreatitis [24]. Expanding to a diameter of 8–10 mm, it is hoped that incorporation of the metal strut into the bile duct wall as well as the significant increment in luminal diameter when compared with polyethylene prostheses, will be associated with prolonged patency rates.

Unproven Endoscopic Therapies

Because ligation of the PD in animals causes glandular atrophy and fibrosis without inducing either pancreatitis or islet cell destruction [3], an attempt has been made to occlude the PD of painful chronic pancreatitis patients. Following an alcohol-prolamine solution injected at ERCP, 24%–40% of the 73 patients reviewed by Rösch had long-term clinical improvement [52]. Additional data by Pap et al. have shown little impairment of pancreatic function tests in these patients, suggesting either slough of the glue solution or inadequate ductal occlusion [53]. Nor are there data, despite initial promising reports [54], that balloon dilation of the PD sphincter either decreases episodes of relapsing pancreatitis or affects the pain of chronic calcific pancreatitis. Data to the contrary suggest an unacceptable incidence of procedure-related pancreatitis, implying that this procedure is currently unwarranted [55].

Conclusions

Although indications and techniques are evolving, the endoscopic approach to patients with chronic pancreatitis appears promising. Clearly more useful in patients with relapsing attacks of pancreatitis as opposed to those with chronic pain, viable techniques to remove obstructive lesions include PD sphincterotomy, stone extraction, stricture dilation, and endoprosthesis placement, alone or in combination. Treatment of ductal disruptions to include pseudocysts, pancreatic ascites, pancreaticothoracic fistulas, and ongoing leaks with slowly resolving peripancreatitis are also amenable to endoscopic therapy, although such treatment must be placed in the perspective of competing technologies and local subspecialty expertise. The author awaits with interest further data and, hopefully, controlled studies utilizing endoscopy in the treatment of chronic pancreatitis.

References

1. Sarles H (1974) Chronic calcifying pancreatitis – chronic alcoholic pancreatitis. Gastroenterology 66:604–615
2. Gyr KE, Singer MV, Sarles H (1985) Pancreatitis: concepts of classification. Elsevier, New York
3. Axon ATR (1986) Endoscopy in the diagnosis and therapy of pancreatic disorders. Clin Gastroenterol 15:279–303
4. Grimm H, Meyer WH, Nam VC et al. (1989) New modalities for treating chronic pancreatitis. Endoscopy 21:70–74
5. Bradley EL III (1982) Pancreatic duct pressure in chronic pancreatitis. Am J Surg 144:313–316
6. Bradley EL III (1987) Long-term results of pancreaticojejunostomy in patients with chronic pancreatitis. Am J Surg 153:207–213
7. Nealon WH, Townsend CM Jr, Thompson JC (1988) Operative drainage of the pancreatic duct delays functional impairment in patient with chronic pancreatitis. Ann Surg 208:321–329
8. Drake DH, Fry WJ (1989) Ductal drainage for chronic pancreatitis. Surgery 105:131–140
9. Frey CF, Bodai BI (1984) Surgery in chronic pancreatitis. Clin Gastroenterol 13:914–940
10. Venu RP, Geenen JE, Hogan WJ et al. (1989) Idiopathic recurrent pancreatitis: an approach to diagnosis and treatment. Dig Dis Sci 34:55–60
11. Sarles H, Bernard JP, Gullo L (1990) Pathogenesis of chronic pancreatitis. Gut 31:629–632
12. Ammann RW, Muench R, Otto R (1988) Evolution and regression of pancreatic calcification in chronic pancreatitis: a prospective long-term study of 107 patients. Gastroenterology 95:1018–1028
13. Fuji T, Amano H, Harima K et al. (1985) Pancreatic sphincterotomy and pancreatic endoprosthesis. Endoscopy 17:69–72
14. Sherman S, Lehman GA, Hawes RH et al. Pancreatic ductal stones: frequency of successful endoscopic removal and improvement in symptoms. Gastrointest Endosc (in press)
15. Ponsky JL, Duppler DW (1987) Endoscopic sphincterotomy and removal of pancreatic duct stones. Am Surg 10:613–616
16. Huibregtse K, Schneider B, Vrij AA, Tytgat GNJ (1988) Endoscopic pancreatic drainage in chronic pancreatitis. Gastrointest Endosc 34:9–15
17. Cremer M, Toussaint J, Dunham F (1980) Endoscopic management of chronic pancreatitis. Gastrointest Endosc 26:65–69
18. Schneider MV, Lux G (1985) Floating pancreatic duct concrements in chronic pancreatitis. Endoscopy 17:8–10
19. Sauerbruch T, Holl J, Sackmann M, Paumgartner G (1989) Extracorporeal shock wave lithotripsy of pancreatic stones. Gut 30:1406–1411
20. Delhaye H, Vadermeeren A, Gabbrielli A, Cremer M (1990) Lithotripsy and endoscopy for pancreatic calculi: the first 104 patients. Gastroenterology 98:A216 (abstr)
21. McCarthy J, Geenen JE, Hogan WJ (1988) Preliminary experience with endoscopic stent placement in benign pancreatic disease. Gastrointest Endosc 34:16–18
22. Kozarek RA, Patterson DJ, Ball TJ, Traverso LW (1989) Endoscopic placement of pancreatic drains and stents in the management of pancreatitis. Ann Surg 209:261–266
23. Cremer M, Deviere J, Delhaye M et al. (1990) Non-surgical management of severe chronic pancreatitis. Scand J Gastroenterol 25(suppl 175):77–84
24. Cremer M, Sugai B, Delhaye M et al. (1990) Expandable pancreatic metal stent (Wallstent) for chronic pancreatitis: first world series. Gastroenterology 98:A215 (abstr)

25. Neuhaus H, Hagenmeuller F, Griebel M, Classen M (1991) Percutaneous cholangioscopic or transpapillary insertion of self-expanding biliary stents. Gastrointest Endosc 37:31–37
26. Kleitsch WP (1955) Anatomy of the pancreas: a study with special reference to the duct system. Arch Surg 71:795–803
27. Cotton PB (1980) Congenital anomaly of pancreas divisum as a cause of obstructive pain and pancreatitis. Gut 21:105–114
28. Warsaw AL, Richter JM, Schapiro RH (1983) The cause and treatment of pancreatitis associated with pancreas divisum. Ann Surg 198:443–450
29. Delhaye M, Engelholm L, Cremer M (1985) Pancreas divisum: congenital anatomic variant or anomaly? Contribution of endoscopic retrograde dorsal pancreatography. Gastroenterology 89:951–958
30. Cotton PB (1985) Pancreas divisum – curiosity or culprit? Gastroenterology 89:1431–1435
31. Sherman S, Lehman G, Nisi R et al. (1990) Results for endoscopic sphincterotomy of the minor papilla for pancreas divisum. Gastrointest Endosc 36:198A (abstr)
32. Siegel JH, Ben-Zvi JS, Pullano W, Cooperman A (1990) Effectiveness of endoscopic drainage for pancreas divisum: endoscopic and surgical results in 31 patients. Endoscopy 22:129–133
33. Liguory C, Lefebvre JF, Canard JM et al. (1986) Pancreas divisum: therapeutic results in 12 patients. Dig Dis Sci 31:530S (abstr)
34. Soehendra N, Kempeneers I, Nam VC et al. (1986) Endoscopic dilatation and papillotomy of the accessory papilla and internal drainage in pancreas divisum. Endoscopy 18:129–132
35. Kozarek RA (1990) Pancreatic stents can induce ductal changes consistent with chronic pancreatitis. Gastrointest Endosc 36:93–95
36. Sahel J, Bastid C, Pellat B et al. (1987) Endoscopic cystduodenostomy of cysts of chronic calcifying pancreatitis: a report of 20 cases. Pancreas 2:447–453
37. Cremer M, Deviere J, Engelholm L (1989) Endoscopic management of cysts and pseudocysts in chronic pancreatitis: long-term follow-up after 7 years of experience. Gastrointest Endosc 35:1–9
38. Hershfield NB (1984) Drainage of a pancreatic pseudocyst at ERCP. Gastrointest Endosc 30:269–270
39. Kozarek RA, Brayko CM, Harlan J et al. (1985) Endoscopic drainage of pancreatic pseudocysts. Gastrointest Endosc 31:322–328
40. Henkinbrant A, Davaux A (1986) Drainage d'un pseudo-kyste du pancreas. Acta Gastroenterol Belg 49:341–347
41. Delmott JS, Mosquet L, Brunetaud JM, Paris JC (1983) Drainage d'un pseudokyste du pancreas par anastomose kysto-gastrique perendoscopiqe au laser. Acta Endosc B:221–223
42. Rogers BHG, Cicurel NJ, Seed RW (1975) Transgastric needle aspiration of pancreatic pseudocyst through an endoscope. Gastrointest Endosc 3:133–134
43. Spinelli P, Meroni E, Prada A (1988) Endoscopic treatment of a pancreatic pseudocyst by nasocystic tube. Endoscopy 20:27–29
44. Knecht G, Kozarek RA (1991) Use of double channel fistulotome for transgastric pseudocyst drainage. Gastrointest Endosc 37:356–357
45. Kozarek RA, Ball TJ, Patterson DJ et al. (1991) Endoscopic transpapillary therapy for disrupted pancreatic duct and peripancreatic fluid collection. Gastroenterology 100:1362–1370
46. Wilson C, Auld CD, Schlinkert R et al. (1989) Hepatobiliary complications in chronic pancreatitis. Gut 30:520–527
47. Warshaw AL, Schapiro RH, Ferrucci JT, Galdabini JJ (1976) Persistent obstructive jaundice, cholangitis and biliary cirrhosis due to common bile duct stenosis in chronic pancreatitis. Gastroenterology 70:562–567
49. Hollands MJ, Little JM (1989) Obstructive jaundice in chronic pancreatitis. HPB Surg 1:263–270

50. Deviere J, Devaere S, Baizo M, Cremer M (1990) Endoscopic biliary drainage in chronic pancreatitis. Gastrointest Endosc 36:96–100
51. Waxman I, Huibregtse K (1992) Endoscopic therapy for chronic pancreatitis. Gut (in press)
52. Rösch W (1983) The value of endoscopic occlusion of the pancreatic duct. Endoscopy 15:175–177
53. Pap A, Flautner L, Tihanyi T et al. (1985) Pancreatic function after endoscopic and surgical occlusion of the pancreatic duct in patients with chronic pancreatitis. Endoscopy 17:60–63
54. Siegel JH, Guelrud M (1983) Endoscopic cholangiopancreatoplasty: hydrostatic balloon dilation in the bile duct and pancreas. Endoscopy 29:99–103
55. Kozarek RA (1988) Balloon dilation of the sphincter of Oddi. Endoscopy 20:207–210

Extracorporeal Lithotripsy of Pancreatic Stones

T. SAUERBRUCH,[1] J. HOLL, M. SACKMANN, and P. PAUMGARTNER

Introduction

Obstruction of the pancreatic duct together with an increased outflow pressure for the pancreatic juice proximal to an obstacle is believed to be one pathogenic factor of persistent pain in patients with chronic calcifying pancreatitis. Obstruction may be caused by stenoses and/or calcified stones in the pancreatic duct. It has been shown that surgical or endoscopic drainage procedures may lead to allevation of pain [2–4, 6, 7]. However, endoscopic extraction of pancreatic calculi may be prevented by their size in relation to the duct anatomy. Therefore, a combined approach of extracorporeal shock wave lithotripsy (ESWL) together with endoscopic drainage procedures was described some years ago [1, 5, 8, 9].

Patients and Methods

In the past 3 years we treated 23 patients (18 men, 5 women; mean age 47 ± 12 years) with chronic pancreatitis, ductal calcifications, and recurrent pain. Of these, 11 had predominantly solitary stones and 12 multiple stones. The largest stone measured on average 12 ± 6 mm. Etiology of pancreatitis was alcoholic in 14, nonalcoholic in 5, and unknown in 4 patients. In the majority of patients ESWL was performed after an endoscopic sphincterotomy of the pancreatic orifice. The stones were crushed with a water tank lithotripter normally used for kidney stones (HM3, Dornier Medizintechnik). On average a total of 1780 ± 880 shock wave pulses were applied within 30–60 min. Of the 23 patients 17 received one ESWL session and 6 two or more sessions.

Results

Fragmentation of the stones was achieved in 20 patients. It failed in three with tightly impacted stones where access to the calculi was prevented by very narrow duct stenoses. Stone fragmentation by ESWL allowed complete

[1] Medical Department II, Klinikum Großhadern, Marchioninistraße 15, W-8000 München 70, FRG. Current address: Department of Internal Medicine, Sigmund-Freud-Str. 25, W-5300 Bonn 1, FRG

Beger/Büchler/Malfertheiner (Eds.)
Standards in Pancreatic Surgery

clearance of the pancreatic ducts in nine patients (40%) and partial clearance in seven (30%). Clearance was insufficient in seven patients.

ESWL was tolerated without major adverse effects. Only two patients exhibited a mild increase in serum amylase together with slight pain attacks the day following lithotripsy. Ten patients (44%) showed considerable improvement or relief of pain. Improvement of pain attacks, but still requiring analgesics from time to time, was achieved in a further seven patients (30%). In six patients (26%) symptoms were not influenced by the combination of endoscopic sphincterotomy and ESWL. Relief or improvement of pain occurred more often in patients with complete stone clearance than in those with partial or no clearance (88% vs 64%). Abdominal surgery was necessary in two patients, one with cholangitis and a bile duct stenosis and the second in a patient with diffuse peritonitis due to an abscess in the bursa omentalis of unknown origin several months after the last lithotripsy session. There was no death.

Conclusion

Our results confirm that ESWL together with an endoscopic drainage procedure of the pancreatic duct system is a safe novel approach to patients with chronic calcifying pancreatitis. It leads to considerable allevation or relief of symptoms in approximately every second patient. Since the rate of adverse effect is small, and up to now no death has been reported, this approach should have first priority for patients with chronic calcifying pancreatitis and recurrent pain. On the other hand, the complex nature of chronic pancreatitis with its difficult duct anatomy and multifactorial pathogenesis of pain may explain why a conservative approach is not successful in every patient.

References

1. Cremer M, Vandermeeren A, Delhaye M (1988) Extracorporeal shock wave lithotripsy (ESWL) for pancreatic stones. Gastroenterology 94:A80 (abstr)
2. Cuilleret J, Guillemin G (1990) Surgical management of chronic pancreatitis on the continent of Europe. World J Surg 14:11–18
3. Fuji T, Amano H, Hariman K et al. (1985) Pancreatic sphincterotomy and pancreatic endoprosthesis. Endoscopy 17:69–72
4. Greenlee HB, Prinz RA, Aranha GV (1990) Long-term results of side-to-side pancreaticojejunostomy. World J Surg 14:70–76
5. Grimm H, Meyer WH, Nam VC, Soehendra N (1989) New modalities for treating chronic pancreatitis. Endoscopy 21:70–74
6. Huibregtse K, Schneider B, Vrij AA, Tytgat GNJ (1988) Endoscopic pancreatic drainage in chronic pancreatitis. Gastrointest Endosc 34:9–15
7. Ihse I, Borch K, Larsson J (1990) Chronic pancreatitis: results of operations for relief of pain. World J Surg 14:53–58

8. Sauerbruch T, Holl J, Sackmann M, Werner R, Wotzka R, Paumgartner G (1987) Disintegration of a pancreatic duct stone with extracorporeal shock waves in a patient with chronic pancreatitis. Endoscopy 19:207–208
9. Sauerbruch T, Holl J, Sackmann M, Paumgartner G (1989) Extracorporeal shock wave lithotripsy of pancreatic stones. Gut 30:1406–1411

Indications for Surgical Treatment in Chronic Pancreatitis

R.C.G. Russell[1]

Introduction

Surgical treatment of chronic pancreatitis has centered on the technical aspects of the operation itself, and on the immediate hospital outcome. Little attention has been given to the indications for surgery or to the long-term benefits of patients who have had an operation. Indeed, little is known of the long-term outlook or natural history of chronic pancreatitis with the result that valid comparisons cannot be made between conservative and operative management. Further, the benefits of careful supervised medical management were discarded until Ammann et al. [1] brought to the attention of pancreatologists the natural resolution of symptoms with time, and the loss of exocrine and endocrine functions of the pancreas.

In contrast to this increasing awareness of the natural history of the disease and the effect of conservative management has been the slow realisation that if defined operative procedures are performed for the correct indications by specialised surgeons the operation will carry an extremely low risk for the patient and can offer good long-term results with a quality of life similar to the best achieved by prolonged conservative management. Further, the indications for surgery and the type of operation performed is no longer an opinion, but beginning to be based on careful imaging delineating the exact pathological problem facing the surgeon, and a limited understanding of the outcome of an operation in particular circumstances.

Unfortunately, what is lacking are clear guidelines and a baseline so that accurate comparisons can be made between different groups studying the patients with this disease. To add to this difficulty is the feeling that each group studying this disease is dealing with a disease process that has been altered by the local environment best illustrated by the so called "tropical pancreatitis" which is found in Kerala, India [5]. Difficulties are further aggravated by the comparative rarity of the disease, and the varying willingness of referral of such cases by physicians to centres with a special interest in the disease, such that the number of patients seen even in specialist centres bears little relationship to the prevalence of the disease. The basic

[1] The Middlesex Hospital, London W1, U.K.

Beger/Büchler/Malfertheiner (Eds.)
Standards in Pancreatic Surgery

lack of definitions and markers of the severity of the disease together with the poor relationship between the disease severity as shown by the pathologist and clinical symptoms increases the innate suspicion amongst surgeons that good results may merely indicate wide selection criteria rather than success of a particular therapy or operative intervention.

Pancreatic surgery has moved from the era of the surgical entrepreneur to that of the accountant whereby a calculated assessment of the problem is made on sound data which enable comparison between selection and outcome. Unfortunately, our methods lack the precision required, and with newer therapies on the immediate horizon, such as the role of somatostatin analogues and the possibilities provided by the interventional radiologist, the baselines are changing. Yet, a start must be made and a consensus in the presentation of the indications for surgery would be helpful in further evaluation. Unfortunately, most surgeons have a philosophical attitude with a pendulum approach, such that small whims and fancies can push the scale for or against operation in the management of a particular patient. This is best illustrated by the "patient first" approach whereby a decision is made individually which sounds to be "caring" yet often pays little attention to well known criteria.

Criteria for Surgical Intervention

The indications for pancreatic surgery must primarily depend on the symptoms of which the patient complains; there is no evidence that pancreatic surgery has a preventative role, and thus what the patient complains of must be high in the list of indications. To a large extent the pathogenesis of the disease is unknown yet of the common causes, alcohol is known to influence the disease process. Simple events such as transection of the pancreas after trauma [2] can be revealed by investigation, and guide therapy. The particular pathology may give a guidance about the appropriateness of surgical treatment such as chronic pancreatitis secondary to an obstruction by a benign tumour for example [3]. Further the timing of surgery bears consideration, and whether the patient should "earn" his operation as was the popular dogma in the days of peptic ulcer surgery. Finally, it is pointless operating in a patient who is relatively unfit for operation and this must be taken into account in any decision algorithm.

Indications

Pain

This is the prime symptom; it is doubtful whether pancreatic surgery should ever be undertaken in the absence of pain unless there is an impending life threatening complication. Unfortunately, pain is extremely difficult to measure, and is not related to any other feature of the disease. Pain is subjective, and thus its severity difficult to determine; however, its frequency and length can be recorded and are important for there is a relationship between outcome and type of pain in that better results are found in patients with intermittent pain.

Narcotic Abuse

A measure of pain is the number and strength of analgesic doses taken over a time period or in the presence of an attack. These should be recorded. Unfortunately, tolerance and addiction prevent this measure being an appropriate comparison. Further, patients who avoid opiates appear to do better, and withstand pain longer. On occasion it seems that opiates aggravate the pain and may even increase the severity of the disease.

Weight Loss

Such may be the severity of the disease process that the patient loses weight rapidly, and is below his height weight percentile. Rapid weight loss with the amount of lost weight should be recorded and taken into account when assessing disease severity and the need for surgery.

Complications

All the complications associated with acute disease are found in chronic pancreatitis and will require appropriate therapy. Thus, this forms a defined group which may override all other factors under consideration. Hence, haemorrhage, abscess or necrosis require immediate measures to control their sequelae, while pseudocysts, fistulae or stones may be better treated by surgery than continued conservative measures. Such factors should be recorded for the presence, in any series, of a larger number of patients with complications such as major bleeding undoubtably affect the mortality and morbidity of the series.

Aetiology

The influence of the cause of the pancreatitis on the longer term results will be great; thus, if the series contains a larger number of patients with alcohol as the probable aetiology and these patients continue to drink alcohol, the outcome will be bad. Similarly, if a large number of patients who have chronic symptoms after an attack of gallstone pancreatitis are included, a good result almost invariably follows the appropriate procedure (for example distal pancreatectomy for duct stricture) provided that the gallstones are also removed. Hence in considering the indications for surgical treatment it is important to define the aetiology, and to treat it if possible. Thus, surgery on the pancreas is likely to fail if hypercalcaemia and hyperlipidaemia are left untreated, while recurrent attacks of pain associated with a congenital abnormality such as annular pancreas is unlikely to respond to conservative measures, yet a well executed operation early in the course of the disease will save years of discomfort.

Pathology

The changes within the gland at microscopic level are unlikely to influence surgical decision making as insufficient is known about the relationship of pathology at the microscopic level to the progress and clinical course of the disease; however, the macroscopic appearance influences surgical decision making in relationship to the timing of the operation and to the type of operation performed. These pathological changes to a large extent are related to the main pancreatic duct and the effect of the fibrosing process on the duct. For instance, if the duct is large there seems to be good circumstantial evidence that the enlarged duct with its increased pressure is related to pain, and a decrease in that pressure will relieve pain. Further, if there is a stone in the duct which is likely to cause obstruction, removal of that stone is associated with a relief of symptoms. Thus, evidence of obstruction provides a goal for the surgeon, namely to relieve the obstruction. Similarly, if there is an obstruction at any point within the duct system, removal of the pancreas distal to that obstruction is likely to relieve the symptoms. The role of obstruction at the major and minor papillae is a subject within itself, but if there is a disorder of function of the papilla then relief of that obstruction will overcome the pathology causing the obstruction and relieve symptoms. The macroscopic appearance of the gland is important for there is no doubt that the disease process affects the gland in a less than uniform manner, thus the surgeon in planning the operation must bear in mind the site of maximum involvement. The Longmire school of thought suggests that in many instances of pancreatitis it is the pathology within the head of the gland that creates the symptoms and progressive worsening of the disease, so removal of the head of the gland is in many instances of diffuse disease the preferable approach. However, if the head is normal and all the pathological changes are confined to the body and tail of the pancreas there is little point in undertaking any surgical procedure but resection of the body and tail of the gland. On occasion, the symptoms are associated with diffuse changes of a mild degree throughout the gland with normal duct anatomy; in such cases there is no lesion amenable to surgical correction, and hence it is difficult to plan a logical approach except ablation of the whole gland. Surgical procedures treat best, defined pathologies by the technique of ablation or relief of obstruction; ignoring this simple philosophy may well lead to failure of the procedure and progression of the disease.

Role of Investigation

With the techniques of imaging at the surgeon's disposal it is now possible to define the macroscopic appearance of the gland, and to outline both the pancreatic duct and the bile duct to determine whether or not obstruction is present. Further, the presence or absence of the complications of pancreatitis can be defined. The role of radiology can be further extended with the interventional techniques which are available and these must undoubtably be considered before surgery is planned. For instance, a stone in the pancreatic duct can be defined by radiology, broken by lithotripsy and the debris removed by the endoscopist with the use of balloon catheters following endoscopic sphincterotomy of the major papilla.

Fitness for Surgery

For benefit to be gained by a surgical procedure, the patient must be sufficiently well to improve his quality of life after an operation. This is rarely a problem in pancreatic surgery for the median age of patients having an operation in most series is around 40 years of age. Provided the operation is successful in relieving the symptoms, a good quality of life can usually be achieved. However, in the elderly patient or those with major coexistent disease the risk of the operation is markedly higher with an increase in morbidity and mortality of the procedure such that the benefits possible are outweighed by the risk. This is particularly apposite in the patient who develops multiple complications. Further, the patient who is addicted to narcotics, to alcohol or is psychologically disturbed may continue with his major problems even though he no longer has a pancreatic problem – a good surgical outcome but a very poor result. The high percentage of failures after a total pancreatectomy bears testimony to this problem, and the poor selection of certain patients for surgery.

Timing of Surgery

In chronic pancreatitis, the patient is suffering from a continuing process with peaks and troughs. If the surgeon ignores the peaks and looks only at the troughs when the patient's disease is well controlled, then there is no indication for surgery; on the other hand, if the physician is a "peak" man looking only at the times when the patient is admitted then the pressure to "do something" is great. The attitude of the physician thus becomes important because of the resources that these patients consume either by frequent "call-outs" or admissions, and this can lead to an inappropriate operation for an inappropriate pathology. On the other hand, if an operation is postponed indefinitely and the patient given inadequate care, increasing amounts of analgesics, especially opiates, can be consumed and the patient becomes drug addicted. The surgeon must choose carefully between the dangers of operating too early and performing unnecessary procedures, and the danger of postponing an operation too long so creating the problems of complications of the disease or addiction.

Role of Medical Therapy

It is not possible to consider the indications for surgical intervention without passing reference to the merits of medical management which is discussed elsewhere in this book. Each group dealing with patients with pancreatic disease must have some protocol of medical management, for some patients can be managed conservatively without resort to surgery. Before surgery is undertaken conservative management should have been showed to have failed as one of the prime indications for operation. My own practice is to assess each patient carefully, to follow their treatment as an outpatient and to consider inpatient care with intestinal rest on one or two occasions depending on the type of disease with which one is dealing. A proper trial of medical management is a prerequisite to a surgical approach.

Role of Surgical Treatment

The threshold of operative intervention is much influenced by the pathology and type of chronic pancreatitis from which the patient suffers. Surgery treats well-localised disease and obstruction, but poorly general disease of the pancreas.

Drainage Operations

If there is incontrovertible evidence that there is an abnormality of the sphincter mechanism, either of the duct of Wirsung or that of Santorini, an endoscopic or surgical sphincterotomy has a place in the management of that patient, and such procedures are best performed early in the course of the disease before severe changes of chronic pancreatitis develop. Similarly, if the patient has dilatation of the pancreatic duct which is greater than 8 mm with or without the presence of stones in the duct, a drainage procedure early in the course of the disease is preferable to prolonged conservative management. The drainage must be effective and relieve all obstruction and all debris be they stones or protein plugs from the duct; occasionally stones and protein plugs can be removed with a combination of endoscopic sphincterotomy and lithotripsy, but most patients are better treated by a Puestow-type procedure with a complete laying open of the duct, and application of a jejunal patch to the opened duct. Again such procedures are preferably performed early in the course of the disease before the onset of continous pain, and further damage to the endocrine and exocrine functions of the pancreas.

Gallstone Pancreatitis

There is some doubt whether gallstones ever cause chronic pancreatitis. This is a problem of semantics, but in clinical practice there are patients who have recurrent attacks of acute pancreatitis, who have changes in the pancreas indicative of chronic pancreatitis and may as a result of a severe attack of pancreatitis have damage to the duct system with complications arising subsequently. A cholecystectomy can be an extremely effective procedure for such patients to prevent subsequent attacks or even continous pain. Any complication arising in such patients should be dealt with by the least invasive procedure as once the initiating factor has been removed resolution usually occurs.

Resection

Removal of part of the pancreas increases the risk of diabetes and exocrine deficiency so such a step should be approached with deliberation. It is not possible to plan resection without good imaging. Distal resection, that is removal of the body and tail of the pancreas, has the lowest operative morbidity and best long-term result functionally, but is only appropriate if the head of the pancreas is normal on pre-operative imaging and at operation. Distal pancreatectomy is ideal in the patient who has a disrupted duct secondary to acute pancreatitis, to trauma or to chronic pancreatitis; the operation gives very poor results if the head of the gland is inflammed. Such patients should be treated by a proximal pancreatectomy; if in doubt, it is preferable to remove the head of the gland, and conserve the body ensuring good drainage of the pancreatic stump to conserve exocrine and endocrine function. Total pancreatectomy is an operation rarely to be undertaken for benign disease; it is necessary to fulfil criteria that are strict and agreed by a team who have experience in managing patients with pancreatic disease and who are prepared to continue caring for these patients after the operation for a long period of time. Medical treatment must have been prolonged and the pain intractable, unrelieved by other therapy. It should rarely be performed as the first operation unless the patient has both endocrine and exocrine deficiency. Before it is undertaken, the patient must be fully aware of its consequences. The commonest indication is for patients who are both endocrine and exocrine deficient and who have continued to have significant symptoms following previous surgery.

Conclusion

There are no fixed criteria for pancreatic surgery, but rather a weighing up of factors involved in the care of the patient, with the balance weighted in favour of medicine. It is well to remember that the divergent results may well be related to different selection criteria, and that the late mortality apparent in many series may well be aggravated by the surgery and its sequelae, although non-operative mortality of patients with pancreatitis is associated with a late mortality of 30% [4]. Nevertheless, defined and circumscribed lesions of the pancreas, particularly those with an obstructive component should be treated early by well planned and appropriate surgery, while disease which is diffuse causing continous pain should be managed with a greater degree of conservation. The balance weighs up aetiology, the pathology, the clinical features and the condition of the patient; as yet a scoring system for such assessment is not possible but as our knowledge of these factors and the outcome of surgery becomes more complete the indications will become even more clearly defined and true comparison of the results between different approaches attained.

References

1. Ammann RW, Akovbiantz A, Lardiader F et al. (1984) Course and outcome of chronic pancreatitis: longitudinal study of a mixed medical-surgical series of 245 patients. Gastroenterology 86:820–828
2. Carr ND, Cairns SR, Lees WR, Russell RCG (1989) Late complications of pancreatic trauma. Br J Surg 76:1244–1246
3. Lowes JR, Rode J, Lees WR, Russell RCG, Cotton PB (1988) Obstructive pancreatitis: unusual causes of chronic pancreatitis. Br J Surg 75:1129–1133
4. Strum WB, Spiro HM (1971) Chronic pancreatitis. Ann Intern Med 74:264–277
5. Thomas PG, Augustine P, Ramesh H, Rangabashyam N (1990) Observations and surgical management of tropical pancreatitis in Kerala and southerm India. World J Surg 14:32–42

Inflammatory Mass in the Pancreatic Head Associated with Chronic Pancreatitis

M.H. SCHOENBERG,[1] M. BÜCHLER, P. MALFERTHEINER, H. FRIESS, and H.G. BEGER

It is widely accepted that chronic alcoholic pancreatitis generally involves the whole pancreas [2, 12]. There is, however, a subgroup of patients (approximately 5%–10%) suffering from focal lesions of chronic pancreatitis. Mainly, in the surgical literature, preponderant lesions of the head and/or the left side of the pancreatic gland have been described in patients undergoing surgery for pain and other complications [1, 9]. Surprising few data, however, exist concerning the prevalence of preponderant pathological lesions involving the head, body or tail of the pancreas which then lead to specific complications of the disease. Due to the improved techniques for imaging, especially computed tomography (CT) scan, which is used on a routine basis in patients with chronic pancreatitis, we are able to observe and evaluate patients with these focal lesions. There are several reasons for the enhanced interest especially in the inflammatory mass in the head of the pancreas.

An inflammatory process in the head, unlike other parts of the pancreas, seems to influence the course of disease due to local complications such as obstruction of the pancreatic and/or extrahepatic bile duct and obstruction of the dudoenum. Sometimes even the major intestinal vessels such as the superior mesenteric vein and/or artery are involved [13]. The resection of this inflammatory tumor, either by Whipple procedure or by duodenum-preserving pancreas resections, leads to excellent pain relief and other favorable long-term results [4, 8, 15] in chronic pancreatitis, suggesting that the resection of this inflammatory mass interrupts the so-called natural course of chronic pancreatitis [3, 5]. Therefore, it might be hypothesized that inflammatory head enlargement is not only the preponderant lesion of a progressive chronic pancreatitis but constitutes a special pathophysiological entity. The aim of this investigation was therefore to evaluate the prevalence and clinical picture of inflammatory head enlargement in patients suffering from chronic pancreatitis.

[1] Department of General Surgery, University Ulm, Steinhövelstraße 9, W-7900 Ulm, FRG

Beger/Büchler/Malfertheiner (Eds.)
Standards in Pancreatic Surgery

Table 1. Age and sex distribution of patients with and without pancreatic head enlargement

	Patients with pancreatic head enlargement		Patients without pancreatic head enlargement	
	(*n*)	(%)	(*n*)	(%)
Men	110	79	108	77
Women	28	21	33	23

Mean age: patients with pancreatic head enlargement 44.5 years (range 22–76 years); patients without pancreatic head enlargement 42.2 years (range 19–76 years).

Materials and Methods

From 1982 to 1990 279 patients (216 men, 63 women) suffering from chronic pancreatitis were treated in the Surgical or Gastroenterological Department of the University of Ulm. The mean age of the patients was 42 years (range 19–76 years). The diagnosis of pancreatitis was based on at least one imaging procedure (endoscopic retrograde cholangiopancreaticography, ERCP; ultrasonography; contrast-enhanced computed tomography, CT), and one exocrine and endocrine function test (exocrine: pancreolauryl test in urine or serum; endocrine: oral glucose load test). Additionally, due to the fact that 159 out of 279 study patients were undergoing surgery the histological confirmation of chronic pancreatitis was available.

The pancreatic head was considered to be enlarged if its vertical diameter exceeded 40 mm as measured by ultrasonography, contrast-enhanced CT scan or intraoperative findings. Patients with solid, cystic, or mixed solid and cystic inflammatory enlargement of the head of the pancreas were included. Vertical pancreatic head diameter of 20.8 ± 0.6 mm ($\bar{x} \pm$ SEM) had been found previously in healthy volunteers by ultrasonography [6]. This investigation supports the findings of Weill [14], who described normal human pancreatic head diameter to be between 25 and 30 mm using ultrasonographic criteria.

Results

Based on above definition, 138 (49%) of 279 patients with chronic pancreatitis had inflammatory pancreatic head enlargement as shown by imaging procedures or intraoperative findings. There were no differences in terms of age and sex distribution between patients with and without head enlargement (Table 1).

Table 2. Duration of symptoms until diagnosis

	Head enlargement (n = 138)	No head enlargement (n = 141)
	(%)	(%)
Less than 24 months	58	63
24–48 months	15	13
More than 48 months	27	24

Table 3. Pain in patients with and without pancreatic head enlargement

Stage level of pain	Head enlargement (n = 138)	No head enlargement (n = 141)
I Slight or no pain	6%	17% } 60%
II Frequent pain attacks	27%	43% } 60%
III Daily pain attacks	33% } 67%	32%
IV Daily severe pain	34% } 67%	8%

In 82% of our patients the cause of pancreatitis was overindulgence in alcohol, with no differences between patients with and without pancreatic head enlargement. Twelve percent of the patients had a biliary etiology, the rest an undetermined etiology of chronic pancreatitis. Interestingly, the time period from the first symptoms to diagnosis of chronic pancreatitis was comparable in patients with and without pancreatic head enlargement. Approximately 60% of all patients suffering from chronic pancreatitis were diagnosed within 2 years of the first symptoms. In contrast, the time between first symptoms and surgery was 70% longer (54 months) in patients who did not have an inflammatory mass in the pancreatic head (Table 2). The reason for this early admittance to the hospital of patients with inflammatory mass in the pancreatic head was mainly due to pain and complications of the disease. Retrospective analysis of pain reveals that patients with and without an inflammatory head enlargement differ significantly. Two-thirds of the patients with head enlargement suffer from daily (in 34% severe) pain attacks. In contrast, 60% of patients without an enlarged head report only slight symptoms combined with periods without any pain or discomfort (Table 3). Moreover, as expected, the patients with head enlargement suffered more frequently from complications of chronic pancreatitis. Of the patients with head enlargement, 46% suffered from cholestasis, versus only 11% in the group without an enlarged head. Moreover, more than half of the patients with an inflammatory mass in the

Table 4. Complications of chronic pancreatitis

	Head enlargement (%)	No head enlargement (%)
Cholestasis	46	11
Pancreatic duct stenosis	53	32
Duodenal obstruction	30	7
Cysts	60	64
Vascular involvement	15	8

pancreatic head also had a pancreatic duct stenosis and 30% a duodenal obstruction. In contrast, only 32% of the patients without an enlarged head showed similar stenosis in the pancreatic duct and only 7% had a stenosis of the duodenum. Prevalence of the other more frequent complications such as pseudocysts or vascular stenosis was comparable in the two groups (Table 4).

Pancreatic Function

In order to determine the pancreatic function of the patients we performed a urine pancreolauryl test in 43 patients and a serum pancreolauryl test in 90 patients [10]. The median T/K ratio (test day/control day) of the urine pancreolauryl test was 37%, ranging from 4% to 76%, in patients with head enlargement and only 16%, ranging from 0.2% to 7.5%, in patients without an inflammatory mass. Concomitantly, the serum pancreolauryl test revealed that both patient groups had an impaired exocrine function. The patients with head enlargement, however, showed a significant higher serum fluorescein concentration curve than those patients without an enlarged head. Similarily, exocrine pancreatic function, analyzed by administrating an oral glucose load test, revealed that only 18% of the patients with an inflammatory mass suffered from insulin-dependent diabetes, whereas 30% of the patients without an inflammatory mass in the head showed a severely pathological glucose test ($p < 0.05$). Apparently, the exocrine and endocrine pancreatic function of patients with head enlargement was better preserved than in those suffering from chronic pancreatitis without an inflammatory mass in the pancreatic head.

Treatment

Due to this constellation, 38% of the patients with an enlarged pancreatic head were operated on, versus 51% without an inflammatory head enlargement. The surgical procedures performed depended not so much on the underlying disease but on the complications the patients suffered. One hundred and twenty-nine patients were treated with a duodenum-preserving head resection, 35 patients received a cystojejunostomy, only 11 patients were treated with a resection of the left pancreas, and 9 patients with Puestow procedure.

Summary

Patients with an inflammatory pancreatic head enlargement constitute a special clinical entity. These patients show a higher pain score, more typical complications of chronic pancreatitis and at the time of clinical presentation a better preserved pancreatic endocrine and exocrine function than patients without an enlarged pancreatic head. The clinical prevalence of an inflammatory pancreatic head in our patient population was about 50%. This is very high and probably due to the fact that most patients have been referred to us for duodenum-preserving pancreas head resection not only from the Upper Swabia region but also from other parts of Germany. On the other hand, it would be worthwile to compare the Ulm population with other large patient populations to clarify the real prevalence of this specific variation of chronic pancreatitis. The question of whether this head enlargement constitutes a special pathological entity cannot be answered with certainty. Since the patients with head enlargement are admitted to our hospital earlier, they might suffer from a complicated yet possibly earlier phase of chronic pancreatitis. This is mirrored by the shorter duration of symptoms until surgery, as revealed by the medical history of these patients. Patients who do not develop an inflammatory mass in the head of the pancreas are treated later. Therefore, one can speculate that the differences in function and the clinical picture of this disease are related only to the time course. In contrast, however, the inflammatory head enlargement could also be regarded as a pacemaker of the disease. This is supported by the observation that resection of the enlarged head not only relieves the pain and other complications but also leads to favorable long-term results, apparently interrupting the natural course of the disease chronic pancreatitis [7].

References

1. Adson MA, Mellrath DC (1986) Surgical treatment of chronic pancreatitis. In: Go VLW, Gradner JD, Brooks FP, Lebenthal E, DiMagno EP, Scheele GA (eds) The exocrine pancreas: biology, pathobiology, and diseases. Raven, New York, pp 587–599
2. Becker V (1984) Chronische Pankreatitis, Klinische Morphologie, In: Bartelheimer H, Kühn HA, Becker V, Stelzner F (eds) Gastroenterologie und Stoffwechsel, vol 21. Thieme, Stuttgart
3. Beger HG, Büchler M (1990) Duodenum-preserving resection of the head of the pancreas in chronic pancreatitis with inflammatory mass in the head. World J Surg 14:83–87
4. Beger HG, Krautzberger W, Bittner R, Büchler M, Limmer J (1985) Duodenum-preserving resection of the head of the pancreas in patients with severe chronic pancreatitis. Surgery 97:467–473

5. Beger HG, Büchler M, Bittner R, Oettinger W, Roscher R (1989) Duodenum-preserving resection of the head of the pancreas in severe chronic pancreatitis – early and late results. Ann Surg 209:273–278
6. Büchler M, Malfertheiner P, Frieß H, Seitz J, Rolle K, Nustede R, Schafmayer A, Beger HG (1989) Pancreatic and GI-hormone adaptation following long-term camostate treatment in man. Pancreas 5:612
7. Büchler M, Malfertheiner P, Frieß H, Senn T, Beger HG (1990) Chronic pancreatitis with inflammatory mass in the head of the pancreas: a special entity? In: Beger HG, Büchler M, Ditschuneit H, Malfertheiner P (eds) Chronic pancreatitis. Springer, Berlin Heidelberg New York, pp 41–46
8. Greenlee HB, Prinz RA, Aranha GV (1990) Long-term results of side-to-side pancreatico-jejunostomy. World J Surg 14:70–76
9. Howard JM (1987) Surgical treatment of chronic pancreatitis, principles, applications, results. In: Howard JM, Jordan GL Jr, Reber HA (eds) Surgical diseases of the pancreas. Lea and Febiger, Philadelphia, pp 496–521
10. Malfertheiner P, Büchler M, Müller A, Ditschuneit H (1987) Fluorescein dilaurate serum test: a rapid tubeless pancreatic function test. Pancreas 2:53–60
11. Münch R, Ammann RW (1989) Entwicklungsstadien der chronischen Pankreatitis. Internist 30:738–746
12. Reber HA (1987) Chronic pancreatitis, etiology, pathology, and diagnosis. In: Howard JM, Jordan GL Jr, Reber HA (eds) Surgical diseases of the pancreas. Lea and Febiger, Philadelphia, pp 475–495
13. Traverso LW (1990) Preservation of the pylorus during pancreaticoduodenectomy for chronic pancreatitis. In: Beger HG, Büchler M, Ditschuneit H, Malfertheiner P (eds) Chronic pancreatitis. Springer, Berlin Heidelberg New York, pp 505–516
14. Weill FS (1978) Ultrasonography of digestive diseases. Mosby, St. Louis
15. Zirngibl H, Gall FP (1990) Results of the Whipple procedure in combination with pancreatic duct occlusion. In: Beger HG, Büchler M, Ditschuneit H, Malfertheiner P (eds) Chronic pancreatitis. Springer, Berlin Heidelberg New York, pp 481–489

Pancreatic Duct Drainage in Chronic Pancreatitis

R.A. Prinz[1]

Chronic pancreatitis is a progressive inflammatory disease characterized by permanent morphologic and functional damage to the pancreas. The destruction of the pancreatic parenchyma that occurs with this disease may be surprisingly asymptomatic or may result in intractable abdominal pain, steatorrhea and/or diabetes mellitus. Chronic pancreatitis is not primarily a surgical disease, and it should be managed medically until a surgically correctable complication develops. Those complications that require surgical treatment include the development of pancreatic ascites, pancreatic fistula, fixed fibrotic obstruction of the intrapancreatic portion of the common bile duct or of the duodenum, hemorrhage secondary to splenic vein thrombosis, and inability to differentiate the disease from pancreatic cancer. However, most patients are referred to a surgeon because of unrelenting abdominal and/or back pain. In addition to being refractory to medical therapy, this incapacitating pain often leads to narcotic addiction.

Pain relief in chronic pancreatitis is a difficult and challenging problem. In dealing with these patients, the surgeon must realize that pain is the end product of a wide spectrum of pathologic changes in the pancreas. Since the gross and microscopic features of chronic pancreatitis that cause pain are not uniform, no one operation can be appropriate for all patients with this disease. The surgeon must be flexible and consider the particular anatomy and level of pancreatic function in each patient when choosing the operation that is best suited for that individual. Surgeons must also realize that abstinence from alcohol and narcotics is just as important if not more so than the type of operation in determining overall patient rehabilitation and benefit.

The therapeutic goal of surgery in chronic pancreatitis is to relieve intractable pain while preserving as much exocrine and endocrine function as possible. Two types of operations have proven success in relieving pain in chronic pancreatitis. These are drainage of a dilated pancreatic duct and resection of the diseased pancreas. Pain relief is achieved in 65%–85% of patients with chronic pancreatitis with either of these procedures [1–4]. However, the cost of ameliorating pain with pancreatic resection is a much

[1] Loyola University Medical Center, 2160 South First Avenue, Maywood, ILL 60153, USA

Beger/Büchler/Malfertheiner (Eds.)
Standards in Pancreatic Surgery

higher rate of exocrine and endocrine insufficiency [5]. Insulin-dependent diabetes is particularly hazardous in these patients since many are non-compliant and continue to use excessive amounts of alcohol. For this reason and because decompression of the pancreatic duct is a less formidable procedure than pancreatic resection, we have favored pancreatic drainage with a defunctionalized loop of jejunum in patients with a dilated duct.

Since our choice of operation hinges on the presence of distention and dilation of the pancreatic duct, it is important to have accurate knowledge of its anatomy before surgery. The best way to demonstrate obstruction of the pancreatic duct is with endoscopic retrograde cholangiopancreatography (ERCP). Formerly, we believed this was an absolutely essential part of the preoperative workup of these patients. However, computed tomography (CT) can delineate a dilated pancreatic duct in a substantial number of patients with chronic pancreatitis. Since ERCP is an invasive procedure and carries a small risk, we omit it if the necessary information is obtained with CT.

A lateral side-to-side pancreaticojejunostomy allows complete drainage of the duct of Wirsung and the duct of Santorini from the duodenum to the splenic hilum and is our preferred method of decompressing the pancreatic duct system. The abdomen is entered through an upper abdominal transverse curvilinear (bucket handle) incision that transects both rectus muscles. In patients with a narrow costal margin or a previous midline scar, an upper abdominal midline incision gives adequate exposure and may be preferable. A thorough exploration of the peritoneal cavity is performed. The entire anterior surface of the pancreas is exposed by dividing the gastrocolic omentum and mobilizing the stomach superiorly and the transverse colon inferiorly. Frequently, the posterior surface of the stomach is adherent to the anterior surface of the pancreas from previous inflammation. These adhesions are divided with sharp dissection staying close to the anterior surface of the pancreas. The hepatic flexure of the colon is mobilized inferiorly so that a wide Kocher maneuver can be performed. This enables evaluation of the entire head of the pancreas.

The anterior surface of the pancreas is then palpated, and the pancreatic duct is located by feeling fluctuation of fluid under pressure. This is confirmed by needle aspiration of water clear pancreatic exocrine fluid (Fig. 1). If palpation is not successful, intraoperative ultrasound can reliably identify the presence and location of a dilated duct. This can also be confirmed by needle aspiration. In both cases, we leave the needle in the pancreatic duct and use it as a guide to cut down and enter the ductal system. When the duct is not palpable and intraoperative ultrasound is not available, an incision is made perpendicular to the expected course of the main pancreatic duct in an area away from major vessels. The incision is carried posteriorly a short distance at a time and absolute hemostasis is maintained so the duct is not obscured. Once the duct is entered, its precise course is determined by using a right-angled clamp or a probe.

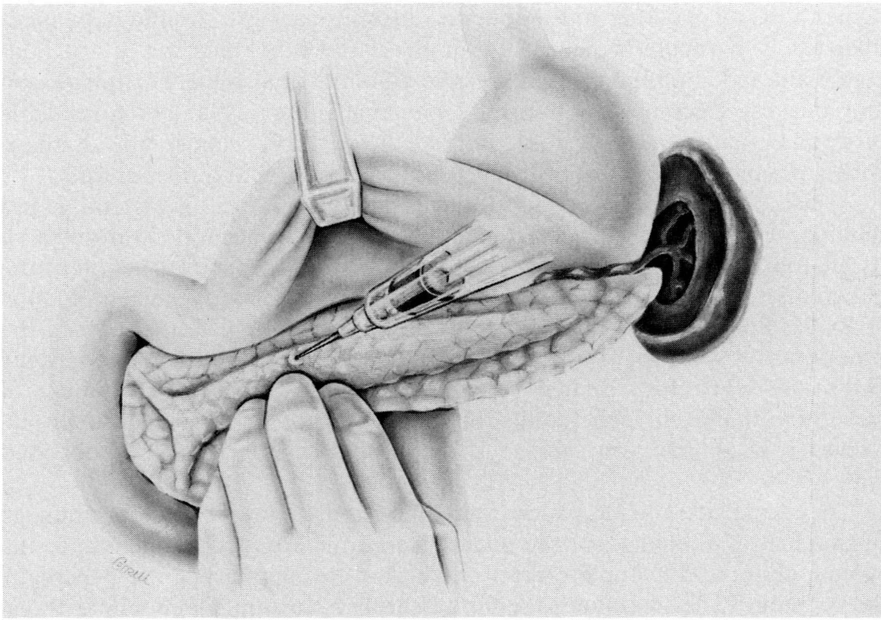

Fig. 1. The pancreatic duct is located by feeling fluctuant fluid under pressure and is confirmed by needle aspiration of water-clear pancreatic fluid

The overlying pancreatic tissue is incised with a scalpel or electrocautery, and both the duct of Wirsung and the duct of Santorini are unroofed from as close as possible to the duodenum out to the splenic hilum (Fig. 2). Bleeding from the cut edge of the pancreas is controlled by electrocautery or suture ligatures. Brisk bleeding is unusual except in the head of the gland where branches of the pancreaticoduodenal artery may be encountered. If intraductal calcifications or stones are encountered, all of these that are accessible are removed. It is not possible to remove calcifications or stones in the secondary branches of the pancreatic ductal system or in the parenchyma itself. After the ductal system is completely opened, the pancreas is palpated to be certain that all diseased areas are drained. Any suspicious areas are biopsied to rule out an underlying carcinoma. This remains a dilemma since a prominent area of fibrosis and scarring may mimic a tumor while a pancreatic cancer may be obscured by the diffuse changes of chronic pancreatitis. In spite of practicing routine biopsy to confirm the diagnosis of chronic pancreatitis and to rule out carcinoma, 4 of the 195 patients who have had pancreatic duct drainage at our institution have died within 1 year of operation from an unsuspected pancreatic carcinoma.

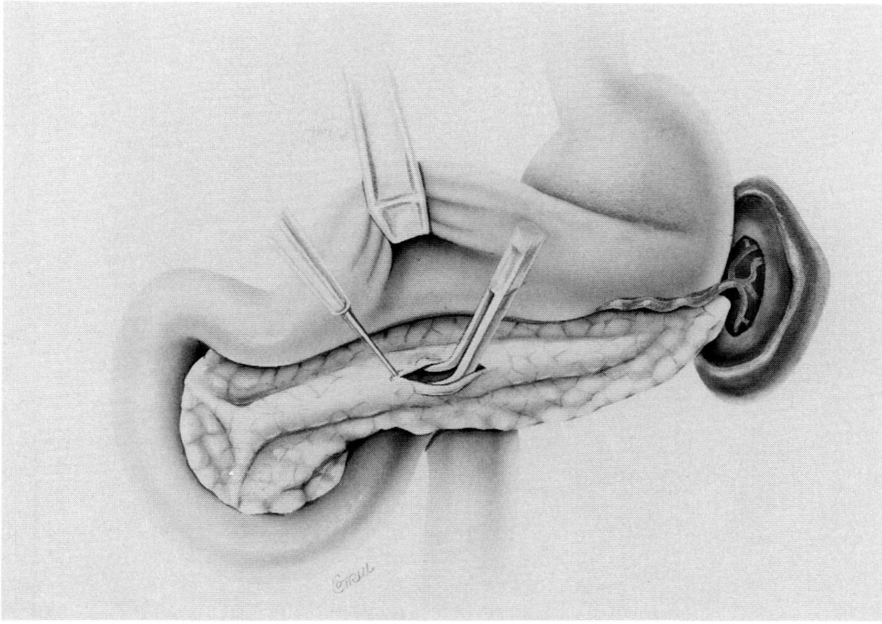

Fig. 2. The overlying pancreatic tissue is incised, and both the duct of Wirsung and the duct of Santorini are unroofed from as close as possible to the duodenum out to the splenic hilum

Often a portion of overlying pancreas has to be removed in the head of the gland where the duct runs posteriorly to enter the duodenum and the pancreatic parenchyma is most thickened by inflammatory fibrosis. The bulk of pancreatic tissue in this area of the head may prevent adequate anterior ductal drainage unless this tissue is resected. Failure to achieve adequate decompression in the juxtaduodenal head of the gland has been the most common cause for failure of pancreatic duct drainage in our experience. We have reported 14 patients with undrained segments of dilated pancreatic duct remaining in the head of the gland after a prior drainage procedure [6]. Redrainage and decompression of these obstructed segments resulted in substantial pain relief in 71% of these patients.

After the entire pancreatic duct system has been unroofed, the jejunal limb is prepared for Roux-en-Y drainage. The jejunum is divided a short distance from the ligament of Treitz where its mesentery is mobile enough to reach the pancreas. We use a stapling instrument to transect the jejunum and oversew the staple line in the distal segment with interrupted non-absorbable Lembert sutures. This distal limb is brought through an avascular area in the transverse mesocolon to the anterior surface of the pancreas. The closed end of the limb is positioned in the splenic hilum. This is the

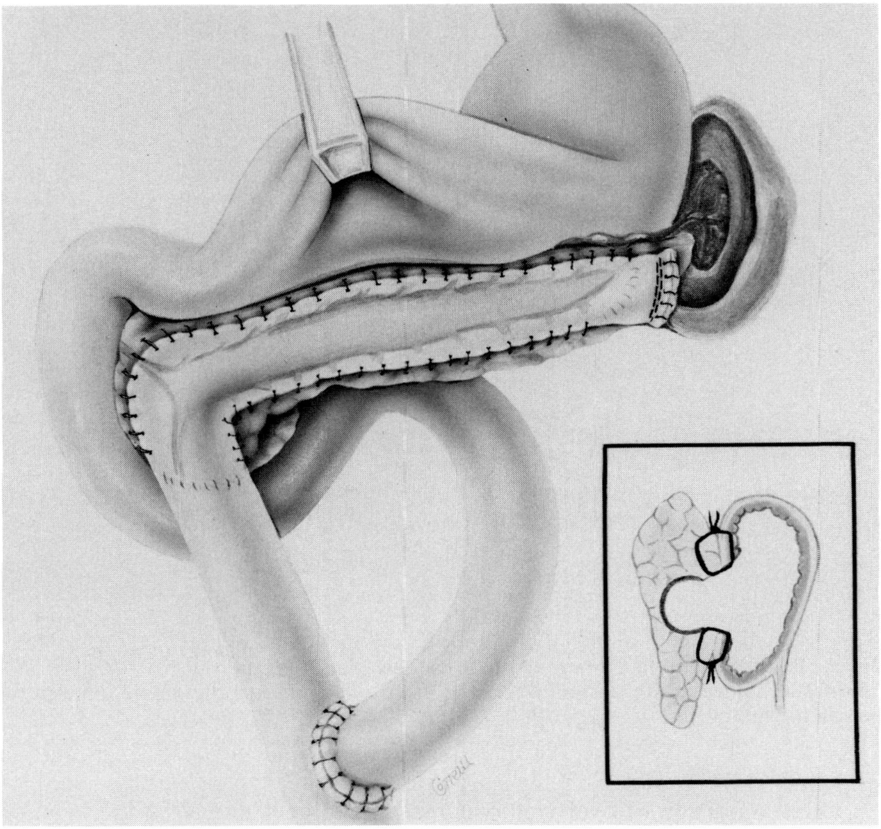

Fig. 3. A side-to-side pancreaticojejunostomy is performed with a single layer of sutures approximating the opened jejunum to the tough fibrous capsule of the pancreas

most difficult area for exposure so we prefer to begin our anastomosis rather than end it at this point. Beginning approximately 5 cm from the oversewn end of the jejunum, a single row of interruped nonabsorbable sutures is placed between the antimesenteric surface of the jejunum and the tough fibrous capsule of the pancreas just inferior to be opened duct. The sutures are passed through the serosa, muscularis, and the mucosa of the jejunum. However, no attempt is made to bring the mucosa of the jejunum down to the mucosa of the pancreatic duct since there is no evidence that long-term patency of this anastomosis is enhanced by mucosa to mucosa apposition. In areas of ductal stricture or stenosis, bringing the mucosa of the jejunum down to the narrowed mucosa of the pancreatic duct may even compromise the overall patency of the anastomosis. The jejunal limb is then opened adjacent and parallel to the opened pancreatic duct. The anastomosis is completed with interrupted sutures passed through the entire wall of the jejunum and the fibrotic tissue and capsule on the superior edge of the pancreatic duct (Fig. 3).

Intestinal continuity is reestablished with an end to side jejunojejunostomy placed approximately 40 cm distal to the pancreaticojejunostomy. Defects in the mesentery of the small and large intestine are closed. External drainage of the pancreas is usually not required after lateral pancreaticojejunostomy for chronic pancreatitis. Postoperative care is similar to that for any other abdominal operation involving anastomosis of the small intestine. Nasogastric suction is maintained until gastrointestinal function returns. The patient's diet is then advanced as tolerated.

Pancreatic duct drainage has been used to treat symptomatic chronic pancreatitis in 195 patients with an operative mortality of 3.6% and a complication rate of 20%. Long-term follow-up has been reported on the first 100 patients to undergo pancreaticojejunostomy at our center [4]. Follow-up ranged from 1 to 25 years with a mean period of 7.9 years. Pancreatic duct drainage gave complete or substantial pain relief to 82% of patients available for long-term evaluation. Although some authors have suggested that patients with pancreatic calcifications have a better likelihood of symptomatic relief, this has not been the case in our experience. There was essentially no difference in pain relief after pancreaticojejunostomy in patients with or without calcifications. When calcifications were present, 79% of patients benefited.

Even though chronic pancreatitis is associated with progressive deficits in endocrine and exocrine function, diabetes, and steatorrhea have not been inevitable consequences after pancreaticojejunostomy. Ten of the 34 patients who were diabetic prior to operation required insulin. Only 6 of the 24 non-insulin-dependent diabetics have required insulin management following pancreatic duct drainage. Of the 53 nondiabetic patients, 11 developed diabetes and of these 8 were treated with insulin. Thus, almost half of these patients never became diabetic, and only 28% ever required insulin.

The findings for pancreatic exocrine function were similar. Steatorrhea requiring oral pancreatic enzyme replacement was present in 17 patients before operation and developed in 12 patients after pancreaticojejunostomy. Thus, only one-third of the patients ever developed clinically important pancreatic exocrine insufficiency. These findings indicate that pancreatic duct drainage exerts little or no deleterious effect on pancreatic function. In contrast, the incidence and severity of diabetes and steatorrhea are markedly increased by pancreatic resection and correlate with the amount of tissue removed. Preservation of functioning pancreatic tissue is the major advantage of pancreatic duct decompression. Three of our patients have died from complications related to diabetes management following pancreatic resection for chronic pancreatitis but only one has died from this problem after pancreaticojejunostomy.

One of the most distressing points in chronic pancreatitis is the poor long-term survival rate with either operative procedure. Almost 40% of our patients survived less than 5 years after pancreaticojejunostomy. Continued alcoholism was the most important factor we could identify affecting survival. Three-fourths of the patients who quit drinking remained alive and well while two-thirds of the patients who continued to drink had died during the period of our evaluation. Obviously, greater efforts are needed to convince these patients to quit drinking.

In addition to causing pancreatic duct obstruction, the fibrosis of chronic pancreatitis can cause mechanical obstruction of the intrapancreatic portion of the common bile duct and the duodenum. Fixed biliary tract and duodenal obstruction has been present in 30% and 15%, respectively, of patients undergoing lateral pancreaticojejunostomy for chronic pancreatitis at our institutions [7]. Biliary tract and duodenal obstruction can cause persistent symptoms if they are not dealt with at the initial operation or recurrent pain if they develop after lateral pancreaticojejunostomy. In patients with fixed obstruction, biliary tract decompression may be accomplished by either choledochoduodenostomy or choledochojejunostomy using either the Roux loop draining the pancreas or a second isolated Roux loop. The extent of disease and variations in individual anatomy dictate which of these alternatives is most appropriate. Duodenal obstruction can be relieved by gastrojejunostomy. These various surgical bypasses can be combined with pancreatic duct drainage to handle the multiple complications that can occur with chronic pancreatitis. We have shown that drainage of the biliary tract and/or stomach in combination with pancreatic duct decompression does not increase the morbidity and mortality of lateral pancreaticojejunostomy alone [7].

Another complication of chronic pancreatitis that can and should be treated at the time of pancreatic duct decompression is pseudocyst. The prevalence of pseudocysts in patients undergoing lateral pancreaticojejunostomy at our institution is 39% [8]. Patients with chronic pancreatitis undergoing pseudocyst drainage alone are likely to require reoperation for intractable pain or pseudocyst recurrence. Of 81 patients treated surgically for pseudocyst that have been reported from our center, 15 needed reoperation. The cause for reoperation was unrelenting pain in seven and recurrent pseudocysts in seven. Since a pseudocyst may signal underlying chronic pancreatitis, patients with a long history of alcohol abuse, pancreatic calcifications, and exocrine or endocrine insufficiency should have a thorough evaluation of their pancreatic duct system before operation. If the pancreatic duct is dilated, it should be decompressed at the time of cyst drainage with a lateral pancreaticojejunostomy. Intrapancreatic cysts can be drained by extending the pancreatic duct incision to include the pseudocyst and incorporating the opening into the overlying Roux-en-Y limb. Larger extra pancreatic pseudocysts can be drained by opening a dependent portion of the cyst and extending the Roux-en-Y limb over this opening for a separate anastomosis. In our experience, combining pseudocyst drainage with lateral pancreaticojejunostomy has not increased the morbidity or mortality of either procedure. We have yet to identify a patient with chronic pancreatitis who has had a recurrent pseudocyst after undergoing complete pancreatic duct drainage. We believe this experience can be extended to other complications of chronic pancreatitis. In patients with pancreatic fistulas or pancreatic ascites who have not responded to medical management, the area of leakage can be incorporated into the open area of the pancreatic duct and drained internally into the Roux-en-Y loop of jejunum.

Complete drainage of the pancreatic duct with a side-to-side pancreaticojejunostomy is the preferred method of treating intractable pain of chronic pancreatitis in patients with a dilated pancreatic duct. Functioning pancreatic tissue is not sacrificed and the natural tendency in chronic pancreatitis to develop endocrine or exocrine insufficiency is not exacerbated. Other complications of chronic pancreatitis such as obstruction of the biliary tract or upper gastrointestinal tract, pseudocyst, pancreatic fistula, and ascites can treated concurrently without an increase in morbidity or mortality.

Acknowledgements. I appreciate the help of Linda Wahrer in preparing the manuscript and Sue Cottrill, Pamela Wielgos, and Sharon Arizzi in preparing the illustrations.

References

1. Beger HG, Büchler M, Bittner RR, Oettinger W, Roscher R (1989) Duodenum-preserving resection of the head of the pancreas in severe chronic pancreatitis. Ann Surg 209:273–278
2. Keith RG, Saibil FG, Sheppard RH (1989) Treatment of chronic alcoholic pancreatitis by pancreatic resection. Am J Surg 157:156–162
3. Prinz RA, Greenlee HB (1990) Pancreatic duct drainage in chronic pancreatitis. Hepatogastroenterology 37:295–300
4. Prinz RA, Greenlee HB (1981) Pancreatic duct drainage in 100 patients with chronic pancreatitis. Ann Surg 194:313–320
5. Eckhauser FE, Strodel WE, Knol JA, Harper M, Turcotte JG (1984) Near total pancreatectomy for chronic pancreatitis. Surgery 96:599–600
6. Prinz RA, Aranha GV, Greenlee HB (1986) Redrainage of the pancreatic duct in chronic pancreatitis. Am J Surg 151:150–156
7. Prinz RA, Aranha GV, Greenlee HB (1985) Combined pancreatic duct and upper gastrointestinal and biliary tract drainage in chronic pancreatitis. Arch Surg 120:361–366
8. Munn JS, Aranha GV, Greenlee HB, Prinz RA (1987) Simultaneous treatment of chronic pancreatitis and pancreatic pseudocyst. Arch Surg 122:662–667

Comprehensive Treatment: Resection and Drainage in the Management of Patients with Chronic Pancreatitis

L. FERNANDEZ-CRUZ,[1] A. SAENZ, E. ASTUDILLO, and C. BAGUR

Pain is the predominant symptom that brings patients with chronic pancreatitis to the surgeon. The surgical treatment of patients with chronic pancreatitis is based on the preservation of as much pancreatic function as possible, while attempting to improve the patient's symptoms. Most operations performed are designed to treat the complications of this disease. Since anatomical complications vary widely, the availability of several operative approaches is essential.

It is widely accepted that the operative approach depends on the anatomy of the pancreatic duct. Approximately 40%–50% of patients develop a dilated pancreatic duct, the remainder develop a scarred contracted duct, which has been compared to a leafless tree in winter. The big-duct pattern, when the Wirsung duct is greater than 7 mm in diameter, allows for long side-to-side pancreaticojejunostomy, usually of the modified Puestow type using a Roux-en-Y loop of jejunum [1]. However, when the duct pattern is of the small caliber type, resection of the gland is the only option. Some 10%–20% of patients develop an inflammatory enlargement of the head of the pancreas; in these patients, the surgical options are pancreaticoduodenectomy [2] (Whipple type) or duodenum-sparing resection of the pancreatic head [3] (Beger type).

Management of Patients Without a Mass and Without Ductal Dilatation

In this paper we will discuss the more controversial management of those patients without a mass of the head of the pancreas and without ductal dilatation for whom the surgical alternatives are more or less extensive resection with or without drainage [4–6].

The operation of left pancreatectomy has been associated with poor results for the following reasons: Inadequate resection leading to recurrence of symptoms, inappropriate indications, lack of a drainage procedure to the pancreatic remnant, and endocrine/exocrine dysfunction. Our own clinical

[1] Department of Surgery, University of Barcelona. Hospital Clinic. Barcelona, Spain

Beger/Büchler/Malfertheiner (Eds.)
Standards in Pancreatic Surgery

Table 1. Signs and symptoms of chronic alcoholic pancreatitis in 33 patients

Presentation	Patients	
	(*n*)	(%)
Pain	33	100
Recurrent attacks	18	55
Biliary obstruction	3	9
Pancreatic ascites	2	6
Endocrine dysfunction	8	24
Exocrine dysfunction	10	30

Patients' median age 38 years (range 28–61 years).

experience will try to demonstrate that better patient selection based on morphological and surgical findings, combined with a drainage procedure to the pancreatic remnant, will give much better results.

Over the past 9 years we have performed left pancreatectomy in 33 male patients with chronic pancreatitis, mainly associated with alcohol abuse, and ages ranging from 28 to 61 years (median age 38 years).

The complications of pancreatitis were identified before surgery on clinical and radiological grounds. Routine biochemical tests were performed including assessment of hepatic function in all patients before and after surgery.

The severity of the underlying pancreatitis as assessed by the presenting symptoms is shown in Table 1. Pain was the dominant indication for resection and was present in all patients. Recurring attacks of severe pancreatic pain requiring hospital admission occurred in 55% of the patients. A study of the complications of pancreatitis showed 6% pancreatic ascites, 9% biliary obstruction, 24% endocrine dysfunction, and 30% exocrine dysfunction. Ultrasonography and computed tomographic scanning were undertaken routinely. Since our operative approach depends on the anatomy of the pancreatic duct, ERCP is the crucial radiographic study for planning the operative procedure.

The indications for pancreatic resection in these patients were ductular stenosis without dilatation in 11 patients and strictures of the pancreatic duct in 15 patients, associated in eight of them with a pseudocyst in the body, in six of them with a pseudocyst in the tail, and in one of them with multiple pseudocysts. Isolated involvement of the tail was seen in four patients and three patients had an obstructed pancreatic duct at the mid portion of the head (Table 2) (Figs. 1–5).

The extent of distal resection ranged between 60% (when the gland is divided to the right of the portal vein) and 80% (when the gland is divided at the level of the gastroduodenal artery). Among 15 patients with pancreatic pseudocysts, in only one did on-table cystography show absence of

Table 2. CT and ERCP findings in chronic pancreatitis no mass in head and duct not dilated (<8 mm)

CT and ERCP Findings	Number of patients
Diffuse pancreatitis	11
Diffuse pancreatitis + pseudocyst in the body	8
Diffuse pancreatitis + pseudocyst in the tail	6
Diffuse pancreatitis + multiple pseudocysts	1
Isolated involvement of the tail	4
Obstructed pancreatic duct at the mid-portion of the head	3

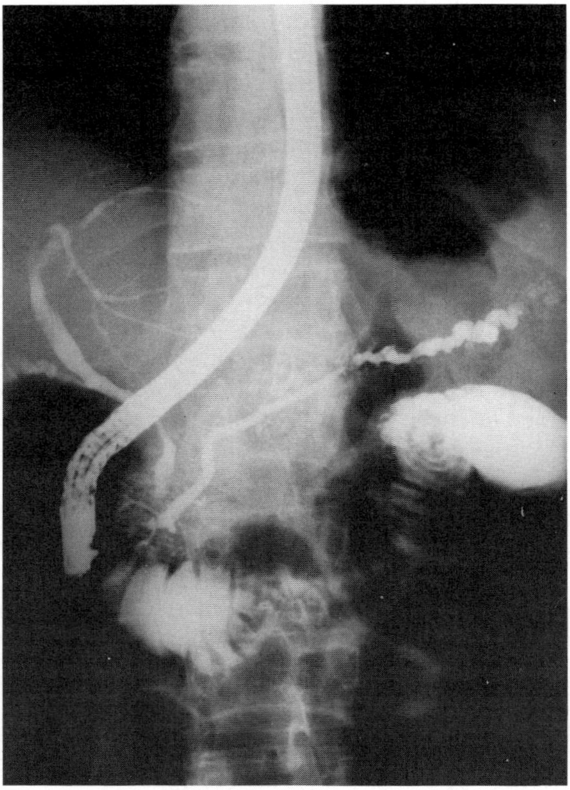

Fig. 1. ERCP showing typical picture of true focal disease in the tail of the pancreas

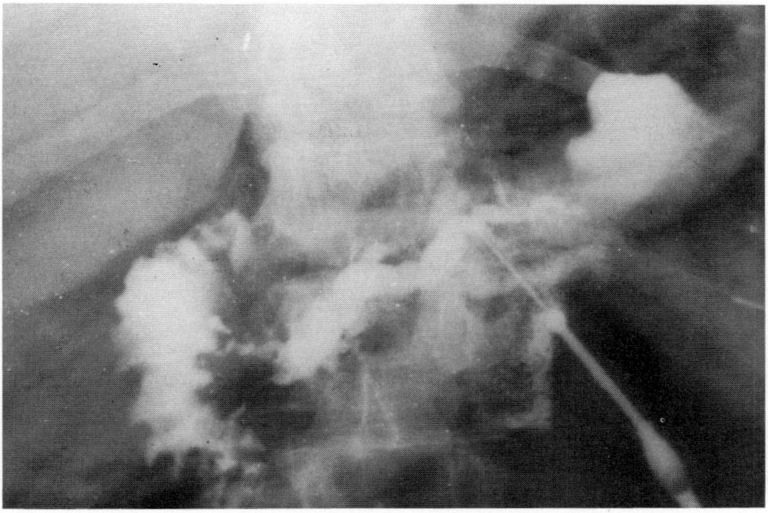

Fig. 2. Operative ambigrade pancreatography showing communication of the Wirsung duct and the pseudocyst in the tail of the pancreas

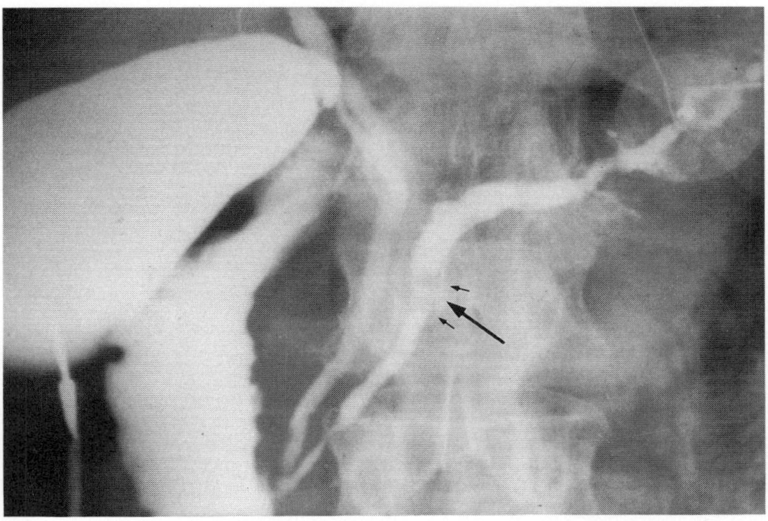

Fig. 3. Combined operative cholangiography (gallbladder injection) and ambigrade pancreatography showing normal common bile duct and 5-mm Wirsung duct dilatation with filling defects in the neck of the pancreas

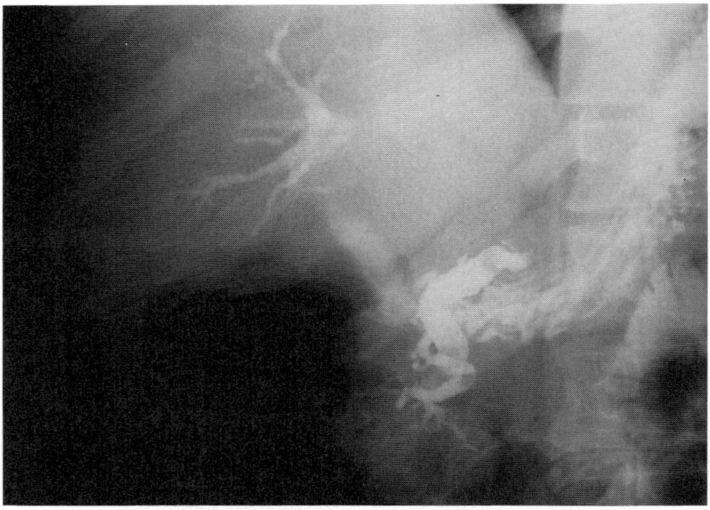

Fig. 4. ERCP showing intraductal filling defects in the head and complete obstruction of the Wirsung duct in the neck of the gland

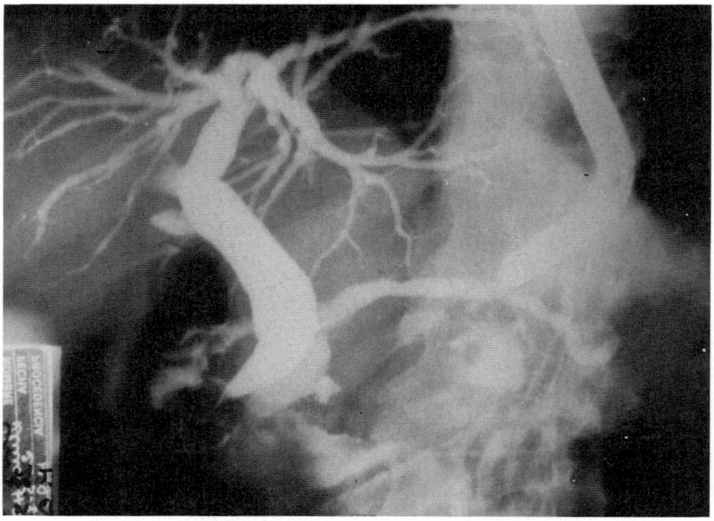

Fig. 5. ERCP showing obstruction of the distal end of the common bile duct; 6-mm Wirsung duct dilatation and multiple pseudocysts communicating with the main duct in the head, body, and tail of the pancreas

communication with the main pancreatic duct. In all cases the patency of the pancreatic duct was assessed by operative prograde pancreatography via the duct in the head of the pancreas after distal pancreatectomy, and serial radiographs confirmed free flow of the contrast into the duodenum. We also probed the duct (Fogarty catheter and Dormia basket) to make sure that the catheter is able to pass through the duct into the duodenum (Fig. 6). We remove all accessible stones present in the head as they may cause persistent or recurrent obstruction. ERCP was performed 1 year after the operation in ten patients, showing a good patency of the pancreaticojejunostomy (Fig. 7).

In 25 patients 80% distal resection was performed and in two patients the body and tail of the resected pancreas were autotransplanted intraperitoneally and revascularized via the hypogastric artery and iliac vein (Figs. 8, 9). Sixty percent pancreatectomy was performed in seven patients and in one patient the Roux-en-Y loop of jejunum draining the stump of the pancreas was also anastomosed side-to-side to an extrapancreatic pseudocyst in the head of the pancreas. One patient with a pseudocyst in the body of the pancreas was managed with a segmental pancreatectomy including only the body of the pancreas and drainage of both the head and the tail pancreatic remnants (after removal of all pancreatic stones) with an on-lay pancreaticojejunostomy using a Roux loop (Table 3). A concomitant splenectomy was performed in all cases.

We have achieved complete relief of pain after different degrees of resection (60%–80%) in 94% of patients and partial relief, occasionally requiring analgesics, in 6% of patients (Table 4).

There were septic complications in nine patients (six respiratory and three catheter sepsis). There were no pancreatic fistulas. The postoperative hospital stay had a median duration of 18 days (range 10–28 days).

Patients were followed-up in our pancreatic clinic at 6-month intervals. The median follow-up period was 3.5 years (range 1–9 years). Diabetes already present in eight patients was apparent in eight additional patients; 16 patients had steatorrhea requiring enzyme supplementation. Five patients did not gain weight. The remaining 28 gained between 3 and 6 kg above pretreatment weight (mean 4 kg).

Management of the Cut End of the Pancreas

Our preferred technique has been to drain the stump of the pancreas into a Roux-en-Y loop of jejunum. Others prefer to find and ligate the pancreatic duct and then to oversew the stump with non-absorbable sutures. The purpose of performing a pancreaticojejunostomy is to avoid the effects of leakage from the pancreatic stump and to achieve better drainage by enabling the pancreatic juice to escape both proximally and distally. Although it has never been proven that pain is a consequence of abnormally

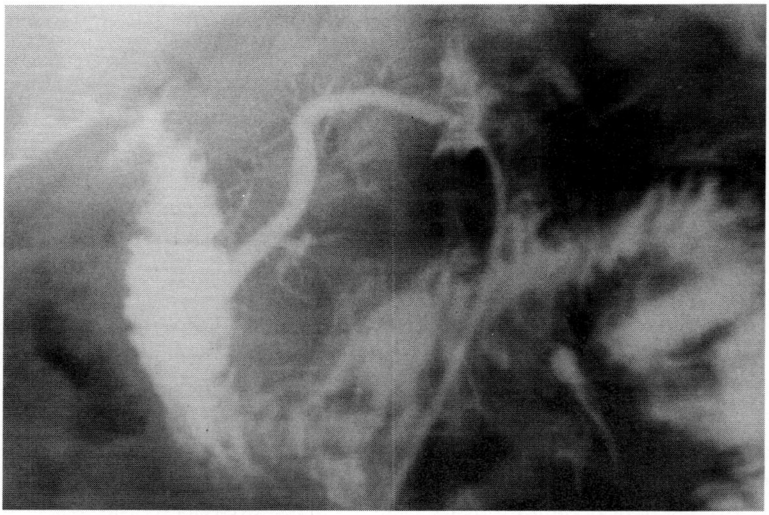

Fig. 6. Prograde pancreatography via the duct in the neck showing free flow of the contrast into the duodenum

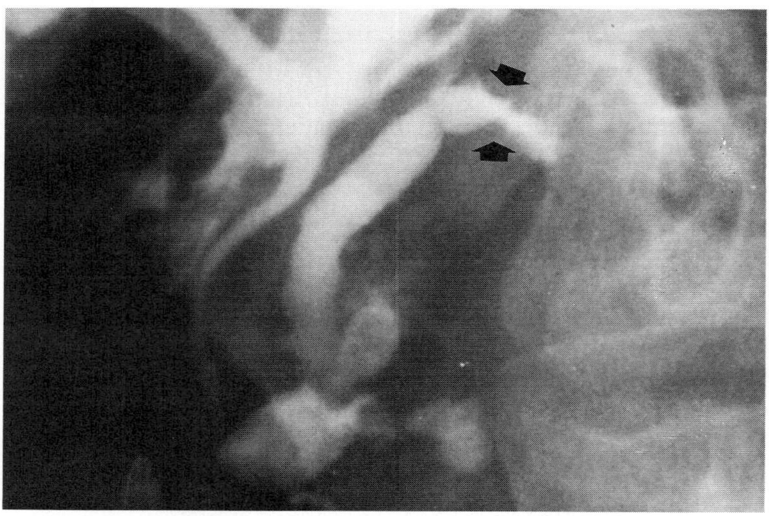

Fig. 7. ERCP 1 year after 80% pancreatectomy and pancreaticojejunostomy showing filling defect in the proximal Wirsung duct, small cyst, and free flow of the contrast to the jejunum

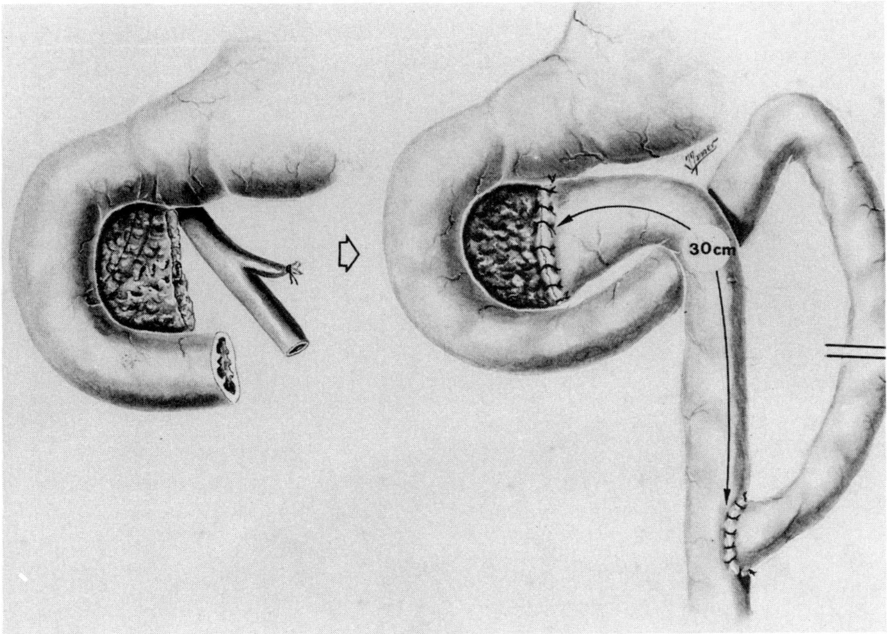

Fig. 8. Diagram of 80% distal pancreatectomy. The pancreatic stump is drained into a Roux-en-Y loop of jejunum

increased intraductal pressure, pancreaticojejunostomy may prevent recurrent attacks of pancreatitis as a result of diminishing the outflow resistance to pancreatic secretion.

Bearing in mind that strictures and stones are frequently located in the head of the pancreas it seems logical to support the choice of an operation dealing with the drainage of these area.

The effect on functional results of pancreaticojejunostomy associated with distal pancreatectomy increases the rate of good results from 40% to 75% in the experience of Leger et al. [7] and from 65% to 75% in that of the Association Française de Chirurgie [8]. However, Shankor et al. [9] have shown, in a large retrospective analysis of 113 patients who had a distal pancreatectomy, that lateral pancreatic drainage confers no benefit following distal pancreatic resection. But, in this study, pancreatic fistula was observed in 2% in the drainage group vs 6% in the non-drainage group; 79% of patients were pain free in the drainage group vs 68% in the non-drainage group; following the operation only 7% of patients in the drainage group had pain controlled by potent analgesia vs 24% in the non-drainage group. Nevertheless, there were an equal number of failures in each group requiring total pancreatectomy. The main criticism of this study is the

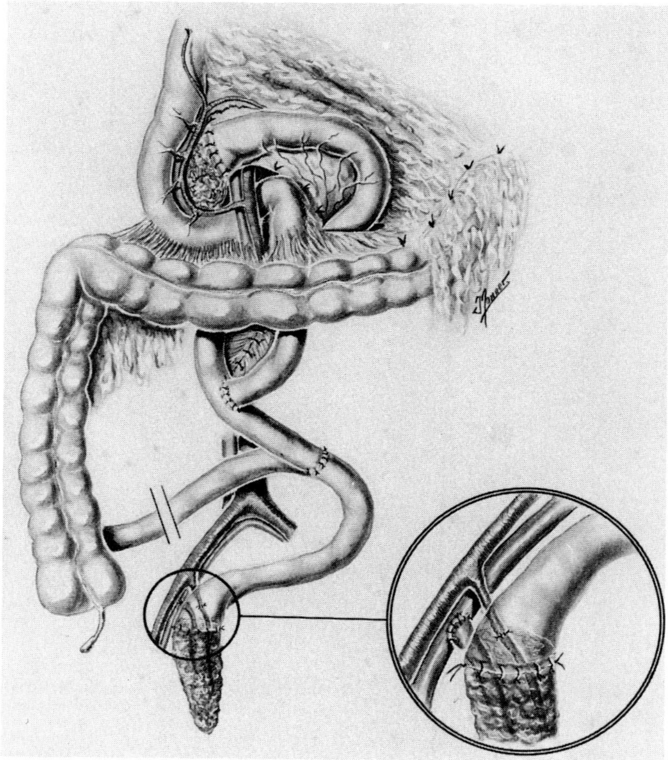

Fig. 9. Diagram of 80% pancreatectomy and segmental autotransplantation. The pancreas is transected at the level of the gastroduodenal artery. Posterior to divided pancreas, the splenic artery and vein are isolated, ligated, and divided near the celiac axis and portal vein, respectively. The splein artery is flushed with EuroCollins. The autograft is revascularized by anastomosis of the splenic vessels to the hypogastric artery and iliac vein. Both the stump of the pancreas in the head of the pancreas and the autograft are drained to two separate Roux-en-Y loops of jejunum

Table 3. Magnitude of the left resection + pancreaticojejunostomy (Roux-en-Y)

Pancreatectomy	Number of patients
80%[a]	23
60%[b]	6
80% + Segmental autotransplant	2
60% + Cystojejunostomy (head)	1
Body (pseudocyst)	1

[a] The gland is divided at the level of the gastroduodenal artery.
[b] Line of resection to the right of the portal vein.

Table 4. Results of resection + Roux-en-Y pancreato-jejunostomy in 33 patients

	Patients	
	(*n*)	(%)
Pain relief		
Complete	31	94
Partial	2	6
Hospital mortality	0	0
Exocrine dysfunction		
Preoperative	10	30
Postoperative	16	48
Endocrine dysfunction		
Preoperative	8	24
Postoperative	16	48

Median follow-up period 3.5 years (range 1–9 years).

limited pancreatic resection performed (1 cm to the right of the portal vein) in all cases, and that the number of surgeons were involved in the surgery and in the survey between May 1976 and June 1988 is not stated.

In analyzing our own series of patients, the surgical objectives of draining the cut surface of the pancreas were to avoid the effects of leakage from the pancreatic stump, and to achieve better drainage by enabling the pancreatic juice to escape both proximally and distally. The overall objective, relief of pain, was achieved in 94% of patients.

The Problem of Postoperative Diabetes

The problem of postoperative diabetes is controversial. The rate of development or aggravation of diabetes varies from 30% to 69% of cases [8]. We should keep in mind, however, that the incidence of postoperative diabetes is not only a consequence of pancreatic excision; it also depends on the natural evolution of the disease. Therefore, the incidence of diabetes after resection varies in proportion to preoperative insufficiency and to the extent of reduction in pancreatic endocrine mass. Two approaches have been developed for surgical diabetes prophylaxis: autosegmental transplantation of the resected pancreas with immediate revascularization at an ectopic site, and, alternatively, islet cells processed from the resected specimen autotransplanted as a free graft [10, 11]. Rossi et al. [12] recently gave long-term follow-up results (median 62 months) on the largest reported series of patients treated with extensive pancreatectomy and segmental autotransplantation; six of 13 patients are currently insulin-independent.

Management of the pancreatic duct and planning the location of the autotransplantation have been the major technical controversies in the small reported experience [12–18] (24 cases) and the two cases described here. The transplant site chosen in the majority of autotransplants, except in our own and the report of Dafoe et al. [18], was a subcutaneous pocket in the groin. This location has several important disadvantages: infection or delayed healing of groin incisions, which may predispose to life-threatening vascular complications; little room to adjust the orientation of the pancreas to avoid kinking of its vessels (which may have contributed to vascular thrombosis in five out of 24 patients); difficulty in accommodating hematoma or extravasation of lymph or pancreatic secretions, which frequently occur. The peritoneal cavity is our preferred site, since it readily allows absorption of fluid (lymph and/or pancreatic juice), which frequently collects around the grafts.

Different methods have been used to handle the exocrine pancreatic secretion. Ligation of the duct, first used by Hogle and Reemtsma [13], may predispose to fistula formation because transected pancreatic lymphatics function as small accessory ducts when the major duct is ligated. Pancreatic duct injection with a polymer was used in 14 patients in a review of previously reported segmental autografts. Although only one patient died as a result of the procedure (4.5%), 11 suffered significant morbidity. Five developed graft necrosis, presumably from vascular thrombosis, four developed abscesses at the transplant site and four had fistulas from the autograft. The main objection to this approach can be summarized in one particularly interesting case reported by Soon Shiong et al. [17]. In this patient, following total pancreatectomy the splenic vessels of the body and tail of the pancreas were revascularized in the groin and the pancreatic duct was ligated. Postoperatively the patient developed pain in the groin, probably from swelling of the graft, which on the pancreatogram was found to have a dilated duct. She also developed a persistent pancreatic fistula and symptoms of severe pancreatic exocrine dysfunction (diarrhea and fatty food intolerance). In an effort to relieve pain and restore exocrine function a Roux loop was tunnelled above the inguinal ligament into the groin and a pancreaticojejunostomy was performed, with postoperative relief of symptoms (pain and malnutrition).

Thus, maintenance of physiological drainage of the exocrine duct is probably desirable and may contribute to long-term function of the endocrine system. In two of our patients after 80% distal pancreatectomy the body and tail of the autografts were placed in the peritoneal cavity and revascularized via the iliac vessels (hypogastric artery and iliac vein). The autograft and the remnant of the head of the pancreas were drained to two separate Roux jejunal loops. Both patients are pain free, insulin-independent, without enzyme therapy and have returned to gainful long-term employment (as an airline pilot and a businessman) 2 and 3 years after distal pancreatectomy and autotransplantation.

When a patient remains normoglycemic after subtotal pancreatic resection and autotransplantation it is difficult to determine whether the autotransplant or the unresected portion of the pancreas (or both) is responsible.

Conclusion

In highly selected patients with disabling pain, a non-dilated pancreatic duct, and disease lateralized to the left of the gland, pancreatic resective procedures become a consideration. Limited distal resection is associated with a low incidence of endocrine and exocrine insufficiency; however, the recurrence rate of pain has been high. More extensive resection, such as total or nearly total pancreatectomy, increases the success rate for relief of pain compared to limited distal resection. However, these procedures are associated with a higher incidence of metabolic complications. When extensive resection is required, techniques of segmental or islet autotransplantation should be considered to prevent or delay the onset of diabetes.

Some of the current distal resective operations have shown relief of pain in 50%–80% of patients [7, 8, 19, 20]. Specific indications include:

1. Disease predominantly affecting the body and the tail of the pancreas
2. Severe disease of the body and tail with duct obstruction at the level of the pancreatic neck
3. A pseudocyst in the body or in the tail, not communicated with the main pancreatic duct

The decision on whether to perform limited or extensive pancreatic resection should be based on (1) morphological investigation (CT, ultrasound and ERCP) for the distribution of calcification, ductal strictures and inflammation, and (2) surgical findings after on-table pancreatography. Operative pancreatograms are invaluable in patients with pancreatic pseudocysts to show whether or not there is communication with the main pancreatic duct. Prograde pancreatography via the duct in the head of the pancreas after distal pancreatectomy will help to confirm free flow of the contrast into the duodenum. An obstructing stone indicates the need to remove it as it may cause persistent or recurrent pancreatitis.

The association of distal resection and a drainage procedure (pancreaticojejunostomy) is essential to decrease intraductal pressure by enabling the pancreatic juice to escape both proximally and distally. When adequately selected, different degrees of left resection can achieve acceptable results in the management of patients with non-dilated ducts and without a mass in the head of the pancreas.

References

1. Prinz RA, Greenlee HB (1990) Pancreatic duct drainage in chronic pancreatitis. Hepatogastroenterology 37:295–300
2. Traverso LW, Longmire WP (1980) Preservation of the pylorus in pancreaticoduodenectomy. A follow-up evaluation. Ann Surg 192:306–310
3. Beger HG, Büchler M, Bittner R, Uhl W (1990) Duodenum-preserving resection of the head of the pancreas. An alternative to Whipple's procedure in chronic pancreatitis. Hepatogastroenterology 37:283–289
4. Frey CF, Child CG III, Fry W (1976) Pancreatectomy for chronic pancreatitis. Ann Surg 184:403–414

5. Frey LF (1981) Role of subtotal pancreatectomy and pancreaticojejunostomy in chronic pancreatitis. J Clin Res 31:361–370
6. Willianson RCN, Cooper MJ (1987) Resection in chronic pancreatitis. Br J Surg 74:807–812
7. Leger L, Leurist JP, Lemaigre G (1974) Five to twenty year follow-up after surgery for chronic pancreatitis in 148 patients. Ann Surg 180:185–191
8. Gauthier-Benoit C, Perissat J (1987) Le traitment des pancreatites chroniques. Rapport du 89ême Congrès de l'Association Française de Chirurgie. Masson, Paris
9. Shankor S, Their B, Russell REG (1990) Management of the stump of the pancreas after distal pancreatic resection. Br J Surg 77:541–544
10. Morrow CE, Cohen JI, Sutherland DER, Najarian JS (1984) Chronic pancreatitis: long-term surgical results of pancreatic duct drainage, pancreatic resection, and near-total pancreatectomy and islet autotransplantation. Surgery 96:608–616
11. Farney AC, Najarian JS, Nakhleh RF, Lloveras G, Field J, Gores PF, Sutherland DER (1991) Autotransplantation of dispersed pancreatic islet tissue combined with total or nearly-total pancreatectomy for treatment of chronic pancreatitis. Surgery 110:427–439
12. Rossi RL, Soeldner JS, Braasch JW, Heiss FW, Shea JA, Watkins E Jr, Silverman ML (1990) Long-term results of pancreatic resection and segmental pancreatic autotransplantation for chronic pancreatitis. Am J Surg 159:51–58
13. Hogle HH, Reemtsma K (1978) Pancreatic autotransplantation following resection. Surgery 83:359–360
14. McDonald JC, Rohr MS, Tucker WY (1983) Recent experiences with autotransplantation of the Kidney, jejunum and pancreas. Ann Surg 197/6:678–687
15. Tossati E, Valente V, Campisi G, Barabino G, Pozzati A (1980) Segmental pancreas autotransplantation in man following total or near total pancreatectomy for serious recurrent chronic pancreatitis. Transplant Proc 12/4 (Suppl 2):15–18
16. Terzigni R, Toledo-Pereyra H, Falluca F, Cavallini M, Capece G, Giagrande L, Capua G, Stipa S (1983) Transplantation of irradiated human pancreas. Ann Surg 49:502–505
17. Soon-Shiong, Swafford PG, Levin S (1987) Successful long-term exocrine and endocrine function of the autotransplanted pancreas in humans. Pancreas 2:357–361
18. Dafoe DC, Naji A, Perloff LJ, Barker CF (1990) Pancreatic and islet autotransplantation. Hepatogastroenterology 37:307–315
19. Morel P, Rohner A (1987) Surgery for chronic pancreatitis. Surgery 101:130
20. Cuilleret J, Guillemin G (1990) Surgical management of chronic pancreatitis on the continent of Europe. World J Surg 14:11–18

Standard Whipple in Chronic Pancreatitis

H.D. SAEGER,[1] G. SCHWALL, and M. TREDE

Introduction

Physicians and surgeons essentially agree today that chronic pancreatitis must primarily be treated conservatively. However, complications of the disease can require operative intervention. The aim of surgery in chronic pancreatitis is the treatment of symptoms; perhaps the progress of the disease can be delayed thereby, but surgical management cannot be a causal therapy for chronic pancreatitis. Various operative techniques have been discussed. The surgical objectives in chronic pancreatitis can be summarized in four points: (a) low operative morbidity and mortality, (b) persisting pain relief, (c) preservation of the (remaining) pancreatic function, and (d) long-term survival.

Whipple was the first surgeon to resect the pancreatic head for chronic pancreatitis in 1946 [18]. Only during the past 20 years has this operation come to be performed frequently. In this period the initially high rates of operative mortality decreased from over 10% to less than 2% [5, 8, 9, 17]. The improvement in the early results was encouraging. If surgery was indicated at all, Whipple's operation therefore became the standard procedure for the (benign) chronically inflamed tumor of the head of the pancreas.

Patients and Indications

From 1972 to 1990, 685 patients suffering from chronic pancreatitis were referred for operation to the Mannheim Surgical University Department. In 42% of cases (n = 286) we felt that conservative therapy had not yet been carried out intensively enough and so advised our patients to avoid any operation at that time. In the other 58% various operative procedures were individually selected for each case: 32% drainage (n = 221) and 26% resection (n = 178). In addition to 50 distal pancreatectomies and 17 total pancreatectomies, we performed 111 duodenopancreatectomies according

[1] Klinikum Mannheim, Chirurgische Univ.-Klinik, Theodor-Kutzer-Ufer, W-6800 Mannheim 1, FRG

Beger/Büchler/Malfertheiner (Eds.)
Standards in Pancreatic Surgery

Table 1. Complications in chronic pancreatitis: indications for duodenopancreatectomy in 111 patients

	n	%
Intractable pain	98	88.3
Bile duct stenosis	69	62.2
Duodenal compression	47	42.3
Portal vein stenosis	6	5.4

to Whipple's operation (92 men, 19 women; median age 42 years, range 19–71). The principal goals of surgical therapy in this context were: (a) removal of mechanical obstacles due to a tumor of the pancreatic head, (b) elimination of the suspicion of cancer, and (c) treatment of conservatively uncontrollable pain.

Pain was the leading symptom in 98/111 of our patients (88.3%). The history of complaints lasted an average of 3.6 years (4 weeks–40 years). In all patients pancreatitis was mainly located within the pancreatic head. This was the reason for common bile duct stenosis in 62%. Not all of these patients presented with an obstructive jaundice, but alkaline phosphatase was always increased above normal and did not show a tendency to normalize. We saw stenoses of the prepapillary pancreatic duct in 90%. In 42% duodenal stenoses were detected radiologically, but these very rarely led to symptoms (Table 1). More than 50% compression of the portal or mesenteric vein was evident in only six patients. In our opinion, thrombosis of these veins is a contraindication to any operation for chronic pancreatitis. The existence of a cavernous transformation of collateral veins makes every surgical intervention – resection and even bypass techniques – a dangerous procedure.

The definitive preoperative elimination of suspicion of cancer can be a dilemma that is impossible to resolve despite a broad diagnostic evaluation. Of 100 patients who had been operated on with the preoperative diagnosis of chronic pancreatitis, 15 had a histologically confirmed pancreatic carcinoma. On the other hand, of 311 patients with the preoperative diagnosis of "cancer" of the head of the pancreas 14% only had an inflammatory tumor due to chronic pancreatitis (Table 2). This rather high rate of uncertain preoperative diagnoses can be explained by the long period of investigation (sonography and computed tomography were not available in the early years). It may also be related to the unsafe fine-needle cytology. Even in excellent series with ultrasound- or CT-guided biopsies, a certain rate of findings remains unclear. This rate, even if demonstrating false-negative results below 10%, is too large to be neglected [4, 6, 10, 12, 13].

In our opinion, in these cases Whipple's procedure is justified if the tumor of the pancreatic head is symptomatic, and if the general operative risk is low.

Table 2. Preoperative differentiation of pancreatic head tumors in 411 duodenopancreatectomies: chronic pancreatitis or pancreatic carcinoma?

Preoperative	Postoperative	
	Pancreatic carcinoma	Chronic pancreatitis
Pancreatic carcinoma? ($n = 311$)	268	43 (14%)
Chronic pancreatitis? ($n = 100$)	15 (15%)	85
Total	283	128

Operative Technique

The operation starts with a horizontal laparotomy of the upper abdomen. For the assessment of the pancreas the lesser sac is opened up by dividing the greater omentum from the transverse colon. Duodenum and pancreatic head are mobilized by the Kocher maneuver. The gallbladder is separated from the liver by orthograde preparation. The common hepatic duct is divided proximally to the cystic duct junction. After preparation of the hepatic artery the gastroduodenal artery is identified and divided between ligatures. The pancreas is then separated from the ventral part of the portal vein.

The distal stomach is skeletonized and divided at the border of the antrum. The pancreas is then divided in front of the portal vein, and the pancreatic head, including the uncinate process, is dissected from the portal and superior mesenteric veins. After having isolated the duodenojejunal flexure, the proximal jejunum is divided and the specimen removed en bloc.

The reconstruction is performed after retromesenteric transposition of the proximal jejunal loop into the upper abdomen. The end-to-end pancreatojejunostomy is performed according to the telescope technique in two layers. About 12 cm from this anastomosis a terminolateral hepaticojejunostomy is performed in one layer. We introduce a Völker stent into this anastomosis. The stent leaves the jejunal loop a further 10 cm distally through a Witzel channel. After closing the medial part of the gastric stump, an antecolic, lateral gastrojejunostomy is performed. Finally, Braun's enteroanastomosis is performed. The operation is finished after having positioned a subhepatic drain [17].

Results

Since 1972 the rate of duodenopancreatectomies for chronic pancreatitis – five or six operations/year – has not changed. During the same period the frequency of Whipple operations for carcinoma patients significantly in-

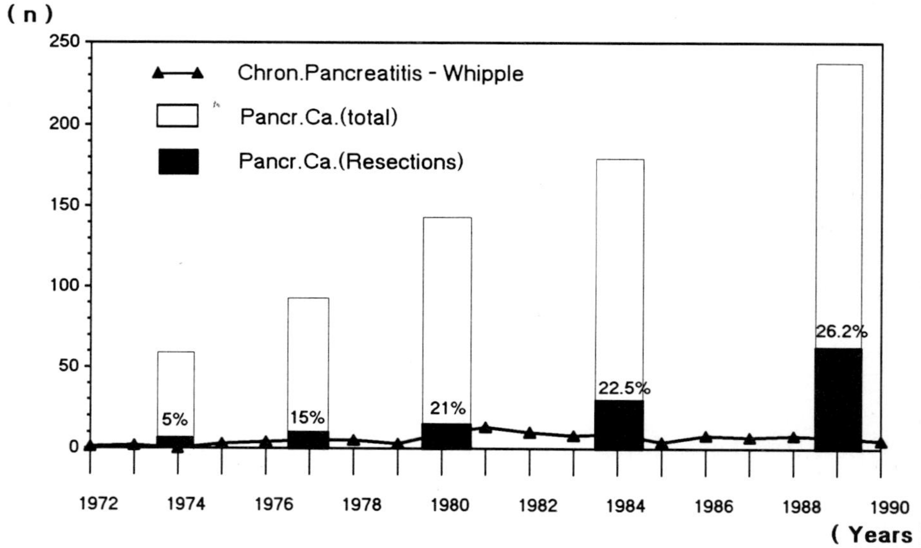

Fig. 1. Duodenopancreatectomies in chronic pancreatitis and resection rates of pancreatic carcinomas over the past 19 years

creased for various reasons (Fig. 1). The average hospitalization time was 21 days. There was one death; hospital mortality was less than 1%.

There were a number of postoperative complications. Bleeding from the gastroenterostomy occurred in five cases and could be stopped three times endoscopically and twice by relaparotomy. Two patients with postoperative bleeding into the abdominal cavity had to be reoperated. One patient died 10 years ago of an anastomotic leak despite relaparotomy. One pancreatic fistula healed after conservative treatment with somatostatin. Another fistula in a symptom-free patient closed spontaneously. One intraabdominal abscess was drained successfully by introduction of a sonographically guided drain. In 91% of the patients the postoperative course was without any surgical complications (Table 3).

For the assessment of late results, follow-up examinations were performed in 79 patients in whom the operation was performed 6 months to 16 years previously. The evaluation period extended from 1972 to January 1, 1989. Of these patients 77% gained weight (median of 12 kg); 79% were completely free of complaints, and only 6% suffered from persisting, intractable pain. Two-thirds went back to work (Table 4).

Examination of endocrine function (including oral glucose test, HbA1, C-peptide) showed diabetes occurring postoperatively in only 12% of patients. Of these only 48% needed insulin. Nearly two-thirds of the patients were free of diabetes. Exocrine function (chymotrypsin, steatorrhea) after the Whipple operation also showed good results. Only 24% of

Table 3. Postoperative surgical complications after duodenopancreatectomy for chronic pancreatitis (in 11 of 111 patients)

Complication	*n*
Gastrointestinal bleeding	5
Intraabdominal bleeding	2
Anastomotic leak	1
Pancreatic fistula	2
Peritoneal abscess	1

Table 4. Late results (6 months–16 years) in duodenopancreatectomy for chronic pancreatitis (79 evaluable patients)

Gained weight	77%
Free of pain	79%
Occasional pain	15%
Pain unchanged	6%
Back at work	66%

the patients developed exocrine insufficiency postoperatively (Table 5). Four of 111 patients developed peptic ulceration (3.6%). One patient had to be reoperated because of a dumping syndrome 2 years after a Whipple resection.

Late mortality (as of Jan. 1, 1991) for all patients was 10.8% (12/111), with a median survival time of 32 months. The causes of death were in 7 out of 12 cases persistent alcoholic abuse. Any other operative method probably would not have prevented the incidence of liver cirrhosis in six patients or an alcohol-toxic cardiomyopathy. Three of the 12 patients died of myocardial infarction, one after acute gastrointestinal bleeding and one other from unknown reasons (Table 6).

Conclusions

These results compare favorably to the spontaneous course of chronic pancreatitis. According to Ammann's report, 56% of conservatively treated patients developed an endocrine insufficiency within 6 years [1]. The distal resection even of 80%–95% of the organ does not always lead to complete pain relief and moreover is associated with a high rate of endocrine and exocrine insufficiencies [7, 11].

Drainage of the pancreatic duct system alone does not compete with duodenopancreatectomy but is rather an alternative treatment. As others, we feel that this operative procedure should be considered only in patients

Table 5. Endocrine and exocrine function before and 6 months to 16 years after duodenopancreatectomy (79 evaluable patients)

Insufficiency	Endocrine	Exocrine
Preoperative	27%	16%
Postoperative	12%[a]	24%
None	61%	60%

[a] 48% requiring insulin.

Table 6. Operative and late mortality after duodenopancreatectomy (111 evaluable patients)

Operative and hospital mortality	1 (0.9%)
Late mortality (median survival 32 months)	12 (10.8%)
Cause of death	
Alcoholism	7
Liver cirrhosis	6
Toxic cardiomyopathy	2
Myocardial infarction	3
Bleeding	1
Unknown	1
Total	12

with a dilatation of the pancreatic duct of at least 8 mm. This finding, however, occurs in about only 20% of patients [4, 14]. Total pancreatectomy in chronic pancreatitis is almost never indicated. In the past 6 years we have no longer performed this operation for benign disease. In this case the large tumor of the pancreatic head and corpus resembled suspiciously a carcinoma.

As chronic pancreatitis very often is concentrated in the pancreatic head, duodenopancreatectomy according to the Whipple procedure seems to be a good operation both for pain relief and concerning late results. The operative technique is well standardized today, so that operative morbidity and mortality have significantly decreased. Therefore this Whipple operation is justified even for chronic pancreatitis – a benign disease. Similar results have also been reported after pylorus- and duodenum-preserving resection of the pancreatic head. Especially preservation of the duodenum is a technically demanding operation, which shows excellent results in the hands of specialized surgeons [2, 3]. There are theoretical advantages, but compared to Whipple's resection there are no clinical differences [2, 15, 16].

Finally, for the surgical treatment of chronic pancreatitis the following will probably still be valid in the future: (a) no operation can improve pancreatic function, (b) there is no ideal operation for all cases, and (c) the *indication* for operation is more important than the operative *technique*.

References

1. Ammann RW, Akovbiantz A, Largiader F, Schueler G (1984) Course and outcome of chronic pancreatitis: longitudinal study of mixed medical-surgical series of 245 patients. Gastroenterology 86:820–828
2. Beger HG, Bittner R (1987) Die duodenumerhaltende Pankreaskopfresektion. Chirurg 58:7–13
3. Beger HG, Büchler M (1990) Duodenum-preserving resection of the head of the pancreas in chronic pancreatitis with inflammatory mass in the head. World J Surg 14:83–87
4. Carter DC (1990) Pancreatico-duodenectomy for chronic pancreatitis. In: Trede M, Saeger HD (eds) Aktuelle Pankreaschirurgie. Springer, Berlin Heidelberg New York, pp 149–157
5. Cuilleret J, Guillemin G (1990) Surgical management of chronic pancreatitis on the continent of Europe. World J Surg 14:11–18
6. Deixonne B, Pignodel C, Chazelet C, Joujoux JM, Raffanel C, Bamuel H (1989) Small carcinomas of the pancreas with associated chronic pancreatitis: two case reports. Eur J Surg Oncol 15:265–270
7. Eckhauser FE, Strodel WE, Knol JA, Harper M, Turcotte G (1984) Near total pancreatectomy for chronic pancreatitis. Surgery 96:599–606
8. Gall FP (1990) Die partielle Duodenopankreatektomie in Kombination mit der Pankreasgangokklusion durch Ethibloc. In: Trede M, Saeger HD (eds) Aktuelle Pankreaschirurgie. Springer, Berlin Heidelberg New York, pp 158–164
9. Howard JM, Zhang Z (1990) Pancreaticoduodenectomy (Whipple resection) in the treatment of chronic pancreatitis. World J Surg 14:77–80
10. Ihse I (1990) Chronic pancreatitis: clinical. Curr Opinion Gastroenterol 6:769–774
11. Imrie CW (1990) Management of recurrent pain following previous surgery for chronic pancreatitis. World J Surg 14:88–93
12. Jennings PE, Donald JJ, Coral A, Rode J, Lees WR (1989) Ultrasound-guided core biopsy. Lancet 17:1369–1371
13. Kocjan G, Rode J, Lees WR (1989) Percutaneous fine needle aspiration cytology of the pancreas: advantages and pitfalls. J Clin Pathol 42:341–347
14. Prinz RA, Greenlee HB (1981) Pancreatic duct drainage in 100 patients with chronic pancreatitis. Ann Surg 194:313–320
15. Trede M (1987) Kommentar auf Einladung zu HG Beger, R Bittner, M Büchler "Pankreaskopfresektion mit Erhaltung des Duodenums". Chir Gastroenterol 3:91–92
16. Trede M (1987) Therapie der chronischen Pankreatitis – Schlußkommentar. Langenbecks Arch Chir 372:379–382
17. Trede M, Schwall G, Saeger HD (1990) Survival after pancreatoduodenectomy. 118 consecutive resections without an operative mortality. Ann Surg 211:447–458
18. Whipple AO (1946) Radical surgery for certain cases of pancreatic fibrosis associated with calcareous deposits. Ann Surg 124:991–1006

Left Resection in Chronic Pancreatitis

C. GEBHARDT[1]

Ten to twenty years ago pancreatic left resection was the standard operation in the treatment of diffuse chronic pancreatitis with minor or no dilatation of the ductal system. In recent years, however, various forms of resection of the pancreatic head have gained more and more importance in the operative therapy. Therefore it seems useful to evaluate the present significance of pancreatic left resection in the treatment of chronic pancreatitis.

Results of Left Resection

Operative Mortality

The average operative mortality in more than 1000 cases is around 6% [1, 6–8] (collected series in [2]). It must be kept in mind, however, that in most hospitals with considerable experience in pancreatic surgery today the results are much better. In our own series of 32 left resections during the past 6 years there has been no postoperative death.

Pain Relief and Rate of Recurrence

Pancreatic left resection leads to a considerable improvement of pancreatitis-associated symptoms in almost 70% of cases. In almost 30%, however, there is no improvement, or there is recurrence of pancreatic pain [1, 7, 8] (collected series in [2]). In analyzing our own series of patients we found that late results depend mainly on the extent of pancreatitis and on the extent of resection [3, 4]. In diffuse pancreatitis was saw poor results in 67% of the partial left resections and in 49% of the subtotal pancreatectomies. A different situation existed in patients with isolated segmental pancreatitis of the pancreatic tail. Here, disappointing results were found, depending on the extent of resection – in 33% with partial resection and in 9% with subtotal resection (Table 1). The subtotal pancreatectomy in these patients

[1] Zentrum für Chirurgie, Stadt Nürnberg Klinikum, Flurstraße 17, W-8500 Nürnberg 90, FRG

Beger/Büchler/Malfertheiner (Eds.)
Standards in Pancreatic Surgery

Table 1. Late results after left resection for chronic pancreatitis (from [4])

	Number of patients	No improvement or recurrence	
		n	%
Left-side pancreatitis (*n* = 58)			
Partial resection	24	8	33.3
Subtotal resection	34	3	8.8
Diffuse pancreatitis (*n* = 67)			
Partial resection	24	16	66.7
Subtotal resection	43	21	48.8

corresponded to an 80% resection of the organ with the resection line above or just to the right side of the portal vein.

Carbohydrate Metabolism

With regard to carbohydrate metabolism, pancreatic left resection leads to an average postoperative increase in the rate of insulin-dependent diabetes of 50%. This is considerably higher than after drainage procedures or even after partial duodenopancreatectomies. In our own 121 patients the rate of diabetics increased by 41% during the late postoperative course. It is of interest that in this series there was no difference between partial and subtotal resection. This can be explained by the fact that there were almost no true 95% subtotal resections in our patients; it also proves the importance of the cauda pancreatis for carbohydrate metabolism. Different results have been reported by Morrow et al. [7]. In cases with 40%–80% resection the results are similar to ours, with an increase in the incidence of diabetes of 38%. The 95% resections, however, resulted in the occurrence of postoperative insulin-dependent diabetes in all cases. Eckhauser and coworkers [1] found that an 80%–95% left resection increased the rate of diabetes by 50%. Of special importance is the fact that 82% of the 44 patients who developed insulin-dependent diabetes in the postoperative period had a normal carbohydrate metabolism preoperatively. Based on these reports it can be expected that in general left pancreatic resection leads to an increase in the incidence of diabetes by about 40%, and that this rate increases to nearly 100% if the resection is very extensive.

Survival Rates

The cumulative, age-corrected 5-year survival rate of our patients excluding the operative mortality was 78%. These results are quite similar to those which can be achieved with drainage procedures. The survival does not seem to depend as much on the type of procedure performed as on the

Table 2. Cumulative 5-year survival rate after left resection for chronic pancreatitis (operative mortality excluded) (from [5])

	Number of patients	5-year survival rate ± 2 SE (%)
Calcifying pancreatitis	47	71 ± 15
No calcifying pancreatitis	113	81 ± 9
Preoperative diabetes mellitus	64	73 ± 12
No preoperative diabetes mellitus	96	82 ± 9
Alcoholics	64	72 ± 13
Nonalcoholics	96	83 ± 9

primary severity and extent of the disease and on the postoperative behavior of the patients. Continued consumption of alcohol is of great importance. Alcoholic patients with calcifying pancreatitis and preoperatively manifest diabetes mellitus had considerably lower 5-year survival rates than nonalcoholics without diabetes and without calcifications (Table 2). The negative influence of continued alcohol consumption on survival after pancreatic left resection is especially evident in the series of patients reported by Eckhauser et al. [1].

Conclusions

An optimal indication with good late results in more than 90% of cases seems to be the segmental pancreatitis with more or less isolated involvement of the tail of the pancreas. However, these good results can be expected only if an 80% resection is performed; this means dividing the organ in the region of the portal vein. We do not recommend more extensive resections because of the significant increase in metabolic problems in these patients. In addition to segmental pancreatitis of the tail region, we consider an indication to be given in persisting or bleeding pseudocysts and in chronic pancreatitis with splenic hypertension in splenic vein thrombosis.

Chronic pancreatitis of the diffuse type is not an indication for left resection because a low recurrence rate can be achieved only with a "near-total" pancreatectomy, which in turn results in an extremely high rate of postoperative diabetes.

References

1. Eckhauser FE, Strodel WE, Knol JA, Harper M, Turcotte JG (1984) Near-total pancreatectomy for chronic pancreatitis. Surgery 96:599–607
2. Gebhardt C (1984) Chirurgie des exokrinen Pankreas. Thieme, Stuttgart
3. Gebhardt C (1987) Indications, techniques and results of surgical or endoscopic pancreatic duct occlusion in chronic pancreatitis. Tijdschr Gastroenterol 17:349–358
4. Gebhardt C, Zirngibl H, Gossler M (1981) Pankreaslinksresektion zur Behandlung der chronischen Pankreatitis. Langenbecks Arch Chir 354:209–220
5. Metzner K (1989) Spätsterblichkeit nach Eingriffen wegen chronischer Pankreatitis. Dissertation, University of Erlangen
6. Morel P, Rohner A (1987) Surgery for chronic pancreatitis. Surgery 101:130–135
7. Morrow CE, Cohen JI, Sutherland DER, Najarian JS (1984) Chronic pancreatitis: long term surgical results of pancreatic duct drainage, pancreatic resection, and near-total pancreatectomy and islet autotransplantation. Surgery 96:608–616
8. Ribet M, Quandalle P, Giard-Lefevre S, Pruvot FR, Watine O (1986) Traitement chirurgical de la pancréatite chronique. Étude rétrospective de 221 cas. J Chir (Paris) 123:559–562

The Pylorus-Preserving Whipple Procedure for Severe Complications of Chronic Pancreatitis

L.W. Traverso[1]

Introduction

This chapter examines the clinical indications for removal of the head of the pancreas in patients with severe complications of chronic pancreatitis. Several methods can be utilized to remove the pancreatic head. These procedures include pancreaticoduodenectomy with hemigastrectomy [1], pancreaticoduodenectomy with preservation of the pylorus [2], excision of the pancreatic head with duodenal preservation [3], or resection of the ventral pancreatic head [4]. This report examines the mortality, morbidity, and short- and long-term results of the author's preferred method to excise the pancreatic head in patients with severe complications of chronic pancreatitis, i.e., pancreaticoduodenectomy with pylorus preservation (PDPP).

The surgical treatment of chronic pancreatitis can obtain safe and superlative relief of abdominal pain with the support of the rapidly progressing technologies of therapeutic endoscopy, interventional radiology, and anesthesiology. Therefore, only the past 5 years of experience with PDPP for chronic pancreatitis will be reviewed in the personal series of the author. Utilizing modern diagnostic and therapeutic techniques combined with proper patient selection, the procedure of PDPP results in solution of the severe problems that cause abdominal pain. These problems include the expanding pseudocyst in the head with or without contained arteriovenous fistula; the duct blow-out with penetration into the pleural cavity or leaves of omentum; and the pseudotumor of calcified fibrosis with bile duct, pancreatic duct, and/or duodenal obstruction. With PDPP every patient in this series obtained pain relief with little gastrointestinal sequelae. The mortality rate of PDPP in this series was zero.

[1] Virginia Mason Medical Center, 1100 Ninth Avenue, Seattle, WA 98111, USA

Beger/Büchler/Malfertheiner (Eds.)
Standards in Pancreatic Surgery

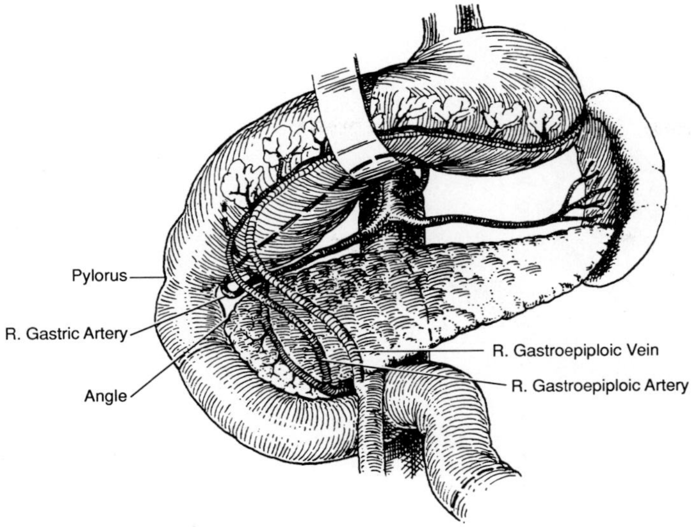

Fig. 1. *Dashed lines*, area of the pancreas, duodenum (parts 2, 3, and 4), and jejunum resected during the pylorus-preserving Whipple procedure. The stomach has been elevated off the pancreas. Ligation of the right gastric (superior pancreatic border) and gastroepiploic vessels (inferior pancreatic border) at their origin preserve the vascular arcade on the lesser and greater curvatures of the stomach. An intact neurovascular supply to the pylorus and first portion of the duodenum is mandatory for a functioning pylorus. A vagotomy or history of vagotomy precludes pylorus preservation

Materials and Methods

Technique of Preserving a Functioning Pylorus

Instead of antrectomy or hemigastrectomy during pancreaticoduodenectomy (Whipple's procedure), the pylorus is widely dissected free of the hepatoduodenal ligament (Fig. 1). The right gastric artery (if present) in the hepatoduodenal ligament at the superior pancreatic border and the right gastroepiploic artery and vein at the inferior border of the pancreas are divided at their origins and remote from the pylorus. With this wide dissection technique the neurovascular supply to the pylorus is protected and preserved. Dissection of the duodenal bulb is continued until the area where the first and second parts of duodenum join. This area is also where the duodenum and pancreas merge forming an "angle." Many shared blood vessels are observed at this point. About 5 cm of duodenum will have been freed, and the GIA stapling device is used to divide the duodenum at the junction of the first and second parts. Wide dissection of the pylorus and

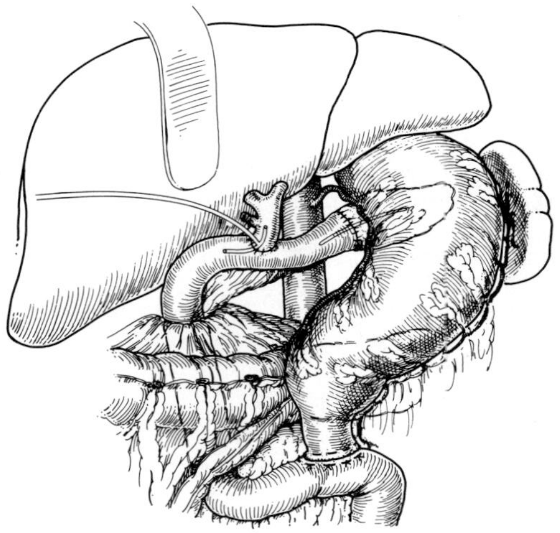

Fig. 2. Reconstruction with retrocolic anastomosis of the pancreatic duct and then bile duct. The pancreatic duct connection should be made with a side-to-side technique if a "chain of lakes" type of ductal dilatation is present. Otherwise an end-to-end mucosa-to-mucosa stented pancreatojejunostomy is shown. The end-duodenal to side-jejunal anastomosis is made antecolic over the left transverse colon to isolate the duodenal anastomosis from the other anastomoses which have leakage potential and could cause gastric outlet obstruction

duodenum adjacent to the head of the pancreas makes PDPP less than ideal for en bloc resection of duodenal or pancreatic cancer, but uniquely suited for chronic pancreatitis. The stomach and stapled-over first part of the duodenum is now mobile and is placed in the left upper quadrant until reconstruction.

The entire vagus nerve supply to the stomach is mandatory to preserve a functioning pylorus. A vagotomy or history of vagotomy does not allow preservation of the metering function of the pylorus. After excision of the pancreatic head, remaining duodenum, and distal common bile duct, the anastomoses are positioned to isolate potential leakage of the bile and pancreatic duct connections from the duodenojejunostomy. This maneuver may help to prevent gastric outlet dysfunction. The proximal jejunum is directed toward the pancreatic and bile duct remnants by a retrocolic route and the stomach with preserved pylorus and duodenum are brought antecolic to the left transverse colon, allowing for a remote duodenojejunostomy (Fig. 2).

If the chain-of-lakes type ductal dilatation is present in the pancreatic tail, the pancreatic anastomosis may be constructed with a longitudinal side-to-side technique. Many patients will have a duct in the pancreatic remnant with a diameter of 2–3 mm because the pain problem is not due to complete pancreatic ductal obstruction but is associated with an expanding pseudocyst or arteriovenous fistula in the head. The small pancreatic duct is reconstructed with an end-to-end mucosa-to-mucosa pancreaticojejunostomy as illustrated in Figs. 2 and 3. A 3- to 5-F polytetrafluoroethylene radiodense stent is utilized that has multiple holes throughout the stent (Wilson-Cook Medical).

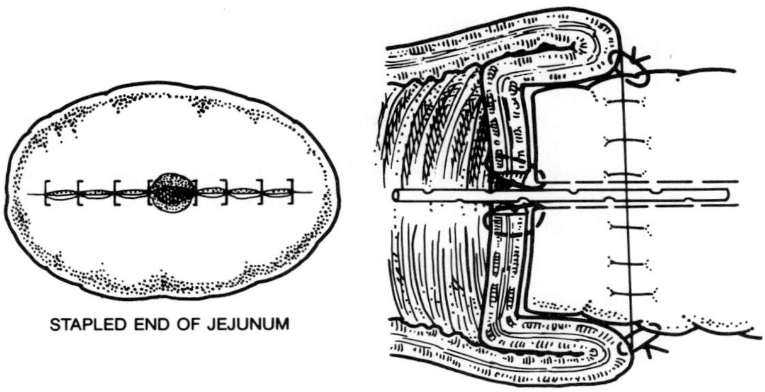

Fig. 3. The proximal jejunum has previously been divided from the surgical specimen with the GIA stapling device (U.S. Surgical). A staple is removed from the middle of the staple line (*left*) and an end-to-end mucosa-to-mucosa pancreaticojejunostomy with 5/0 Maxon (Davis and Geck). A polytetrafluoroethylene 3-, 4-, or 5-F radiodense stent is attached to the anastomosis with absorbable suture. The outer layer is completed with 3/0 silk providing a seromuscular envelope to prevent pancreatic fluid leakage. (From [10])

Patient Data

Between January 1986 and May 1991, 16 patients with chronic pancreatitis required excision of the head of the pancreas. One of these patients (LC) had undergone a vagotomy and antrectomy and therefore underwent standard pancreaticoduodenectomy. The remaining 15 patients underwent PDPP.

Patient characteristics are illustrated in Fig. 4 while the operative status of the bile duct, pancreatic duct, and pancreatic head is shown in Fig. 5. All patients were studied with endoscopic retrograde cholangio-pancreatography (ERCP) and computed tomography (CT) and some received preoperative endoscopic placement of bile or pancreatic duct stents. Percutaneous drainage of pancreatic fluid collections was also utilized.

Visceral arteriography with portal venous phase was obtained in 15 patients. The importance of understanding the frequent presence of hepatic

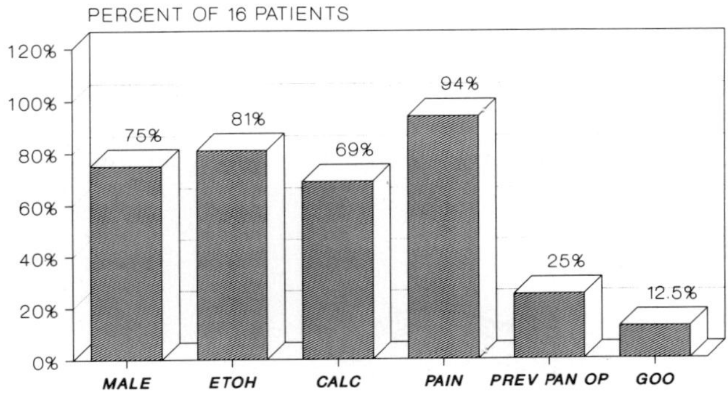

Fig. 4. Characteristics of 16 patients showed younger men with alcohol-induced chronic pancreatitis were frequent. (Mean age 46 years; range 37–65). Also, the glands were chronically involved with the majority calcified. Abdominal pain was the most common reason for operation. *PREV PAN OP*, Previous pancreatic operation; *GOO*, preoperative gastric outlet obstruction

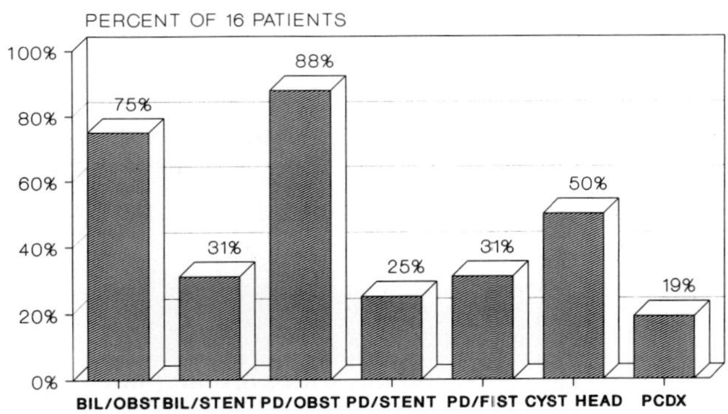

Fig. 5. Every patient underwent ERCP and most demonstrated biliary (*BIL/OBST*) and/or pancreatic duct (*PD/OBST*) obstruction. *BIL/STENT*, Biliary stent; *PD/STENT*, endoscopic transpapillary pancreatic stent; *FIST*, cutaneous fistula; *CYST HEAD*, one or more pseudocysts in or around the head; *PCDX*, percutaneous drainage preoperative

artery anomalies under the pancreatic head and their significance to prevent biliary fistula cannot be overemphasized when the Whipple procedure is performed for any disease [5]. When chronic pancreatitis is present additional vital information is frequently obtained as was the case in 60% of these cases (Fig. 6) with 20% having more than one abnormality (Fig. 7).

Case Histories

An overview of indications for excision of the pancreatic head in these patients is listed in Table 1. More specific details are presented below regarding the events leading to resection in five selected cases.

Case 1: R.R.

This hard-working man had a long history of heavy alcohol use. After a 4-month history of right upper quadrant abdominal pain, radiating to the back, he was hospitalized for sepsis, jaundice, and abdominal bloating. An arteriogram showed a hypervascular mass in the head of the pancreas

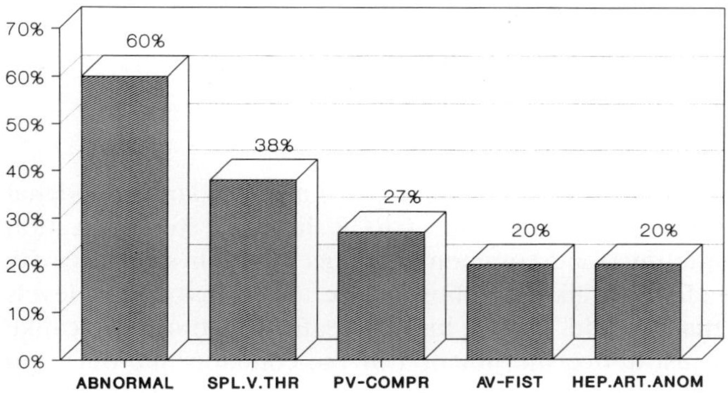

Fig. 6. Results (n = 15) of superior mesenteric plus celiac arteriography with portal venous phase; the majority were abnormal. *SPL V THR*, Splenic vein thrombosis; *PV-COMPR*, portal vein compression; *AV-FIST*, arteriovenous fistula; *HEP ART ANOM*, hepatic artery anomaly

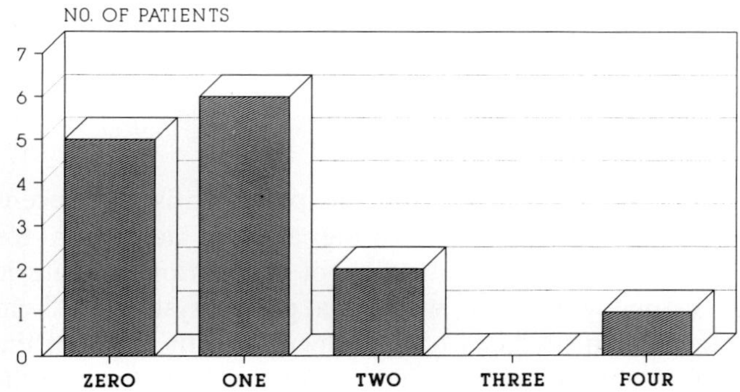

Fig. 7. Number of abnormalities per patient. Three of 15 patients had more than one abnormality: combinations of arteriovenous fistula, clotted vein, hepatic artery anomaly

Table 1. Reason for resection ($n = 16$)

	n
Expanding pseudocyst in head – pain	5
Pancreatic duct blow-out −4	
Arteriovenous fistula −3	
Biliary obstruction −3	
Pleural fistula −1	
Multiple pseudocysts in head – pain	3
Pancreatic and bile duct obstruction −3	
12-cm pseudotumor −1	
Pancreatic duct blow-out −1	
Biliary, pancreatic, gastric outlet obstruction – pain	2
Pancreatic fistula −1	
Pancreatic duct obstruction – pain	5
Diffuse calcified and enlarged head −4	
Biliary obstruction −1	
Cutaneous fistula	1
From pancreatic duct blow-out −1	

thought to be an endocrine tumor. Endoscopy showed a large duodenal ulcer just proximal to the ampulla of Vater. ERCP showed a communication between the pancreatic duct and common bile duct through a 3-cm cavity in the pancreatic head. Both alkaline phosphatase and transaminase levels were elevated more than tenfold. During his pancreatic resection a cloacalike cavity [6] was found just above the junction of the common bile duct and the pancreatic duct that communicated freely with both structures (Fig. 8). The cavity had enlarged to cause local necrosis of the duodenum (as seen by the duodenal ulcer). Bile was present in the pancreatic duct when the pancreas was divided over the portal vein. Histologic examination of the resected specimen showed the intense inflammation to be benign. A 14-h PDPP Whipple procedure with 2300 ml blood loss was required to resolve the problem. Postoperative ventilator dependence occurred because of adult respiratory distress syndrome (ARDS). No gastrointestinal or endocrine sequelae were present 5 years and 4 months postoperative.

Case 2: L.C.

This patient had a long history of alcohol-related pancreatitis and recent abdominal pain with biliary obstruction. During a prior admission for abdominal pain, he had undergone embolization of a superior mesenteric artery to portal vein fistula within the wall of a pseudocyst. The 3-cm necrotic cyst was located within the head of the pancreas to the right of the portal vein. Resolution of abdominal pain led to discharge, but 6 months later, he was readmitted for increasing abdominal pain, jaundice, nausea, and vomiting. A percutaneous transhepatic biliary stent was placed. An arteriogram showed absence of mesenteric-portal fistula. CT scan showed

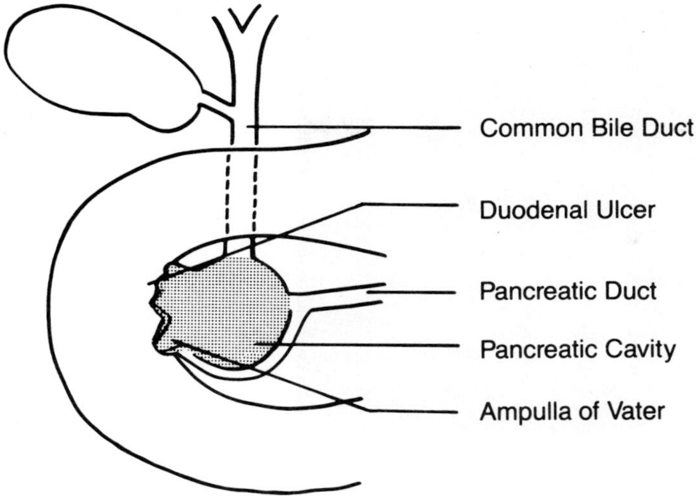

Fig. 8. Schematic summary of the pancreaticobiliary "cloacalike" chamber in patient RR as obtained from preoperative studies and the surgical specimen. (From [6])

persistent pseudocyst. The abdominal pain had to be managed with a chronic epidural catheter. After total parenteral nutrition for 10 days, the patient underwent standard pancreaticoduodenectomy (past history of antrectomy). The medial wall of the pseudocyst was the portal vein. An 11-h Whipple procedure with 2800 ml blood loss was required to solve the problem. Postoperative abscess around the pancreatic anastomosis required percutaneous drainage. No pain or gastrointestinal sequelae were present 3 years and 4 months postoperative. He began using 5 U/day insulin 1 year postoperative.

Case 3: R.S.

A long history of alcohol use resulted in an enlarged pancreatic head with multiple calcifications. Abdominal pain and shortness of breath was associated with an amylase rich pleural effusion and a contrast enhancing pseudocyst in the head (Fig. 9). ERCP showed a PD blow-out filling the cyst and another blow-out communicating with the hepatoduodenal ligament (Fig. 10). An arteriogram showed a clotted portal vein and splenic vein plus an arteriovenous fistula off the gastroduodenal artery in the wall of the pseudocyst (Fig. 11). A replaced right hepatic artery was seen from the superior mesenteric artery (Fig. 12). A 19-h PDPP Whipple procedure with 10 000 ml blood loss was required to resolve the problem. Tracheostomy was necessary for 30 days of ventilator dependence because of ARDS and *Pseudomonas* pneumonia. No pain, gastrointestinal, or endocrine sequelae were present 1 year and 4 months postoperative.

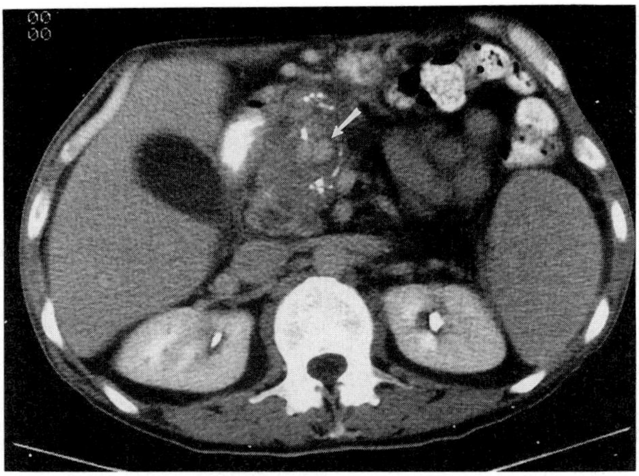

Fig. 9. Contrast-enhanced CT scan of patient RS showed a calcified head with pseudocyst (*arrow*) plus an adjacent contrast-enhanced area which was shown to be an arteriovenous fistula

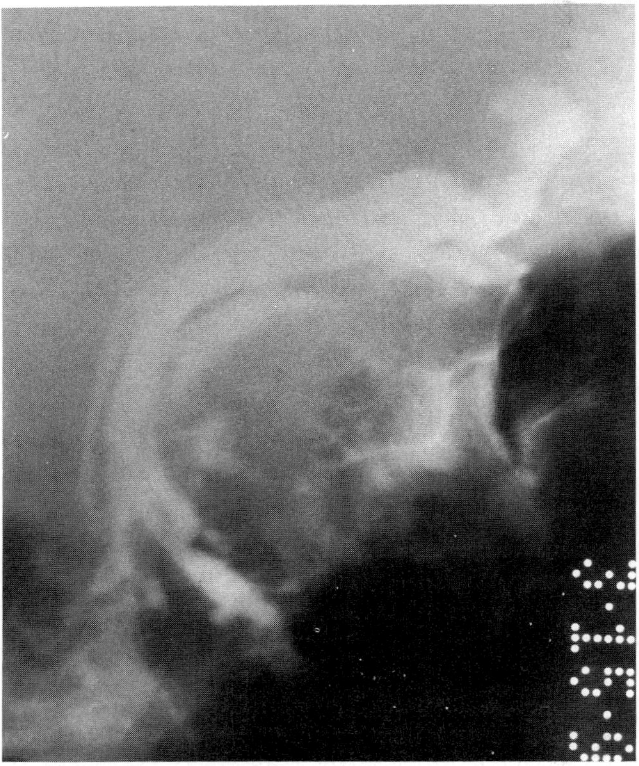

Fig. 10. ERCP of patient RS showed a pancreatic ductal blow-out in the right upper portion of this slide plus a crescent-shaped leak filling the pseudocyst. The latter structure is compressing the main pancreatic duct from below

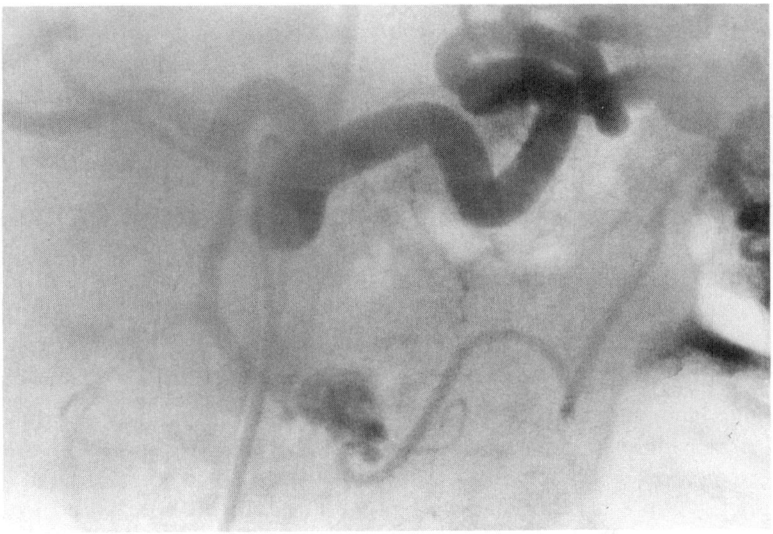

Fig. 11. Arteriogram of patient RS shows an arteriovenous fistula off the gastroduodenal artery (Lower Portion of Figure). This AV fistula was in the wall of the expanding pseudocyst

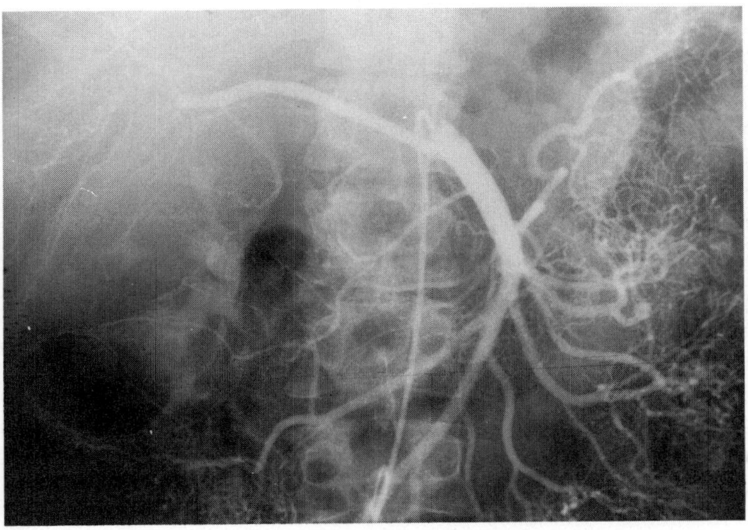

Fig. 12. A replaced right hepatic artery in patient RS that passed underneath the pancreatic head and bile duct as it coursed from the superior mesenteric artery

Case 4: V.A.

The patient developed abdominal pain and a 10 × 12 cm mass in the pancreatic head (Fig. 13) after many years of three drinks of alcohol per day. The mass contained many 1 mm–2 cm pseudocysts. Both bile and pancreatic ducts were strictured. An 11-h PDPP Whipple procedure with 1400 ml blood loss solved the problem. Pathology showed intense fibromatosis throughout the mass which was the entire head of the pancreas. "The pseudotumor" contained multiple cystic spaces not connecting to the main duct. No pain, gastrointestinal, or endocrine sequelae were present 10 months postoperative.

Case 5: W.M.

A 65-year-old man who drank heavily 40 years ago during military duty developed increasingly frequent abdominal pain. ERCP showed a blow-out of the pancreatic duct dorsally between portal vein and aorta connecting to a 2-cm pseudocyst. An 8-h PDPP Whipple procedure with 1100 ml blood loss solved the problem. A wound infection developed on the 7th postoperative day. No pain or gastrointestinal sequelae were present 6 months postoperative. Preoperatively he took high doses of an oral hyperglycemic drug. Now he takes the lowest dose possible.

Results

Short Term

The results are divided into the following groups: "ALL" operations combined, only the PDPP "Whipple," and only the PDPP "total" pancreatectomy. Short-term operative results are presented (Table 2) in regard to the length of operation, estimated blood loss, intraoperative or subsequent need for blood transfusion, use of a chronic epidural catheter during the operation and postoperatively, and the 30-day hospital mortality rate. Morbidity in the postoperative period was seen in seven of 16 patients. The most common complication resulting in delay of hospital discharge was gastric outlet obstruction seen in 4/16 patients (Whipple, three; total, pancreatectomy, one). All were associated with intra-abdominal abscess that required percutaneous drainage. Elevated amylase was found in each collection. Within several days after drainage the gastric outlet obstruction resolved. Drainage was temporary eliminating the abscess without pancreatic fistula. Two patients developed ARDS and ventilator dependence for ten and thirty postoperative days. There was one wound infection. No instances of new diabetes were observed during the postoperative hospital stay.

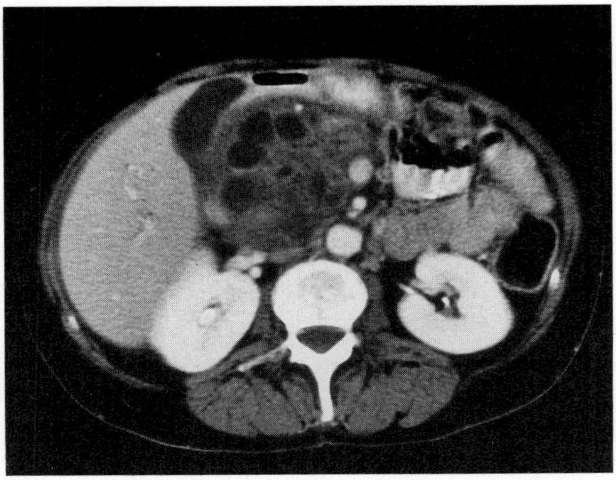

Fig. 13. Contrast-enhanced CT scan of patient VA showed a 10 × 12 cm "pseudotumor" in the head of the pancreas. Multiple pseudocysts are present throughout the head while the normal-sized CBD is in the center of the head

Long Term

Long-term results are valuable after the patient has resumed regular physical activity and diet. This stage has occurred in all patients by 6 months. Twelve patients were over 6 months postoperative for an average follow-up of 26.5 months (6–64). All patients were alive, and 11 (92%) were interviewed. Physical activity and habits are shown in Fig. 14. All patients had returned to full activity, work, or school.

Gastrointestinal, exocrine, and endocrine function status is shown in Fig. 15. Every patient indicated they were eating "everything" to "no problem." Every patient's weight was stable, except two complained of being overweight. One patient developed a marginal ulcer 9 months postoperative. He had had a history of peptic ulcer disease and was treated with omeprazole. No patient complained of persistent diarrhea, but five (45%) indicated that diarrhea occurred when they did not take pancreatic enzyme supplements. Two patients indicated they had had postprandial diarrhea for 6 months and 1 year postoperatively. Each patient's diarrhea had resolved. One patient described dumping syndrome prevented by avoiding a high-carbohydrate meal, particularly milkshakes or chocolate. This resolved 1 year postoperative. Insulin-dependent diabetes was present in five patients preoperatively and seven postoperative.

The sequelae of preserving the pylorus during pancreaticoduodenectomy were assessed by examining potential symptom complexes from either excision of the duodenum and distal common bile duct or the preserved pylorus.

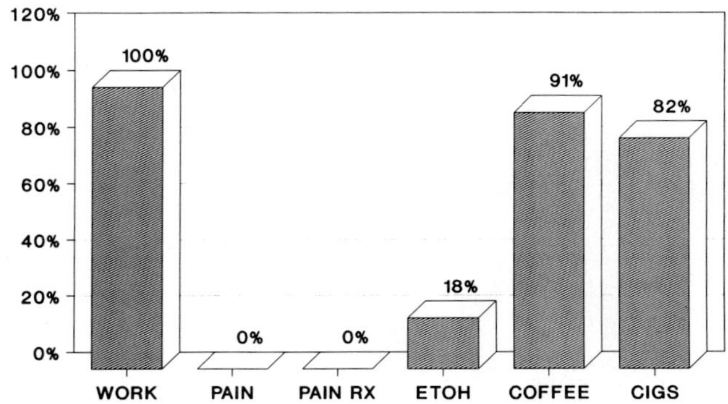

Fig. 14. Long-term follow-up (6–64 months; mean 26) was available in 92% of the 12 eligible patients. *WORK*, Return to physical activity, school, or employment; *PAIN RX*, taking any pain medication for abdominal pain; *ETOH*, use of any alcoholic beverage; *CIGS*, cigarette use

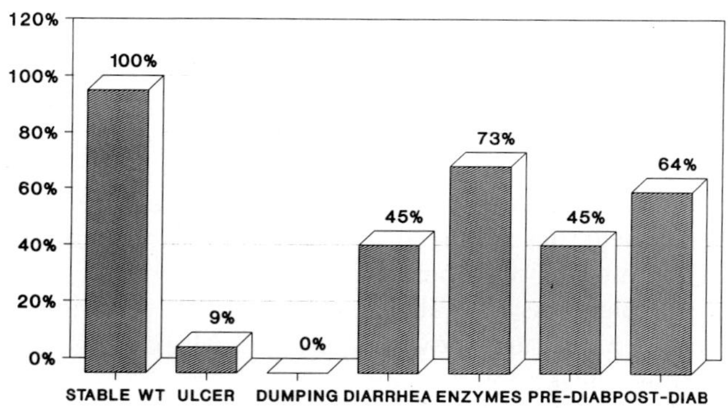

Fig. 15. Long-term gastrointestinal, exocrine, and endocrine function in the patients of Fig 14. *STABLE WT*, Able to regain and maintain preoperative weight; *ULCER*, marginal ulcer; *DIARRHEA*, any loose bowel movements on a regular basis; *ENZYMES*, oral pancreatic exocrine enzyme replacement; *PRE-DIAB* and *POST-DIAB*, pre- and postoperative diabetes

In regards to the excision of the duodenum and the distal common bile duct, there had been no episodes of cholangitis, biliary fistula, unavoidable dumping, or permanent diarrhea in patients receiving PDPP.

Those patients not developing gastric outlet obstruction resumed a diet on an average of the 11th postoperative day. Gastric outlet obstruction developed in three of 15 PDPP patients in the postoperative period, and they were able to resume a regular diet 20 days postoperatively. In all patients with gastric outlet obstruction, a CT scan showed a retrogastric or peripancreaticojejunostomy fluid collection, which was percutaneously drained. All collections were associated with an elevated amylase. All patients began eating with several days of percutaneous drainage. The remaining gastric outlet obstruction patient (L.C.) had had prior antrectomy and a similar CT finding of peripancreatic fluid collection. Effective drainage resulted after repositioning a nearby drain on the 22nd postoperative day, however, he did not resume a diet until the 36th postoperative day.

In regards to sequelae of pyloric preservation, one patient with a prior history of peptic ulcer developed a marginal ulcer (9%) with the lack of hemigastrectomy. This patient had undergone percutaneous drainage of a postoperative abscess that contained amylase. The patient continued with intermittent abdominal pain which resolved when a marginal ulcer was discovered at 9 months postoperative, and omeprazole was begun.

Discussion

Excision of the head of the pancreas was required in these patients for abdominal pain resulting from one of two situations: progressive disease in the pancreatic head (pseudocyst, duct blow-out, AV fistula), or significant fibrosis in the pancreatic head resulting in an enlarged, usually extensively calcified head with the pancreatic duct obstructed with or without bile and/or duodenal obstruction.

These cases emphasize that the head of the pancreas was the pacemaker of chronic pancreatitis. A continuous smoldering inflammatory process within the head of the gland results in persistent symptoms even after major ductal decompression procedures. The latter procedure is incapable of draining the multiple ductal connections within the head of the gland, and therefore, cannot interrupt the process. The current report indicates that excision of the head of the gland relieved symptoms in all patients, was associated with zero mortality, and little permanent gastrointestinal dysfunction. Pain relief was immediate. In addition, PDPP solved distressing clinical problems of sepsis, jaundice, or dependence on parenteral nutrition. No patient reported attacks of recurrent pancreatitis or reoperations. Previous experience with pain relief following a Whipple procedure has been superior if patients abstained from alcohol [7]. These latter patients also had statistically superior results (as compared to pseudocyst drainage) with fewer readmissions and recurrent pancreatitis. Follow-up in the latter study was 3.2 years and 2.2 years in the current series. Beger and colleagues [3] reported a 14% recurrent pancreatitis rate after a median follow-up of 24 months following duodenal preservation and pancreatic head excision. Chronic pain relief was complete or near complete in 93%. As the advantages of this operation approach those of PDPP future randomized comparison studies should be considered.

Marginal ulceration was seen in one patient associated with intra-abdominal abscess and a history of peptic ulcer disease. Five years may be necessary to follow patients to reliably assess the incidence of marginal ulceration [8]. No higher incidence has been observed after PDPP when compared to standard pancreaticoduodenectomy [9, 10]. Patients with a prior history of peptic ulcer disease should be just as susceptible to acid associated ulceration after PDPP as before this surgery. In this case the advantages and disadvantages of H_2 blockers versus hemigastrectomy should be reconsidered.

There is a significant morbidity, however, as with any series of pancreaticoduodenectomy. In contrast to excision of the head for periampullary tumors, the patient with chronic pancreatitis has a marked inflammatory or fibrotic process with frequent portal venous compression or thrombosis. An obligate intraoperative blood loss results. Blood transfusions were therefore, the rule in treating these chronic pancreatitis patients with excisional procedures. The operative difficulty with this inflammatory process is also significant, as explained by the increased operating time. However, the major cause of morbidity was not related directly to chronic pancreatitis-associated inflammation, but rather to pulmonary complications or presence of pancreatic juice in the peritoneal cavity. The latter complication accounts for the increased morbidity with the Whipple as compared to total pancreatectomy.

Utilizing the end-to-end mucosa-to-mucosa PTFE stented anastomosis (described in Fig. 3), the last five patients with a pancreatic anastomosis have not leaked or developed an abscess. A canine study using this stented anastomosis observed no leaks in 24 experiments [11]. In these chronic pancreatitis patients the association of leakage with gastric outlet obstruction is seen in Table 2. The morbidity was greater return, to GI function was slower, and hospital stay was longer in the Whipple versus the total pancreatectomy group primarily due to a minimal leaking anastomosis. The use of somatostatin analogue in patients with the Whipple procedure should be considered [12]. The only gastric outlet obstruction seen in the total pancreatectomy group had a fragment of residual pancreatic tail remaining which resulted in a left upper quadrant abscess, gastric outlet obstruction, and marginal ulcer.

The major cause of morbidity was abdominal abscess near a pancreatic anastomosis with secondary gastric outlet obstruction. Investigation with CT scanning found peripancreatic fluid collections in all patients with delayed return to gastrointestinal function. Once the fluid was percutaneously drained, the obstruction resolved. PDPP has been reported to have a high incidence of delayed gastric function [13], but the only patient in the current series with pancreaticoduodenectomy *without* pylorus preservation also had this problem. The common factor appears to be an inflammatory process (temporary or subclinical leak from the pancreatic anastomosis) locally

Table 2. Short-term results

	All (n = 16)	Whipple (n = 11)	Total (n = 5)
Duration of operation (h)	10.3 (7–19)	10.6 (7–19)	9.8 (7–15)
Estimated blood loss (ml)	1762 (300–10 000)	2060 (300–10 000)	1110 (450–2000)
Proportion of patients transfused	81%	82%	80%
Units transfused	4 (0–20)	3.5 (0–20)	4.4 (0–11)
Epidural catheter	81%	73%	100%
Mortality	None	None	None
Morbidity	44%	54%	20%
Return to GI function (days)	14.3 (8–36)	15.7 (10–36)	11.4 (8–18)
Hospital stay (days)	21 (12–68)	24 (12–68)	14.4 (12–20)

irritating the new gastric connection. The pancreatic anastomosis techniques associated with gastric outlet obstruction were reviewed. One lateral pancreaticojejunostomy and two end-to-side pancreaticojejunostomy procedures were utilized. The latter two were performed with silicone rubber stents, a technique I have found in the dog pancreas to be associated with a 40% leak rate as compared to no leaks using the Wilson-Cook stent. The stented end-to-end pancreaticojejunostomy in the chronic pancreatitis patients has not leaked.

Advances in anesthesia through the use of epidural catheters have significantly decreased the amount of inhalation anesthetics to obtain adequate anesthesia. The epidural catheter is utilized for excellent pain control in the postoperative period, although it may prolong postoperative ileus. Improved postoperative pain control with regional administration of narcotics undoubtedly improves the patients' respiratory function in these chronically debilitated and usually tobacco-smoking (89%) individuals. No episodes of persistent atelectasis or pneumonia were seen in these patients. The two pulmonary complications (ARDS) were related to large volume changes associated with the operative blood loss.

The advances of interventional radiology and therapeutic endoscopy are evident in the case histories of these patients. Preoperatively, three patients underwent percutaneous drainage of pseudocysts while one underwent embolization of an arteriovenous fistula contained within a pseudocyst. Biliary obstruction was seen in 75% of cases, and five of these individuals underwent preoperative biliary stent placements, either endoscopically or transhepatically. Pancreatic duct obstruction was common (88%), with four patients having an endoscopically placed pancreatic stent. The PD stent allows time for nutritional support while inflammation subsides [14]. One patient underwent endoscopic transduodenal decompression of a large pseudocyst, utilizing a pancreatic stent placed from the duodenum through the pancreatic duct in the body of the gland and the stent allowed resolution of the pseudocyst and ultimate operative management. Four patients required postoperative percutaneous drainage of fluid collections around the pancreatic anastomosis.

Because of significant inflammation, fibrosis, and ductal obliteration or blow-out in the head of the gland, the pathology in these patients resulted in stenosis of the duodenum and/or common bile duct. Even disruption of the bile duct resulted in one case. Therefore, a procedure that preserved the duodenum and distal common bile duct was felt not indicated, and PDPP was performed without mortality. In this series, no significant or permanent sequelae from removal of the duodenum and preserving the pylorus were seen, while all patients experienced relief of symptoms.

The concept of conserving portions of the gastrointestinal tract traditionally removed during the standard Whipple procedure deserves attention by pancreatic surgeons. Future studies are required to compare the results of PDPP to the duodenal preserving resection of the head of the pancreas, a procedure which also removes the "pacemaker of the pancreatitis."

References

1. Child CG, Frey CF (1966) Pancreaticoduodenectomy. Surg Clin North Am 46:1201–1213
2. Traverso LW, Longmire WP (1978) Preservation of the pylorus during pancreaticoduodenectomy. Surg Gynecol Obstet 146:959–962
3. Beger HG, Krautzberger W, Bittner R, Büchler M, Limmer J (1985) Duodenum-preserving resection of the head of the pancreas in patients with severe chronic pancreatitis. Surgery 97:467–473
4. Frey CF, Smith GJ (1987) Description and rationale of a new operation for chronic pancreatitis. Pancreas 2:701–702
5. Traverso LW, Freeny PC (1989) Pancreaticoduodenectomy: the importance of preserving hepatic blood flow to prevent biliary fistula. Am Surg 55:421–426
6. Miller BM, Traverso LW (1988) Intrapancreatic communication of bile and pancreatic ducts secondary to pancreatic necrosis. Arch Surg 123:1000–1003
7. Traverso LW, Tompkins RK, Urrea PT, Longmire WP (1979) Surgical treatment of chronic pancreatitis. Twenty-two years experience. Ann Surg 190:312–319
8. Grant CS, Van Heerden JA (1979) Anastomotic ulceration following subtotal and total pancreatectomy. Ann Surg 190:1–5
9. Itani KM, Coleman RE, Akwari OE, Meyers WC (1986) Pylorus-preserving pancreaticoduodenectomy. Ann Surg 204:655–665
10. Traverso LW, Longmire WP (1980) Preservation of the pylorus in pancreaticoduodenectomy. A follow-up evaluation. Ann Surg 192:306–310
11. Biehl TA, Traverso LW (1991) The pancreatic anastomosis. Is stenting necessary? Am J Surg 163:530–532
12. Büchler M, Friej H, Hermanek P, Sulkowsky U, Becker H, Klemps I, Schafmayer A, Dennler HJ, Beger HG (1992) Role of octreotide in the prevention of postoperative complications following pancreatic resection. Am J Surg 163:125–131

13. Warshaw AL, Torchiana DL (1985) Delayed gastric emptying after pylorus-preserving pancreaticoduodenoscopy. Surg Gynecol Obstet 160:1–4
14. Kozarek RA, Patterson DJ, Ball TJ, Traverso LW (1989) Endoscopic placement of pancreatic stents and drains in the management of pancreatitis. Ann Surg 209:261–266

The Role of Pylorus-Preserving Duodenopancreatic Head Resection

W. Kozuschek,[1] H.B. Reith, and W. Haarmann

Introduction

In 1909 Kausch [21] performed the first successful radical duodenopancreatic head resection with preservation of the gastric antrum and pylorus [22], following the suggestions of Desjardins 1907 [7] and Sauve 1908 [29], which referred to the surgical procedure developed by Krönlein [25]. Kausch performed the operation in two stages. For years he was the only one to be successful with the procedure, and only very few cared to copy the method. The surgical procedure developed for lesions of the duodenum and pancreas by Whipple and colleagues in 1935 did not intend partial gastric resection. In both procedures the duodenum was transected, the stump closed blindly, and the antropyloric passage bridged by gastroenterostomy [39, 40]. Watson reported a duodenopancreatectomy in the case of a carcinoma of the papilla in 1942, in which the antrum, pylorus, and 2.5 cm of the duodenum were preserved. Watson believed that preservation of an intact stomach would be beneficial for digestion and thus improve the state of nutrition [38].

In 1942 Whipple published the first successful radical duodenopancreatic head resection with en bloc removal of the distal third of the stomach. Since then various modifications of the original procedure have been developed. In the resectional phase of the operation it was attempted to remove as much of the stomach with or without vagotomy as possible because the percentage of gastric ulcers following resection of the pancreatic head was high [4, 37, 39]. Whipple's duodenopancreatic head resection involved the following adverse appearances: high postoperative mortality rate, poor digestive function after this deep operation and a low 5-year survival rate in the case of carcinoma. In 1984 Fortner suggested extensive resections, similar to a disembowelment of the upper abdomen to increase the 5-year cure. With eight anastomoses and duration of the operations up to 31.5 h the perioperative mortality was very high, and from then on the postoperative survival was measured in weeks and months – not in years [13].

In the past the high mortality rate could be attributed to the dangerous pancreatic anastomosis and the surgeons' lack of experience. These factors

[1] Chirurgische Universitäts-Klinik Bochum-Langendreer, Knappschaftskrankenhaus, In der Schornau 23, W-4630 Bochum 7, FRG

Beger/Büchler/Malfertheiner (Eds.)
Standards in Pancreatic Surgery

Table 1. Reports on pylorus-preserving duodenopancreatectomy

	Partial	Total
Itani [20][a]	224	28
Grace 1986 [16]	37	–
Crist 1987 [6]	14	–
Sharp 1989 [30]	9	–
McAfee 1989 [27]	29	4
Braasch 1991 [3]	170	16
Present study	52	–

[a] Review of the literature.

have been corrected since. Dumping, diarrhea, or dyspeptic complaints are known to occur as late complications following Whipple's operation, as well as peptic ulcer. To improve the postoperative digestive function following duodenopancreatic head resection Traverso and Longmire in 1978 [34] as well as Watson in 1948 [38] recommended preservation of the stomach, pylorus, and proximal duodenum. In the meantime almost 400 duodenopancreatectomies with preservation of the pylorus (PDP), performed because of inflammatory or tumorous alterations of the duodenum and pancreas, have been published in the literature (Table 1).

Materials and Methods

Patients

Between February 1985 and December 1990 we performed the modified Whipple's procedure with pylorus preservation in 52 patients. There were 28 men and 27 women. The youngest patient was 37 and the oldest 84 years old; the median age was 62.8 years. Of the 52 patients 41 presented a neoplasm, and 11 had chronic pancreatitis of the pancreatic head. The most frequent neoplasms were adenocarcinomas of the pancreatic head (24), followed by carcinomas of the papilla (six) and the periampullary region (six). Carcinoma of the duodenum occurred twice, and a carcinoid and a malignant insulinoma occurred once each. The second recurrence of a retroperitoneal sarcoma with infiltration of the pancreatic head and in pars II of the duodenum was the cause of this palliative procedure. We operated on only six a T1 tumors; the other 35 patients were resected in advanced stages.

Thirty-seven patients had obstructional jaundice, 17 had diabetes mellitus, and 11 had undergone previous surgery (correction of the bile ducts in six cases, coronary bypass in two, myocardial pacemaker implantation in three).

In patients with a malignoma of the pancreatic head a duodenopancreatic head resection with preservation of the pylorus was performed if the initial dissection showed no positive lymph nodes below the pylorus or no tumor infiltration of the large retropancreatic veins ("carcinomatous umbilication"). The patients with chronic pancreatitis selected for the operation had advanced lesions of the pancreatic head, generally with bile duct and duodenal stenoses.

Surgical Technique in Pylorus-Preserving Duodenopancreatic Head Resection

The procedure is similar to the standard operation, with the exception that the duodenum is dissected 2–4 cm from the pylorus. As the right gastroepiploic artery, inferior pancreatoduodenal artery, and right gastric artery must be ligated during resection of the pancreatic head, the arterial supply of the duodenal stump succeeds via the left gastric artery along the small curvature of the stomach and the pylorus. It is thus imperative that this vasculature be preserved, as suture disruption can easily develop. A second group of important structures which must be preserved is the nerve plexus of Latarjet, which innervates the antrum and pylorus. Destruction of these structures could lead to impairment of the emptying function of the stomach.

After construction of the pancreatojejunal and biliodigestive anastomoses the duodenum is anastomosed end-to-side with a pulled-up jejunal loop.

The risk of disruption of the pancreatic anastomosis can be avoided to a large extent by forming a broad plication of the jejunum.

Depending on the consistency of the pancreatic parenchyma and the morphology of the duct in the rest of the pancreas either a terminoterminal anastomosis using a telescope technique or a terminolateral pancreatojejunal anastomosis with a broad intestinal plication is constructed.

Occlusion of the ductal system with Ethibloc in the remaining pancreas was not performed in our patient series.

Postoperative Course

The postoperative treatment according to the described surgical procedure is held as simple as possible. Close clinical monitoring of the patient in the surgical intensive care unit is of utmost importance. After surgery extubation of the patient is strived for as soon as possible. In spite of ensuing peristalsis the gastric tube remains inserted for an average of 5–8 days. The indwelling gastric tube was never necessary for more than 10 days after the operation.

Postoperative medication is reduced to perioperative antibiotics and the usual prophylaxis of stress ulcer and thromboses. Hourly determination of blood glucose levels with possible substitution of insulin is performed as long as the patient receives parenteral nutrition, including glucose solutions. Later, insulin medication depends on the development of postoperative diabetes mellitus, if it did not already exist prior to surgery.

Results

Complications

Postoperative complications in our series were rare. Most complications were controllable by conservative measures. The rate of relaparotomy was 6%. Complications in the area of the pancreatic anastomosis, the "Achilles' heel" of this procedure, are feared most.

In 6 of the 52 PDP procedures temporary pancreatic fistulas occurred. In one patient there was a serious incident. The most important complication of this surgical procedure – acute pancreatitis of the remaining pancreas – was recognized too late, so that this patient succumbed to multiorgan failure in spite of pancreatectomy of the remaining pancreas.

Hemorrhages from the operational site are particularly dangerous, especially when they arise from enzyme digestion of large visceral blood vessels, for example, during pancreatitis of the remaining pancreas or due to suture disruption [6]. Vascular sutures and pancreatectomy of the remaining pancreas were not able to control the massive hemorrhage caused by the splenic blood vessels in a female patient described here.

Comparatively harmless are biliary fistulas subsequent to duodeno-pancreatic head resections. These occurred only five times. As long as they are adequately drained, it is justified to wait patiently until the leak closes spontaneously. Reoperation was not necessary in our series.

Early and Long-Term Results

The published early results after duodenopancreatectomy show a recent worldwide improvement over to the reported operative mortality rates of 10%–30% [1–3, 23, 33, 35]. This rate now lies under 10% in a great number of series [1, 18, 33]. Several authors [3, 6, 35] also report an operational mortality of less than 5%. In our own series we lost four patients after the operation. There were no deaths among the last 34 consecutive PDP patients. This favorable outcome of surgery has unfortunately not resulted in an improved long-term prognosis in cases of malignomas. The vital thing in evaluation of a surgical procedure of a malignant disease is the survival rate.

The long-term results of the Bochum series are presented below for all of the 38 malignomas of the duodenum and pancreas (after PDP). The 5-year survival rate is 18%. In 28 of the 48 patients the nutritive situation was examined more closely. Eleven of the 20 patients who could not be evaluated remained exclusively in the care and follow-up of their family physicians. These examination data were not taken into consideration. In the nine remaining patients no nutritional or digestive data could be assessed because in four tumor patients there was local recurrence, and in five patients with pancreatitis exocrine pancreatic insufficiency was manifest.

In 21 of the 28 patients the capacity for food uptake was normal; seven others reached 50%–90% of normal. An average body weight of 93% of the weight prior to onset of the disease or 106% of the preoperative weight was the standard set as a sign of optimal nutrition. The dumping syndrome was not observed. In the period of follow-up (8–34 months) none of the patients presented with peptic jejunal or gastric ulcers. Medical substitutional treatment of evident exocrine pancreatic insufficiency was necessary in two cases.

The hydrogen-breathanalytic function test showed identical orocecal passage duration in 12 subjects as opposed to a control group (114 ± 3.8 versus 105 ± 2.4 min, respectively; $n = 12$ both groups). In all patients the operation was at least 4 months past [18].

The secretory capacity of the endocrinium upon gastrointestinal stimulation, the presentation of the so-called incretin effect, ensued via a biostator (artificial beta cell). Comparison of the dynamics of insulin and C-peptide secretion under isoglycemic stimulation resulted in a similar profile of secretory capacity for a group of patients who underwent the classic Whipple's procedure without occlusion and in patients with pylorus preservation. In contrast to these, an earlier series of patients who underwent the classic Whipple's procedure with ductal occlusion presented flat curves for insulin and C-peptide secretion.

By means of the pylorus-preserving Whipple procedure functional stabilization and improvement in regard to the endocrine secretion of insulin and C-peptide was evident, which is obvious even upon comparison of pre- and postoperative results (which unfortunately is not always possible).

Results in Ductal Carcinomas

Similarly to the study of Grace et al. [16], we compared PDP and Whipple procedure operations. We operated on 43 patients with ductal carcinoma – 24 with the pylorus-preserving technique and 19 in the classical way. Age and TNM classification did not differ between the two groups (Table 2).

The long-term results between PDP and Whipple operations show a 5-year survival rate of 19% for PDP and 11% for the Whipple operation (Fig. 1). We conclude, with Grace et al. [16], that the pylorus-preserving method is a feasible alternative among oncological therapeutic procedures.

Discussion

Upon follow-up examinations our patients showed almost no signs of maldigestion or malabsorption after PDP. Functional tests over several days

Table 2. Characteristics of patients receiving PDP and Whipple procedure

	PDP (n = 24)	Whipple (n = 19)
Age		
<40 years	0	1
41–50 years	4	3
51–60 years	2	4
61–70 years	12	7
71–80 years	4	2
>80 years	2	2
TNM		
T1 N0	2	2
T2 N0	8	5
T3 N0	3	2
T2 N1	8	7
T3 N1	3	3

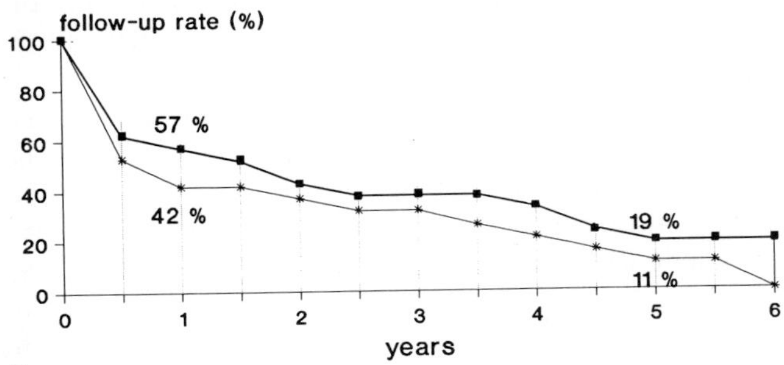

a

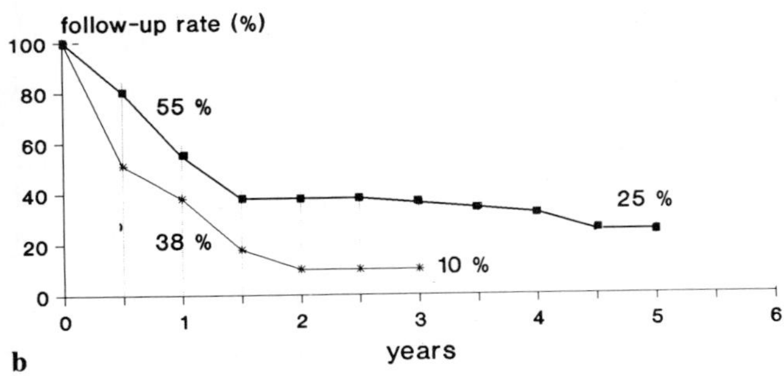

b

Fig. 1a,b. Comparison of 5-year survival rates following PDP (■) and Whipple procedure (*) for ductal carcinoma. **a** Present study. PDP, n = 21; Whipple, n = 19. **b** Grace et al. [16]. PDP, n = 13; Whipple, n = 13

on the patients with Whipple's classic operation versus those with PDP showed that preservation of the antrum, pylorus, and bulbus unit maintained a high degree of the digestion-promoting mechanisms. In most cases it was demonstrated that the exocrine functional unit was not completely destroyed, and that the release of enterogastron, secretin, and cholecystopancreaticokinin was still allowed by the 2- to 3-cm-long remaining cuff of the proximal duodenum.

Principally from research in the United States we know that considerable digestive losses, especially regarding fat and protein uptake result after gastrectomies and duodenopancreatectomies with subtotal gastric resection [9, 10, 12, 41]. In our series the patients reached almost 100% of their preoperative weight in an average of 3 months after the operation with pylorus preservation.

The fear has also been expressed that with gastric and pyloric preservation the number of peptic ulcers could increase. The incidence of peptic ulcers after the classical Whipple's procedure varies between 6% and 20% [8, 15, 17, 19]. According to the literature, the ulcer rate is very low after pylorus-preserving procedure – 2%–3% [20, 23, 33]. Ulcers arose mainly in patients who had undergone total pancreatectomy. That the development of ulcers can be attributed to the missing protective effect of the pancreatic juice in these cases was shown in studies by Gall in 1979 [14] and Gebhardt et al. in 1982 [15], who reported an ulcer rate of 39% in patients with PDP and occlusion of the ductal system of the remaining pancreas.

The complication rate is due mainly to deficient anastomoses [3, 11, 19, 27, 30, 35, 36]. The anastomosis between duodenum and jejunum is technically simple. Careful attention must be paid to the vascular supply. The gastroepiploic artery should be ligated close to its origin at the gastroduodenal artery. In agreement with others, we found that the right gastric artery is nonexistent or only rudimentary in nature in most patients [25]. In these cases there is generally a good vascular supply via a strong branch from the left gastric artery which runs along the small gastric curvature to the proximal duodenum. Utmost care must be taken to protect this blood vessel during preparation of the pyloroduodenal region. Despite our care in this regard we once had to accept suture disruption in the duodenojejunal anastomosis as the result of focal necroses of the wall.

The overall low complication rate in our series and those of other studies is evidence of the improved anastomoses technique in the vicinity of the pancreatojejunostomy. The terminoterminal telescope anastomosis in fibrosed and terminolateral pancreatojejunostomy with broad jejunoplication in the case of soft remaining pancreas prevent a considerable degree of the clinically manifest and life-endangering suture insufficiencies [19, 30].

Our long-term results after pancreatic resection with pylorus preservation because of malignant disease show that the survival rate of carcinoma patients undergoing this surgical procedure is just as good or even better compared with those receiving standard operations. A study by Grace et al.

[16], who concentrated mainly on patients with carcinoma of the pancreatic head, demonstrated that the survival rate with the pylorus-preserving method was similar to that in patients after a classic Whipple resection (see Fig. 1).

Prerequisites for the successful use of this procedure are exact intraoperative diagnosis and knowledge of the lymphatics of the pancreatic region.

In 1978 Cubilla and colleagues [5] published a paper pertaining to metastases and involvement of the various lymph nodes in tumors of the pancreatic region. This paper shows that the adenocarcinoma of the pancreatic duct in the head area tends to metastasize early to the local lymph nodes as well as to those more distant (in 88% of the examined cases). Periampullary adenocarcinomas and duodenal tumors metastasized in 33% to the posterior and anterior pancreatoduodenal groups of lymph nodes. None of the 33 examined resection specimens from the classical Whipple procedure showed metastases in the lymph nodes along the small and great curvatures of the stomach. In only 5% of the pancreatic ductal adenocarcinomas were the pyloric group of lymph nodes involved.

Manabe and colleagues [26] found in their study of resection specimens that the antral lymph nodes were not involved in cases of carcinoma. In 6%–8% the subpyloric lymph nodes were affected. Both surgical procedures (PDP and standard Whipple) probably fail because the carcinoma has extended beyond the resected region [27, 36].

In 1980 Edis and colleagues showed that in a series of 124 patients who underwent Whipple's operation because of pancreatic ductal carcinoma more than 50% of the present lymph nodes contained metastases. The prognosis of these patients was comparable to that of patients in whom no lymph node metastases were found. This leads to the corresponding average periods of survival [11].

These results show preservation of the pylorus to be of value in carcinomas not extending beyond the organ, especially when the lower postoperative complication rate and the comparable period of survival are taken into consideration.

Sharp and colleagues [30], however, warn against the use of PDP in tumor surgery. They reported three cases in which PDP did not represent an adequate surgical procedure for carcinoma. The pancreatic carcinoma had infiltrated the duodenum and showed submural and perineural spread to the duodenal resectional margin in two cases. In another patient a submucosal relapse was removed from the pylorus 5 months subsequent to a PDP. The last cases also had extensive cancerous growth beyond the resection area, so that any form of duodenopancreatectomy would primarily have been inadequate.

In view of this question we asked our pathologist to analyze the histology of the Bochum pancreatic resection specimens once again. Retrospectively no intramural growth could be found in either the PDP or the standard operation series. Since the publication of Sharp et al. [30] this question is being treated prospectively. The results so far do not indicate intramural growth in the duodenoantral area.

Conclusion

The advantages of the PDP procedure are: (a) the operation is limited to the right upper abdomen, and thus (b) the surgical trauma is less, and the duration of the operation is shorter, and (c) digestion and nutrition are not impaired when the antrum-pylorus unit is preserved.

The debate about the role of the preserved pylorus and antrum in pancreatic resection has yet not come to an end. Final evaluations as to the gastroduodenal integrity are lacking because of the paucity of comparative studies.

The advances in surgery of pancreatic carcinoma do not result from the modified surgical procedures, which surely are to be seen as an advantage, but from early diagnosis of these tumors and the search for adjuvant forms of therapy.

References

1. Bittner R, Roscher R, Safi et al. (1989) Der Einfluß von Tumorgröße und Lymphknotenstatus auf die Prognose des Pankreascarcinoms. Chirurg 60: 240–245
2. Braasch JW, Rossi RL, Watkins E, Deziel D, Winter P (1986) Pyloric and gastric-preserving pancreatic resection. Experience with 87 Patients. Ann Surg 204 4:411–417
3. Braasch JW, Gaguer M (1991) Pylorus-preserving pancreatoduodenectomy – technical aspects. Langenbecks Arch Chir 376:50–58
4. Catell RB, Warren KW (1953) Surgery of the pancreas. Saunders, Philadelphia, pp 262–336
5. Cubilla AL, Fortner J, Fitzgerald PJ (1978) Lymph node involvement in carcinoma of the head of the pancreas area. Cancer 41:880–887
6. Crist DW, Sitzmann JV, Cameron JL (1987) Improved hospital morbidity, mortality and survival after the Whipple procedure. Ann Surg 206:358–373
7. Desjardines A (1907) Technique de la pancrèatéctomie. Rev Chir (Paris) 35:945
8. Edelmann M, Kozuschek W (1986) Preservation of the pylorus in pancreatoduodenectomy. 9th world congress collegium internationale digestivae, Jerusalem, 31 August–5 September. Dig Surg 2:88 (abstr)
9. Edelmann M, Sonntag D (1989) Funktionsuntersuchungen des endokrinen Pankreas nach Resektion. In: Kozuschek W, Reith HB (eds) Pankreaserkrankungen. TM, Hameln, pp 37–50
10. Edelmann M, Kozuschek W, Edelmann A, Sonntag D (1987) Die endokrine Pankreasrestfunktion nach unterschiedlicher Pankreasresektion von Patienten mit chronischer Pankreatitis. Langenbecks Arch Chir 372:877
11. Edis AJ, Kiernan PD, Taylor WF (1980) Attempted curative resection of ductal carcinoma of the pancreas. Review of Mayo clinic experience 1951–1975. Mayo Clin Proc 55:531–536
12. Fish JC, Smith LB, Williams RD (1969) Digestive function after radical pancreaticoduodenectomy. Am J Surg 117:40–45

13. Fortner JG (1984) Regional pancreatectomy for cancer of the pancreas, ampulla and other related sites. Ann Surg 199:418–425
14. Gall FP (1980) Die partielle Duodenopankreatektomie mit Gangokklusion und Erhaltung des Magens. In: Häring R (ed) Die Chirurgie der akuten und chronischen Pankreatitis. TM, Hameln, pp 201–205
15. Gebhardt C, Gall FP, Rösch W, Schackert HK (1982) Anastomosenulcus nach Whipple-Operation mit Magenerhaltung. Zentrabl Chir 107:952–959
16. Grace PA, Pitt HA, Longmire WP (1986) Pancreatoduodenectomy with pylorus preservation for adenocarcinoma of the head of the pancreas. Br J Surg 73: 647–650
17. Grant CS, van Heerden JA (1979) Anastomic ulceration following subtotal and total pancreatectomy. Ann Surg 190:1–5
18. Haarmann W (1991) Die pyloruserhaltende Pankreaskopfresektion – Funktionsuntersuchungen zur erhaltenen gastro-intestinalen Integrität. Habilitationsschr (Bochum)
19. Hollender LF, de Manzini N (1992) Pankreasschwanzversorgung nach partieller Duodenopankreatektomie. In: Kozuschek W, Paquet KJ (eds) Pankreas – Diagnostik und Therapie. Karger, Basel, Germezing, pp 363–374
20. Itani KMF, Coleman RE, Akwari OE, Meyers WC (1986) Pylorus-preserving pancreatoduodenectomy. A clinical and physiological appraisal. Ann Surg 204: 655–664
21. Kausch W (1909) Die Resektion des mittleren Duodenum. Eine typische Operation. Vorläufige Mittelungen. Zentrabl Chir 39:1350–1353
22. Kausch W (1912) Das Carcinom der Papilla duodeni und seine radikale Entfernung. Beitr Klin Chir 3:439–486
23. Kozuschek W (1989) Duodeno-Kephalopankreatektomie mit Pyloruserhaltung. Zentrabl Chir 114:745–754
24. Kozuschek W (1989) Kommentar auf Einladung zu L.W. Traverso: Pyloruserhaltung bei Pankreatikoduodenektomie wegen Pankreaskarzinom. Chir Gastroenterol 5:375–377
25. Krönlein M (1895) Klinische und topographisch-anatomische Beiträge zur Pankreaschirurgie. Bruns' Beitr Klin Chir 14:663
26. Manabe T, Suzuki T, Tobe T (1985) Evaluation of en bloc radical pancreatectomy for carcinoma of the head of the pancreas involving the adjacent vessels. Dig Surg 2:27–30
27. McAfee MK, van Heerden JA, Adson MA (1987) Is proximal pancreato-duodenectomy with pyloric preservation superior to total pancreatectomy? Surgery 105:347–351
28. Mielke F, Beger HG, Schirop T (1975) Digestive und inkretorische Funktion nach partieller Duodeno-Pankreatektomie. Dtsch Med Wochenschr 100:171–176
29. Sauvé L (1908) Des pancréatéctomies et spécialement de la pancréatéctomie céphalique. Rev Chir 37(113):335
30. Sharp KW, Ross CB, Halter SA et al. (1989) Pancreatoduodenectomy with pyloric preservation for carcinoma of the pancreas: a cautionary note. Surgery 105:645–653
31. Siedek M, Birtel F, Mitrenga I (1985) Pankreasanastomose und Pankreato-jejunoplication nach Rechtsresektion. Langenbecks Arch Chir 366:610
32. Stotz W (1951) Radikaloperation von Pankreastumoren. Langenbecks Arch Chir 267:540–544
33. Traverso LW (1989) Die pyloruserhaltende Duodenopankreatektomie zur Behandlung des Pankreaskarzinoms. Chir Gastroenterol 5:351–366
34. Traverso LW, Longmire WPJ (1978) Preservation of the pylorus in pancreatico-duodenectomy. Surg Gynecol Obstet 146:959–962
35. Trede M, Schwall G (1989) Chirurgische Therapie des Pankreaskarzinoms: Standardverfahren. Chir Gastroenterol 5:351–366

36. van Heerden JA (1984) Pancreatic resection of carcinoma of the pancreas: Whipple versus total pancreatectomy – an institutional perspective. World J Surg 8:880–888
37. Warren KW, Choe DS, Plaza J, Relihan M (1975) Results of radical resection for periampullary cancer. Ann Surg 181:534–540
38. Watson K (1942) Carcinoma of ampulla of Vater: successful radical resection. Br J Surg 31:515–526
39. Whipple AO (1942) Present day surgery of the pancreas. N Engl J Med 226: 515–526
40. Whipple AO, Parsons WB, Mullins CR (1935) Treatment of carcinoma of the ampulla of Vater. Ann Surg 102:763–779
41. Wollaeger EE, Comfort MW, Clagett OF, Osterberg AE (1948) Efficiency of gastrointestinal tract after resection of head of pancreas. JAMA 137:838–848

Pancreatic Head Resection with Complete or Partial Preservation of the Duodenum

A.A. Shalimov[1] and Y.Z. Lifshits

Different resection techniques are important when choosing a method of surgical treatment for patients with chronic pancreatitis, periampullary tumors, and tumors of the pancreatic head. At present, the progress in diagnostic techniques enables small tumors to be revealed in the early stages of disease and differentiated preoperatively from inflammatory processes by means of target punctures and histologic study of a pathologic focus.

The detection of pancreatic head tumors of less than 2.0 cm in diameter without the involvement of parapancreatic lymph nodes revised the indications for the conventional Whipple operation (pancreatoduodenal resection) in favor of less radical techniques. Proper definition of the indications for pancreatic head resection with complete or partial preservation of the duodenum improves the functional results of surgical treatment without decreasing the radicality of the operation.

Our clinic has experience of more than 500 different pancreatic head resections performed for chronic pancreatitis, tumors of the pancreatic head, and periampullary tumors (Table 1).

When choosing the type of operative intervention, we considered the nature, extent, and location of the pathologic process, and whether it had spread to the duodenum, bile ducts, portal vein, or mesenteric vessels. In employing different modifications of the operations we noted the advantage of the resections that permit duodenum preservation. Comparative analysis of the state of carbohydrate metabolism in patients after Whipple operation and in those after pancreatoduodenal resection with preservation of part of the duodenum has shown the expediency of wide use of the duodenum-preserving interventions. After Whipple resection the state of carbohydrate metabolism was normal in 7.0%, latent diabetes was present in 44.2%, and insulin-dependent in 48.8%.

We perform the following modified pancreatic head resections with complete or partial preservation of the duodenum. The pancreatic head resection with complete preservation of the duodenum developed by Dr. Hans Beger we perform only in patients with chronic pancreatitis.

[1] Institute of Clinical and Experimental Surgery, Kiev, Ukraine

Beger/Büchler/Malfertheiner (Eds.)
Standards in Pancreatic Surgery

Table 1. Pathologic changes which served as indications for pancreatic head resections

Pathologic changes	No. of patients	Deaths	
		(*n*)	(%)
Pancreatic head cancer	301	40	13.3
Periampullary cancer	124	12	9.7
Chronic pancreatitis	89	5	6.0
Total	514	57	11.0

Table 2. Types of pancreatic head resections performed with complete or partial preservation of the duodenum (1976–1990)

Type of operation	No. of patients	Deaths	
		(*n*)	(%)
Pancreatic head resection with complete preservation of the duodenum (Beger's modification)	23	1	4.3
Pancreatic head resection with partial preservation of the duodenum (our technique)	27	2	7.4
Pancreatic head resection with preservation of the stomach and part of the duodenum	36	2	5.5
Total	86	5	5.8

For oncologic patients with tumors under 2.0 cm in diameter, located in the pancreatic head, or periampullary organs (T1N0M0), we have developed a procedure for pancreatic head resection with partial preservation of the duodenum.

In patients with chronic pancreatitis and secondary inflammatory affection of the duodenum, or in T1N0M0 tumors we perform a pancreatoduodenal resection with preservation of the stomach and part of the initial and terminal duodenum (Table 2).

In our opinion, preservation of even a small duodenal portion (hormonally active mucosa) can have an influence on the subsequent functional results of the operation. Such an operation is contraindicated for patients with high gastric acidity, or ulcer history. As this operation is rather widely used in various clinics, it is not described in detail in our report.

Let us now turn to the duodenum-preserving pancreatic head resection developed by Beger and the technique of pancreatic head resection with partial preservation of the duodenum suggested by us.

Table 3. Types of intervention on a duct in duodenum-preserving pancreatic head resection

Type of intervention	Patients	
	(*n*)	(%)
Longitudinal pancreaticoenterostomy	8	34.8
End-to-end pancreaticoenterostomy	10	43.5
Duct occlusion	5	21.7

Since 1980, the duodenum-preserving pancreatic head resection has been performed in 23 patients for chronic pancreatitis. The age of the patients ranged from 21 to 56 years. The majority of patients (20) were men (86.9%). As for the etiology of the disease, alimentary causes or alcohol addiction were revealed in 19 (82.6%) of the patients. In 4 (17.4%), morphologic changes in the pancreatic head were associated with the biliary system pathology. In establishing indications for the operation, the clinical course of the disease – pronounced pain syndrome in the epigastrium or upper abdomen, weight loss of 8–27 kg within 3–6 months, presence of obstructive jaundice, impaired passage at the duodenal level – was considered. The diagnosis was verified by instrumental investigations. Ultrasonography was performed in 23 patients, including 8 with target puncture of a pathologic focus for cytologic study. Computed tomography (CT) was performed in 21 patients (in 4 with puncture), and endoscopic pancreatoduodenography was performed in 23. Carbohydrate metabolism and exocrine pancreatic function were studied in all the patients.

The final decision about the technique for pancreatic resection was made at operation. The volume and size of the changed pancreatic head, involvement of an inflammatory infiltrate of the portal vein, and the presence of a technical possibility of separating the posterior pancreatic surface from it were assessed. In all the cases at operation, immediate histologic diagnosis of pancreatic tissue from the site of gland dissection and from the sites most suspicious for tumorous degeneration (no fewer than three) was performed.

In four patients, who were not in the group studied, the tumor cells were revealed in a removed specimen. This was the reason for extension of the operation to pancreatoduodenal resection.

The technique of duodenum-preserving pancreatic head resection is well described by Beger, and we followed his procedure in the majority of cases. However, at the reconstructive stage of an operation we made certain changes.

The wound surface of the paraduodenal pancreas was treated with hemostatic sutures with mandatory separate ligation of the pancreatic stump duct. The duct of the distal pancreatic stump was sewn into the jejunum, which was isolated according to Roux in 18 patients and occluded with a polymer in 5 patients (Table 3).

Table 4. Complications which developed postoperatively

Complication	No. of patients	Died	
		(*n*)	(%)
Postoperative peritonitis	7		
Acute gastric ulcers, peritonitis, sepsis	1	1	4.3
External pancreatic fistula	1		
External biliary fistula	1		
Duodenitis with impaired passage	3		
Abdominal abscess	1		

In patients with stenosed areas of the pancreatic duct, a side-to-side anastomosis was performed. In the absence of such changes, an end-to-end anastomosis with external duct drainage was created. Occlusion of the main pancreatic duct was undertaken in patients with disorders of the carbohydrate metabolism. Thus, our observations have shown that the pancreatic duct occlusion had the most favorable long-term effect on the state of carbohydrate metabolism.

The common bile duct stenosis was present in nine patients, including eight (34.8%) with an increased preoperative bilirubin level in the blood. In five patients, after removal of a pathologically changed pancreatic head, internal drainage of the common bile duct was performed.

In three patients, a supraduodenal choledochoduodenal anastomosis was created. In four patients, after the pancreatic head resection, revision of the distal common bile duct by means of a 3 mm diameter probe has shown its patency. The intervention in these patients was limited to temporary external duct drainage. In two patients, during pancreatic head removal, iatrogenic injuries were inflicted on the intrapancreatic portion of the common bile duct. In both cases we performed closure of a defect in transverse direction and temporary external duct drainage. After the operation one patient died (4.3%). This was caused by multiple acute gastric ulcers with perforation, which developed against a background of postoperative pancreatitis with subsequent septic state and polyorganic failure. There were the following postoperative complications. Transient leakage of the pancreatic secretion was noted in one patient, transient biliary fistula after plasty of the bile duct in its iatrogenic injury in one patient, and duodenitis with impaired passage through the duodenum in three patients. Conservative measures in combination with nutrition via a tube introduced below the narrowed site have proved to be sufficient. In one patient, an abscess in the subhepatic space was drained (Table 4).

The long-term results after the operations were assessed in 21 patients. The period of follow-up was from 2 to 10 years. In 16 (76.2%) patients,

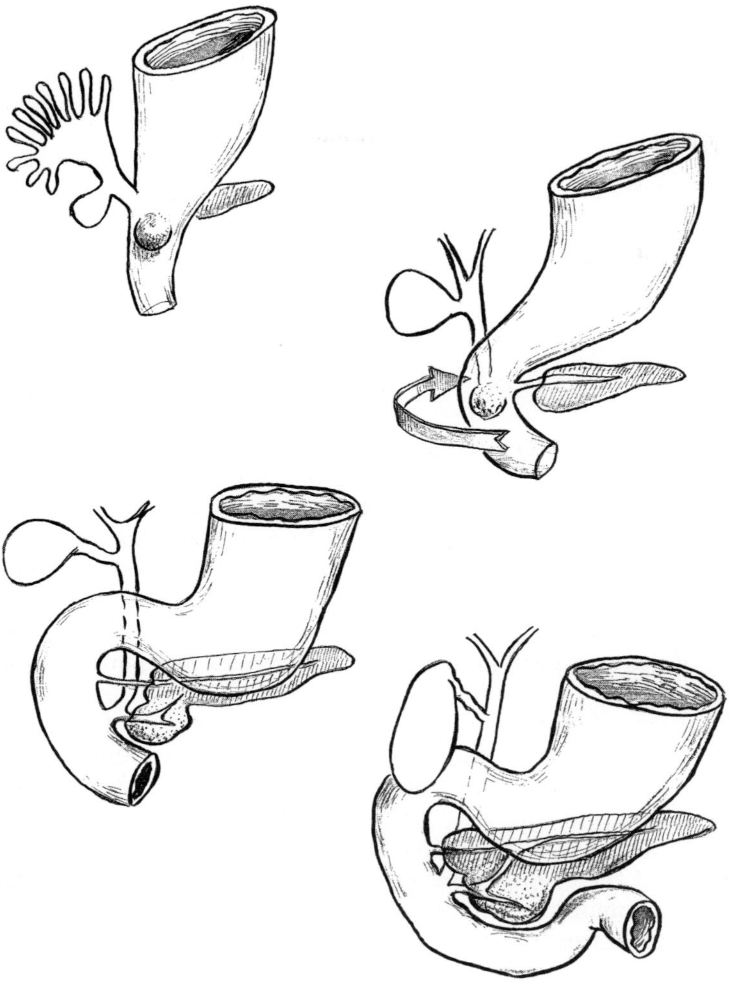

Fig. 1. Embryonic development of the pancreas. (H. Tuchmann-Duplessis and P. Haegel, 1974)

significant improvement and absence of pain were noted after the operation. Four (19%) patients had periodic pain attacks requiring conservative treatment 1–3 times a year. However, these patients noted that after the operation their state was significantly better than before, and the pain was less intensive and responded better to conservative treatment. One (4.8%) noted no improvement after the operation.

With the aim of employing the sparing and physiologic modification of pancreatoduodenal resection in the treatment of small (under 2 cm in diameter) tumors of the pancreatic head and periampullary region, we have

Table 5. Pathologic changes which served as indications for pancreatic head resection with partial preservation of the duodemum (our technique)

Pathologic changes	Patients (*n*)	Died	
		(*n*)	(%)
Adenocarcinoma of the major duodenal papilla	19	1	5.3
Adenocarcinoma of the pancreatic head under 2 cm in diameter	8	1	12.5
Total	27	2	17.8

developed a technique of pancreatoduodenal resection of a portion of the pancreatic head which develops at the period of embryonic development from the ventral germinal layer. The proximal pancreatic duct, part of the head, and a segment of the uncinate process are formed from this (Fig. 1).

Tumors of the major duodenal papilla, parapillary portion of the common bile duct, and corresponding part of the pancreas that are under 2 cm in diameter can be radically removed by means of resection of the affected portion of the organ within the limits of ventral germ separated by a connective layer.

Our modification of pancreatoduodenal resection formed from the ventral germ was employed in 27 patients. The age of patients ranged from 32 to 76 years. Tumor location and number of the patients operated on are presented in Table 5.

The technique of operation was as follows (Fig. 2). The operation includes the stages of removal of a pancreatic portion developed from the ventral germ, with a tumor and adjacent part of the duodenum, biliary and pancreatic ducts. Reconstruction consists of restoration of the passage of the bile, pancreatic secretion and alimentary tube patency.

The operation was performed in the absence of signs of parapancreatic lymph node involvement. In doubtful cases intraoperative morphologic study was performed. Mobilization of the duodenum according to Kocher and transection of a ligament of the duodenojejunal junction are necessary for intraoperative review of the process extent and limits of the tumor.

The anterior pancreatic surface is freed, and the portal vein is exposed under the gland. To the left of the portal vein, the descending duodenum is freed to the extent of 2.0–2.5 cm. A site for division of the duodenum in its descending and low horizontal part is determined. In eight patients we managed to expose the connective layer between the dorsal and ventral gland and remove a pathologically changed portion of the pancreas within the limits of the part which had developed from the ventral germ, together with adjacent structures – distal choledochus, major duodenal papilla and

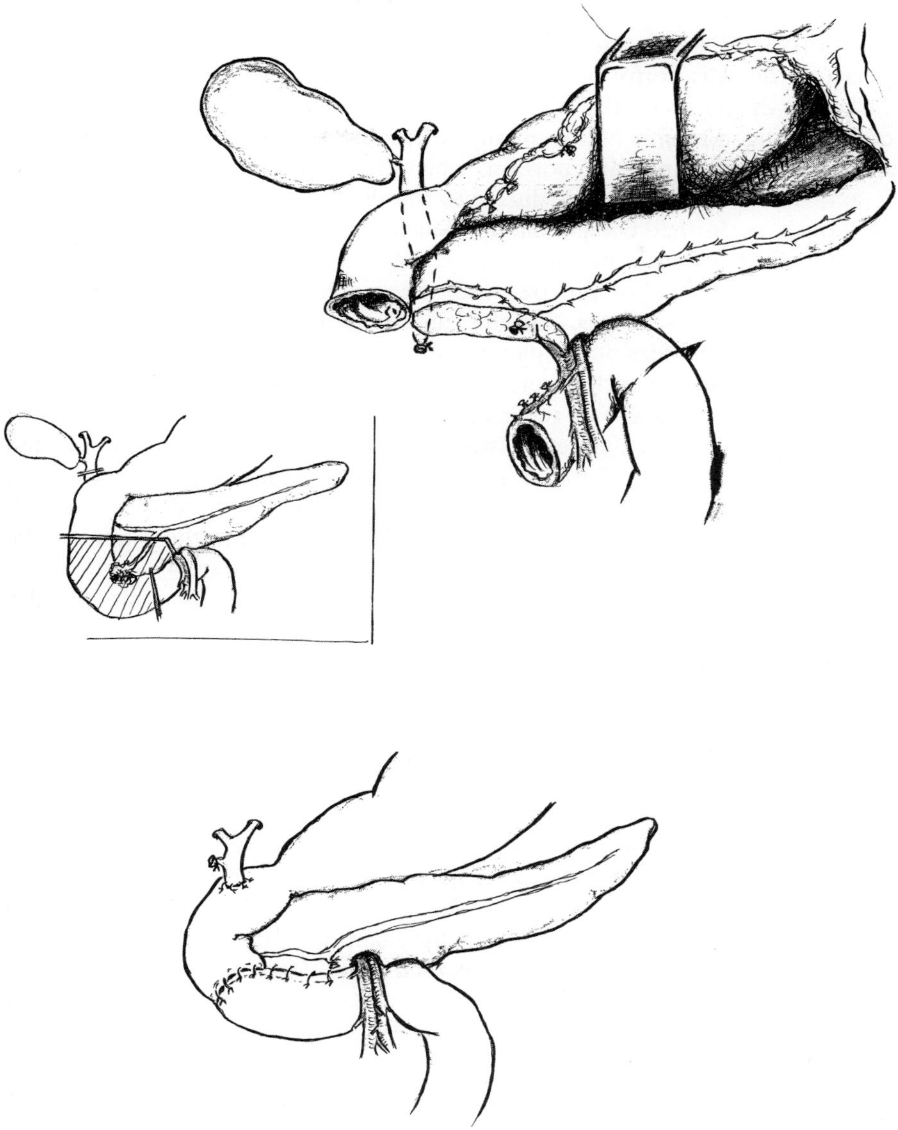

Fig. 2. Resection of the pancreatic head with partial preservation of the duodenum

adjoining part of the duodenum. In 19 patients, resection of the ventral portion of the organ was performed without identification of a boundary layer because of fibrous degenerative changes in pancreatic parenchyma. After resection, the reconstructive stage of the operation was performed.

Firstly, the main duct of the pancreatic stump was sewn into the low horizontal portion of the duodenum on the side of its internal wall. Anastomosis was performed on the external drain. In two patients, due to sufficient diameter of the Santorini's duct (3.0 mm), no anastomosis was created, and a stump of the main pancreatic duct was ligated. Thus, the secretion of the pancreatic portion, which developed from the dorsal germ, is drained via the Santorini's duct into the duodenum. In one patient, after previously performed choledochoduodenostomy, drainage was accomplished via the distal choledochus into the choledochoduodenal anastomosis and duodenum (Fig. 3). For this purpose, the gaping main pancreatic duct was dissected lengthwise for a distance of 2.0 cm to achieve correspondence between the diameters of the pancreatic and common bile ducts. They were then anastomosed to each other.

At the second stage of reconstruction, anastomosis between the lower and upper parts of the duodenum was created by means of single interrupted sutures. In two of the 27 patients, anastomosis was not feasible because of the considerable distance between the duodenal portions to be anastomosed. To preserve the passage through the distal duodenum, the isoperistaltic jejunal segment was interposed for a distance of 15 cm (Fig. 4).

At the third and final stage of reconstruction, a choledochoduodenal a nastomosis at the supraduodenal portion of the bile duct was created to divert bile into the duodenum.

Recently, in two patients with T0N0M0 cancer of the distal choledochus without involvement of the major duodenal papilla ampulla, the local pancreatoduodenal resection was performed with preservation of the ventral part of pancreatic head. The main pancreatic duct and major duodenal papilla were preserved.

When analyzing the results of operation, we assessed: 1) postoperative lethality, 2) incidence and character of postoperative complications, 3) state of exocrine and endocrine pancreatic function, 4) restoration of working ability after the operation, 5) time of the main disease recurrence.

After the operation, two patients died. One death was caused by acute cardiac failure aggravated by the background of postoperative pancreatitis and the other by aggravating hepatorenal failure in a patient with prolonged preoperative obstructive jaundice.

In 6 (22.2%) patients in the early postoperative period, inflammation of the duodenoduodenal anastomosis was observed, which impaired gastric emptying. In all the patients the conservative therapy in combination with enteral feeding via a tube passed beyond the anastomosis removed this complication by 7–18 days after the operation. A transient external pancreatic fistula in the postoperative period was noted in 2 (7.4%) patients. The fistula was eliminated by conservative treatment.

Endocrine function was studied in 25 patients before and after the operation. As a result of the operation normalization of carbohydrate metabolism was noted in some patients. The number of patients with

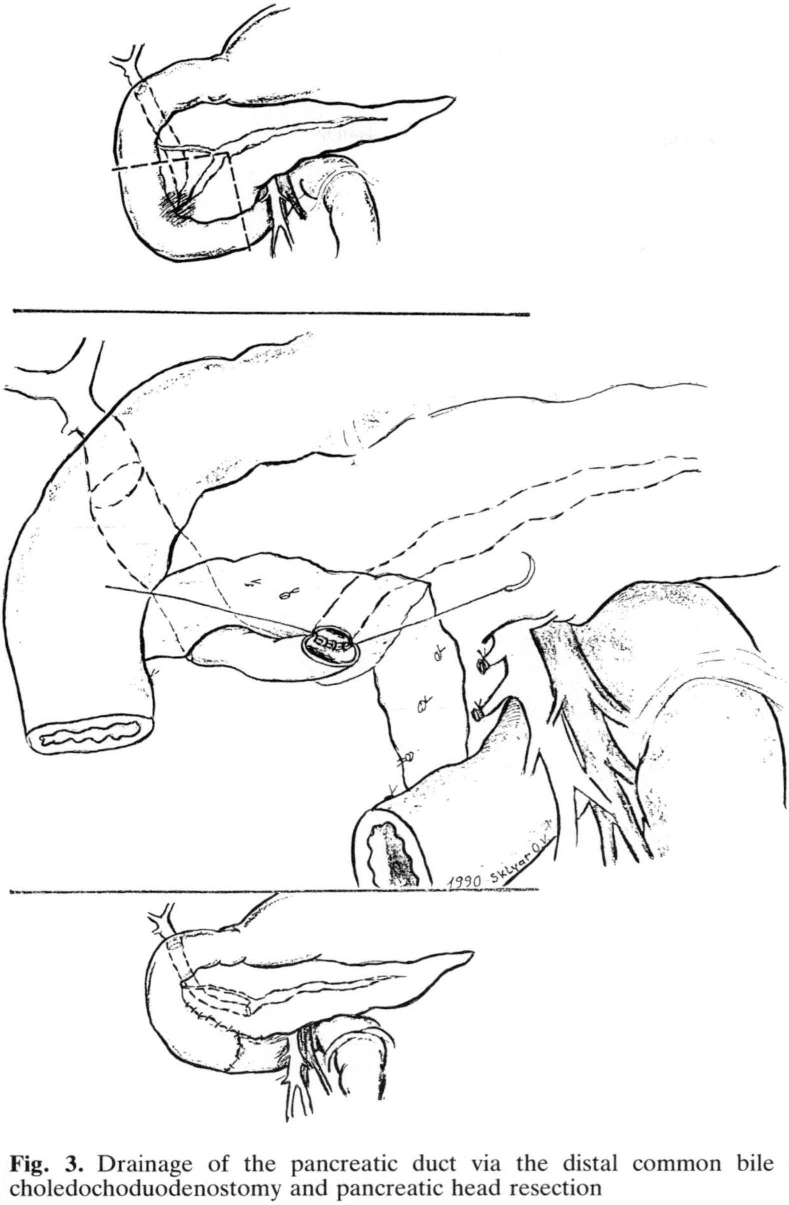

Fig. 3. Drainage of the pancreatic duct via the distal common bile duct after choledochoduodenostomy and pancreatic head resection

diabetes mellitus decreased owing to an increase in the number of patients with impaired glucose tolerance, or normal carbohydrate metabolism (Fig. 5). Thus, sparing resection has a favorable effect on the prognosis of carbohydrate metabolism after the operation. Exocrine postoperative

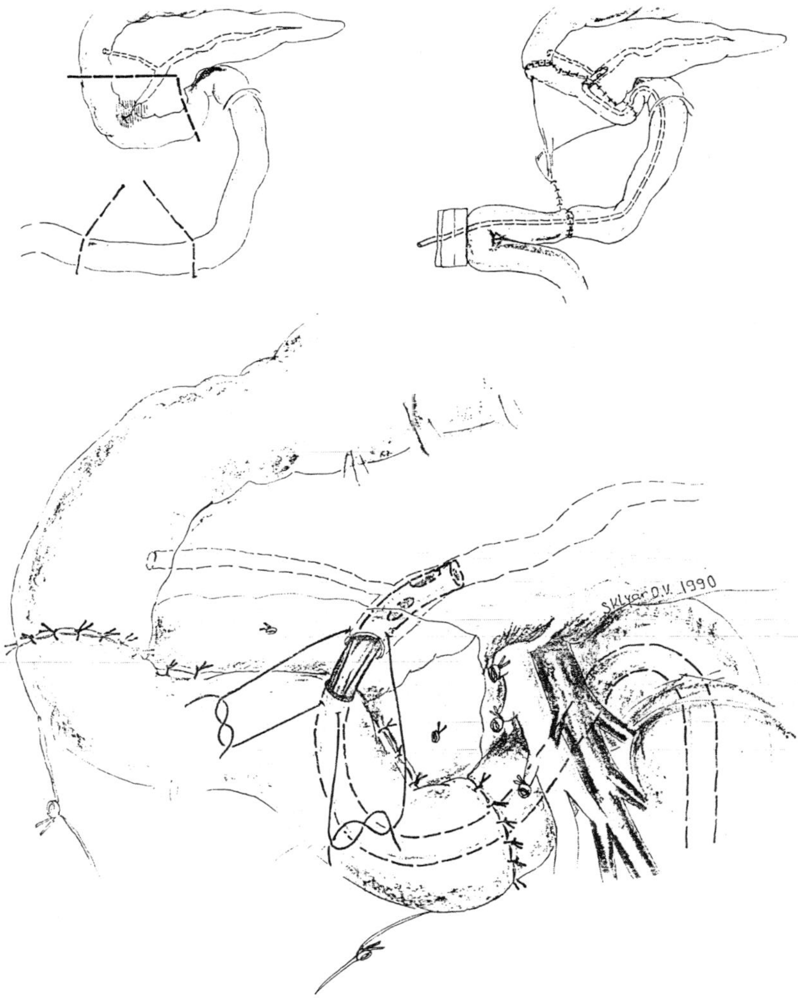

Fig. 4. Pancreatoduodenal resection with partial preservation of the duodenum (our technique). Forming the isoperistaltic insert between the proximal and distal duodenal portions for preservation of duodenal patency

function was studied in 18 patients. Before the operation, normal exocrine activity was noted in 25% of the patients. Three months after the operation normal exocrine activity was noted in 55%, and 24 months after in 35% (Fig. 6).

Of the patients operated on, 18 preserved their working ability postoperatively. In two patients control studies (ultrasonography and CT) revealed liver metastases after removal of pancreatic adenocarcinoma, 18

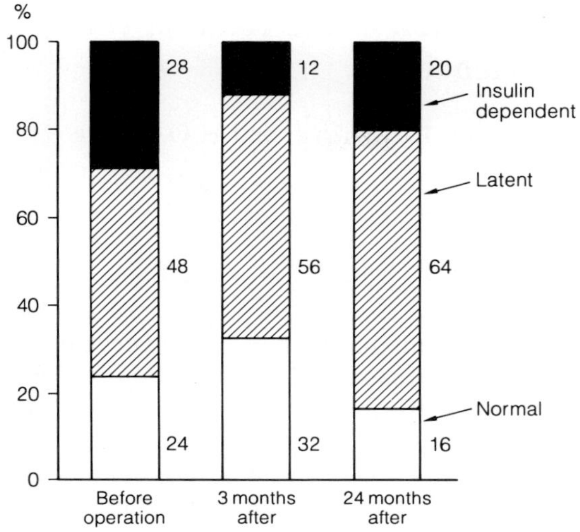

Fig. 5. Pancreatoduodenal resection with partial preservation of the duodenum (our technique): pre- and postoperative carbohydrate metabolism

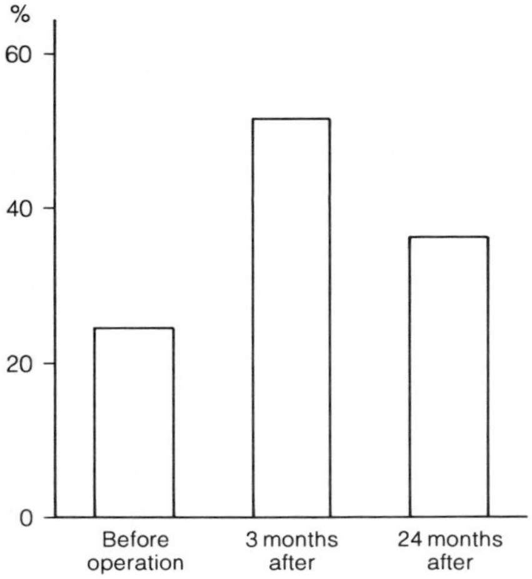

Fig. 6. Pancreatoduodenal resection with partial preservation of the duodenum (our technique): proportion of patients with normal exocrine function of the pancreas before and after operation

and 26 months later. In the remaining patients operated on there were no signs of disease recurrence after follow-up for 4–36 months.

Thus, in local forms of pathological process pancreatic head resections have functional advantages over the Whipple operation without detriment to the radicality of the intervention.

Duodenum-Preserving Resection of the Head of the Pancreas: The Ulm Experience

M. Büchler,[1] H. Friess, R. Jseumann, R. Bittner, and H.G. Beger

Up to one third of patients suffering from chronic pancreatitis develop an inflammatory mass in the head of the pancreas [1, 2]. Upper abdominal pain and recurrent attacks of acute pancreatitis are the leading symptoms and determine the clinical picture in these patients. This inflammatory enlargement of the head of the pancreas leads to a compression of the common bile duct and occlusion or stenosis of the main pancreatic duct. Furthermore an obstruction of the duodenum and a compression of the portal vein and major intestinal vessels may be observed [1–5]. From a morphological point of view, parenchymatic calcifications, pancreatic duct stones, pseudocystic cavities, and even areas of parenchyma necrosis are frequently found within the inflammatory mass in the head of the pancreas. Histologically, atrophy of the exocrine pancreas with a focal nodular increase of fibrotic tissue is common.

With regard to pain generation and the continuation of a painful condition, the nerve tissue reveals typical alterations within the area of the inflammation of the pancreas [6]. These chances can be classified as a pancreatitis-associated neuritis. Recent investigations have shown that in addition to an increase in pressure within the ductal system and in the parenchyma, the local release of sensory (pain) neurotransmitters such as substance P and calcitonin gene-related peptide (CGRP) in the inflammatory mass plays a crucial and causative role in the generation of pain in chronic pancreatitis [7, 8]. Even nowadays, partial duodenopancreatectomy, the so-called Whipple's procedure is the surgical procedure of choice in chronic pancreatitis with an inflammatory mass in the head and local complications [9]. Since neither stomach, nor duodenum, nor the extrapancreatic common bile duct are involved in the inflammatory process of the pancreas, the use of Whipple's procedure goes far beyond the requirements for optimal treatment of chronic pancreatitis. Furthermore, as we know, partial pancreatoduodenectomy is associated with a considerable hospital mortality together with a high late morbidity and mortality rates [10–16]. Recently, these generally accepted disadvantages of the Whipple's procedure have encouraged the development and use of organ-preserving surgical pro-

[1] Department of Surgery, University of Ulm, Steinhövelstr. 9, W-7900 Ulm, FRG

Beger/Büchler/Malfertheiner (Eds.)
Standards in Pancreatic Surgery

cedures in chronic pancreatitis. Duodenum-preserving resection of the head of the pancreas was introduced in 1972 and has since been regularly employed in patients with chronic pancreatitis and an inflammatory enlargement of the head of the pancreas [1–5]. The aim of duodenum-preserving pancreatic head resection is to achieve a local resection of the inflammatory mass via preserving surrounding organs such as the duodenum, the extrahepatic bile duct, and the stomach as well as by protecting the pancreatic parenchyma to a large extent.

Indication for Duodenum-Preserving Pancreatic Head Resection

Generally surgical treatment in chronic pancreatitis is mandatory if chronic abdominal pain occurs in combination with typical complications of the disease. An absolute surgical indication is the development of obstruction of the common bile duct with persisting cholestasis syndrome or even jaundice, severe stenosis of the duodenum with clinical relevant obstruction of gastric emptying, and compression of the retropancreatic major intestinal vessels such as superior mesenteric vein, splenic vein or portal vein, or a thrombosis developing into a portal hypertension. Still nowadays despite sophisticated diagnostic approaches including imaging techniques such as endoscopic retrograde cholangiopancreatography (ERCP) or CT scanning surgical therapy is necessary, when the inflammatory mass in the pancreatic head cannot be unequivocally differentiated from a malignant process in chronic pancreatitis.

The duodenum-preserving pancreatic head resection has become the standard procedure in Ulm for patients with inflammatory enlargement of the head of the pancreas leading to complications of chronic pancreatitis. So far 258 patients underwent duodenum-preserving pancreatic head resection for chronic pancreatitis.

Surgical Techniques

Three major phases during duodenum-preserving pancreatic head resection must be described.

Exposure Phase

The pancreatic head is exposed by dividing the gastrocolic ligament with careful handling of the vessels of the transverse colon. Subsequently the duodenum is mobilized, as described by Kocher, as is the pancreatic head dorsally, which requires a special dissecting cut to achieve decompression of the duodenum in patients in whom the duodenum is stenosed. This stenosis generally is caused by broad and fibrous tissue bands at the anterior wall of the suprapapillary duodenum that is frequently edematous. Removal of the

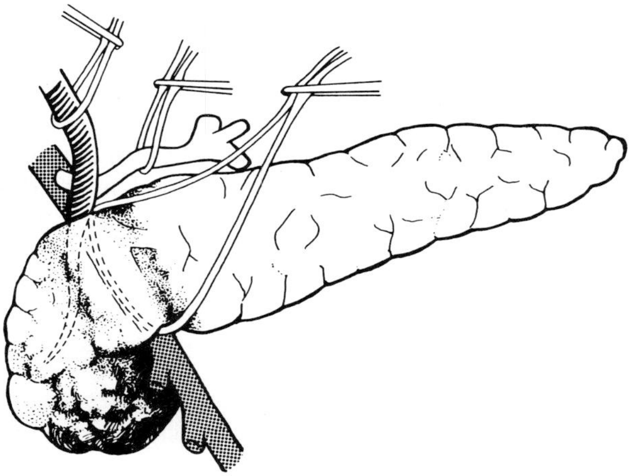

Fig. 1. Exposure of the head of the pancreas in chronic pancreatitis with an inflammatory mass in the head of the pancreas; banding of the pancreas at the level of the portal vein, the hepatic artery, and the common bile duct

fibrous layers from the front wall results in restoration of a normally wide duodenal lumen, and simultaneously exposes the plane between the head of the pancreas and the duodenal wall. Then follows the preparation of the portal vein and the superior mesenteric vein at the lower margin of the pancreas (Fig. 1). A tunnel is prepared between the portal vein and the pancreatic head, extending to the upper margin of the pancreas just above the portal vein, even in severe cases of inflammatory and edematous alterations of the head of the pancreas. Through this tunnel, the pancreas is then snared with a small rubber band at the transition from the head to the body. In patients with a cholestasis syndrome and severe choledochostenosis it is preferable to expose and tie off the common bile duct at the upper margin of the pancreas coming from the hepatoduodenal ligament.

Resection Phase

Resection of the inflammatory mass in the pancreatic head begins with the transverse division of the head at the duodenal edge of the portal vein. At the point of determining the resecting border, it is important to place the cut adjacent to the duodenum in order to preserve the pancreatic parenchyma. At the cut surface of the left pancreas, subtle hemostasis is performed using monofilament sutures (Fig. 2).

For subtotal resection, the head of the pancreas is rotated at the ventrodorsal level. This can easily be achieved by freeing the head of the pancreas from the portal vein. Small branches entering the portal vein directly must be ligated and divided. The head of the pancreas is removed

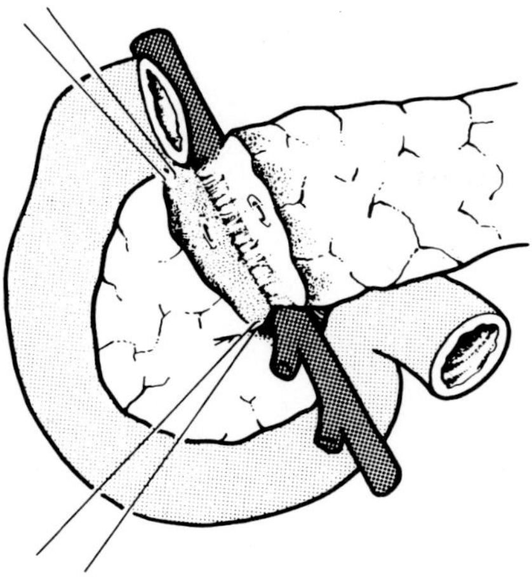

Fig. 2. Transection of the pancreas between the head and body

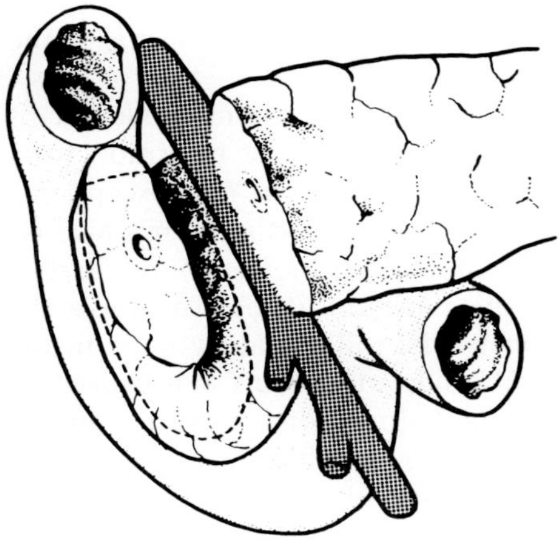

Fig. 3. After ventrodorsal rotation of the pancreatic head, subtotal resection of the inflammatory enlarged head of the pancreas is carried out

from the retroportal region after individual dissection of the vessels opening into the portal vein. The resection of the pancreatic head, which is then carried out, is preceded by marking the resection line at the dorsal surface of the pancreatic head by means of stay sutures (Fig. 3). It has not proved necessary to preserve the gastroduodenal artery for the purpose of ensuring an optimal blood supply to the duodenal wall, since the supraduodenal vessels and the dorsal duodenopancreatic arcade together with the meso-duodenal vessels suffice for this purpose. The excision is performed on the

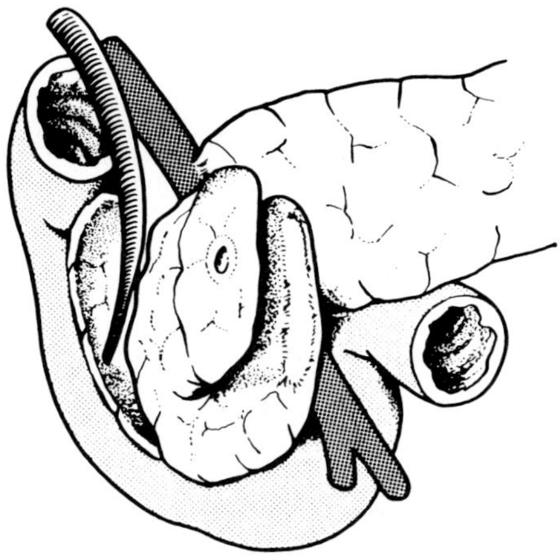

Fig. 4. Subtotal resection of the head of the pancreas results in decompression of the intrapancreatic segment of the common bile duct, which in most patients is narrowed by compression due to an inflammatory mass

ventral side of the head of the pancreas at a distance of about 5–8 mm to the duodenal wall, parallel to the duodenal C-line (Fig. 4).

The dissection of the intrapancreatic segment of the common bile duct is started at the upper margin of the pancreatic head at the transition from the hepatodudoenal ligament to the head. With only a few exceptions, decompression has been successfully achieved by dissecting along a loose tissue border between the pancreatic parenchyma and the common bile duct wall. In the majority of patients with chronic pancreatitis, obstruction of the common bile duct is due to compression by the inflammatory mass in the head of the pancreas, and only in a small group of patients is it caused by inflammatory infiltration of the choledochal wall. After completion of the dorsally pit-shaped subtotal resection of the pancreatic head, an orange peel-like, 5- to 8-mm wide remnant of the tissue of the pancreatic head is left (Fig. 5).

Reconstruction Phase

Jejunal Interposition and Pancreatico-Jejunal Anastomosis

Reconstruction after subtotal resection of the head of the pancreas is initiated by dissecting the uppermost jejunal loop 40 cm distally to the ligament of Treitz. The aboral jejunal loop is brought up via a retrocolic mesenteric cleft, and a two-row, layered, end-to-end anastomosis is carried out between the left pancreas and the jejunum (Fig. 6). If the pancreatic duct is not dilated, it can be quite difficult to anastomose the mucosa to the duct. In patients with a widely dilated pancreatic duct or fibrous stenosis of

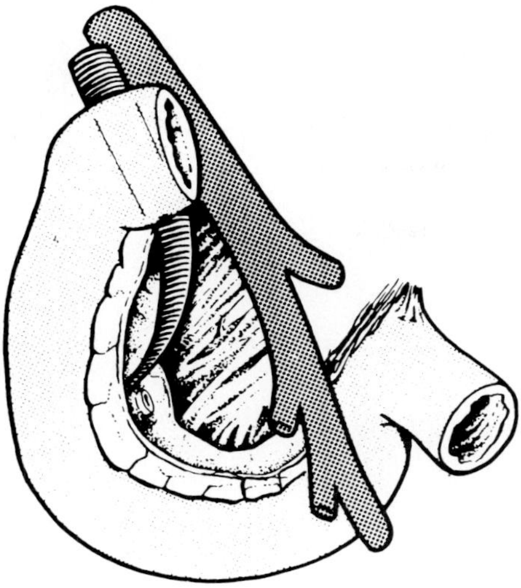

Fig. 5. After subtotal resection of the pancreatic head, a shell-like remnant of the pancreatic head between the common bile duct and the duodenal wall, and a 5- to 8-mm remnant of the uncinate process is preserved

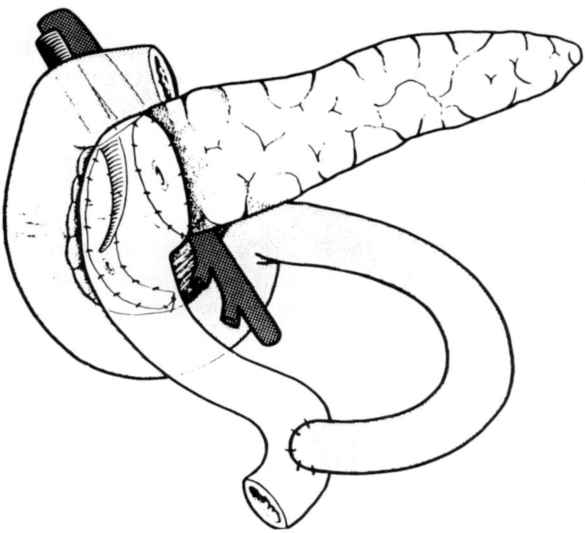

Fig. 6. Restitution of pancreatic secretory flow is accomplished by interposing the upper jejunal loop between the left pancreas and the jejunum. Two pancreatic anastomoses are carried out

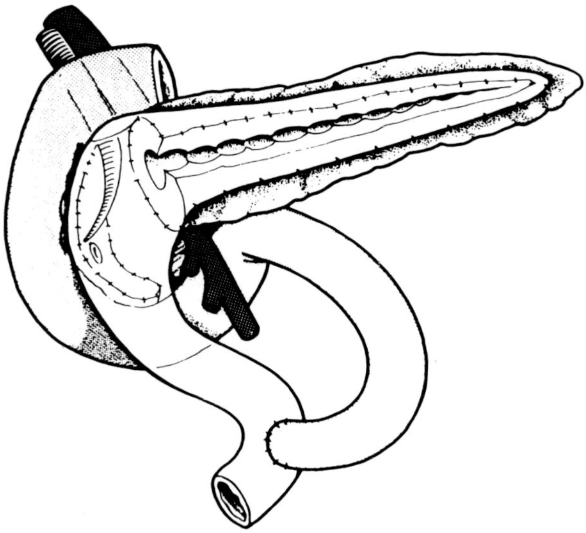

Fig. 7. In the case of a dilated and stenosed pancreatic main duct in the left pancreas, a side-to-side anastomosis like the Puestow procedure is performed instead of an end-to-end anastomosis between the pancreas and the jejunal loop

the pancreatic duct, the pancreatic main duct is incised longitudinally at its anterior surface up to the tail. In these patients, the anastomosis performed is a kind of side-to-side anastomosis between jejunum and longitudinally incised pancreas (Fig. 7).

Anastomosis with the Remnant of the Pancreatic Head

After very carefully accomplishing hemostasis, a side-to-side anastomosis between the jejunal loop and the remnant of the pancreatic head is carried out at a distance of 5–8 cm. The jejunal incision for this anastomosis has a length of 3–5 cm. A single layer suture between the jejunum and pancreas along the incision line serves as the interior layer. The outer layer is created between the dorsal pancreatic capsule and the seromuscularis of the jejunum (Figs. 6–8).

Anastomosis with the Common Bile Duct

An additional anastomosis between the prestenotic common bile duct and jejunal loop is mandatory in cases in which subtotal resection of the head of the pancreas has not led to complete decompression of the intrapancreatic segment of the common bile duct, and also when intra-operative gross examination has revealed wall infiltration in the common bile duct proximal to the papilla. The side-to-side anastomosis between the common bile duct

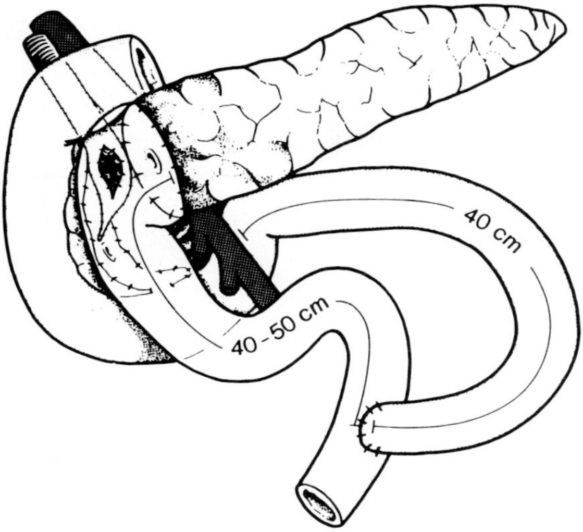

Fig. 8. In the case of stricture of the common bile duct, an additional common bile duct jejunum anastomosis is necessary to restore bile flow in the upper intestine

and the jejunum is sutured to the jejunal loop using a single-layer technique. In these patients, cholecystectomy is necessary (Fig. 8).

Restoration of the Intestinal Transit

For restoration of food transit a typical Roux-en-Y anastomosis is carried out 40 cm distally to the pancreaticojejunal anastomosis between the efferent and afferent jejunal loops (Figs. 6–8).

Puestow Modification

A Puestow modification of the duodenum-preserving resection of the head of the pancreas, with side-to-side pancreaticojejunal anastomosis was performed in 7% of the 258 patients (Fig. 7).

Bile Duct Anastomosis

An additional choledochojejunal anastomosis had to be done in 36 patients (14%) to restore regular bile flow (Fig. 8).

Patients

So far 258 patients (217 men, 41 women) have undergone operation with the duodenum-preserving pancreatic head resection (Table 1). The indication for surgery was abdominal pain in 95% (245/258) of the patients in combina-

Table 1. Preoperative morbidity in 258 patients undergoing duodenum-preserving resection of the head of the pancreas

	Number of patients (n = 258)	Percentage
Abdominal pain	245	95
Frequent	111	43
Daily	106	41
Daily, severe	80	31
Pancreatic main duct stenosis (head)	154	60
Common bile duct stenosis	129	50
Duodenal stenosis	79	31
Vascular obstruction	38	15

Table 2. Early postoperative complications after duodenum-preserving resection of the head of the pancreas

	Patients (n = 258)	Percentage	Reoperation (n)
Cardiopulmonary dysfunction	30	11.6	–
Bleeding (>3 blood units/24 h)	5	1.9	3
Pancreatitis	12	4.6	–
Ischemia of the duodenum	1	0.4	1
Anastomotic leakage	5	1.9	4
Sepsis	3	1.2	1
Pancreatic fistula	8	3.1	–
Intraabdominal abscess	7	2.7	2
Common bile duct stenosis	1	0.4	1
Ileus	3	1.2	2
Others	1	0.4	1
Total			15 (5.8%)
Hospital mortality			2 (0.8%)

tion with cholestasis syndrome in 50% (129/258) of the patients. Obstructive jaundice occurred in 14% (36/258). Sixteen (7%) were found to have severe stenosis of the suprapapillary duodenum, and 15% (38/258) had signs of portal hypertension caused by obstruction of the portal vein.

Early and Late Postoperative Results

Median hospitalization time was 13 days. Of the 258 patients, 15 had to undergo reoperation (Table 2). Two patients died, one of a fulminant embolism of the pulmonary artery on the ninth postoperative day, the second on the basis of a sepsis syndrome caused by leakage of the pancreatic

Table 3. Late results in patients undergoing a duodenum-preserving resection of the head of the pancreas[a]

	Patients	
	n	%
Abdominal pain		
None	172	79
Seldom	25	11
Frequent	22	10
Professional rehabilitation		
Complete	138	63
Unemployed	14	6
Retired	41	19
Others	26	12
Body weight		
Increased	118	54
Reduced	42	20
Attacks of acute pancreatitis	40	18
Late mortality	11	4.2

[a] Median follow up 3.5 years, range 3 months–18 years.

anastomosis. Hospital mortality amounted to 0.8%. During the follow-up period of between 3 months and 18 years, the late mortality amounted to 4.2%. The eleven deaths that we were able to register were related directly or indirectly to the underlying disease. In both the early and late post-operative phases, the pain syndrome was clearly and lastingly improved in 90% of the patients. Some 79% were completely relieved of pain. Ten percent of the patients complained of persistent mild epigastric pain. In the median follow-up period of 3.5 years, 40 of 219 (18%) patients required further hospital treatment for an attack of acute pancreatitis (Table 3). Around 80% of our patients experienced a marked increase or stabilization in weight during the postoperative course. At the time of the follow-up study 63% had returned to work, 6% were unemployed, and 31% were in either temporary or permanent retirement (Table 3).

Endocrine Function After Duodenum-Preserving Pancreatic Head Resection

Duodenum-preserving resection of the head of the pancreas in patients with chronic pancreatitis does not impair glucose tolerance. As compared with the preoperative status, the glucose metabolism was unchanged in 75% of the patients, improved in 16%, and had deteriorated in only 9% (Table 4). Follow-up examinations in the late postoperative period have revealed that

Table 4. Endocrine pancreatic function (oral glucose tolerance test) before and following duodenum-preserving resection of the head of the pancreas

	Number of patients	Normal		Diabetes mellitus			
				Subclinical		Insulin dependence	
		n	%	*n*	%	*n*	%
Preoperatively	251	132	53	57	23	62	24
Postoperatively	211	102	48	46	22	63	30

Table 5. Endocrine pancreatic function in 15 patients with chronic pancreatitis, before and 3 months after duodenum-preserving resection of the head of the pancreas

	Preoperatively	Postoperatively		*p* value
		10 days	3 months	
Disappearance of glucose (K value)	1.5	1.9	2.3	0.001
C-peptide peak (μU/ml)	4.05	5.06	4.8	ns
Insulin peak (μU/ml)	27	17	23	ns
Glucagon baseline (pg/ml)	820	444	336	0.001
Somatostatin baseline (pg/ml)	71.8		47.3	0.05
PP peak (pg/ml)	191	116	134	0.01

ns, not significant; PP, pancreatic polypeptide.

the percentage of patients with normal glucose regulation diminishes owing to the underlying disease.

In 15 patients we were able to analyze endocrine pancreatic function pre- and postoperatively according to a standardized protocol. Duodenum-preserving resection of the pancreatic head led to a marked increase in the median K value in the early postoperative period, and to a significant rise of the K value in the late postoperative period as compared with the preoperative data (Table 5) [17, 18]. It therefore appears that, as a result of duodenum-preserving pancreatic head resection, the glucose tolerance likely undergoes an improvement or normalization in the late postoperative phase. Preoperative and late postoperative insulin secretion was almost identical. In view of the improved glucose tolerance in the late postoperative period, this is an apparent contradiction that can be explained by the fact that the operation resulted in a normalization of the glucagon, somatostatin, and pancreatic polypeptide concentration in the peripheral blood that had risen significantly preoperatively.

Comments

Duodenum-preserving pancreatic head resection has been introduced to clinical practice to take out the inflammatory mass in the head of the pancreas while preserving important peripancreatic organs [1–5]. Therefore this procedure was inaugurated to replace standard pancreaticoduodenectomy or Whipple's procedure [9]. With duodenum-preserving pancreatic head resection comparable results are achieved as have been demonstrated for the Whipple procedure with respect to postoperative pain relief. Also this organ-saving operation overcomes the problem of common bile duct compression or obstruction as well as duodenal stenosis. Therefore, with regard to the true goals of surgery, namely to relieve pain and treat chronic-pancreatitis-associated pancreatic head complications, the duodenum-preserving pancreatic head resection delivers results comparable to those achieved with the Whipple procedure.

In contrast, hospital mortality (0.8%) as well as late mortality (4.2%) within 3.5 years (median follow-up) are considerably lower than those reported in the literature for the Whipple procedure in chronic pancreatitis [10–16]. Furthermore, the isolated resection of the inflammatory mass in the head of the pancreas preserves the endocrine capacity of the pancreas and duodenum to a large extent [17, 18].

Surgery of chronic pancreatitis nowadays is increasingly concentrating on draining or small resectional procedures. This is mainly because late mortality following major resectional procedures such as pancreatico-duodenectomy or subtotal left resection was unacceptably high in several series [10–16, 19, 20]. On the one hand, duodenum-preserving pancreatic head resection achieves the goal of treating pancreatic-head-related complications of chronic pancreatitis, and on the other hand it preserves endocrine function and the interegulation of upper gastrointestinal organs with exocrine and endocrine pancreatic function, therefore preserving normal food passage and pancreaticocibal synchronization. This is why the long-term results, particularly with regard to late mortality, are superior following duodenum-preserving pancreatic head resection. The most important problem in chronic pancreatitis surgery is how to achieve pain relief. We recently found that there is an increase in the proportion of the sensory nerve fibers in chronic pancreatitis that are neuroimmunologically characterized by the neurotransmitters substance P and CGRP [7, 8]. As the sensory autonomous nervus system consists mainly of pain fibers, the increase in neuropeptides in the sensory segment could additionally explain the complex pain syndrome in chronic pancreatitis. It might, therefore, be assumed that the characteristic upper abdominal pain of chronic pancreatitis, which lasts for many years, is mainly caused by the inflammation and the changes in the nerves in and around the head of the pancreas. Therefore a limited resection of this portion of the head of the pancreas as performed in duodenum-preserving pancreatic head resection might explain the long-lasting pain relief following this operation. It might also explain why simple drainage procedures are unable to achieve long-lasting pain relief if there is an inflammatory mass in the head of the pancreas [20, 21].

In summary, duodenum-preserving resection of the head of the pancreas is a low-risk operation for patients with chronic pancreatitis and an inflammatory mass in the head of the pancreas. Owing to the limited nature of this intervention, hospital and late mortality rates are low. More than 80% of patients with chronic pancreatitis have experienced long-lasting pain relief. In comparison with the Whipple operation, the duodenum-preserving resection of the head of the pancreas spares the patient a gastrectomy, a duodenectomy, and resection of the extrahepatic bile duct.

References

1. Beger HG, Büchler M, Bittner R, Oettinger W, Roscher R (1989) Duodenum preserving resection of the head of the pancreas in severe chronic pancreatitis – early and late results. Ann Surg 209:273–278
2. Büchler M, Malfertheiner P, Senn T, Beger HG (1990) Chronic pancreatitis with inflammatory mass in the head of the pancreas: a special entity? In: Beger HG, Büchler M, Ditschuneit H, Malfertheiner P (eds) Chronic pancreatitis. Springer, Berlin Heidelberg New York
3. Beger HG, Witte C, Kraas E, Bittner R (1980) Erfahrung mit einer das Duodenum erhaltenden Pankreaskopfresektion bei chronischer Pankreatitis. Chirurg 51:303–309
4. Beger HG, Büchler M (1990) Duodenum-preserving resection of the head of the pancreas in chronic pancreatitis with inflammatory mass in the head. World J Surg 14:83–87
5. Büchler M, Beger HG (1989) Neue Indikationen und Operationsverfahren bei chronischer Pankreatitis. Internist (Berl) 30:747–751
6. Bockman DE, Büchler M, Malfertheiner P, Beger HG (1988) Analysis of nerves in chronic pancreatitis. Gastroenterology 94:1459–1469
7. Büchler M, Weihe E, Frieß H, Malfertheiner P, Bockman DE, Müller S, Beger HG (1992) Changes in peptidergic innervation in chronic pancreatitis. Pancreas 7:183–192
8. Weihe E, Büchler M, Müller S, Frieß H, Zentel HJ, Yanaihara N (1990) Peptidergic innervation in chronic pancreatitis. In: Beger HG, Büchler M, Ditschuneit H, Malfertheiner P (eds) Chronic pancreatitis. Springer, Berlin Heidelberg New York, pp 83–105
9. Whipple AO, Pearson WB, Mullins CR (1935) Treatment of carcinoma of the ampulla of Vater. Ann Surg 102:763–769
10. Gall FP, Mühe E, Gebhardt C (1981) Results of partial and total pancreaticoduodenectomy in 117 patients with chronic pancreatitis. World J Surg 5: 269–275
11. Guillemin G, Cuilleret J, Michel A, Berard P, Foroldi J (1971) Chronic relapsing pancreatitis. Surgical management. Including 63 cases of pancreaticoduodenostomy. Am J Surg 122:802–807
12. Hoffmeister WH, Trede M (1982) Chronische Pankreatitis. Chirurgische Therapie individuell planen. Klinikarzt 2:272–280
13. Howard JM (1987) Surgical treatment of chronic pancreatitis. In: Howard JM, Jordan GL Jr, Reber HA (eds) Surgical disease of the pancreas. Lea and Febiger, Philadelphia, pp 496–521
14. Leger L, Lenriot JP, Lemaigre G (1980) Lhypertension et la stase postale ségmentaire dans les pancréatites chroniques. J Chir (Paris) 95:599–608

15. Warren KW (1976) Changing patterns in surgery of the pancreas. Surg Clin North Am 56:615–629
16. Warren KW (1969) Surgical management of chronic relapsing pancreatitis. Am J Surg 117:24–30
17. Bittner R, Beger HG (1979) Significance of the duodenum for carbohydrate metabolism. In: Herfarth C (ed) Gastric cancer. Springer, Berlin Heidelberg New York, pp 242–246
18. Bittner R, Butters M, Büchler M, Nägele S, Roscher R, Beger HG (1988) Glucose homeostasis and endocrine pancreatic secretion in patients with chronic pancreatitis before and after surgical therapy. Biomed Res 9:28
19. Frey CF (1981) Role of subtotal pancreatectomy and pancreaticojejunostomy in chronic pancreatitis. J Clin Res 31:361
20. Leger L, Lenriot JP, Lemaigre G (1974) Five to twenty-five year follow up after surgery for chronic pancreatitis in 148 patients. Ann Surg 180:198
21. Howard JM (1981) The treatment of chronic pancreatitis. 1978. Ann Surg 194:319

Preservation of the Duodenum in Total Pancreatectomy for Chronic Pancreatitis

R.C.G. Russell[1]

Introduction

The surgical options in the management of pancreatic disease are limited by the macroscopic disease which the surgeon faces as he assesses the pancreas during the initial laparotomy in conjunction with the pre-operative investigations. There is no procedure suitable for all patients and there are only a few patients suitable for duodenal preservation either as part of a resection of the head or as part of total ablation of the pancreas. The interest shown in preservation procedures such as the Beger operation (Büchler, this volume), the Frey procedure (Frey, this volume), the pylorus-preserving operations (Traverso, this volume) is indicative of the importance of preserving pancreatic function. The need to preserve as much duodenum as possible has arisen because the technical challenges of pancreatic surgery have largely been overcome with a very low morbidity and mortality [14], with the result that surgeons are now becoming more aware of the long-term implications of the ablation of the pancreas. On purely physiological grounds many feel that preserving the pylorus and if possible, as much duodenum as possible will give a better long-term result [13]. Preserving the duodenum should preserve gastric emptying, duodenal and small intestinal motility and bile mixing by preserving the hormonal release from the antrum and duodenum, and maintaining the antropyloric emptying mechanism as well as the duodenal pacemaker with coordinate duodenal and jejunal contractions as a result of the undisturbed myenteric plexus. As a result, the clinical outcome should be improved with a better weight gain, due to better absorption, better diabetic control as a result of more predictable absorption pattern and less diarrhoea due to a more coordinate intestinal activity with less undigested food reaching the caecum.

It was Whipple, in one of his original articles, who said it was necessary to resect the duodenum because "complete removal of the pancreas so compromises the blood supply to the duodenum as to favour necrosis and fistula formation." Nevertheless, experience in the surgery on children who have nesidioblastosis has shown that 98% pancreatectomy can be per-

[1] The Middlesex Hospital, London W1, U.K.

Beger/Büchler/Malfertheiner (Eds.)
Standards in Pancreatic Surgery

formed with preservation of the duodenum. Animal work performed during the early studies on pancreatic transplantation showed that the duodenum survived following meticulous dissection of the pancreas off the duodenum. This simplified the animal model as it avoided the usual duodenal resection and major reconstruction involved. Biochemical studies of the animals showed no detectable insulin or insulin activity, thereby indicating that the pancreatectomy was complete. Further, the duodenum appeared vascularized and appeared to function normally.

Harken et al. in 1971 [4] described a total pancreatectomy performed in infants with idiopathic hypoglycaemia in whom a 50% pancreatectomy had failed to control the symptoms. All the identifiable pancreatic tissue within the C loop of the duodenum was removed. The spleen was preserved, relying on the blood supply via the short gastric vessels. It was apparent that the duodenum in the neonate would survive after sacrifice of both the superior and inferior pancreatoduodenal arteries. Subsequent description of this procedure by Gough [3] confirmed that this operation was safe in infants, and in fact was the only procedure which would satisfactorily relieve the symptoms of infantile hyperinsulinism. My own experience in ten infants [11] confirmed that the duodenum could be well separated from the pancreas in the infant, and that a plane of cleavage could be developed along the pancreatic border of the duodenum by careful dissection. In the infant, the colour of the duodenum was completely normal at the end of the operation. Further, the growth of these children has remained normal over a 7-year observation period indicating that there are no major long-term sequelae to this procedure.

Injection studies in the human suggest that there is an arcade of vessels within the mucosa of the duodenum similar to those of vessels in the stomach [12]. These injection studies suggested that contrast injected at the superior pancreatoduodenal artery would perfuse through this submucosal plexus down to the fourth part of the duodenum [7]. Subsequent experience in the adult has confirmed that the duodenum will survive devascularization extending from the first to the fourth part and that presumably the duodenum is preserved by this submucosal plexus. Nevertheless this anastomosis is tenuous for the duodenum is a dusky cyanotic colour by the end of the procedure, and thus the older patient or those in whom there has been previous surgery to the duodenum should be approached with the greatest care being more suited for a duodenal resection.

Indications

To justify duodenal preservation during a resection of the head of the pancreas whether or not it is part of a total removal of the pancreas requires most careful selection. First, it is necessary to determine that the patient requires pancreatic surgery to relieve his symptoms (this volume) and second, that resection with duodenal preservation is the correct procedure. To justify the operation of total pancreatectomy for which I have done all but three of my duodenal preserving procedures, it is necessary to fulfil criteria that are strict and agreed by a team who have experience in managing patients with pancreatic disease and who are prepared to continue caring for these patients after the operation for a long period of time. First, medical therapy must have failed after an adequate trial of conservative therapy. Second, the pain, which is the major indication for this type of conservative procedure, must be intractable and unrelieved by other therapy. Third, operations of a lesser severity such as drainage procedures or a partial resection must have been previously undertaken and deemed to have failed as a result of the persistence or recurrence of the symptoms. It is doubtful whether a total pancreatectomy should be performed in the absence of either endocrine or exocrine deficiency. Fourth, patients who have severe pancreatic fibrosis often in relationship to pancreatic calculi who are both insulin and enzyme deficient may be better treated by a total resection than a pancreas preservation procedure. Fifth and finally, there are a few patients in whom there is no ductal abnormality, but who suffer from repeated episodes of pain of pancreatic origin. These patients inevitably develop recurrent pain after lesser procedures and can be appropriately managed by total pancreatectomy. This group requires most careful assessment.

At operation, a most careful assessment of the pancreatic disease from which the patient suffers must be undertaken. The ideal candidate for duodenum preservation is the patient who has severe fibrosis such that the pancreas contracts away from the duodenum, while the most unsuitable patient has the swollen, inflammed, oedematous and expanded pancreatic head with no line of cleavage or visible vessels. Judgment is required; it is well to remember that the safety of the patient is paramount, and the advantages in the longterm of duodenal preservation will be quickly outweighed by a stormy post-operative recovery.

Pre-Operative Preparation

Once the decision has been taken to offer the patient a duodenum-preserving pancreatectomy, it is necessary to inform the patient of the consequences of the procedure. If the patient has neither pancreatic enzyme deficiency nor the need for insulin, it is essential to start the enzyme replacement to ensure that the rather unpalatable capsules are taken with good compliance. It is essential that the implications of diabetes are fully discussed, and correct instruction given before the procedure. Because many of the patients are malnourished, it is preferable to improve their nutritional status by means of parenteral feeding, as rehabilitation in the post-operative period is hastened by an adequate lean body mass. Further, the intestinal rest associated with parenteral nutrition enables the narcotics, on which these patients usually are, to be reduced and hopefully stopped, as it is easier if not essential to stop the narcotic abuse pre-operatively rather than in the post-operative period. Such pre-operative care has the added attraction of reducing peripancreatic inflammation, and often allowing duodenum preservation which in the presence of severe inflammation would have been impossible.

Before operation it is appropriate to repeat the computed tomography of the pancreas and to obtain a cholangiogram. This will alert the surgeon to technical problems, ensure that a lesser procedure is not appropriate and ensure that the bile duct is normal thus being suitable for preservation. Angiography has not proved to be of value.

Operative Technique

The pancreas is approached through a long transverse upper abdominal incision and a full laparotomy undertaken to assess the extent of disease and its complications. During assessment, it is important not to mobilize the duodenum by a Kocher manœuvre as the duodenum may well draw some blood supply from the peritoneal attachments. If this assessment suggests that disease is localised to the pancreas with no evidence of complication and that the operation of duodenal preservation is technically satisfactory then the pancreas is exposed further by dividing the gastrocolic omentum within the epiploic arch and so opening the lesser sac. If a distal pancreatectomy has not previously been performed, the body and tail of the pancreas are mobilized in the usual way. Having assessed and mobilized the distal pancreas, attention is turned to the head of the pancreas and an assessment made whether the vessels to the pancreas can be clearly identified and separated from the duodenum. The superior mesenteric vein and the portal vein should be clearly identified at this stage. The middle colic and left colic vessels should be defined and separated from the inferior border of the pancreas and uncinate process so that they do not get damaged or compromised during the procedure.

The omentum is cleared from the head of the pancreas by dividing the right gastroepiploic artery. The hepatic flexure of the colon and its mesocolon is dissected easily inferiorly, well away from the operating field. The front of the pancreas and the whole of the duodenum should now be clearly exposed and dissection commenced. Before commencing dissection it is essential not to mobilize the head of the duodenum by dividing the peritoneum on the lateral surface of the C loop. Further assessment is made of the pancreas to ensure that a preservation procedure is technically possible and that there is no inflammatory mass preventing dissection between the duodenum and the pancreas itself.

In order to ease the dissection, if the body and the tail is still present it is useful to divide the neck of the pancreas with a GIA stapler so that the portal vein is clearly exposed. The portal vein and superior mesenteric vein are divided free of their branches to the pancreas so further exposing the vessels and defining their relationship to the pancreatic tissue. The uncinate process of the pancreas at the junction of the duodenum with the mesenteric vessels is inspected and all adhesions from this area divided. A clamp is placed on the apex of the pancreas which is then lifted forwards. With mosquito forceps, each vessel between the pancreas and the duodenum or the pancreas and the mesenteric vessels is dissected out and tied as near to the pancreas as possible. Ties are preferable to ligaclips as they are less prone to slip during handling. The dissection is continued posteriorly to ensure that the duodenum is free from the pancreatic tissue but this posterior dissection should not be sufficiently deep as to destroy the vessels running on the surface of the posterior aspect of the pancreas and conveying blood from the superior mesenteric artery to the duodenum. The tip of the uncinate process can be brought further fowards and a finger inserted onto the posterior surface of the uncinate process. With the finger lifting the pancreas forward and tensing the vessels it is more easy to dissect out the small vessels passing from the pancreas directly to the superior mesenteric and portal veins. This dissection is continued until the upper border of the pancreas is reached. The dissection is now continued along the fourth part of the duodenum continuing with the left hand to lift forward the pancreas and individual vessels divided up to the point of the entry of the ampulla of Vater. Dissection is difficult near the ampulla of Vater for the tissue planes at this point between the pancreas and the duodenum are obliterated. When near the ampulla, it is wise to lift the pancreas forward and inspect the posterior part of the pancreas for occasionally the bile duct lies superficial. Otherwise, in the angle between the first part of the duodenum and the portal vein a dissection is made until the bile duct is found. It is dissected away from both structures. The bile duct is traced down to the ampulla of Vater gently teasing the pancreas off the bile duct and entering the tunnel around the biliary tree. Once the ampulla is reached, it is easy to define the pancreatic duct and continue working the pancreas off the duodenum. Attention is now turned to the attachment of the pancreas to the first and second part of the duodenum. By careful dissection, avoiding the bile duct and the main pancreato-duodenal artery, which is tied as far from the duodenum as possible, the dissection is continued down to the second part of the duodenum at which point the accessory duct may be present. This is dissected out, tied and oversewn. All that remains attaching the pancreas to the duodenum is the segment of tissue between the accessory and main pancreatic ducts. Careful removal by sharp dissection enables a clear dissection of the structures to be achieved.

The duodenum is now carefully inspected to ensure that there are no perforations present. If there is bleeding from the medial wall of the duodenum it is wise to oversew rather than to diathermy. The bile duct is inspected to ensure that there are no perforations present: if there are, accurate suture with 6-0 Prolene is advised. Packs are now placed on the duodenum and the colour assessed after five minutes in which no handling takes place. There is usually a normal colour of the fourth and second parts of the duodenum but the third part will be a dusky hue. With time this colour resolves and the duodenum remains viable. Once meticulous haemostasis has been achieved a drain is placed within the C loop.

The procedure takes between 2.5 and 4.5 h to complete. Intraoperative blood loss varies between 200–900 ml (median 550 ml). In two patients, the bile duct has been opened during dissection and in one the duodenum was opened. The bile duct was repaired with 6-0 Polydioxanone and the duodenum with two layers of 3-0 Polydioxanone. In the post-operative period patients are monitored carefully and the arterial PO_2 maintained at a high level of ensure adequate tissue oxygenation. A period of gastric stasis may be encountered post operatively and for this gastric aspiration is advised with intravenous infusion. The median time before a return of emptying occurs is 14 days and has been as long as 34. The post-operative appearances of the duodenum on barium examination suggests ischaemia, but this appearance returns to normal after a variable period of 2–4 weeks. In one patient, a cannula placed in the gallbladder to monitor the appearance of the bile duct showed gross oedema around the ampulla of Vater with narrowing of the terminal portion of the bile duct, yet returning to a normal appearance within a 6-week period.

Results

Recent data on total pancreatectomy for chronic pancreatitis continue to be sparse, and there are few large series from which to glean information. In a review by Frey and colleagues [2] which included all published data between 1972 and 1988, the information on total pancreatectomy was limited as the original papers lacked "vital" information. The largest recent study is a retrospective report describing collected data on 83 patients from six centres in the United Kingdom [1]; this article included little information on follow-up. The largest series from Mannheim describes 52 patients who had a total pancreatectomy, but only 17 of these were for chronic pancreatitis [14]. Smaller experience from Kiviluoto et al. [6] (10 patients), Keith et al. [5] (7 patients) and McAfee et al. [10] (4 patients) support the general conclusions from the larger studies that total pancreatectomy for benign disease is a safe operation with comparatively low morbidity, yet with major longer term problems.

In the review by Frey and colleagues [2] the mortality was 31 deaths out of 324 resected patients (9.6%). The more recent publications have shown a lower mortality ranging from 0% to 6%. The morbidity is high with as many as 40% developing complications [14] in the postoperative period. The complications were varied with sepsis being the most common, a biliary or

Table 1. Age, length of history and aetiology of patients with duodenum-preserving total pancreatectomy or standard total pancreatectomy

	Duodenum preserving (n = 32)	Standard total (n = 26)
Median age (years; range)	34 (14–52)	39 (22–51)
Median history (years; range)	6 (1–26)	6 (0.1–15)
Aetiology		
Alcohol	9	14
Pancreas division	5	4
Familial	2	3
Trauma	2	2
Gallstone	2	1
Minimal change	9	2
Other	3	0

enteric leak next, and a delayed haemorrhage in a small number. Details on the long-term outlook of total pancreatectomy are sparse, but early experience [16] suggested that there was an increased early mortality, and major complications from diabetes.

Personal Results

Since 1976, 290 patients have had a resection for chronic pancreatitis. Of these 125 have had a proximal pancreatectomy, 152 have had a distal pancreatectomy and, 13 have had a total pancreatectomy primarily. Of the 125 patients who have had a proximal pancreatectomy 13 have proceeded to a distal pancreatectomy so ablating the pancreas, whilst of the 152 distal pancreatectomies (12 performed elsewhere), 32 patients have proceeded to a proximal pancreatectomy so ablating their pancreas. Thus, 58 patients have had a total pancreatectomy, and of these 32 have had a duodenum-preserving procedure and 26 have had a total pancreatectomy with excision of the duodenum.

In the presentation of the results, the outcome of the standard resections are given alongside those of the duodenum-preserving procedures in order to compare the merits of the operations. Table 1 shows that the median age of the duodenum-preserving patients was similar to those who had a standard procedure. Length of history was similar in both groups and the aetiology comparable. Many of the unknown aetiology patients had a minimal change pancreatitis [15] with previous documented evidence of raised amylase levels following which pancreatic pain started with great severity. Most of the patients whose pancreatitis was due to alcohol had been weaned off alcohol by the time they had their total pancreatectomy performed; indeed, this was a prerequisite in our selection of patients. Many patients had had previous procedures both operative and non-operative

Table 2. Previous operative procedures performed on patients with duodenum-preserving total pancreatectomy or standard total pancreatectomy

	Duodenum preserving (n = 32)	Standard total (n = 26)
Distal pancreatectomy	22	10
Proximal pancreatectomy	3	10
Cholecystectomy	13	12
Cyst drainage	2	6
Sphincteroplasty	7	3
Biliary procedure	5	2
Duct drainage	3	2
Laparotomy, other	21	14

Table 3. Previous non-operative procedures performed on patients with duodenum-preserving total pancreatectomy or standard total pancreatectomy

	Duodenum preserving (n = 32)	Standard total (n = 26)
None	3	6
Parenteral feeding	24	12
Coeliac plexus block	13	8
Endoscopic	6	6
Percutaneous	3	2

(Tables 2, 3). 15 patients who had a duodenum-preserving pancreatectomy were diabetic pre-operatively, and 19 of the standard total patients were already diabetic. Steatorrhoea was present in 13 of the duodenum-preserving patients, and 16 of the standard total pancreatectomy patients.

Perioperative Complications

The mortality among the 32 patients who had a duodenum-preserving total pancreatectomy was nil, while three patients who had a standard total pancreatectomy died, each as a consequence of the severe complications of an attack of pancreatitis in patients with the complications of chronic pancreatitis. One patient died of the adult respiratory distress syndrome, whilst the other two died as a consequence of sepsis. The complications for both procedures are outlined in Table 4, sepsis being the commonest complication. In the nine patients who had sepsis following a duodenum-preserving procedure three had chest infections necessitating treatment with

Table 4. Peri-operative complications following duodenum-preserving total pancreatectomy or standard total pancreatectomy

	Duodenum preserving (n = 32)	Standard total (n = 26)
Mortality	0	3
Sepsis	10	9
Leak		
Bile	1	
Enteric	3	
Haemorrhage		
Major (≥4 g/dl)		
Minor (<4 g/dl)	1	1
Gastric stasis	6	
Other	1	5
None	14	12
Length of stay		
Median	21	21
Range	10–49	11–98

antibiotics, two had infection of their central venous feeding line which resolved following removal of the line, and one had a urinary tract infection. A duodenal leak occurred in three patients, but in none was this serious and in each it settled with conservative management without re-operation. The single biliary fistula was transitory, and resolved within a few days without intervention. The delayed gastric emptying was a problem and accounts for the prolonged in-patient stay in some patients. In time it invariably resolves.

The length of stay was similar in the two groups of patients with a mean of 21 days. Apart from the delayed gastric emptying, the reason for the prolonged post-operative hospital stay was the policy not to discharge patients until their diabetes was under control, their steatorrhoea treated with enzyme tablets and their analgesic requirements reduced to nil or a minimal quantity. It has been found that if patients are discharged on pethidine or other similar major analgesics then they tend to remain on narcotics for a long period of time.

Long-Term Assessment

An appropriate yardstick by which to assess the success of a procedure is to determine the number of times such patients are readmitted to hospital. Few patients avoided such readmissions, and in some many hospital admissions were not necessarily in order to solve their medical problems. The vast majority of these patients were admitted on account of narcotic abuse and nutritional difficulties, with poor diabetic control, being a frequent reason.

There have been four late deaths; three of these occurred in the standard total pancreatectomy group whilst one occurred in the duodenum-preserving patients. In one patient, a carcinoma of the oesophagus developed requiring an oesophagogastrectomy at his local hospital from which he died. One patient died at 9 months of sepsis, a further patient died of alcohol intoxication at 24 months, while a final patient died some 74 months after the original operation of a perforated duodenal ulcer.

Bile Duct Stricture

The major late surgical complication associated with duodenum-preserving procedures has been the development of a bile duct stricture which has occurred in seven patients. In two patients an endoscopic sphincterotomy, at 14 months and 29 months has been sufficient to control the problem. In a further patient insertion of stents has been found to be suitable and these remained patent on a long-term basis, but were later removed when the stricture resolved. Four patients have required a choledochojejunostomy. These operations have been performed at 5, 12, 15 and 30 months after the original procedure. Predisposing factors to bile duct stricture include damage at the time of the original operation and ischaemia; those related to ischaemia invariably required a surgical bypass procedure. Subsequent follow-up of these seven patients has been good, with normal liver function tests.

Long-Term Follow-up

It is our standard practice to see all patients following duodenum-preserving pancreatectomy in a special pancreatic clinic. At this clinic standard questions are asked such as pain, analgesic requirements, bowel function, pancreatic enzyme supplements and requirement and level of activity. Pain is divided into nil or minimal, moderate and severe, while the analgesics required for their pain sub-divided into minor (acetaminophen, codeine), intermediate (pentazocine or buprenorphine) and major which is a continual requirement for a narcotic.

Taking the 1-, 3- and 5-year results (Table 5) it is noted that after duodenum-preserving pancreatectomy 16 of 32 patients had minimal or no pain with a further one requiring only moderate analgesics. This good response continued throughout the 3- and 5-year follow-up periods. A similar proportion had pain relief following a standard total pancreatectomy. Nevertheless, 13 duodenum-preserving patients still had severe pain with six of these requiring major analgesics. From the point of view of pain relief, there was no significant difference between those patients that had had a duodenum-preserving procedure and those patients who had had a standard total pancreatectomy.

Table 5. Late follow-up results on patients after duodenum-preserving total pancreatectomy or standard total pancreatectomy

	Duodenum preserving (n = 32)			Standard total (n = 26)		
Years post-operatively	1	3	5	1	3	5
Pain						
Nil	8	6	6	1	4	4
Minimal	8	3	4	9	4	2
Moderate	1	4	1	1	1	1
Severe	13	14	7	8	5	1
Analgesics						
None	14	7	8	6	4	5
Minor	1	1	2	1		
Moderate	9	10	2	5	5	2
Narcotic	6	9	6	7	5	1
Bile duct stricture		7			0	
Length of follow-up (months)						
Median		64			54	
Range		6–120			3–145	

Diabetic Status

The patients are all managed by "normal" – that is, twice daily injection of a combination of rapidly absorbed and intermediate insulins – with the exception of two patients who are controlled using an insulin pump. One of these patients was an anorexic, and one is a young fit man. Patients routinely monitor their blood glucose with a reagent strip and also test their urine. One patient who has been insulin dependent since 1977 and had a total pancreatectomy performed in 1983 had peripheral neurophathy; this was represented only by loss of the ankle jerks. A further patient who had only been diabetic since a total pancreatectomy in 1984 has possible peripheral neuropathy, the diagnosis being complicated by the carpal tunnel syndrome. Neither of these patients has any history of alcohol abuse.

There were no other long-term complications of diabetes, but the follow-up period was too short to draw conclusions. The frequency of hypoglycaemic episodes tends to occur more frequently in those who have had a standard total pancreatectomy than in the duodenum-preserving group. Although mild hypoglycaemic episodes are not routinely recorded by the patients. Many of these mild episodes of hypoglycaemia are associated with diarrhoea and malabsorption.

In patients who have had a duodenum-preserving procedure, good control was achieved in 11 patients, while 15 had poor control, whereas after a standard total pancreatectomy 8 of 15 patients had good control and the remaining 7 poor control.

Table 6. Comparison of ideal body weight at operation and at 1, 3 and 5 years post-operatively

	% Ideal body weight		Post-operative weight change (kg)	
	Duodenum preserving	Standard total	Duodenum preserving	Standard total
At operation				
n	21	14		
Median	99.5	83		
Range	75–138	64–129		
At 1 year				
n	21	14	21	14
Median	105	89	+1.5	+3.2
Range	72–143	70–112	−8.2–+9.2	118.5–+12.1
At 3 years				
n	17	8	17	8
Median	108	88	+3.8	+3.5
Range	74–142	63–117	−3.2–+14.1	−13.5–+15.0
At 5 years				
n	3	6	3	6
Median	116	82	+4.4	−1.6
Range	106–121	67–103	+2.3–+9.0	−15.0–+2.5

It is of interest that the overall requirement of insulin was 38 U in the duodenum-preserving group and 33 units in the standard total pancreatectomy group rising to 43 U (range 14–80) and 44 (range 10–90) 3 and 5 years after surgery in the duodenum-preserving group, while in the standard total pancreatectomy group the insulin requirement was 34 U (range 18–96) and 35 (range 18–96) at 3 and 5 years respectively. The greater requirement for insulin in the duodenum-preserving group was interpreted as indicating a more normal absorption of food.

Pancreatic Enzyme Replacement Therapy

In the management of patients after a total pancreatectomy, the control of steatorrhoea appears important and many patients have a less than optimal outcome because they do not master sensible control of their pancreatic enzyme supplements. The amount of enzyme replacement varies markedly between individuals as illustrated by the range of capsules in the duodenum-preserving pancreatectomy group from 4 to 100 with a mean of 60 capsules/day. However, for those who have had a standard total pancreatectomy the median requirement is only 30 capsules/day with a range of 9–150 capsules/day. The increased requirement of enzyme capsules in association with the increased requirement of insulin suggests that the diet in these patients was more normal and better absorbed than in the standard total pancreatectomy group.

In order to test this hypothesis the weight of the patients was compared with that at their original operation. As is seen in Table 6 that there is a far higher weight gain in the patients who have had a duodenum-preserving procedure than in those that have the standard excisional procedure. It is apparent that the patients who had a standard total pancreatectomy were thinner compared to their height than those who where selected for a duodenal preservation. Therefore, the weight difference may merely indicate that a more severe form of pancreatitis was chosen for those who had larger surgical procedure. This fact is indisputable but the continued weight gain of the duodenum-preserving group suggests that this operation is compatible with a more normal life-style and is achieving the desired outcome, namely a normal diet, good insulin control and normal weight.

In the maintainence of these patients the importance of overcoming pancreatic enzyme insufficiency cannot be over emphasised. Our current practice is to use only three enzyme replacement products, standard enteric coated capsule preparation (Nutrizym-GR, Merck), and enteric coated granular preparation (Creon, Duphar), and an enteric coated microsphere preparation (Pancrease, Cilag). Patients are usually started on the standard preparation as it is cheaper and increase the dose until diarrhoea is controlled. If the control is not possible with reasonable doses, the enteric coated preparation is substituted at the same dose. If this fails to control the diarrhoea, then the enteric coated microsphere preparation is used. A reasonable dose is determined by the patient after guidance.

Conclusions

Duodenal preserving pancreatectomy can be performed safely in the right patients. Selection is important and the procedure should only be performed in those patients in whom technical risks of doing the operation are reasonable. Whether this rather tedious dissection is appropriate and preferable to a standard total pancreatectomy is at present difficult to determine. Certainly, there are no more immediate complications and the only specific complication related to duodenal preserving pancreatectomy is an incidence of biliary stricture in 7 of 32 patients. Undoubtedly this complication could be reduced by a more careful dissection of the bile duct and after a difficult dissection with perhaps perforation of the biliary tree, performing an elective choledochoduodenostomy at the time of the original procedure.

The advantages of this procedure are fewer longterm complications with improved gastrointestinal function and diabetic control. The work of Linehan et al. [8] (Table 6), has shown that patients with duodenum-preserving total pancreatectomy have a more normal weight than those after a standard total pancreatectomy and a better control of their diabetes. Further, Linehan et al. [9] have shown that no dumping occurs with this operation. These are all factors which suggest that gastrointestinal function is more normal after this procedure, but assessment is so difficult in these patients and only prolonged studies with large numbers of patients will determine the merit of the procedure. Nevertheless, the argument is strong that the duodenum's alkaline tide and pacemaker function may well provide a more physiological setting for long-term management. Finally, this study has shown on contra-indication to perform the procedure and it is felt that as this operation may have advantage over the standard duodenal resection, it should be tried in appropriately selected patients as a way of offering a better quality of life in the long-term.

References

1. Cooper MJ, Williamson RCN, Benjamin IS et al. (1987) Total pancreatectomy for chronic pancreatitis. Br J Surg 74:912–915
2. Frey CF, Suzuki M, Isaji S, Zhu Y (1989) Pancreatic resection for chronic pancreatitis. Surg Clin North Am 69:499–528
3. Gough MH (1984) The surgical treatment of hyperinsulinism in infancy and childhood. Br J Surg 71:75–78
4. Harken AH, Filler RM, Auruskin TW, Crigler JF (1971) The role of total pancreatectomy in the treatment of unremitting hypoglycaemia of infancy. J Pediatr Surg 6:284–289
5. Keith RG, Saibil FG, Sheppard RH (1989) Treatment of chronic pancreatitis by pancreatic resection. Am J Surg 157:156–162
6. Kiviluotu T, Schröder T, Lempinen M (1985) Total pancreatectomy for chronic pancreatitis. Surg Gynaecol Obstet 160:223–227
7. Lambert MA, Linehan IP, Russell RCG (1987) Duodenum preserving total pancreatectomy for end stage chronic pancreatitis. Br J Surg 74:35–39
8. Linehan IP, Lambert MA, Brown DC, Kurtz AB, Cotton PB, Russell RCG (1988) Total pancreatectomy for chronic pancreatitis. Gut 29:358–365
9. Linehan IP, Russell RCG, Hobsley M (1988) The dumping syndrome after pancreatoduodenectomy. Surg Gynaecol Obstet 167:114–118
10. McAfee MK, van Heerden JA, Adson MA (1989) Is proximal pancreato-duodenectomy with pyloric preservation superior to total pancreatectomy? Surgery 105:347–351
11. Murphy JP, Russell RCG (1988) Operative treatment of nesidioblastosis. Br J Surg 75:930
12. Thomas LM, Langford RM, Russell RCG, Le Quesne LP (1978) The anatomical basis for gastric mobilisation in total oesophagectomy. Br J Surg 65:356–360
13. Traverso LW, Longmire WP (1979) Preservation of the pylorus in pancreatico-duodenectomy. A follow-up evaluation. Ann Surg 190:312–316
14. Trede M, Schwall G (1988) The complications of pancreatectomy. Ann Surg 207:39–47
15. Walsh TN, Rode J, Theis BA, Russell RCG (1991) Minimal change chronic pancreatitis. Gut (in press)
16. Warren KW, Poulantzas JK, Kune GA (1966) Life after total pancreatectomy for pancreatitis. Ann Surg 164:830–834

A New Procedure for Duodenum-Preserving Total Resection of the Head of the Pancreas with Pancreaticocholedochoduodenostomy

T. IMAIZUMI,[1] F. HANYU, and M. SUZUKI

Introduction

Since pancreatoduodenectomy was originally described by Whipple et al. [1] in 1935, the Whipple procedure has long been performed with modifications and refinements. The indications for the Whipple procedure have recently become widened. An extended radical pancreatoduodenectomy has been used for peripancreatic malignant diseases. On the other hand, organ-preserving procedures have been employed for the treatment of benign peripancreatic diseases. Traverso and Longmire [2], in 1978, performed the pylorus-preserving pancreatoduodenectomy for the first time, reporting gratifying results with low incidence of postoperative peptic ulceration. Various other methods for resection of the head of the pancreas were developed in succession. Beger et al. [3] described a subtotal resection of the head of the pancreas for chronic pancreatitis.

We recently developed a new, physiologically reconstructed and function-preserving procedure consisting of total resection of the head of the pancreas with pancreaticoduodenostomy and choledochoduodenostomy [4]. This article deals with the operative methods and with its early post-operative results.

Operative Techniques

The most outstanding feature of this operation is to resect the head of the pancreas completely without sacrificing the duodenum. After resection of the head of the pancreas the blood supply to the duodenum depends upon intramural blood flow. The blood supply to the distal portion (i.e., the infrapapillary and horizontal parts of the duodenum) is maintained by preserving the duodenal branches from the inferior pancreaticoduodenal artery or the so-called mesoduodenal vessels. As Kocher's mobilizing procedure is not performed, branches of the portal vein are drained into the retroperitoneum. Since the entire gland of the head of the pancreas can be

[1] Department of Gastroenterological Surgery, Tokyo Women's Medical College, Tokyo, Japan

Beger/Büchler/Malfertheiner (Eds.)
Standards in Pancreatic Surgery

resected while keeping the ganglion and the second part of the nerve plexus at the pancreatic head intact, and the pancreatic head is transected on the right border of the portal vein, very little damage to the endocrine and exocrine function of the pancreas is expected to result.

Exposure of the Head of the Pancreas

The front surface of the pancreas is exposed by dividing the gastrocolic omentum and opening the lesser sac via an upper median incision. Neither the duodenum nor the head of the pancreas is mobilized. After dissecting the right gastroepiploic artery and vein and tying them flush with the pancreas, the stomach is lifted so as not to injure the vessels. Then, the superior mesenteric vein is exposed at the inferior border of the pancreas. A finger passes along the main trunk of the portal vein from below upward. On the superior border of the pancreas the common hepatic artery is identified and the gastroduodenal artery is ligated and divided.

The pancreas is divided just above or to the right of the portal vein.

Division of the Bile Duct

After cholecystectomy the common bile duct is divided at the junction of the cystic duct. It is of the utmost important to dissect free and divide the bile duct by right lateral approach while taking care not to cause a damage to mesoduodenal vessels and lymphatic as well as nerve branches. The amputated bile duct is passed behind the duodenum, the gastric artery, and gastroduodenal artery.

Resection of the Head of the Pancreas

The head of the pancreas and the common bile duct are dissected out and divided (Fig. 1). While lifting them forwards, the parenchyma of the head of the pancreas is separated from the duodenum, with care being taken not to damage the duodenal wall. Retracting the distal stump of the pancreas anteriorly, all veins emptying into the portal vein are ligated and dissected from the retroperitoneum. Dissection of these veins is made as close to the edge of the head of the pancreas as possible. The uncinate process of the pancreas is resected very carefully so as to preserve the mesoduodenal vessels. This is usually enough to ensure an adequate blood supply to that portion of the duodenum which extends from the third part up to the second part of the duodenum. By separating the head of the pancreas from the duodenum superiorly, interiorly, anteriorly, and posteriorly towards the ampulla of Vater one can expose the accessory pancreatic duct, common bile duct and the pancreatic duct extramurally. Total resection of the head of the pancreas is completed by resection of the common bile duct and ligation of the common bile duct. The color of the mucosa of the preserved

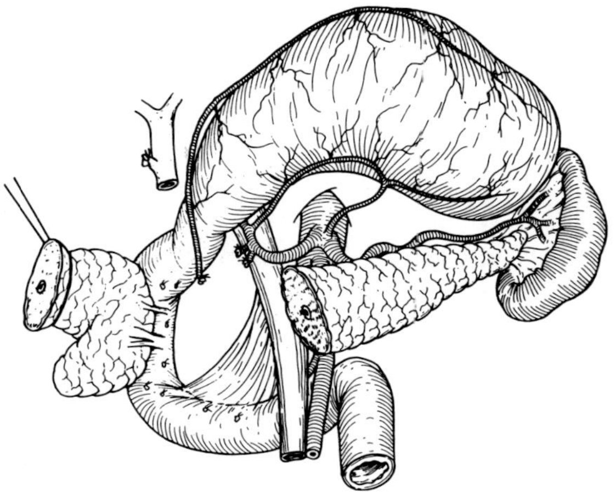

Fig. 1. The right gastric artery, the gastroduodenal artery, and the pancreatic branches of the inferior pancreatoduodenal artery are divided. The pancreas is transected on the right side of the portal vein to preserve as much gland of the body and tail of the pancreas as possible. The common bile duct is divided after cholecystectomy without disturbing the small vessels and branches of the nerves in the hepatoduodenal ligamentum

duodenum can be confirmed by inspection. The main pancreatic duct and the common bile duct are ligated and divided in the extramural portion of the duodenum without resection of the main papilla.

Gastrointestinal Reconstruction

The gastrointestinal reconstruction in our procedure is characterized by an end-to-side anastomosis of the residual pancreas and the common bile duct to the second part of the preserved duodenum (Fig. 2). After this type of the gastrointestinal reconstruction, no blind loop of the jejunum is exited.

It is very important for the pancreaticoduodenal anastomosis to preserve a well-perfused duodenum. As the pancreas is divided just superior to the portal vein, tension to the pancreaticoduodenal anastomosis is not unusual in this procedure. The technique of anastomosis between the pancreatic duct and the duodenal mucosa is basically the same as in ordinary pancreatico-jejunostomy, i.e. end-to-side two-layer suture. Choledochoduodenostomy is done in the usual end-to-side fashion with one-layer suture of the common bile duct to the anterior wall of the duodenum. A decompression tube is usually inserted in the stomach and the duodenum during the perioperative period.

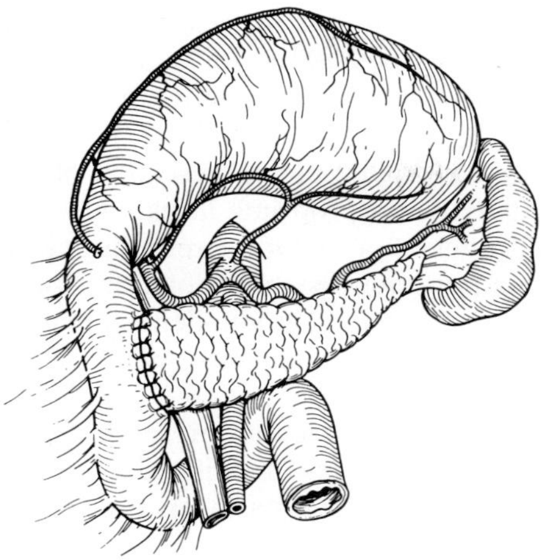

Fig. 2. End-to-side pancreaticoduodenostomy is performed. The blood supply to the duodenum is maintained by the duodenal branches from the inferior pancreatoduodenal artery and small vessels in the duodenal wall. The whole duodenum can be preserved without Kocher's mobilization

Early Postoperative Complications

Eleven patients had duodenum-preserving total resection of the head of the pancreas. No operative death occurred. Two patients experienced minor pancreatic fistulas, and one patient experienced minor bile leakage. No patient required a further operation. The amount of gastric discharge was acceptably small, 250–780 ml/day, mean 550 ml/day. All patients showed adequate construction of the stomach and duodenum on the barium study 7 days after the operation and were able to take solid food. The median follow-up time in the 11 patients was less than 6 months, with a range of 3–13 months. No patient died and no patient required reoperation. All patients attained normal daily activity.

Discussion

A variety of surgical procedures have been performed in the resection of the head of the pancreas. In Whipple's [1] original pancreatoduodenectomy, resection of the duodenum was indicated to avoid ischemic necrosis and fistulation of the duodenum. The head of the pancreas and the duodenum are so closely related to each other, both anatomically and embryologically, that dissection of the head of the pancreas from the duodenum was thought to be impossible. Warren [5] showed that the original Whipple operation was associated with a 17% incidence of anastomotic ulceration postoperatively. He argued that a more radical gastrectomy was necessary, and after his procedure the jejunal ulceration rate was reduced to 7.5%. Ever since then, the standard Whipple procedure includes duodenectomy and partial gastrectomy.

In 1978, Traverso and Longmire [2] argued that radical resection of the stomach following pancreatoduodenectomy is inappropriate in patients with benign peripancreatic disease and introduced a pylorus-preserving procedure, with gratifying results concerning postoperative nutritional function. After the introduction of pylorus-preserving pancreatoduodenectomy by Traverso and Longmire, many surgeons have performed this operation for patients with benign peripancreatic disease.

Recently Beger et al. [3] have reported a duodenum-preserving subtotal resection of the head of the pancreas as a new modification of the pancreatectomy for patients with chronic pancreatitis. It has been augmented to supply an adequate blood flow to the duodenum after the resection of the head of the pancreas. The authors reported that preservation of the gastroduodenal artery is not mandatory for duodenal blood flow and performed subtotal resection of the head of the pancreas, including the uncinate process, but the common bile duct and the rim of the pancreatic tissue remained and both the stomach and the duodenum were preserved. The blood flow of the duodenum depends primarily upon the vessels in the mesoduodenum and retroperitoneum. He also indicated that total resection of the mesoduodenum may produce damage to the duodenal wall and may cause early postoperative complications, such as hemorrhage, intra-abdominal abscess and pancreatic fistula.

In the report by Frey et al. [6], the authors described a 95% distal pancreatectomy with preservation of the rim of the pancreatic tissue along the duodenum wall and the bile duct, stressing the importance of preservation of the superior and inferior pancreatoduodenal arteries and their branches for adequate blood supply to the duodenum.

Lambert et al. [7] performed a total pancreatectomy with preservation of the duodenum and bile duct in 14 patients with end-stage chronic pancreatitis. The blood supply to the duodenum could be maintained through the mesoduodenal vessel and the gastroepiploic artery as well as those vessels from the superior mesenteric artery. After the dissection of these vessels in his procedure, the duodenum usually assumed a dusky blue color but actively contracted on stimulation. Although the postoperative appearance of the duodenum on the barium examination suggested ischemia in some cases, no patients experienced necrosis, fistula or ulceration postoperatively. Only one patient required surgical treatment because of bile duct stenosis.

Ryo et al. [8] have recently succeeded in duodenum-preserving total resection of the head of the pancreas with pancreaticojejunostomy. The blood supply to the third and fourth parts of the duodenum is important in this procedure.

The removal of the uncinate process of the pancreas should be performed to dissect out the vessels which pass from the superior mesenteric artery and vein to the pancreas. Care has to be taken to preserve the branches from the inferior pancreatoduodenal artery to the third part of the duodenum.

Although some patients in our series showed bluish discoloration of the suprapapillary segment of the duodenum, the postpyloric portion of the duodenum could be maintained even by a little intramural blood flow, and no patients required segmental resection of the duodenum. The pancreatic tissue can be dissected off without Kocher's mobilization so as not to damage the small vessels in the connective tissues between the duodenum and the retroperitoneum.

Ryo anastomosed the residual pancreas to the jejunum lifted by Roux-en-Y loop. In our procedure, the residual pancreas is anastomosed to the second part of the duodenum without interrupting the continuity of the gastrointestinal tract. Pancreatic juice and bile are not diverted but can flow into the duodenum to restore its normal function in terms of secretion of the gastrointestinal hormones, motility, and acid neutralization of the duodenum. This type of the gastrointestinal reconstruction can be accomplished most physiologically after the resection of the head of the pancreas.

Intractable gastric stasis after pylorus-preserving pancreaticoduodenectomy has been reported; all patients in our series, however, were able to have solid food early after operation without developing any symptoms.

The strict indications for the duodenum-preserving total resection of the head of the pancreas have not been settled. Benign peripancreatic diseases including chronic pancreatitis, anomalous junction of the pancreatico-biliary ductal system, malformation of the pancreatic duct, and cystic disease of the head of the pancreas might be good indications for this operation. The number of patients who received this operation was not high enough to evaluate its effectiveness. Long-term results after the operation have not yet obtained. It might be said that this procedure can replace pylorus-preserving pancreaticoduodenectomy in some patients with benign peripancreatic disease.

References

1. Whipple AO, Parsons WB, Mullins CR (1935) Treatment of carcinoma of the ampulla of Vater. Ann Surg 102:763–779
2. Traverso LW, Longmire WP (1978) Preservation of the pylorus in pancreaticoduodenectomy. Surg Gynecol Obstet 146:959–962
3. Beger HG, Krautzberger W, Bittner R et al. (1985) Duodenum-preserving resection of the head of the pancreas in patients with severe pancreatitis. Surgery 97:467–473
4. Imaizumi T, Hanyu F, Suzuki M et al. (1990) A new procedure: duodenum-preserving total resection of the head of the pancreas with pancreatico-choledocho-duodenostomy (in Japanese). J Bil Tract Pancreas 11:621–626

5. Warren WD (1969) Surgical management of chronic relapsing pancreatitis. Am J Surg 117:24–32
6. Frey CF, Child CG, Fry W (1976) Pancreatectomy for chronic pancreatitis. Ann Surg 184:403–412
7. Lambert MA, Linehan IP, Russell RCG (1987) Duodenum-preserving total pancreatectomy for end stage chronic pancreatitis. Br J Surg 74:35–39
8. Ryo H, Hanyu F, Watayo T et al. (1990) A new procedure for total resection of the head of the pancreas with duodenal preservation (in Japanese). Operation 44:447–451

Local Resection of the Head of the Pancreas Combined with Longitudinal Pancreaticojejunostomy: An Update

C.F. Frey[1] and B.F. Leary

Introduction

The "ideal" operation for the patient with chronic pancreatitis should have a low mortality and morbidity, be easy to perform, provide pain relief, rectify the structural abnormalities such as common bile duct obstruction, and not augment exocrine and endocrine insufficiency [1].

In 1987, we published a description of a new operation with application to patients with chronic pancreatitis having pain, a multiply strictured main pancreatic duct, and diseased pancreatic head and uncinate process [2] (Figs. 1–4). We envisioned the local resection of the pancreatic head (LRH) combined with longitudinal pancreaticojejunostomy (LPJ) to be particularly useful in patients with a markedly enlarged fibrotic pancreatic head and uncinate process. (Fig. 5) In such patients, the duct of Wirsung, Santorini, and duct to the uncinate process along with their tributary ducts are often impacted with calculi and behind these calculi lie dilated strictured ducts and retention cysts. It was also thought the operation would have application to patients with enlarged fibrotic pancreatic head associated with common duct (Fig. 6) or duodenal obstruction due to fibrosis and inflammation or compression by pseudocysts or retention cysts.

We felt the local resection of the head of the pancreas would contribute to improved drainage of the duct of Wirsung, Santorini, and duct to the uncinate process over and above that provided by LPJ even if properly performed according to the Partington-Rochelle technique [3], i.e., the duct of Wirsung opened from tail of pancreas to duodenum. It has long been recognized that the results of LPJ with regard to pain relief tend to deteriorate overtime, not just from an inadequate opening of the main duct of Wirsung but from unrelieved disease in the head of the pancreas from the obstructed ducts of Santorini and duct to the uncinate process as well as obstruction to their tributary ducts and associated retention cysts [1] (Figs. 7, 8). In patients who had previously had a LPJ who were not relieved of pain or developed recurrent pain, the procedure is easily adapted. The

[1] University of California, Davis Medical Center, Department of Surgery, 4301 X Street, Room 2310, Sacramento, CA 95817, USA

Beger/Büchler/Malfertheiner (Eds.)
Standards in Pancreatic Surgery

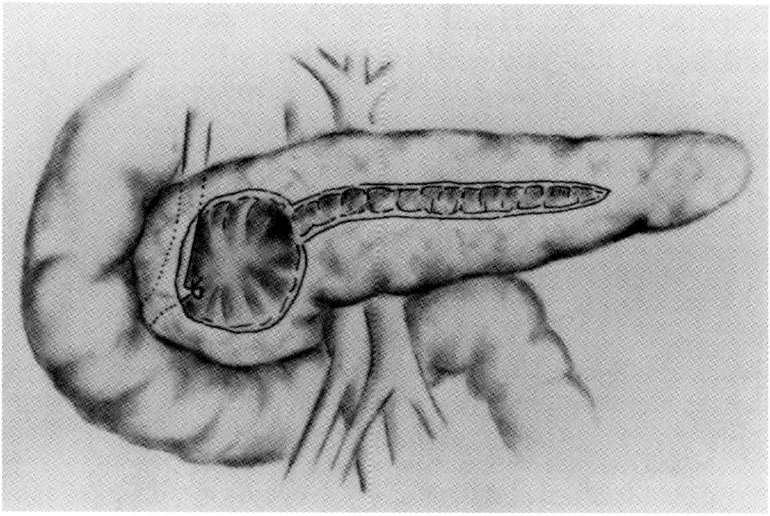

Fig. 1. Coring out the pancreatic head and uncinate process decompresses the common bile duct if obstructed. Most of the major pancreatic duct in the head of the pancreas is excised. The major pancreatic duct is filleted open and remains in continuity in the body and tail of the pancreas as in the Rochelle-Partington modification of the Puestow procedure

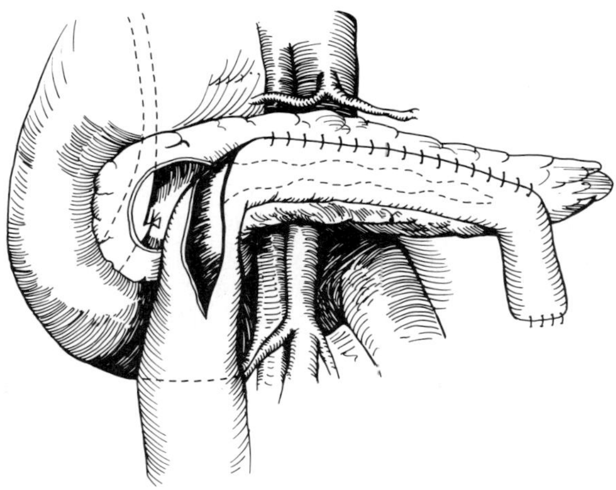

Fig. 2. The cored-out pancreatic head and uncinate process are drained in continuity with the main pancreatic duct by means of a Roux-en-Y limb of jejunum. Exocrine secretion from the pancreatic remnant in the head and uncinate process is drained into the Roux-en-Y limb, rather than into the peritoneal cavity as occurs in the 95% pancreatectomy or Warren procedure

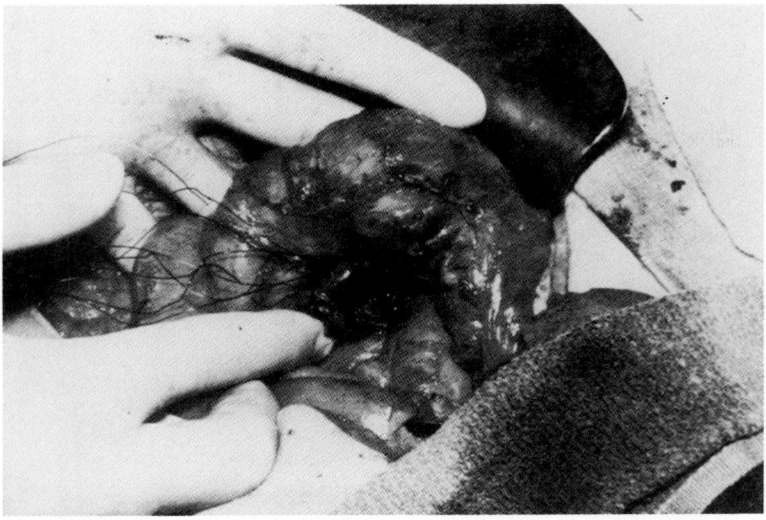

Fig. 3. Cored-out pancreatic head with hemostatic sutures placed along the inner aspect of the duodenal C

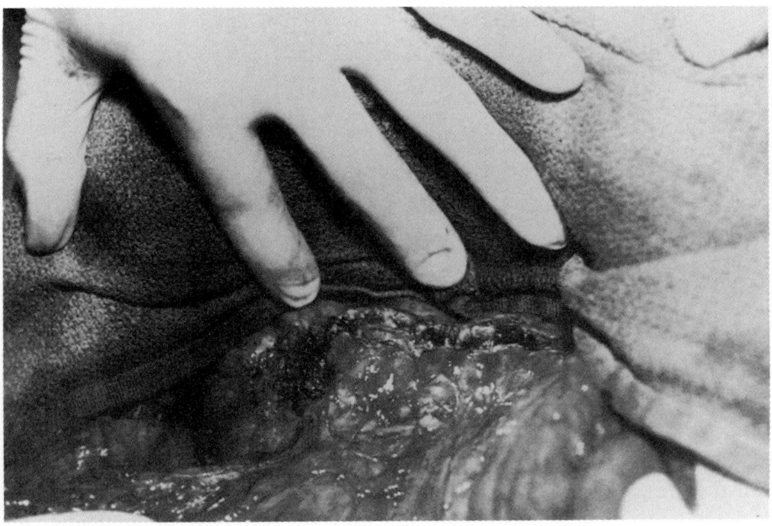

Fig. 4. Cored-out pancreatic head in continuity with dilated main pancreatic duct in body and tail of the pancreas

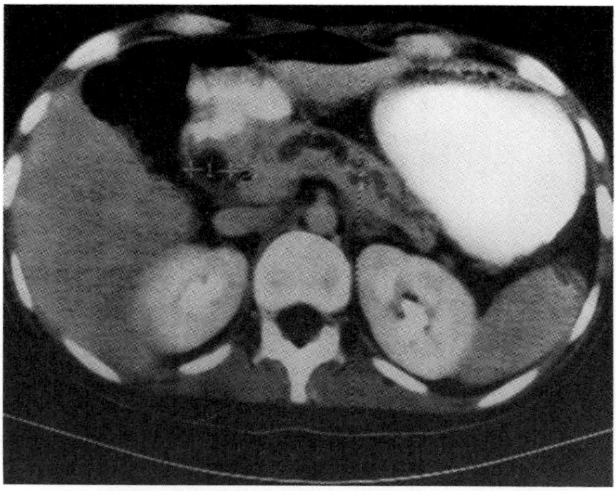

a

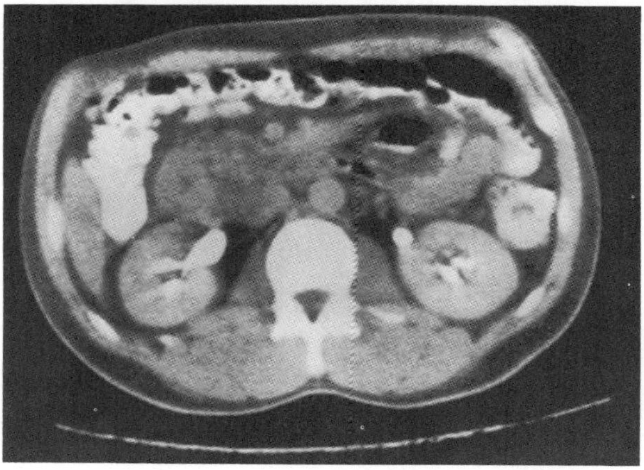

b

Fig. 5. a Dilated common bile duct, enlarged pancreatic head, and "chain of lakes" appearance of pancreatic duct seen on CT scan. **b** Enlarged pancreatic head seen on CT scan

proximal attachment of the Roux-en-Y limb to the head of the pancreas is detached and the head of the pancreas and uncinate process cored out. The Roux-en-Y limb is then reattached to the rim of the pancreas along the inner aspect of the duodenal cuff.

Unlike some surgeons such as Keith et al. [4] who are reluctant to perform a LPJ in patients whose main duct in the body and tail is less than 1 cm in diameter, we will drain ducts as small as 5 mm in diameter. We feel this is feasible as we sew to the capsule of the pancreas. Unlike an end-to-side pancreaticojejunostomy in which we feel a duct to mucosa anastomosis

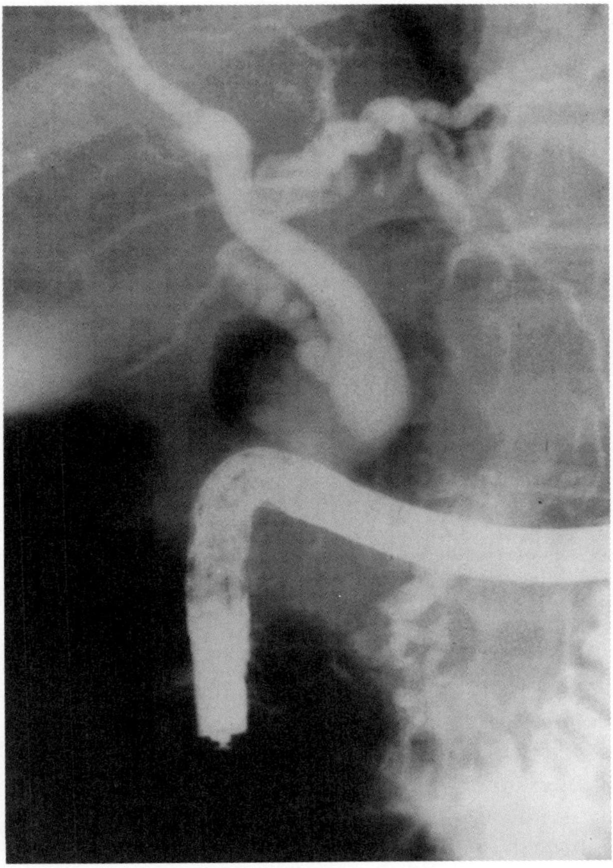

Fig. 6. Dilated common bile duct and proximal stricture of main pancreatic duct

is essential to patency of the anastomosis, we do not feel a duct to mucosa anastomosis is necessary in a side-to-side pancreaticojejunostomy. In fact, a duct to mucosa anastomosis in patients with what some surgeons consider "small" pancreatic ducts (e.g., 5 mm) could be harmful as the potential for obstruction by suture of tributary ducts entering at right angles to the main duct is greater than if the suture lines involve the capsule of the pancreas.

The principal features of the operation are as follows: (a) the obstructed main pancreatic duct in the body and tail of the pancreas is opened fully and drained into a Roux-en-Y limb (b), the head of the pancreas is cored out to the depth of the posterior wall of the main pancreatic duct and a rim of pancreatic tissue is left along the inner aspect of the duodenum, and (c) the Roux-en-Y limb is extended and sutured to the rim of pancreatic tissue on the inner aspect of the duodenum. The Roux-en-Y limb drains the cored out

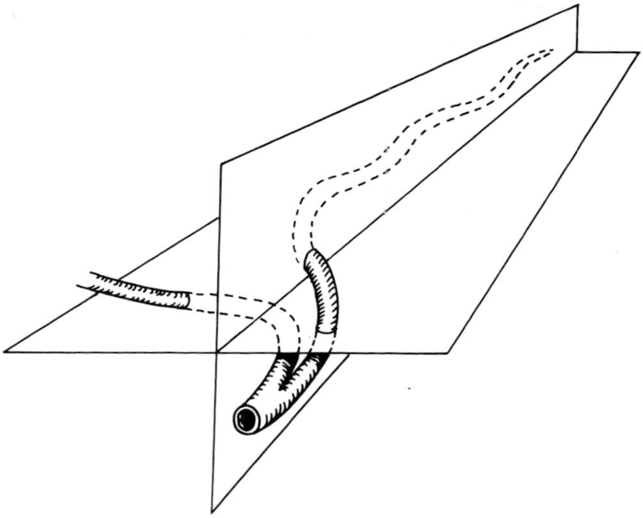

Fig. 7. The major pancreatic duct in the body and tail of the pancreas lies in a horizontal plane while the duct in the head of the pancreas moves in an anteroposterior direction towards the ampulla

head of pancreas and uncinate process as well as the main pancreatic duct in the body and tail. (For details of the procedure see [2].)

The operation was developed with the objective of providing a simpler and less time consuming operation with a lower operative mortality than pancreaticoduodenectomy with or without pyloric preservation and by removing less pancreatic mass than either 80%–95% distal pancreatectomy or pancreaticoduodenectomy reducing the operatively induced incidence of exocrine and endocrine insufficiency.

Our operation combines the advantages of the Beger [5] procedure: (a) In addressing the problem of extensive pancreatic head disease characterized by multiple strictures and retention cysts involving the duct of Santorini, Wirsung, and duct to the uncinate process (a situation in which LPJ is most likely to fail) with decompression of a dilated main duct in the body and tail of the pancreas (5 mm or greater) in which LPJ is usually successful. (b) We feel our operation is easier to perform than the Beger procedure or denervated splenopancreatic flap operation described by Warren et al. [3] both of which require dividing the neck of the pancreas and in the case of the denervated splenopancreatic flap, ligation of the splenic artery and vein. The Warren [3] procedure suffers from the same perioperative complications encountered in the Child 80%–95% pancreatectomy (i.e., a high incidence of short-lived pancreatic fistulas and infected collections emanating from the remaining pancreatic tissue about the inner aspect of the duodenum. Short-lived fistulas and infected collections of pancreatic juice

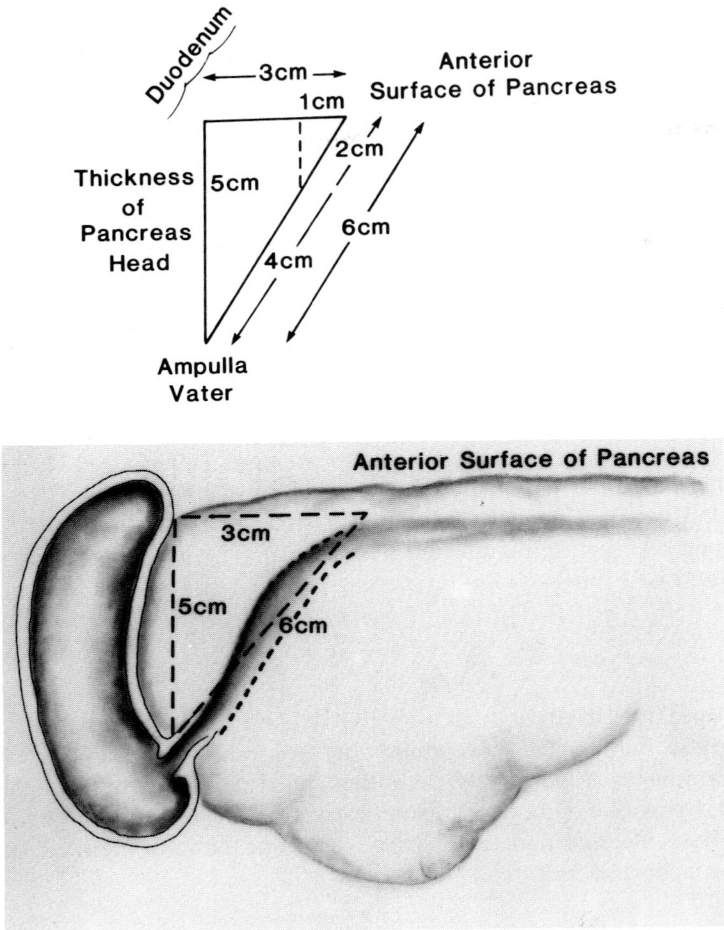

Fig. 8. If the pancreatic head is 5 cm thick, and the distance 3 cm from duodenum to the point on the main pancreatic duct at which the duct courses posteriorly and inferiorly, the distance from the junction of the ventral and dorsal duct to the ampulla of Vater is 6 cm. Filleting open this portion of the main duct in the head of the pancreas toward the duodenum for 1 cm as measured on the anterior surface of the gland leaves 4 cm of the major pancreatic duct in the head of the pancreas undrained and obstructed and 2 cm of duct drained through a 1-cm opening

were described in two of their five patients [6], similar to the incidence of these complications following the 80%–95% resection in the Child procedure [7].

At the time the description of our operation was published in 1987, we reported on six patients in whom the procedure had been performed [2].

We have now performed 30 local resections of the head of the pancreas combined with LPJ.

Patient Population

Of the 30 patients coming to operation, 10 (33.3%) were women and 20 (66.6%) men. Twenty-eight (93.3%) of the patients had a history of alcohol abuse. Symptoms of chronic pancreatitis had been present on the average for 6 years prior to operation. Twenty-nine (96.7%) smoked cigarettes. The number of patients undergoing operation in the years from 1985 to 1991 have been: 1, 5, 2, 1, 6, 11, and 4; since the largest number of operations were performed in 1989, 1990, and 1991, the majority of our patients have had less than a 3-year follow-up (average 2.3 years). Previous pancreatic surgery excluding cholecystectomy had been performed on 11 (36%) of the 30 patients. Six (20%) of the patients had had a previous LPJ, four (13%) a cystgastrostomy, and three patients (10%) a distal pancreatectomy. At the time of operation, two patients had duodenal obstruction, and one patient, common bile duct obstruction manifested by jaundice. The length of follow-up after LRH and LPJ ranges from 0 to 6 years.

Results

There was no operative mortality. There were two late deaths. One patient died from hepatic failure and encephalopathy secondary to cirrhosis of the liver 6 months postoperatively. Another patient died from fungal endocarditis and a stroke 4 months postoperatively. Five patients (16.6%) were found to have infected pancreatic juice, calculi or tissue in the head of the pancreas on operative cultures.

Operative Complications

No patients developed a leak, fistula, or abscess postoperatively. There were four postoperative complications in four patients (13%). Two patients were reexplored 2 and 5 days following operation for signs of sepsis, but no intraabdominal pathology was detected in either patient. One of these two patients later died from fungal endocarditis and a stroke. A third patient was readmitted 3 months post operatively for drainage of infected ascites. This patient later died from hepatic failure encephalopathy secondary to cirrhosis of the liver. A fourth patient who had an intrapancreatic stricture of the pancreatic duct and a elevation of alkaline phosphates, but normal bilirubin developed obstructive jaundice postoperatively. An attempt at endoscopic placement of a stent and transhepatic drainage were not successful necessitating T-tube drainage of the common bile duct on the 5th postoperative day. The common bile duct on cholangiography appeared unchanged in appearance, and the obstruction was presumed to be the result of edema and inflammation associated with the operation.

Late Complications

One of the 30 patients developed duodenal obstruction 2 years after LRH and LPJ. The patient was treated by gastrojejunostomy. The patient had been totally free of pain.

Diabetes

Eight patients (26.6%) prior to operation were diabetic; five required insulin, one oral medication and two dietary control. Postoperatively, nine patients (30%) were diabetic. The two patients whose diabetes was controlled by diet, and the one patient controlled by oral medication preoperatively required insulin postoperatively. One patient who had not been diabetic prior to operation in spite of a distal pancreatectomy prior to LRH and LPJ became diabetic after excision of 6 g tissue in the head of the pancreas and required insulin therapy.

Exocrine Status

Twenty-one (70%) of the 30 patients gave a history of steatorrhea preoperatively. Of these patients, 18 (86%) were treated preoperatively with pancreatic enzyme therapy consisting of enteric coated microspheres, i.e., pancrease of creon and H-2 blocker therapy with cimetidine, ranitidine, or famotidine. Postoperatively, 26 of 27 patients (96.3%) were treated with pancreatic enzymes and H-2 blocker therapy. Steatorrhea was reported in four patients. In two patients, the diarrhea occurred only occasionally, and these patients gained 5–8 lbs, respectively, postoperatively. In two patients, steatorrhea was a significant problem postoperatively in spite of enzyme therapy and in one patient resulted in rehospitalization.

Weight

Insufficient time has elapsed since operation to assess the effect of the operation on the patients' weight in six patients. In the other 24 patients, the data must be considered preliminary. Twelve patients (80%) had a mean weight gain at last follow-up of 12.4 lb. Twelve patients (50%) had a mean weight loss of 4 lb on last follow-up.

Pain Control

Preoperatively all 30 patients were taking oral medication daily, consisting of either Tylenol 3 or Vicodin; 18 of the 30 patients (60%) were also taking more potent narcotics, either Demerol, morphine, or Percocet on a daily basis. Postoperatively, 17 of 28 patients (61%) were occasionally taking Tylenol 3 or Vicodin. Two patients, at one time or another postoperatively, required Demerol, morphine, or Percocet. One of these two patients has not required these more potent narcotics at any time for the last 3 years. Regarding patients' perception of pain, excluding the two patients that died at 4 and 6 months after operation, all but two patients (7%) feel they have significantly benefited with regard to pain relief.

Work Status

No statistically significant change in work status occurred during the period of follow-up. The one-third of patients working preoperatively returned to work postoperatively. There was no evidence of improved work status associated with pain relief.

Continued Alcoholism

Twenty-one of 28 patients (75%) on whom we had good information discontinued alcohol preoperatively. Three additional patients (11%) discontinued alcohol postoperatively. Two patients have continued to abuse alcohol, and two may be continuing to imbibe alcohol.

Drug Addiction

We continue to find drug addiction difficult to assess preoperatively and postoperatively in some patients.

Discussion

In reviewing the results of LRH and LPJ and comparing them with the ideal operation, the following conclusions seem warranted. The operation is associated with a low mortality (0%) and morbidity (13.3%). Operatively induced diabetes is unlikely to occur in patients in the immediate postoperative period in the absence of preoperative diabetes, except when a pancreatic resection has been performed (distal pancreatectomy) previously. The average period of follow-up of our patients is insufficient to assess the impact of ductal decompression on preserving pancreatic endocrine and exocrine function over time. Nealon et al. [8] have reported stabilization of exocrine and endocrine function after LPJ when performed relatively early in the course of chronic pancreatitis. In contrast, our patients all had advanced disease, particularly in the head of the pancreas, so that we anticipate progressive loss of exocrine and endocrine function.

We did not routinely assess pancreatic exocrine function in patients following operation. Patients were usually placed on a regimen of pancreatic enzyme replacement and H-2 blocker therapy. Patients who had persistent steatorrhea in spite of enzyme replacement were studied.

Half of our patients have had significant weight gain postoperatively, with a mean weight increase of 12 lb compared to their preoperative weight. The other half of our patients who did not gain weight or lost weight had a mean weight loss of 4 lb compared to their preoperative weight. There seems to be a period of time needed following the operation to find the dosage of pancreatic enzymes the patient will find acceptable. Many patients complain of constipation with pancreatic enzyme therapy and unilaterally cut back intake of these enzymes in order to have a softer, looser bowel movement even though they know it may affect their weight. When patients fail to gain weight following operation, the cause is usually inadequate consumption of pancreatic enzymes.

Over 90% of our patients have experienced pain relief with the operation. One patient operated on 4 years ago experienced a period of complete pain relief but over the past 6 months has returned with complaints of pain. Objectively, the requirement for pain medication in terms of potency, quantity, and frequency has been markedly reduced in most patients. However, our findings in these patients regarding pain relief based on the relatively short period of follow-up should be considered preliminary. We were asked for the purpose of this conference to update our results on LRH and LPJ which we were happy to do, but we feel constrained to emphasize that the average length of follow-up should be 3–5 years before any legitimate claims can be made for an operation regarding long-term pain relief, work status, and the incidence of late complications [9]. It should be noted not all patients with chronic pancreatitis in whom the pancreatic head seemed the main locus of disease were considered candidates for LRH and LPJ.

We continue to feel there is no one operation which addresses all the complications associated with chronic pancreatitis. We feel some patients will do better with pylorus-preserving resection of the head of the pancreas when there is both duodenal and common bile duct obstruction associated with jaundice, and a less than 5-mm main pancreatic duct, or microabscesses in the head of the pancreas.

During the 1985–1991 interval corresponding to the time period covered in this update, we performed five pancreaticoduodenectomies with pylorus preservation in patients who had a combination of duodenal and common bile duct obstruction and marked disease of the head and a major pancreatic duct less than 5 mm in diameter. Two of the five patients had microabscesses of the pancreatic head and had experienced intermittent fevers preoperatively. An additional patient, suspected of having pancreatic cancer, underwent pancreaticoduodenectomy but was found to have chronic pancreatitis. In patients with main pancreatic ducts less than 5 mm in diameter in whom disease is limited to the body and or tail of the pancreas and the head of the pancreas is normal as determined by computed tomography and ERCP, distal pancreatectomy is the procedure of choice.

The role of LPJ in our hands over the past 3 years has diminished. We are now performing more LRH combined with LPJ than LPJ alone. LPJ is now reserved only for patients with a very thin pancreatic head 2–2.25 cm – in whom we are relatively certain that disease is limited principally to the duct of Wirsung. We have been surprised at the frequency of infection in the diseased pancreatic heads of patients with chronic pancreatitis and feel this finding deserves further study.

Conclusion

We continue to pursue with enthusiasm the role of LRH combined with LPJ in the management of selected patients with chronic pancreatitis, particularly those patients with enlarged fibrotic calcified pancreatic heads and major pancreatic ducts in the body and tail which are enlarged to 5 mm or more. We feel the operation is particularly useful in patients with failed LPJ. The operation is relatively simple to perform and is associated with a low operative morbidity and mortality. Operatively induced diabetes or exocrine insufficiency is unlikely in the patient who is nondiabetic or had no steatorrhea preoperatively. Weight gain after operation largely depends on finding the level of pancreatic enzyme replacement the patient will tolerate.

While pain relief in our patients has been encouraging to date, the length of follow-up of just over 2 years is not sufficient to make any more than preliminary conclusions at this time.

References

1. Frey CF, Suzuki M, Isaji S, Zhu YV (1989) Pancreatic resection for chronic pancreatitis. Surg Clin North Am 69:499–528
2. Frey CF, Smith JG (1987) Description and rationale of a new operation for chronic pancreatitis. Pancreas 2:701–707
3. Partington PF, Rochelle RL (1969) Modified Puestow procedure for retrograde drainage of the pancreatic duct. Ann Surg 152:1037–1043
4. Keith RG, Sabil FG, Sheppard RH (1989) Treatment of chronic pancreatitis by pancreatic resection. Am J Surg 157:156
5. Beger HG, Krautzberger W, Bittner R et al. (1985) Duodenum preserving resection of the head of the pancreas in patients with severe chronic pancreatitis. Surgery 97:467–473
6. Shires GT, Warren WP, Milliken WJ et al. (1986) Denervated splenopancreatic flap for chronic pancreatitis. Ann Surg 203:568–573
7. Frey CF, Child CG, Fry W (1976) Pancreatectomy for chronic pancreatitis. Ann Surg 184:403–413
8. Nealon WH, Townsend CM Jr, Thompson JC (1988) Operative drainage of pancreatic duct delays functional impairment in patients with chronic pancreatitis. A prospective analysis. Ann Surg 208:321
9. Frey CF, Braasch J (1984) Surgical management of chronic pancreatitis: the need to improve our observation and assessment of results. Am J Surg 147:189–190

Comparison of Pancreatic Function and Life Quality After Whipple and Duodenum-Preserving Resection

I. Klempa, J. Menzel, H. Morr, and I. Baca[1]

Introduction

In about half of all cases, chronic pancreatitis is accompanied by severe inflammatory changes in the head of the pancreas [1, 2]. The primary goals of surgical therapy in pancreatitis of this type are pain relief and the avoidance of local complications [3, 7].

Given an indication for surgery, such as distal common bile duct obstruction, duodenal stenosis, or dilated pancreatic duct with stones and congestion, the surgeon must decide the type of operation to perform. A duodenopancreatectomy, the Whipple procedure, is widely considered to be the gold standard [3, 4]. It is highly effective in relieving pain and eliminating the structural abnormalities noted above. However, a duodenopancreatectomy is not appropriate if one desires to change or to improve the functional status of the exocrine pancreas. To improve functional results, we developed our own procedure as early as in the 1970s. This is principally a stomach-preserving duodenopancreatectomy with an additional vagotomy. In 1978 we reported on ten patients who had been operated on according to this concept [5]. In 1979 a quite similar procedure, the pylorus-preserving duodenopancreatectomy, was presented by Traverso and Longmire [9].

In the attempt to obtain the most satisfactory functional results, the duodenum-preserving resection of the head of the pancreas represents the real mainstay – inaugurated in 1972 by Beger. In our opinion this type of operation represents the most significant procedure today for the treatment of pancreatitis of the head of the gland [1, 10]. Nevertheless, the correct treatment for chronic pancreatitis is still open to discussion. Making a decision about the best treatment remains crucial. Although at first glance, the Beger procedure is most promising from a technical point of view and often a rational alternative to the Whipple procedure from a physiological point of view, we still have much to learn. Until now there exists no direct comparison which would allow us to prefer one procedure over the other on the basis of sufficient data, for example, postoperative hormone secretion after a standardized meal.

---

[1] Klinik für Allgemein- und Gefäßchirurgie (Direktor: Prof. Dr. med. I. Klempa), Zentralkrankenhaus, St.-Jürgen-Straße, W-2800 Bremen, FRG

Beger/Büchler/Malfertheiner (Eds.)
Standards in Pancreatic Surgery

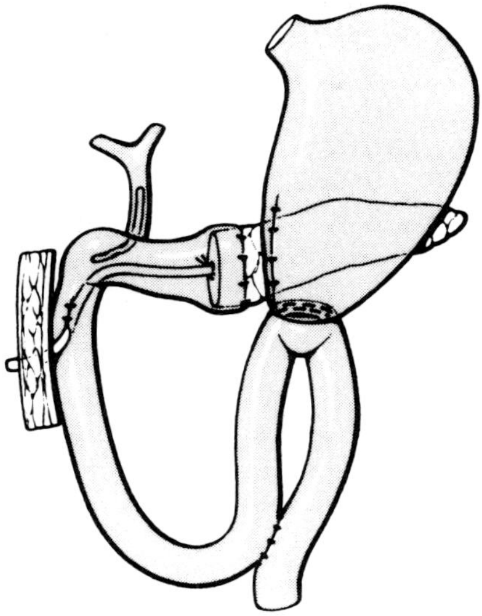

Fig. 1. The standard Whipples procedure. Note: A small silicone catheter is put into the duct of the pancreatic remnant and is brought out through the abdominal wall

Patients and Methods

In an ongoing prospective, randomized clinical trial, we are evaluating the effectiveness of the standard duodenopancreatectomy and the duodenum-preserving resection of the head of the pancreas in patients with chronic pancreatitis. In all cases an indication for a resection is mandatory. We consider the postoperative course, the perioperative mortality, and post-operative complications as parameters for our evaluation. As concerns long-term results, the postoperative hormonal status (insulin, neurotensin, cholecystokinin, and gastrin) is checked with basal and stimulated standard assay kits. Stimulation is performed with a standardized meal.

The following presentation is restricted to the first 20 cases. It is therefore a preliminary report.

In all patients included in this study, a diagnosis of chronic pancreatitis was established at least 3 years prior to surgery. They all underwent the usual medical treatment. Preoperative examinations included the following: history (pain, alcohol), physical examination, plain abdominal X-ray, ultrasound of the abdomen, computed tomography of the abdomen, endoscopic retrograde cholangio pancreatography, and angiography (in cases of suspected carcinoma).

An indication for surgery was based on one or more of the following criteria: pain untreatable with analgesics, bile duct obstruction, duodenal

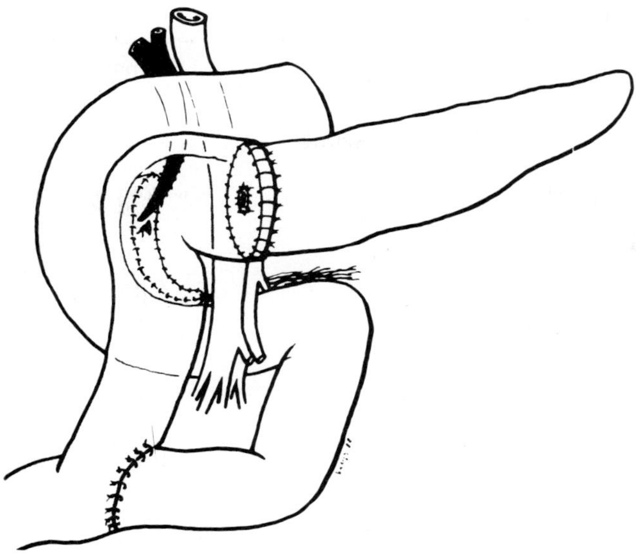

Fig. 2. The duodenum-preserving resection of the pancreatic head

stenosis, symptomatic stones in the pancreatic duct with dilation, obstruction of the pancreatic duct in the head of the gland, and multiple pseudocysts in the head of the pancreas.

The 20 patients were randomly assigned to undergo a standard Whipple procedure (Fig. 1) or a duodenum-preserving resection of the pancreatic head (Fig. 2). In six cases, we had to add a choledochojejunostomy about 10 cm distal to the pancreaticojejunal anastomosis because of subtotal stenosis of the common bile duct. The preoperative status of the patients is described in Table 1.

Results

Unfortunately, we had one fatal outcome in the group treated with the duodenum-preserving procedure. This patient died from sepsis originating from a colonic anastomosis. A transverse colonic resection had to be carried out simultaneously. In the group with the Whipple procedure we encountered two postoperative bleedings, both requiring reoperation. Further, we observed a gastric outlet syndrome in two patients, which was considered a complication. The mean hospital stay was 5 days shorter in the duodenum-preserving group. Over all, their recovery was quicker and easier. The period of postoperative follow-up now ranges from 8 to 30 months. None of the patients needed further surgery. One patient in each group has died

Table 1. Preoperative status of patients

	DPRHP (n = 10)	Whipple (n = 10)
Etiology		
Alcohol	9	8
Idiopathic	1	2
Mean time of manifestation (years)	4.5	3.8
Abdominal pain	10	10
Opioid analgesics	7	6
Obstruction		
Biliary	4	4
Duodenal	2	3
Diabetes mellitus		
No diabetes	8	7
Insulin dependent	–	2
Latent	2	1
Preliminary operation		
Puestow procedure	–	1

DPRHP, duodenum-preserving resection of the head of the pancreas.

Table 2. Late results after operation (patient follow-up 8–30 months)

	DPRHP (n = 8)	Whipple (n = 9)
Abdominal pain		
No pain	7	6
Tolerable	1	1
Strong	–	1
Requiring analgesics	–	1
Diabetes		
Insulin dependent	1	2
Increase in weight (kg)	8.6	5.5
Professional rehabilitation	7	6
Late mortality (24, 27 months postoperatively)	1	1

DPRHP, duodenum-preserving resection of the head of the pancreas.

in the meantime, 2 and 2.5 years after operation, from liver failure due to continuing excessive alcohol consumption and from carcinoma in the pancreatic remnant.

At the time of the last check-up eight patients in the Beger group presented in a good clinical status, not requiring any substitution of pancreatic enzymes. Seven patients were at their regular job. The mean weight gain in this group was 8.6 kg. Seven patients were free of pain; one had complaints closely related to the intake of alcohol. In one case diabetes, was a problem postoperatively. In the Whipple group six of nine patients were free of pain. These six were working at their jobs again. The mean

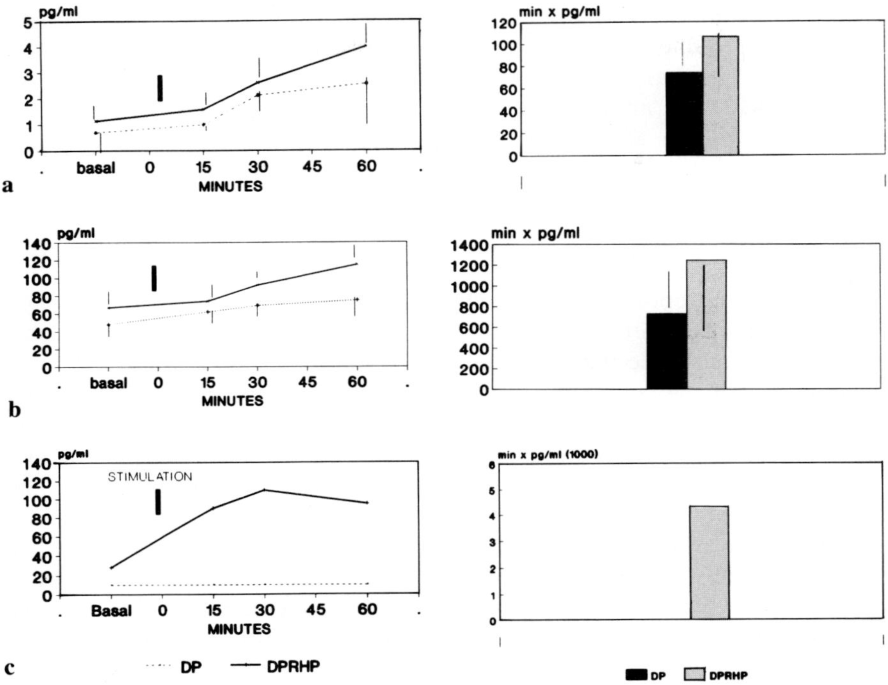

Fig. 3a–c. Secretion of hormones (*left*) and the integrated total response (*right*) after stimulation with a standardized meal. *DP*, Duodenopancreatectomy; *DPRHP*, duodenum-preserving resection of the head of the pancreas. **a** Cholecystokinin. **b** Neurotensin. **c** Gastrin

weight gain in this group was 5.6 kg. Two patients suffered from diabetes postoperatively. Table 2 summarizes the clinical status of the two groups.

Hormonal Status

Figure 3a shows the secretion of cholecystokinin and the total response after stimulation with a standard meal. The values range within normal limits in both groups but are higher in the group with an intact duodenum. This is also true for the total response, with an about 40% higher output of the hormone. A quite similar finding exists for insulin. The secretion and the total response was more favorable in the group with intact duodenum in comparison to the Whipple group. Figure 3b shows the results for neurotensin. In both groups basal values are elevated. After a meal, in the Whipple group there was almost no increase. The integrated total response was about 50% higher in the group with preserved duodenum. Thus for cholecystokinin, insulin, and neurotensin no significant differences existed in secretion or total response; this was not true for gastrin. Theoretically a patient after the Whipple procedure cannot secrete gastrin either from the antrum or from the duodenum, and the values measured were very low. Patients with an intact stomach and duodenum secreted significant amounts of gastrin after a meal in spite of resection of the head of the panreas (Fig. 3c).

Discussion

The preliminary report on a prospective trial such as ours must be interpreted with caution. To prefer one procedure over the other is not acceptable based on the available data. We must keep in mind that repeated examinations of the clinical course revealed satisfying results for both groups in our study. On the other hand, our patients with the Beger procedure had a more rapid recovery, shorter stay in hospital, and better rehabilitation to their jobs. These are parameters which must be considered. Interestingly, no patient who underwent a duodenum-preserving resection needed substitution with pancreatic enzymes. In contrast, after a Whipple procedure, all needed the substitution of pancreatic enzymes. The Whipple procedure is promising for the treatment of tumors, as for pancreatitis confined to the head. The primary goal in cases with chronic pancreatitis is relief from pain [3, 4, 7, 10]. Resection of antrum, duodenum, and a small portion of jejunum, on the other hand, is not a suitable procedure for the correction of a hormonal malfunction, apart from correction of anatomic abnormalities.

This consideration does not apply for a duodenum-preserving procedure. From investigation and our clinical experience we know much about feedback mechanisms which act on the exocrine pancreatic function. This is the same in healthy patients as in those with chronic pancreatitis [8].

The exocrine secretion of the pancreatic remnant is physiologically relevant [6]. With the Beger procedure these mechanisms remain and may entail some benefit for the patient. This benefit does not exist for patients with a Whipple procedure.

References

1. Beger HG, Büchler M, Bittner RR, Oettinger W, Roscher R (1989) Duodenum-preserving resection of head of the pancreas in severe chronic pancreatitis. Ann Surg 209:273
2. Büchler M, Malfertheiner P, Friess M, Senn T, Beger HG (1990) Chronic pancreatitis with inflammatory mass in the head of the pancreas: a special entity? In: Beger HG, Büchler M, Malfertheiner P, Ditschuneit H (eds) Chronic pancreatitis. Springer, Berlin Heidelberg New York, pp 44–46
3. Gall FP, Mühe E, Gebhardt C (1981) Pancreatectomy for chronic pancreatitis. World J Surg 5:269
4. Gall FP, Gebhardt C, Meister R, Zirngibl H, Schneider MU (1989) Severe chronic cephalic pancreatitis: use of partial duodenopancreatectomy with occlusion of the pancreatic duct in 289 patients. World J Surg 13:809

5. Klempa I (1978) Jejunumtransposition und selektive proximale Vagotomie nach Duodenopankreatektomie. Chirurg 49:556–560
6. Klempa I, Baca I, Menzel J, Schuszdiarra V (1991) Auswirkung von Somatostatin auf die basale und stimulierte exokrine Pankreassekretion nach partieller Duodenopankreatektomie. Chirurg 62:293–299
7. Moossa A (1987) Surgical treatment of chronic pancreatitis: an overview. Br J Surg 74:661
8. Owyang C, Louie DS, Tatum D (1986) Feedback regulation of pancreatic enzyme secretion. J Clin Invest 77:2042–2047
9. Traverso LW, Longmire WP (1978) Preservation of the pylorus during pancreatico-duodenotomy. Surg Gnyecol Obstet 146:759
10. Trede M (1984) Pankreaskopfresektion bei chronischer Pankreatitis. Langenbecks Arch Chir 362:227

Segmental Pancreatic Autotransplantation in Management of Patients with Chronic Pancreatitis

R.L. Rossi[1]

Introduction

Disabling pain and complications are common indications for operation in patients with chronic pancreatitis [1]. Surgical therapy has produced limited success, but failures are common. Because of the poor understanding of the basic pathogenesis of pancreatitis and of the mechanisms of pain, the choice of therapy continues to be empirical and directed at treating symptoms, sequelae, and complications. For patients who have a nondilated pancreatic duct or whose previous decompressive operations have failed, different resective procedures may be required. All patients who undergo total pancreatectomy and about 80% of patients who undergo 90%–95% distal resection become diabetic. Poorly controlled diabetes often causes multiple hospital readmissions and late mortality [2].

Since 1981, in attempt to prevent or delay the onset of diabetes, we began performing segmental autotransplantation of the body and tail of the pancreas as a vascularized and denervated graft in patients who were thought to be candidates for extensive distal resection of the pancreas.

Patients and Methods

Our operative technique consists of variable degrees of distal resection (60%–100%) with autotransplantation of the body and tail of the gland (that is, about 50% of the gland) to a subcutaneous pocket in the femoral region with anastomosis of the splenic vessels to the common femoral vessels. The pancreatic duct was injected with 1–2 ml neoprene and ligated. An effort was made to avoid excessive injection of the duct with disruption of secondary branches and extravasation of neoprene in the interstices of the gland. A distal arteriovenous fistula, as described by Calne et al. [3] was used in our early experience but was later abandoned [4]. Patency of graft blood vessels was assessed by Doppler ultrasonographic studies and femoral angiography. Production of insulin was determined by insulin assays of

[1]Department of General Surgery, Lahey Clinic Medical Center, 41 Mall Road, Burlington, MA 01805, USA

Beger/Büchler/Malfertheiner (Eds.)
Standards in Pancreatic Surgery

blood samples from both external iliac veins. Function of the graft and glucose homeostasis were studied by oral and intravenous glucose tolerance tests and by intravenous glucagon stimulation studies with determinations of serum glucose, insulin, and C peptide levels. In some patients, results of late biopsies of the graft were available. For the evaluation of pain, patients served as their own controls with regard to severity of pain, use of narcotics, and disability.

The procedure was performed in 13 patients, ten with idiopathic pancreatitis and three with alcohol-related pancreatitis. All patients had a nondilated pancreatic duct as seen on pancreatography. Earlier biliary pancreatic surgical procedures included sphincteroplasty in six patients, other biliary procedures in four patients, drainage of retroperitoneal pancreatic sepsis in three patients, internal drainage of cysts in two patients, and pancreatoduodenectomy in one patient. The median follow-up time was 62 months, with a range of 21–94 months. Of the patients, nine were observed for more than 5 years or until death [5].

Results

Segmental pancreatic autotransplantation was technically successful in 11 patients (85%). Removal of the graft was required in two patients (15%) at 7 and 9 days after operation because of vascular thrombosis as seen on arteriography.

Early operative complications included eight pancreatic graft fistulas that lasted less than 6 weeks in five patients but lasted 3, 7, and 39 months in the other three. Bleeding from the pancreatic graft occurred in two patients during the early part of the series. Bleeding from branches of the splenic artery at the level of the tail of the pancreas was a complication in one patient, and bleeding from the transected neck of the graft occurred in the other patient. No operative deaths occurred.

Of the two patients with early technical graft failure, the patient who underwent 90% distal resection required 10 U neutral protamine Hagedorn (NPH) insulin daily. The second patient underwent 60% distal resection and remained insulin independent. At 57 months, this patient underwent pancreatoduodenectomy at another institution because of pain.

Successful grafts in 11 patients were evaluated by March 1989 (Table 1). Insulin was not required in six patients. Three of the six patients had undergone 90% distal resection and had been observed for 27, 56, and 71 months, respectively. Initial or staged total pancreatectomy was performed in three patients who had follow-up examinations at 94, 39, and 33 months.

Of 11 patients with successful grafts, five required insulin (Table 1). Of these patients, two had undergone 90% resection and required 20 units and 8 U NPH insulin at 23 and 40 months of follow-up study, respectively, with a total follow-up time of 54 and 43 months each. Initial or staged

Table 1. Glucose homeostasis in 11 patients with technically successful segmental autotransplants

Result	n
Insulin independent	
90% Resection	3[a]
Total pancreatectomy	3[b]
Insulin dependent	
90% Resection	2[c]
Total pancreatectomy	3[d]

[a] Follow-up examination at 27, 71, and 56 months.
[b] Follow-up examination at 94, 39, and 33 months.
[c] Began requiring insulin at 23 months (20 U) and 40 months (8 U), with follow-up examination at 51 and 43 months, respectively.
[d] Began requiring insulin at 0 (10 U), 27 (12 U), and 56 months (0–15 U), with follow-up examination of 21, 64, and 64 months, respectively.

Table 2. Control of pain in 13 patients (from [52])

Initial pancreatic resection	n	Control of pain		Treatment	Improvement of pain
60%	2	Failed	2	Pancreatoduodenectomy 2	2
90%	9	Improved	4		4
		Recurred	5[a]	Pancreatoduodenectomy 3	5
100%	2	Improved	2		2

[a] Recurred at 7, 20, 24, 26, and 54 months.

pancreatectomy was performed in three patients. One patient required 10 U NPH insulin immediately, one required 12 U NPH insulin at 27 months, and one required 0–15 U regular insulin a day at 56 months, with a total follow-up time of 21, 64, and 64 months, respectively.

The results of control of pain are summarized in Table 2. The procedure failed to improve pain in the two patients who had 60% distal resection. Both patients subsequently underwent pancreatoduodenectomy with improvement of pain. All nine patients who had 90% resection and autotransplantation had transient improvement of pain. However, the pain recurred in five patients at 7, 20, 24, 26, and 54 months, respectively. Of the five patients, three underwent pancreatoduodenectomy for completion pancreatectomy with improvement of pain. The two patients who had initial total pancreatectomy had improvement of pain. All 13 patients were taking narcotics before operation and were totally disabled. After operation, six

Table 3. Total pancreatectomy and segmental autotransplantation in six patients (one initial; five staged)

Result	n
Pain improvement	6
Insulin independent[a]	3
Insulin dependent[b]	3

[a] Follow-up examination at 94, 34, and 33 months.
[b] Required insulin at 0 (10 U), 27 (12 U), and 56 (0–15 U) months, with follow-up examination at 21, 64, and 64 months, respectively.

patients returned to active employment. Only six patients required narcotics, but the dose was less than before operation.

The results of initial or staged total pancreatectomy are summarized in Table 3. Of the six patients, all ultimately had improvement of pain. Insulin was not required in three patients who had follow-up examinations at 94, 39, and 33 months, respectively. Insulin was required in three patients at 0, 27, and 56 months in doses of 10, 12, and 10 U, respectively. Review of the glucose clearance rate after intravenous infusion (K value expressed in percent of glucose removed per minute) in the six patients who underwent initial or staged total pancreatectomy and autotransplantation suggests that patients with a higher glucose clearance rate before and after resection were more likely to have a prolonged postoperative insulin-independent state compared with patients who had lower K values for glucose clearance.

Late complications in the groin included delayed abscess in one patient, fluid collection in one patient, and mild thigh and groin discomfort in two patients. The graft was removed in one patient because of progression of pain, recurrent drainage, and the development of insulin-dependent diabetes. The most frequent late operation in this group was pancreatoduodenectomy for completion pancreatectomy (five patients) because of recurrent abdominal pain in patients with subtotal distal resection. Three patients who had 90% distal resection with improvement of pain died. The first patient committed suicide 27 months after operation, and the second patient had fulminating pneumococcal pneumonia at 56 months despite receiving pneumococcal vaccine. The third patient died of human immunodeficiency virus infection at 51 months.

Some reports from the literature on total pancreatectomy show that diabetes develops in all patients and that the late mortality is appreciable (Table 4). In our six patients who had initial or staged total pancreatectomy and segmental autotransplantation, three did not require insulin, and the three who required insulin appeared to have well-controlled diabetes. In these six patients, no late deaths occurred, probably, in part, a reflection of careful patient selection.

Table 4. Reports of total pancreatectomy (from [6] by permission)

Authors	Year	*n*	Mean follow-up (years)	Improvement of pain (%)	Diabetes mellitus (%)	Late mortality (%)
Braasch et al. [2]	1978	26	4.1	62	100	46
Cooper et al. [7]	1987	83	1.5	83	100	13
Stone et al. [8]	1988	15	9.1	67	100	40
Rossi et al. [5]	1990	6	5.0	100	50	0

Table 5. Reports of proximal pancreatic resection (from [6] by permission)

Authors	Year	Resection	*n*	Years of follow-up	Improvement of pain (%)
Frey et al. [10]	1976	Pancreatoduodenectomy	19	+5.0	60
Rossi et al. [9]	1987		73	4.9	79
Stone et al. [8]	1988		15	6.2	80
Gall et al. [11]	1989	With ductal occlusion	289	8.0	88
Beger et al. [12]	1989	Duodenum preserving	128	3.6	89

At the time we were evaluating results with distal resection and autotransplantation, we reviewed our data on proximal pancreatic resection and data reported in the literature. In a report from Lahey Clinic [9] on 73 patients who underwent pancreatoduodenectomy for pancreatitis, 80% of the patients continued to have improvement of pain by 5 years. The incidence in that interval of newly developed diabetes that was easily controlled in most patients was 44%. Similarly, an ongoing review of 45 of our patients with pylorus-preserving pancreatoduodenectomy for pancreatitis, with a median follow-up time of 60 months, has shown improvement of pain in 90% of patients (M. Gagner, R.L. Rossi, unpublished data). The pain score was rated on a scale from 0 to 5 with 0 meaning no pain and 5 representing severe disabling pain with narcotic addiction. The preoperative pain score of this group was 4.5, and postoperative pain score was 1.3 ($p < 0.0001$). The reported results in the literature with proximal pancreatic resection for chronic pancreatitis are shown in Table 5. Most studies showed improvement in about 80% of patients.

In conclusion, segmental pancreatic autotransplantation can prevent or delay the onset of diabetes, and when insulin is required, diabetes is, at least initially, stable. Recurrence of pain is frequent after distal subtotal pancreatic resection (60%–90% resection). Based on our good results with proximal pancreatic resection and on results reported by others [8–12], we favor initial use of pylorus-preserving pancreatoduodenectomy in these patients. Distal resection and autotransplantation is reserved for patients in whom pancreatoduodenectomy failed. In this instance, the technique of autotransplantation described can be used. However, Roux-en-Y pancreatico-jejunostomy with the graft in the iliac fossa may improve the result [13]. Total or near total pancreatectomy is a last resort in selected patients. However, when required, the addition of segmental autotransplantation offers definitive, although sometimes temporary, benefits in glucose homeostasis.

References

1. Rossi RL, Heiss FW, Braasch JW (1985) Surgical management of chronic pancreatitis. Surg Clin North Am 65:79–101
2. Braasch JW, Vito L, Nugent FW (1978) Total pancreatectomy of end-stage chronic pancreatitis. Ann Surg 188:317–322
3. Calne RY, McMaster P, Rolles K, Duffey TJ (1980) Technical observations in segmental pancreas allografting: Observations on pancreatic blood flow. Transplant Proc 12[Suppl 2]:51–57
4. Rossi RL, Soeldner JS, Braasch JW, Heiss FW, Shea JA, Nugent FW, Watkins E Jr, Silverman ML, Bolton J (1986) Segmental pancreatic autotransplantation with pancreatic ductal occlusion after near total or total pancreatic resection for chronic pancreatitis: Results at 5- to 54-month follow-up evaluation. Ann Surg 203:626–636
5. Rossi RL, Soeldner JS, Braasch JW, Heiss FW, Shea JA, Watkins E Jr, Silverman ML (1990) Long-term results of pancreatic resection and segmental pancreatic autotransplantation for chronic pancreatitis. Am J Surg 159:51–58
6. Cooper MJ, Williamson RCN, Benjamin IS, Carter DC, Cuschieri A, Linehan IP, Russell RCG, Torrance HB, Rossi RL (1990) Pancreatic resections for chronic pancreatitis. Hepatogastroenterology 37:279
7. Cooper MJ, Williamson RCN, Benjamin IS, Carter DC, Cuschieri A, Linehan IP, Russell RCG, Torrance HB (1987) Total pancreatectomy for chronic pancreatitis. Br J Surg 74:912–915
8. Stone WM, Sarr MG, Nagorney DM, McIlrath DC (1988) Chronic pancreatitis: results of Whipple's resection and total pancreatectomy. Arch Surg 123:815–819
9. Rossi RL, Rothschild J, Braasch JW, Munson JL, ReMine SG (1987) Pancreatoduodenectomy in the management of chronic pancreatitis. Arch Surg 122: 416–420
10. Frey CF, Child CG III, Fry W (1976) Pancreatectomy for chronic pancreatitis. Ann Surg 184:403–413
11. Gall FP, Gebhardt C, Meister R, Zirngibl H, Schneider MU (1989) Severe chronic cephalic pancreatitis: use of partial duodenopancreatectomy with occlusion of the pancreatic duct in 289 patients. World J Surg 13:809–817
12. Beger HG, Büchler M, Bittner RR, Oettinger W, Roscher R (1989) Duodenum-preserving resection of the head of the pancreas in severe chronic pancreatitis: early and late results. Ann Surg 209:273–278
13. Dafoe DC, Naji A, Perloff LJ, Barker CF (1990) Pancreatic and islet autotransplantation. Hepatogastroenterology 37:307–315

Quality Control Following Surgery for Chronic Pancreatitis*

R.W. AMMANN[1]

Chronic pancreatitis (CP) is characterized by a long-term evolution over 10–20 years or more. Morphologically, CP is a progressive process, leading finally to "cirrhosis" of the pancreas combined with pancreatic dysfunction. The clinical spectrum of CP varies in relation to (a) duration of the disease, (b) progressive pancreatic dysfunction, and (c) the presence of local complications. Three typical clinical patterns can be distinguished:

1. *Uncomplicated CP, early stage* (e.g., recurrent short episodes of "acute" pancreatitis)
2. *Uncomplicated CP, late stage* (e.g., lack of pain, diarrhea, steatorrhea, diabetes)
3. *Complicated CP*, often associated with persistent severe pain, pseudocysts, obstructive jaundice, etc.

Classification and Staging of CP

Despite many attempts, there is no generally accepted terminology for inflammatory pancreatic diseases. Terms such as acute and chronic pancreatitis are used with different meanings by different authors [1, 8]. Accordingly, there are marked semantic problems in the literature on CP [1]. Obviously, the postoperative course has to be analyzed separately for different entities of CP because of differences in the natural history of progressive CP compared with that of "CP" in pancreas divisum or obstructive "CP". Table 1 gives a classification of CP with three main subgroups.

We will focus here on long-term studies of alcoholic progressive CP, particularly because it is the largest and most homogeneous group of patients with CP in our series. It has previously been shown that there are marked differences between alcoholic and nonalcoholic CP in regard to age distribution, clinical symptoms, and natural history [5].

In progressive CP, staging of the disease (early versus late stage, ± presence of local complications) is mandatory for evaluation of the long-

* The study was supported by the A. Waring Foundation, Zurich
[1] Gastroenterology Service, Dept. of Medicine, University Hospital, Zurich, Switzerland

Beger/Büchler/Malfertheiner (Eds.)
Standards in Pancreatic Surgery

Table 1. Types and stages of chronic pancreatitis

Progressive CP	
– Alcoholic	
Early stage	±Complications
Late stage	±Complications
– Nonalcoholic	
– Tropical	
Nonprogressive CP	
– Post-acute pancreatitis	
– Alcoholic nonprogressive pancreatitis	
– Segmental CP	
– Pancreatic fibrosis	
Obstructive CP	

term (and postoperative) course. It should be noted that conclusions based upon the results in progressive CP are not valid for nonprogressive and obstructive CP because in these subgroups persistent pancreatic dysfunction is usually lacking or transitory [1, 2].

These few remarks are meant to emphasize that evaluation of surgical results (and postoperative quality control) in collective series of different types of CP is useless. Such an analysis should be performed separately for the different subgroups of CP (see Table 1).

Quality of Life Following Surgery – Major Factors

The quality of life can not be assessed separately for the period following surgery because the postoperative course and outcome are markedly influenced by three major factors:

1. The disease process (classification, etiology, stage of disease)
2. The patient (pre- and postoperative behavior regarding alcohol and narcotics)
3. The surgical technique (drainage versus resection)

The role of nonsurgical interventional therapy as an alternative to surgery in CP has not yet been defined [3] and will not be discussed here.

The Patient as Important Factor in the Postoperative Outcome

A major factor in the outcome of surgery in CP, but one which is considered least in most publications, is the patient and his behavior. The statement: "The morale of the patient is a more important determinant of outcome after operation than the type of operation itself" [13] emphasizes this aspect. To perform a major pancreatic resection in an unreformed alcoholic or narcotic addict is considered to be a mistake by many experts in surgery [8, 15, 16] (see also below).

The Influence of Surgical Technique on Outcome

In the current literature much emphasis is given to the different surgical techniques and to the short- or middle-term outcome following surgery in CP. However, the role of surgery is still not clearly defined, and controversies persist over drainage procedures and pancreatic resections. In a more general way, the role of surgery in CP is comparable to the therapeutic strategy in Crohn's disease rather than to that in intractable ulcerative colitis. Total colectomy in ulcerative colitis is curative and well tolerated as far as quality of life is concerned. In CP as in Crohn's disease, surgery should be based on four principles:

1. Surgery is not curative.
2. Surgery should treat complications.
3. Surgery should be safe.
4. A minimal amount of pancreatic tissue should be sacrificed.

Marked controversies in the management of CP have persisted over the past few decades, despite important advances in diagnostic accuracy. There is currently no standardized documentation of pre- and postoperative clinical data, and there is a lack of fundamental knowledge: the cause of pain is ill-defined; early diagnosis of CP is difficult, often impossible; and the natural history of CP is largely unknown. One important aspect has been emphasized recently by the statement: "Progress in clinical management is totally dependent on accurate reporting of treatment results. At the present time this reporting is tragically inadequate" [6]. There is one fact which has to be taken into account in this regard: An accurate evaluation of the postoperative outcome relies basically on two factors: (a) a precise staging of the preoperative condition, and (b) a close follow-up for a period of at least 5–10 years postoperatively [6].

Some long-term studies of surgical series of CP are available. However, most of the series started between 1950 and 1970, i.e., before a precise morphological staging by modern imaging techniques was possible [8, 10–12, 14, 16, 19, 20]. Thus, surgical series with both long-term results and precise preoperative staging (particularly morphological) are not yet available.

Criteria of Quality of Life in CP

Pertinent quality-of-life criteria in CP are:

1. Pain
2. Pancreatic dysfunction
3. Life span
4. General physical condition (e.g., weight)
5. Capacity to work

Life span is generally limited in CP, but mainly due to extrapancreatic factors. In our experience, less than 20% of deaths in CP are directly related to pancreatitis and its complications [4]. According to some surgical series, the postoperative life span is markedly shorter in alcoholic than in nonalcoholic CP, particularly after large pancreatic resections [7, 12, 16, 19]. However, in our series with a small rate of pancreatic resections, the postoperative long-term survival was identical for alcoholic and nonalcoholic CP [4].

General condition and working capacity are, in our experience, also primarily influenced by alcohol abuse and its socioeconomic sequelae, rather than by factors directly related to CP. Furthermore, it should be noted that similar data are found in alcoholic CP, regardless of whether or not pancreatic surgery was performed.

Pain and Pancreatic Dysfunction

The major indication for surgery in CP (in ⩾95%) is pain [13, 18]. The following comments on quality control following surgery focus primarily on pain (and pain relief), pancreatic dysfunction (e.g., factors related to the natural history of CP), and alcohol or narcotic addiction (e.g., patient-related factors).

The data which form the basis of discussion derive from our prospective long-term study of patients with strictly defined alcoholic CP, as described in part previously [2, 4, 5]. Only patients with a follow-up (from onset) of at least 8 years are considered. Table 2 summarizes some relevant clinical data from our series. This is a homogeneous group of patients with a clearly defined natural history.

Table 2. Data from our own series of 185 patients with alcoholic CP

Duration of disease	>8 years
Number with calcification (%)	161 (87)
Number with surgery	78
Number without surgery	71
Follow-up (years from onset)	
– with surgery	14.6 ± 4.7
– without surgery	16.2 ± 5.9

About 50% of the patients had pancreatic surgery for pain relief as described previously [1], and the mean follow-up from onset of CP in the surgical and the nonsurgical group is comparable. Patients who underwent surgery for local extrapancreatic complications like splenic vein thrombosis, pancreatic ascites, or duodenal obstruction are excluded from the discussion because any operation performed for pain in CP has to be evaluated separately from that performed for local (painless) complications in CP [13].

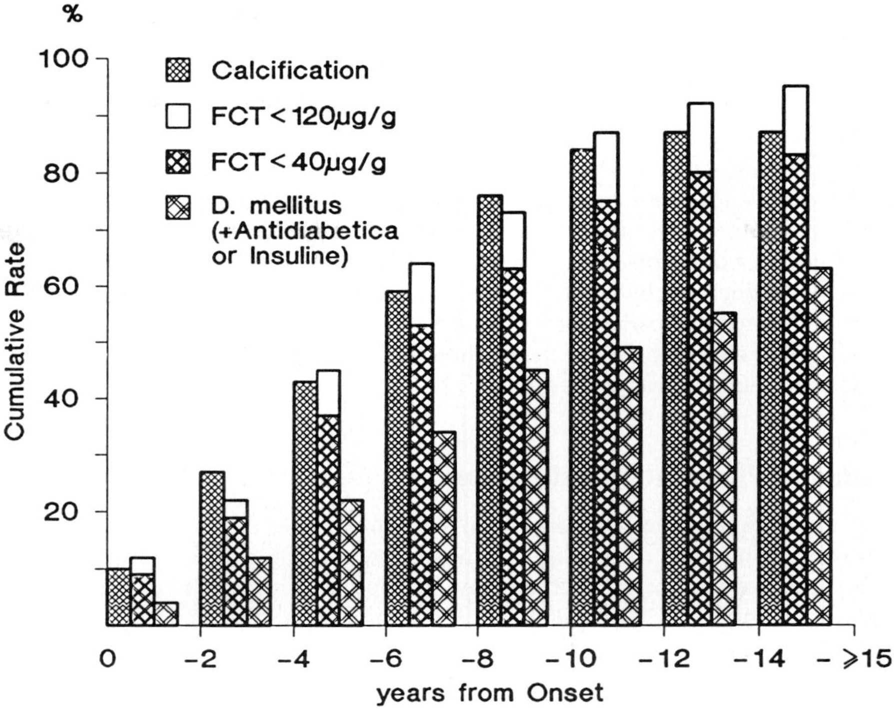

Fig. 1. Evolution of alcoholic CP in 185 patients (161 with calcifying CP) with follow-up ≥8 years. A steady increase of the "markers" of CP (calcification, exocrine and endocrine insufficiency) in relation to duration of CP from onset is noted. (*FCT*, fecal chymotrypsin test, normal values >120 µg/g; FCT <40 µg/g indicates marked exocrine insufficiency)

As shown in Fig. 1, there is a parallel steady progression of calcification, exocrine insufficiency, and diabetes mellitus in relation to duration of CP from onset, which indicates that alcoholic CP is a diffuse progressive process. In Fig. 2 the cumulative rate of persistent pain relief (>2 years without any pancreatic pain) is outlined for patients without and with pancreatic surgery in relation to duration of CP from onset. The data from Figs. 1 and 2 together support the thesis that persistent pain relief occurs progressively in relation to duration of CP and in association with marked pancreatic dysfunction ± pancreatic calcifications. The data suggest that marked pancreatic dysfunction is the price for persistent pain relief in uncomplicated CP. This "burnout" thesis is in opposition to the surgical philosophy which postulates pain relief and preservation of pancreatic function [13]. Thus, many surgical experts have not accepted the "burnout" thesis, and some of them have misinterpreted our data by implying that, according to our thesis, there was no place for surgery in CP [13]. However,

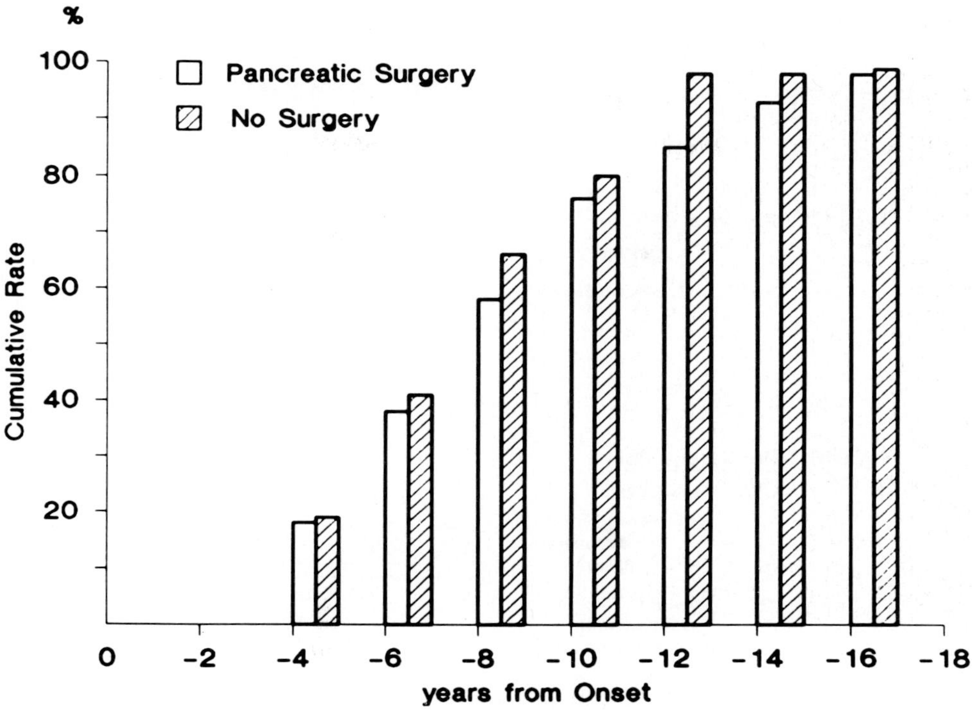

Fig. 2. Persistent pain relief (>2 years) occurs with increasing frequency in relation to duration of CP from onset, both in patients without and in those with pancreatic surgery

about 50% of our patients with alcoholic CP needed pancreatic surgery for short-term pain relief and this fact is not taken into account by such conclusions.

In our experience, surgery (primarily drainage procedure) is indicated in complicated CP with persistent severe pain. Postoperative pain relapses are common in patients with continued alcohol abuse as long as the late (painless) stage of CP is not reached.

Persistent Versus Short-Term Pain Relief in CP and the Role of Surgery

The problem of pain and pain relief by surgery in CP is multifactorial and has to be analyzed under different aspects. The pathomechanism of pain is ill-defined. There are probably different causes of pain, and also the severity of pain is quite variable in CP. Unfortunately, no common generally accepted score system of pain in CP exists, and therefore a comparison of

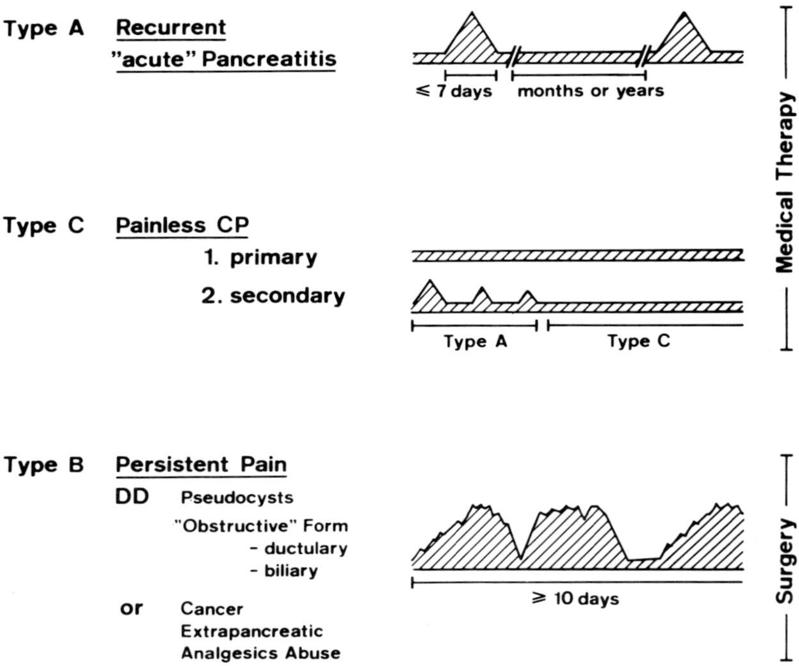

Fig. 3. The three classical pain patterns observed in chronic pancreatitis

data between different series is not possible. Based upon clinical experience, three distinct typical pain patterns can be distinguished [1].

According to Fig. 3, there are two pain patterns of uncomplicated CP (types A and C, in early and late CP respectively) and one typical pain pattern of complicated CP (type B). Persistent severe pain (or repeated episodes of type-A pain without pain-free intervals) is typical for type-B pain. Type-B pain is usually caused by local complications, e.g., pseudocysts, focal inflammatory masses in acute or chronic pancreatitis, and ductal hypertension (pancreatic or biliary duct system) in CP. In cases of type-B pain, pancreatic cancer and extrapancreatic causes of pain (including opiate abuse) have to be considered.

By drainage procedures, immediate short-term relief of type-B pain is achieved in virtually 100% of cases of complicated CP. By the drainage procedure complicated CP is converted back into uncomplicated CP, with a corresponding long-term course postoperatively. This means that type-A pain will recur postoperatively if (a) the late, painless stage of CP is not yet reached, and (b) the patient continues with alcohol abuse.

A major issue of discussion is whether postoperative type-A pain recurrence should be classified as failure of surgery. In the surgical literature, pain recurrences postoperatively are usually classified as surgical failure

Table 3. Results regarding pain relief according to treatment (from [8])

Surgical procedure	Pain relief	
	Good or fair	Poor or recurrence
Pancreaticojejunostomy	478/599 (79.8)[a]	121/599 (20.2)
Distal pancreatectomy	242/328 (73.8)	86/328 (26.2)
Pancreatoduodenectomy	398/448 (88.8)	50/448 (11.2)
Total pancreatectomy	131/158 (82.9)	27/158 (17.5)

[a] Numbers in parentheses represent percentage of total.

[8] (Table 3). This may be the case in few patients with an inadequate drainage procedure or with recurrence of local complications (e.g. pseudocysts, extrahepatic biliary obstruction). In a large percentage of patients the postoperative recurrence is of the type-A pain in the unreformed alcoholic before CP has "burned out" (e.g. patient's failure). In this situation type-A pain will stop spontaneously with "burnout" of CP. Thus, postoperative recurrence of type-A pain is *not* the surgeon's failure but rather the failure of the patient. Recurrence of type-A pain must be treated *not* by extensive resection but by abstinence from alcohol. In the unreformed alcoholic, type-A pain stops with the "burnout" of CP.

Our experience with 185 alcoholic CP patients supports these conclusions (Fig. 4). There are three subgroups of patients:

1. *Uncomplicated CP* (no surgery, $n = 71$). Persistent pain relief is reached after a mean period of 7.5 years from onset in association with a high incidence of calcification and marked exocrine insufficiency (fecal chymotrypsin $<40\,\mu g/g$) in $>80\%$ and diabetes (oral antidiabetics or insulin) in 50%.
2. *Complicated CP* and *late surgery* ($n = 40$). Surgery, mainly drainage procedures, was performed for type-B pain after a mean period of 7.1 years from onset. In these patients prompt and persistent pain relief occurred postoperatively. The incidence of pancreatic calcification and of marked exocrine and endocrine insufficiency at the time of surgery was similar to that in uncomplicated advanced CP (Fig. 4).
3. *Complicated CP* and *early surgery* ($n = 38$). Surgery, mainly drainage procedures, was performed for type-B pain after a mean period of 4.2 years from onset. In this group of patients type-A pain recurrences were observed postoperatively, but persistent pain relief occurred spontaneously after a mean period of 4.6 years postoperatively in association with a high incidence of calcification and of marked exocrine and endocrine insufficiency.

Of the 185 cases, 36 have been excluded for various reasons: analgesic abuse ($n = 6$), postoperative death ($n = 4$), primary painless CP ($n = 6$), and incomplete postoperative follow-up or lost ($n = 20$).

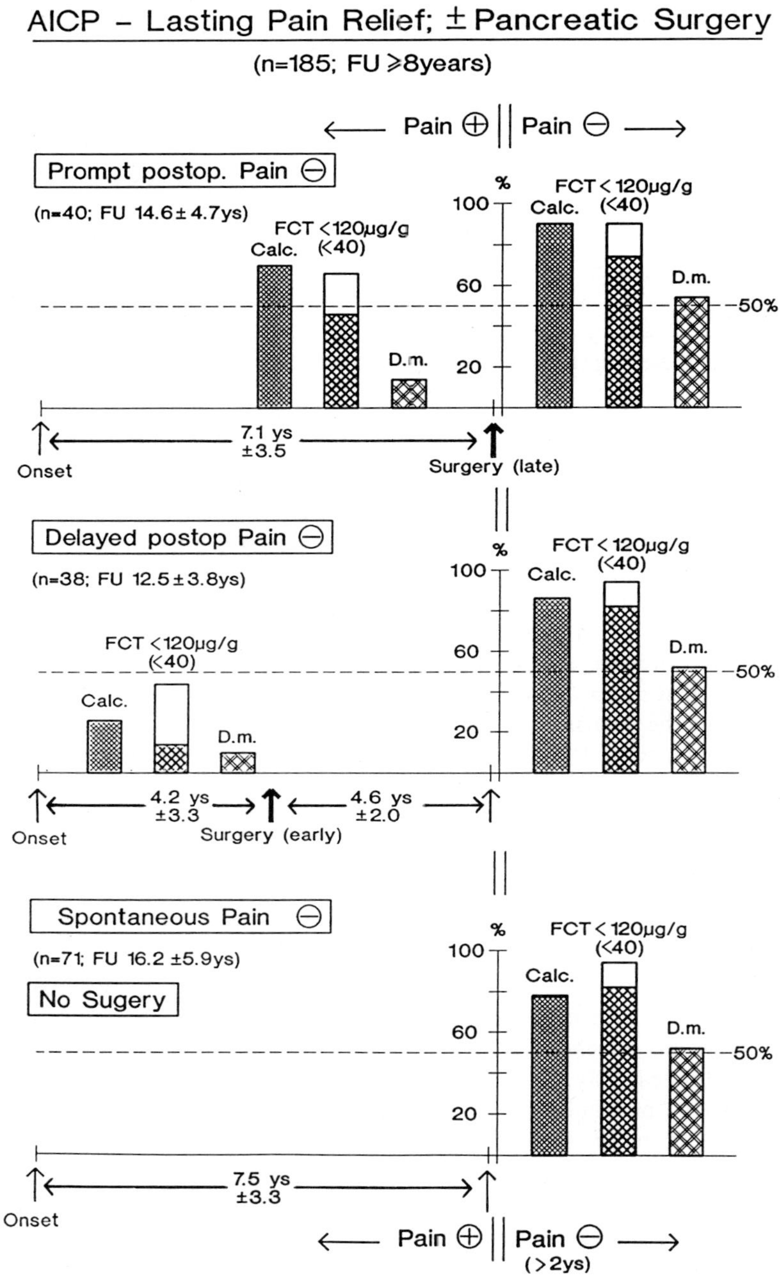

Fig. 4. Long-term course of CP from onset to the late stage of advanced (painless) CP in (a) uncomplicated CP (no surgery) (*lower panel*); (b) complicated CP with late surgery for type-B pain with prompt lasting pain relief postoperatively (*upper panel*); and (c) complicated CP with early surgery for type-B pain with delayed onset of persistent pain relief postoperatively (*middle panel*). In all three groups pain relief persisted on the average 7–9 years from onset in association with marked pancreatic dysfunction (and a high percentage of calcification) (Legend for FCT see Fig. 1)

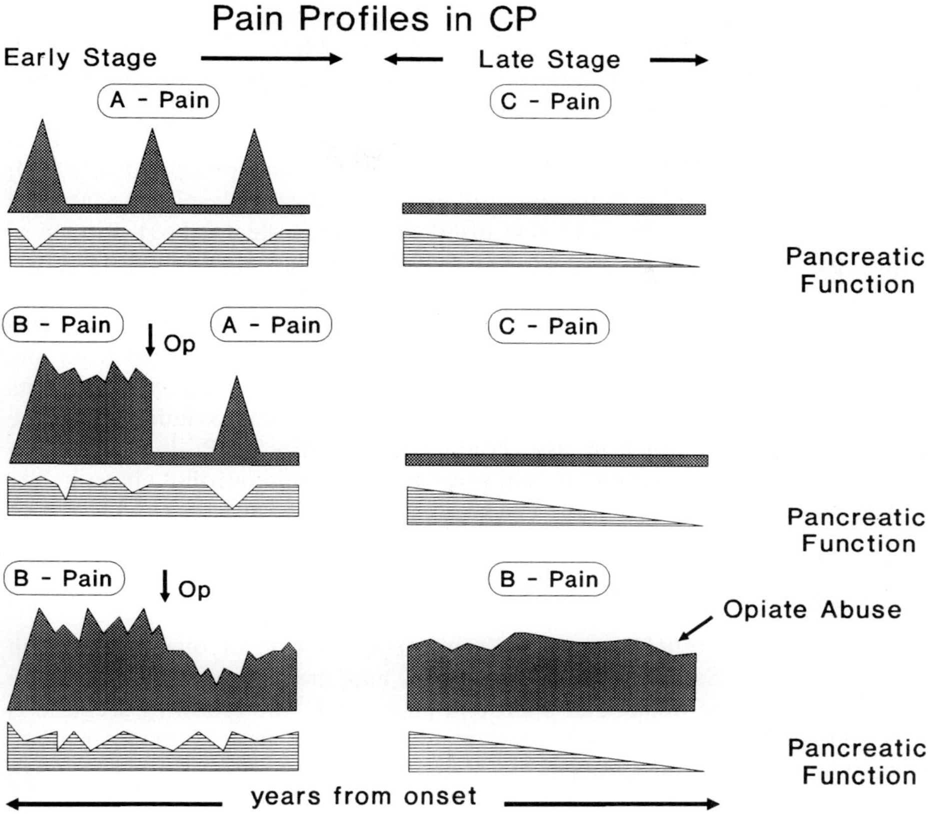

Fig. 5. Typical pain profiles in alcoholic chronic pancreatitis in relation to duration: *upper panel*, uncomplicated CP; *middle panel*, complicated CP with early drainage surgery for type-B pain and type-A pain recurrence postoperatively; *lower panel*, complicated CP with surgery for type-B pain, but no lasting pain relief in relation to opiate addiction (despite marked pancreatic dysfunction)

Alcohol Abuse, Narcotic Addiction, and Postoperative Outcome

In surgical series poor postoperative results regarding pain relief are found in 10%–30% of patients regardless of the surgical technique. These poor results are most often attributed to continued alcohol abuse. That is probably true in early CP (see above), but not in late stages of alcoholic CP. The group of Marks et al. and our group have shown that the pancreas becomes "immune" to alcohol in advanced CP as far as pain recurrence is concerned [1, 9].

In contrast, persistent postoperative pain in uncomplicated late CP is probably often related to narcotic addiction. Unfortunately, narcotic addiction is rarely documented adequately in the literature on CP. According to Warren and Cattell, "No other benign condition leads to such a high incidence of narcotic addiction" [17]. In a surgical series of 160 patients with CP, the authors noted narcotic addiction in 33% of patients. In a recent surgical series of alcoholic CP patients who underwent an 80% pancreatectomy, all 32 patients had been on narcotics preoperatively [11]. Postoperatively, 16 of 31 patients still experienced pain, despite the fact that over 90% had advanced exocrine insufficiency (e.g. steatorrhea). Fifteen of the patients were pain free postoperatively and had abandoned narcotics, whereas 16 patients who still were using narcotics postoperatively complained of continued pain [11]. Accordingly, about 50% of the patients in the series were probably narcotics addicts who will not profit from any pancreatic surgical procedure. In our personal series less than 5% of patients were addicted to narcotics, and these patients were excluded from the analysis of pain relief in association with advanced CP. In contrast to narcotic addiction, persistent pain relief results despite alcohol abuse in late CP, as shown in Fig. 5.

Conclusion

Persistent pain relief is the most important criterion of quality of life in alcoholic CP. Surgery, patient behavior, and the natural history are the major three determinants of persistent pain relief. The following scenario is based upon our experience accumulated over the past 30 years in close cooperation with our surgeons.

Early Stages of CP

In uncomplicated CP, type-A pain recurrence will be prevented through close cooperation between the patient and the physician (e.g., no alcohol, no narcotics, no surgery). In complicated CP (type-B pain), local complications are relieved (primarily by drainage procedures), and alcohol abstinence serves to prevent type-A pain recurrence postoperatively.

In the unreformed alcoholic, relief of local complications (drainage procedure) and patience are necessary, because CP will "burnout" in accordance with its natural history. Large pancreatic resections should be avoided in the unreformed alcoholic or narcotic addict because of severe metabolic sequelae and a high rate of late postoperative deaths.

Late Stages of CP

In uncomplicated CP, persistent pain relief occurs as a rule in association with marked pancreatic dysfunction ± calcification. In complicated CP relief of local complications (primarily drainage of pseudocysts, pancreatic or biliary duct system) will result in prompt and persistent pain relief (despite continued alcohol abuse). Persistent pain relief postoperatively is unlikely in narcotic addicts or in patients with extrapancreatic causes of pain.

Acknowledgements. This study was performed in close cooperation with the Dept. of Surgery, University Hospital, Zurich (Prof. F. Largiadèr); the Surgical Clinic, City Hospital Waid, Zurich (Prof. A. Akovbiantz); the Dept. of Pathology, University Hospital, Zurich (Prof. P. Heitz); and the Dept. of Radiology, University Hospital, Zurich (Prof. W. Fuchs).

References

1. Ammann RW (1989) Klinik, Spontanverlauf und Therapie der chronischen Pankreatitis. Schweiz Med Wochenschr 119:696–706
2. Ammann RW (1991) Zum natürlichen Verlauf der chronischen Pankreatitis. Z Gastroenterol [Verh] 26:53–57
3. Ammann RW (1991) A critical appraisal of interventional therapy in chronic pancreatitis. Endoscopy 23:191–193
4. Ammann RW, Akovbiantz A, Largiadèr F, Schuler G (1984) Course and outcome of chronic pancreatitis. Gastroenterology 86:820–828
5. Ammann RW, Buehler H, Muench R, Freiburghaus A, Siegenthaler W (1987) Differences in the natural history of idiopathic (non-alcoholic) and alcoholic chronic pancreatitis. Pancreas 2:368–377
6. Frey CF, Braasch J (1984) Surgical management of chronic pancreatitis: the need to improve our observations and assessment of results. Am J Surg 147: 189–190
7. Frey CF, Child CG, Frey W (1976) Pancreatectomy for chronic pancreatitis. Ann Surg 184:403–412
8. Frey CF, Suzuki M, Isaji S, Zhu Y (1989) Pancreatic resection for chronic pancreatitis. Surg Clin North Am 69:499–528
9. Girdwood AH, Marks IN, Bormann PC, Kottler RE, Cohen M (1981) Does progressive pancreatic insufficiency limit pain in calcific pancreatitis with duct stricture or continued alcohol insult? J Clin Gastroenterol 3:241–245
10. Holmberg JT, Isaksson G, Ihse I (1985) Long-term results of pancreato-jejunostomy in chronic pancreatitis. Surg Gynecol Obstet 160:339–346
11. Keith RG, Saibil F, Sheppard RH (1989) Treatment of chronic alcoholic pancreatitis by pancreatic resection. Am J Surg 157:156–160
12. Leger L, Lenriot JP, Lemaigre G (1974) Five- to twenty-year follow-up after surgery for chronic pancreatitis in 148 patients. Ann Surg 180:185–191
13. Moossa AR (1987) Surgical treatment of chronic pancreatitis: an overview. Br J Surg 74:661–667
14. Prinz RA, Kaufman BH, Folk FA, Greenlee HB (1978) Pancreaticojejunostomy for chronic pancreatitis. Arch Surg 113:520–524
15. Smith R (1972) Operative management of exocrine pancreatic disease. Clin Gastroenterol 1:239–256
16. Traverso LW, Tompkins RK, Urreas PT, Longmire WP (1979) Surgical treatment of chronic pancreatitis. Ann Surg 190:312–317
17. Warren KW, Cattell RB (1959) Pancreatic surgery. N Engl J Med 261:280–288, 333–340
18. Warshaw A (1990) Indications for surgical treatment in chronic pancreatitis. In: Beger HG, Büchler M, Ditschuneit H, Malfertsheimer P (eds) Chronic pancreatitis. Springer, Berlin Heidelberg New York, pp 395–399

19. White TT, Keith RG (1973) Long-term follow-up of fifty patients with pancreaticojejunostomy. Surg Gynecol Obstet 136:353–359
20. White TT, Slavotinek AH (1979) Results of surgical treatment of chronic pancreatitis. Ann Surg 189:217–224

III. Management of Pancreatic Pseudocysts

Pseudocysts in Chronic Pancreatitis: Natural Course

P.G. LANKISCH[1] and A. LÖHR-HAPPE

Introduction

In contrast to the well-documented natural course of pancreatic pseudocysts in acute pancreatitis [11], data on their natural course in chronic pancreatitis are scarce.

Textbook chapters deal only with the indication for operation in chronic pancreatic pseudocysts, the different operative procedures and the immediate operative results [8, 12]. Individual studies have either excluded chronic pancreatic patients who refused surgery [6] or compared results for acute and chronic pancreatic patients without differentiating between operative and nonoperative treatment of the patients [11].

Therefore, most of the data on the natural course of pseudocysts in chronic pancreatitis, presented here or referred to, are part of our own study of such patients [20].

Design of Our Study

This study included 86 of 335 (25.7%) patients with chronic pancreatitis in whom we examined the natural course of the disease. In these 86 patients, ultrasound examination had revealed a pancreatic pseudocyst.

The diagnosis of chronic pancreatitis was based on case history and at least one abnormal secretin-pancreozymin test (SPT) [13, 21], performed more than 3 months after the last pain attack. Plain abdominal X-ray (n = 81) and fecal fat analysis [31] (n = 86) were also used. Fecal fat analysis was performed at the same time as the SPT. Ultrasound (n = 86), computed tomography (CT) (n = 24) and endoscopic retrograde cholangiopancreatography (ERCP) (n = 42) were performed when indicated and available.

The duration of the disease was defined as the time from the onset of symptoms and/or first hospitalization for pancreatitis until the end of the observation period. Mean observation time was 12.1 ± 8.0 years (median 11.0 years), following operative treatment it was 12.4 ± 8.3 years (median

[1] Medizinische Abteilung, Städtisches Krankenhaus, Bögelstraße 1, W-2120 Lüneburg, FRG

Beger/Büchler/Malfertheiner (Eds.)
Standards in Pancreatic Surgery

11.0 years), and following conservative treatment it was 11.3 ± 6.8 years (median 11.1 years).

A patient was classified as being free from pain ("pain relief") when without pain attacks for more than 1 year.

Severity of pancreatic insufficiency was classified into the following four groups on the basis of SPT and fecal fat analysis: absent = normal; slight = reduced enzyme output; moderate = reduced bicarbonate concentration and enzyme output, fecal fat still normal; severe = abnormal SPT plus steatorrhoea [21].

Diabetes mellitus, in line with the WHO definition, is the equivalent of endocrine pancreatic insufficiency. It was classified according to treatment for diabetes: absent = normal fasted blood glucose and/or normal glucose tolerance test; moderate = diet alone or diet plus oral medication; severe = diet plus insulin.

Finally, the Cambridge classification was used for the results of ERCP examination [7].

The etiology of chronic pancreatitis was alcohol abuse in 71 (82.6%) patients, idiopathic in 14 (16.3%) patients and familial chronic pancreatitis in one (1.2%) patient (Table 1).

Fifty-five of the 86 patients agreed to operative treatment of the pancreatic pseudocyst, whereas 31 patients refused. The latter conservatively treated group of patients included a female patient with painless chronic pancreatitis.

Pancreatic calcifications were present in 52 (64.2%) patients, but the incidence of pancreatic calcifications was higher in the operatively ($n = 37$, 67.3%) than in the conservatively treated ($n = 15$, 48.4%) patients.

Information concerning recurrence of pain and further parameters for follow-up was gathered either during examination in the hospital or by questionnaires sent to the patients. For statistical analysis, the two-tailed Fisher's exact test was used.

Table 1. Patients with pancreatic pseudocysts in chronic pancreatitis

	Operative treatment	Conservative treatment	Patients	
			(*n*)	(%)
Total patients	55	31	86	100.0
Sex				
Male	43	26	69	80.2
Female	12	5	17	19.8
Etiology				
Alcohol-induced	45	26	71	82.6
Idiopathic	9	5	14	16.3
Familial	1	0	1	1.2
Calcifications				
Present	37	15	52	64.2
Absent	16	13	29	35.8

Pain

The Zurich group and others have concluded that pain decreases with the progression of the underlying disease [1, 3, 5, 16], because 84% of their patients with calcifying alcoholic pancreatitis experienced lasting pain relief within a median of 4.5 years from onset. In our own study of 335 patients, including the patients reported here with pancreatic pseudocysts, it was found that even after a follow-up of more than 10 years only 46.7% of the patients became pain free.

In our subgroup of patients with chronic pancreatic pseudocysts, 66.7% of the conservatively treated and 52.7% of the operated patients became pain free during the observation period (Table 2).

Pain patterns in the operatively treated group were differentiated as follows: Pain relief occurred in 37 patients immediately after operation; two patients complained of unchanged severe pain; statements from the remaining 16 patients were not clearly enough articulated to determine the exact time of pain relief. Pain relapse occurred in 14 (37.8%) of the 37 patients with postoperative improvement of pain; in another 14 patients, pain relief was stable, and from the remaining nine no clear statement was obtained. By the end of the observation period, 29 (52.7%) patients were pain free.

Pain relief in the conservatively treated group of patients occurred after 3.4 ± 3.9 years (median 1.8 years). By the end of the observation period, 20 patients (66.7%) were free of pain.

Our results are hardly comparable to those of other studies [10, 18] because ours relate to the pattern of pain not only in operatively but also in conservatively treated patients. The noticeable – although statistically not significant – difference concerning pain relief in our study cannot be explained, but is not due to a difference in pancreatic duct changes as seen by ERCP, since ERCP findings for both groups of patients were similar.

ERCP examinations were performed successfully in 15 operatively and ten non-operatively treated patients, showing similar results for both groups: normal findings in 7% and 10%, slight changes in 7% and 10%,

Table 2. Pain relief following operative/conservative treatment of pancreatic pseudocysts in chronic pancreatitis. One patient with painless chronic pancreatitis who was treated conservatively is not included

Status of pain	Operative treatment (n = 55)		Conservative treatment (n = 30)	
	(n)	(%)	(n)	(%)
Persisting pain	26	47.3	10	33.3
Pain relief	29	52.7	20	66.7

Table 3. Pain relief following operative/conservative treatment and alcohol abstinene in patients with pancreatic pseudocysts in chronic pancreatitis

Treatment	Drinking habits				Patients	
	Continued to drink		Stopped drinking			
	(*n*)	(%)	(*n*)	(%)	(*n*)	(%)
Operative treatment	28		17		45	
Pain relief	13	46.4	12	70.6	25	55.6
Conservative treatment	16		10		26	
Pain relief	11	68.8	7	70.0	18	69.2

moderate changes in 20% and 20%, and severe changes in 67% and 60%, respectively.

Pain and Alcohol Intake

In our previous study [23] we reported that the incidence of pain relief among abstainers was higher than among non-abstainers, but not significant. This is essentially in agreement with two other studies [15, 25]. In contrast, previous studies [5, 17] had suggested that pain decreases with the duration of alcoholic pancreatitis as long as the patient refrains from alcohol. In our study, alcohol abstinence had a noticeable beneficial influence on pain, since 70.6% of the operatively treated abstainers, but only 46.4% of the operatively treated non-abstainers, experienced pain relief (Table 3). This is in agreement with two other studies showing that alcohol abstinence had a beneficial effect on postoperative pain and on the prognosis of pancreatic pseudocysts in general [9, 18]. It remains, however, an open question why in the conservatively treated subgroup of patients with pancreatic pseudocysts there was no noticeably better pain relief for abstainers (Table 3).

Endocrine Pancreatic Insufficiency

Our overall observation in patients with chronic pancreatitis that endocrine pancreatic insufficiency either deteriorates or remains unchanged, but shows no improvement (Table 4), generally agrees with other studies [2, 5, 24, 26, 29], and was also seen in the subgroup of patients with pancreatic pseudocysts. The more frequent deterioration in patients with operatively treated pancreatic pseudocysts (Table 4) cannot be explained, but it is not due to a preoperatively more severe endocrine situation, since test results for both groups were similar in this respect at the beginning of the observation period.

Table 4. Course of endocrine pancreatic insufficiency in 86 patients with pseudocysts in chronic pancreatitis following operative/conservative treatment

Endocrine pancreatic insufficiency	Operative treatment		Conservative treatment		Patients	
	(*n*)	(%)	(*n*)	(%)	(*n*)	(%)
Improvement	0		0		0	
No change	22	40.0	18	58.0	40	46.5
Deterioration	33	60.0	13	42.0	46	53.5
Total	55	100.0	31	100	86	100.0

Exocrine Pancreatic Insufficiency

Two previous studies [22, 29], and our overall evaluation of the natural course of chronic pancreatitis [23], have questioned the inference that chronic pancreatitis leads, in the long run, to progressively deteriorating exocrine pancreatic function. We found an improvement in 11.2% and a standstill in 46.2%. Our finding of improvement of exocrine pancreatic insufficiency agrees with three reports [14, 19, 26], but differs from one report [5] in which severely deteriorating exocrine pancreatic insufficiency was established by fecal chymotrypsin.

Similar percentages were also found in our subgroup of patients with pancreatic pseudocysts (Table 5). The lower percentage of improvement and the higher percentage of deterioration in the operatively treated group cannot be explained by preoperative differences, for the degrees of exocrine pancreatic insufficiency for both patient groups were similar at the start of the observation time. However, the improvement that was found in the operatees is in agreement with a prospective study by Nealon et al. [28], which reported that pancreaticojejunostomy in patients with large ducts, in whom severe morphological changes and exocrine and endocrine pancreatic

Table 5. Course of exocrine pancreatic insufficiency in 46 patients with pancreatic pseudocysts in chronic pancreatitis following operative/conservative treatment

Exocrine pancreatic insufficiency	Operative treatment		Conservative treatment		Patients	
	(*n*)	(%)	(*n*)	(%)	(*n*)	(%)
Improvement	5	14.7	3	25.0	8	17.4
No change	16	47.1	6	50.0	22	47.8
Deterioration	13	38.2	3	25.0	16	34.8
Total	34	100.0	12	100.0	46	100.0

insufficiency had not occurred early, retarded further progression of exocrine and endocrine insufficiency, regardless of whether the patients abstained from alcohol or not. The smaller percentages of deterioration in our conservatively treated patients cannot be compared to any other studies, but the higher rate of deterioration in operatees by comparison may have resulted from the resection performed.

Socioeconomic Situation

Data on the implications of chronic pancreatitis for the socioeconomic status of patients is not forthcoming in most studies of chronic pancreatitis.

At the beginning of the observation period in our study, with one exception, all patients were either employed or worked as housewives/ househusbands. By the end of the observation period, only 32 (50.8%) of the operatively and 21 (67.7%) of the nonoperatively treated patients were still capable of working; four and two patients in the respective groups were unemployed. Eighteen (32.7%) of the operatively and five (16.1%) of the nonoperatively treated patients had retired, retirement being due to pancreatitis in ten (55.6%) and two (40.0%) patients, respectively. Working ability was not affected by etiology. Forty-five (64.3%) of 70 alcoholics and eight (66.7%) of 12 nonalcoholics were still working at the end of the observation time.

Despite the sharp increase in retirement and unemployment among patients in our overall study and in the subgroup of patients with pancreatic pseudocysts, the drop in social status was not as significant as in the study of Pedersen et al. [29]. In this context it is of interest that, in another study, in contrast to our findings, alcohol abstinence in patients with alcohol-induced chronic pancreatitis and pancreatic pseudocysts led to improved working capacity [9].

Mortality

Within the observation period of 11.0 (median) years, about one-third of our patients died (27 of 86 patients). The cause of death remained unknown in ten patients, occurred due to pancreatic disease during postoperative hospital stay in two, and was related to pancreatitis in one conservatively treated patient (diabetes mellitus). Three of 27 died of chronic pancreatitis. In 12 operatively and two conservatively treated patients there was no relationship between death and the underlying disease.

Three of the operatively treated patients died due to an extrapancreatic carcinoma (brain tumor, rectum carcinoma, oral diaphragm carcinoma). Two of the conservatively treated patients died of pancreatic carcinoma.

It is difficult to compare data on mortality as the several studies vary considerably in the length of observation time. In our overall evaluation of the natural course of chronic pancreatitis, we found a mortality rate of 21.8% during a mean follow-up of 11.3 ± 8.3 years (median 9.8 years) [23]. The two other studies, comparable with ours [5, 26], showed similar data. The distinctly higher mortality rate in the subgroup of patients with pancreatic pseudocysts, amounting to about one-third of the patients, possibly reflects either the severity of this complication of the disease or the longer observation period of our study.

The incidence of patients with pancreatic and extrapancreatic carcinoma in chronic pancreatitis is still a matter of debate [4, 25–27, 30]. The number of patients with pancreatic pseudocysts in our study is too small for further conclusions, but the incidence (not higher than in other studies [23]) of patients who died of pancreatic and extrapancreatic carcinomas should remind the clinician that these may occur in chronic pancreatitis complicated by pancreatic pseudocysts.

Conclusions

The limitation of our study is that it is not a proper control study insofar as the patients could not be categorized on a one-to-one basis in all aspects of the disease. The ERCP findings, however, as well as the results of exocrine and endocrine function tests, were similar and, therefore, facilitated comparison between both groups. The only other operation indicator that was not matchable was the pain factor. At present there is, unfortunately, no standardized pain score or a score for chronic pancreatitis including pain, exocrine and endocrine pancreatic insufficiency, ability to work, and general status.

Within these given limitations, we conclude that conservatively treated patients with chronic pancreatitis and pancreatic pseudocysts will perhaps not fare significantly better than patients who undergo surgery for the pancreatic pseudocyst, but may at least show the same results in the long run in respect to pain attacks and the progress of exocrine and endocrine pancreatic insufficiency. A comparison between the two categories of patients would be even more helpful if we had more precise classifications of pain. We hope this study stimulates the development of scores for the various parameters of the diesease which may be used as the basis for controlled studies investigating the course of chronic pancreatitis and its complications.

References

1. Ammann R (1989) Klinik, Spontanverlauf und Therapie der chronischen Pankreatitis. Unter spezieller Berücksichtigung der Nomenklaturprobleme. Schweiz Med Wochenschr 119:696–706
2. Ammann RW, Hammer B, Fumagalli I (1973) Chronic pancreatitis in Zurich, 1963–1972. Clinical findings and follow-up studies of 102 cases. Digestion 9:404–415
3. Ammann RW, Largiadèr F, Akovbiantz A (1979) Pain relief by surgery in chronic pancreatitis? Relationship between pain relief, pancreatic dysfunction, and alcohol withdrawal. Scand J Gastroenterol 14:209–215
4. Ammann RW, Knoblauch M, Möhr P, Deyhle P, Largiadèr F, Akovbiantz A, Schüler G, Schneider J (1980) High incidence of extrapancreatic carcinoma in chronic pancreatitis. Scand J Gastroenterol 15:395–399
5. Ammann RW, Akovbiantz A, Largiadèr F, Schueler G (1984) Course and outcome of chronic pancreatitis. Longitudinal study of a mixed medical-surgical series of 245 patients. Gastroenterology 86:820–828
6. Aranha GV, Prinz RA, Esguerra AC, Greenlee HB (1983) The nature and course of cystic pancreatic lesions diagnosed by ultrasound. Arch Surg 118:486–488
7. Axon ATR, Classen M, Cotton PB, Cremer M, Freeny PC, Lees WR (1984) Pancreatography in chronic pancreatitis: international definitions. Gut 25:1107–1112
8. Beger HG, Büchler M, Ditschuneit H, Malfertheiner P (1990) Chronic pancreatitis. Springer, Berlin Heidelberg New York
9. Bödker A, Kjaergaard J, Schmidt A, Tilma A (1981) Pancreatic pseudocysts. A follow-up study. Ann Surg 194:80–84
10. Bourliere M, Sarles H (1989) Pancreatic cysts and pseudocysts associated with acute and chronic pancreatitis. Dig Dis Sci 34:343–348
11. Bradley EL III, Clements JL Jr, Gonzalez AC (1979) The natural history of pancreatic pseudocysts: a unified concept of management. Am J Surg 137:135–141
12. Carter DC, Warshaw AL (1989) Pancreatitis. Churchill Livingstone, Edinburgh (Clinical surgery international, vol 16)
13. Creutzfeldt W (1964) Funktionsdiagnostik bei Erkrankungen des exokrinen Pankreas. Verh Dtsch Ges Inn Med 70:781–801.
14. García-Pugés AM, Navarro S, Ros E, Elena M, Ballesta A, Aused R, Vilar-Bonet J (1986) Reversibility of exocrine pancreatic failure in chronic pancreatitis. Gastroenterology 91:17–24
15. Gastard J, Joubaud F, Farbos T, Loussouarn J, Marion J, Pannier M, Renaudet F, Valdazo R, Gosselin M (1973) Etiology and course of primary chronic pancreatitis in Western France. Digestion 9:416–428
16. Girdwood AH, Marks IN, Bornman PC, Kottler RE, Cohen M (1981) Does progressive pancreatic insufficiency limit pain in calcific pancreatitis with duct stricture or continued alcohol insult? J Clin Gastroenterol 3:241–245
17. Hayakawa T, Kondo T, Shibata T, Sugimuto Y, Kitagawa M (1989) Chronic alcoholism and evolution of pain and prognosis in chronic pancreatitis. Dig Dis Sci 34:33–38
18. Köhler H, Schafmayer A, Lüdtke FE, Lepsien G, Peiper H-J (1987) Surgical treatment of pancreatic pseudocysts. Br J Surg 74:813–815
19. Kondo T, Hayakawa T, Noda A, Ito K, Yamazaki Y, Iinuma Y, Okumura N, Sakakibara A, Mizuno R, Naruse S (1981) Follow-up study of chronic pancreatitis. Gastroenterol Jpn 16:46–53
20. Lankisch PG, Löhr-Happe A (1991) Natural course of pseudocysts in chronic pancreatitis. Pancreas 6:707
21. Lankisch PG, Schreiber A, Otto J (1983) Pancreolauryl test. Evaluation of a tubeless pancreatic function test in comparison with other indirect and direct tests for exocrine pancreatic function. Dig Dis Sci 28:490–493

22. Lankisch PG, Lembcke B, Wemken G, Creutzfeldt W (1986) Functional reserve capacity of the exocrine pancreas. Digestion 35:175–181
23. Lankisch PG, Löhr-Happe A, Otto J, Creutzfeldt W (1992) Natural course of pain, exocrine and endocrine pancreatic insufficiency in chronic pancreatitis. Digestion (submitted)
24. Linde J, Nilsson LH, Bárány FR (1977) Diabetes and hypoglycemia in chronic pancreatitis. Scand J Gastroenterol 12:369–373
25. Marks IN, Girdwood AH, Bank S, Louw JH (1980) The prognosis of alcohol-induced calcific pancreatitis. S Afr Med J 57:640–643
26. Miyake H, Harada H, Kunichika K, Ochi K, Kimura I (1987) Clinical course and prognosis of chronic pancreatitis. Pancreas 2:378–385
27. Möhr P, Ammann R, Largiadèr F, Knoblauch M, Schmid M, Akovbiantz A (1975) Pankreaskarzinom bei chronischer Pankreatitis. Schweiz Med Wochenschr 105:590–592
28. Nealon WH, Townsend CM Jr, Thompson JC (1988) Operative drainage of the pancreatic duct delays functional impairment in patients with chronic pancreatitis. A prospective analysis. Ann Surg 208:321–329
29. Pedersen NT, Andersen BN, Pedersen G, Worning H (1982) Chronic pancreatitis in Copenhagen. A retrospective study of 64 consecutive patients. Scand J Gastroenterol 17:925–931
30. Rocca G, Gaia E, Iuliano R, Caselle MT, Rocca N, Calcamuggi G, Emanuelli G (1987) Increased incidence of cancer in chronic pancreatitis. J Clin Gastroenterol 9:175–179
31. Van de Kamer JH, ten Bokkel Huinink H, Weijers HA (1949) Rapid method for the determination of fat in feces. J Biol Chem 177:347–355

Diagnosis of Pancreatic Pseudocysts

P. Layer[1] and D. Grandt

Clinical Presentation

Since ultrasound and computed tomography (CT) are available and routinely used in patients with acute pancreatitis, it has become apparent that many small pseudocysts do not cause clinical signs or symptoms. However, large pseudocysts usually are symptomatic and associated with abdominal pain. Nausea and vomiting are also frequent symptoms. A palpable mass is found in approximately half of symptomatic patients. Many patients have a history of weight loss. Ascites, or pleural effusions, jaundice due to common bile duct compression, and gastrointestinal bleeding episodes are encountered occasionally (Fig. 1).

Conventional Radiology

The diagnosis of pancreatic pseudocysts before ultrasound and CT became available relied on the finding of a palpable mass in the abdomen and radiological studies of the upper gastrointestinal tract showing a distortion of structures adjacent to the pseudocyst. Consequently, with these insensitive diagnostic tools only large pseudocysts were detected, which usually caused clinical symptoms (Fig. 1) [13]. Typically, barium meals demonstrated displacement of the stomach and/or duodenum with widening of the duodenal C, or ventral/cranial, or left-lateral displacement of the stomach depending on the location of the pseudocyst in the head, body, or tail region of the pancreas, respectively.

Ultrasound, Computed Tomography

Ultrasound and CT detect cystic lesions in the pancreas larger than 1–1.5 cm in diameter [1, 4, 9, 15]. We now know that pancreatic pseudocysts occur far more often than previously believed and can be found in more than 50% of patients with severe acute pancreatitis [3]. The rate of complications

[1] Medizinische Klinik, Abt. für Gastroenterologie, Universitätsklinikum Essen, Hufelandstraße 55, W-4300 Essen 1, FRG

Beger/Büchler/Malfertheiner (Eds.)
Standards in Pancreatic Surgery

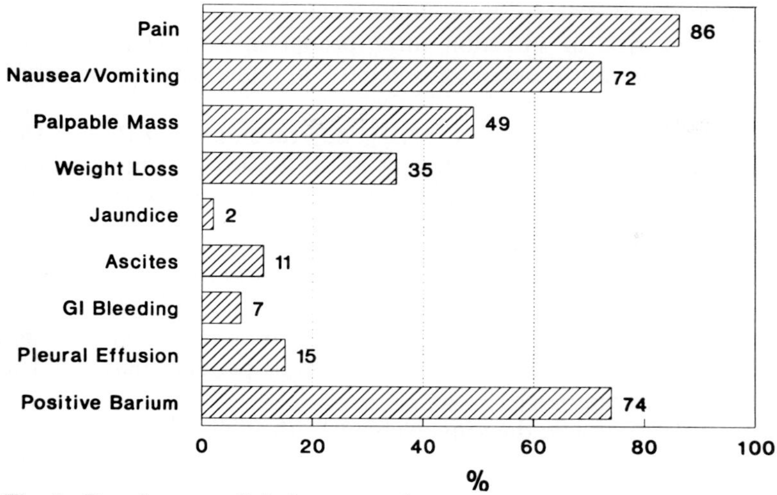

Fig. 1. Pseudocysts: clinical presentation

increases with the size of the pseudocyst, which correlates with the need for intervention [7, 21]. Pseudocysts tend to develop in the course of pancreatitis and should be differentiated from the early peripancreatic fluid collections that are characterized by variable shape, the absence of a defined cyst wall and a high tendency to resolve spontaneously.

For the diagnosis of pseudocysts ultrasound and CT are complementary techniques. Ultrasound is widely available, noninvasive, and inexpensive. A CT scan has superior resolution, yields information even in the presence of abdominal gas, and offers the additional option of using contrast media; thus, localization, size, and internal and wall structures may be documented more reliably [5, 16]. In addition, CT may be helpful in differentiating pseudocysts from necrosis [10]. In essence, CT has advantages in establishing the diagnosis, while ultrasound is an excellent tool for follow-up.

Angiography

Angiography is not considered a routine procedure in patients with pseudocysts, but should be performed in patients with gastrointestinal bleeding in association with pseudocysts.

ERCP

Endoscopic retrograde cholangiopancreatography (ERCP) has not been used as a standard procedure for the evaluation of pancreatic pseudocysts because it carries the potential risk of iatrogenic infection or rupture of the pseudocyst. In a recent retrospective study Kolars et al. reported no significantly increased risk of infection after preoperative ERCP [7], but further studies with greater numbers are needed to address this issue more convincingly.

We, in accordance with others [11, 12, 17, 22], recommend ERCP in the presence of pseudocysts only immediately prior to surgical intervention. Under these conditions, it offers valuable information at a reasonable risk:

- ERCP may reveal anatomical abnormalities of the pancreatic duct.
- ERCP can detect communication of the pseudocyst with the pancreatic duct, other cysts, or adjacent structures. Recurrence of pseudocysts appears to occur more often in patients with a pseudocyst communicating with a stenotic pancreatic duct [12]. Hence these patients may need a different therapeutic approach.
- ERCP can demonstrate bile duct involvement with stenosis and dilatation which occur frequently in patients with chronic pancreatitis [11] and may require biliary decompression [17].
- If pancreatic ascites is present, ERCP is able to localize the site of leakage.

Thus ERCP emerges as a potentially valuable diagnostic tool in those patients who require intervention because of symptomatic or complicated pseudocysts. Nealon et al. published the results of a prospective study using routine preoperative ERCP in their patients. They reported that ERCP findings changed their surgical strategy in 24 out of 41 patients and may have improved outcome [12].

Fine Needle Aspiration

Established indications for fine needle aspiration are suspected infection of a pseudocyst or suspected cystic neoplasm. Analysis of the amylase within the pseudocyst has been suggested to assess the characteristics of the pseudocyst: If amylase is confined to a cystic cavity, deamination leads to a specific degradation product ("old amylase"). Warshaw and Rattner [19] demonstrated that in the presence of old amylase all of 14 pseudocysts were suitable for internal drainage, but in its absence four of five pseudocysts required external drainage. This supports their hypothesis that old amylase is an additional marker for maturation of the pseudocyst and its wall [2, 20, 23].

Differential Diagnosis: Cysts, Cystic Neoplasms

Neither CT nor ultrasound can differentiate with certainty a pseudocyst from a true, congenital cyst or a cystic neoplasm [18]. As pseudocysts are a complication of acute or chronic pancreatitis a history of pancreatitis increases the likelihood of a cystic lesion to be a pseudocyst, whereas in patients without pancreatitis a cystic neoplasm (or a true cyst) must be suspected. True cysts are rare and usually asymptomatic. Therefore, in patients with a cystic pancreatic lesion without history of pancreatitis or trauma a mucinous neoplasm must be excluded [18]. Neither CT nor ultrasound is able to distinguish both entities, and more invasive tests such as angiography and percutaneous biopsy fail in up to one-third of patients [14, 18]. ERCP may be of diagnostic value in these patients: focal, irregular narrowing of pancreatic ducts at the corresponding localization without ductal changes typical of chronic pancreatitis are suggestive of a tumor [14]. If a cystic neoplasm is suspected, a fine needle biopsy can help to establish histological diagnosis in 70% of patients [19]. Moreover amylase concentration has been shown usually to be higher in pseudocysts than in cystic neoplasms [19].

Warshaw and Rudledge have described criteria that may help to distinguish pseudocysts from cystic neoplasms (Table 1) [20]. Even with these criteria the diagnosis may be difficult to establish, and laparotomy may be necessary [8]. If laparotomy is performed, histological confirmation of the diagnosis should always be sought to ensure that no cystic neoplasm is mistaken for a pseudocyst.

Table 1. Differentiating pseudocysts from cystic neoplasms (from [20])

Criterion	Pseudocyst	Cystic neoplasm
Clinical history	Pancreatitis	No pancreatitis
Gender predilection	Male : Female ratio, 1:3	Predominantly middle-aged women
Serum amylase	Elevated in majority	Normal
Ultrasound/CT scan	Single, occasionally multiple pseudocysts	Multiple cysts, septae
ERCP		
– Communication with prancreatic duct	60%	No
– Appearances of ducts	Changes in chronic pancreatitis	Normal ducts
Angiography	Hypovascularity, vessel displacement	Perhaps: hypervascular, tumor vessels, encasement
Gross appearance	Thick-walled, opaque, adherent to viscera	Thin-walled, transparent, not adherent
Cystic fluid amylase	Very high	Equal to serum or lower

References

1. Aranha GV, Prinz RA, Freeark RJ (1982) Evaluation of therapeutic options for pancreatic pseudocysts. Arch Surg 117:717–721
2. Bradley EL, Clements JL (1975) Spontaneous resolution of pancreatic pseudocysts. Am J Surg 129:23–28
3. Bradley EL, Clements JL, Gonzales AC (1979) The natural history of pancreatic pseudocysts: a unified concept of management. Am J Surg 137:135–139
4. Crass JR, Way LW (1981) Acute and chronic pancreatic pseudocysts are different. Am J Surg 142:660–663
5. Gerzof SG, Banks PA, Robbins AH, Johnson WC, Speckler SJ, Wetzner SM, Snider JM, Langevin RE, Jay ME (1987) Early diagnosis of pancreatic infection by computed tomography-guided aspiration. Gastroenterology 93:1315
6. Hessel SJ, Siegelmannm SS, McNeil BJ, Sanders R, Douglass FA, Philip OA, Harris JF, Abrams HL (1982) A prospective evaluation of computed tomography and ultrasound of the pancreas. Radiology 143:129–133
7. Kolars JC, Allen MO, Ansel H, Silvis SE, Vennes JA (1989) Pancreatic pseudocysts: clinical and endoscopic experience. Am J Gastroenterol 84:259–264
8. London NJ, Neoptolemos JP, Lavelle J, Bailey I, James D (1989) Serial computed tomography scanning in acute pancreatitis: a prospective study. Gut 30:397–403
9. Lumsden A, Bradley EL (1989) Pseudocyst or cystic neoplasm? Differential diagnosis and initial management of cystic pancreatic lesions. Hepatogastroenterology 36:462–466
10. Lutz H (1989) 20th anniversary of sonographic diagnosis of the pancreas. Ultraschall Med 10:136–142
11. Mainwaring R, Kern J, Schenk WG, Rudolf LE (1989) Differentiating pancreatic pseudocyst and pancreatic necrosis using computerized tomography. Ann Surg 209:562–567
12. Nealon WH, Townsend CM Jr, Thompson JC (1989) Preoperative endoscopic retrograde cholangiopancreatography (ERCP) in patients with pancreatic pseudocyst associated with resolving acute and chronic pancreatitis. Ann Surg 209:532–538
13. Nordback I, Auvinen O, Airo I, Isolauri J, Teerenhovi O (1988) ERCP in evaluating the mode of therapy in pancreatic pseudocyst. HPB Surg 1:35–44
14. Northrop WF, Sommons RL (1972) Pancreatic trauma: a review. Surgery 71:27–43
15. Pinson CW, Munson JL, Deveney CW (1990) Endoscopic retrograde cholangiopancreatography in the preoperative diagnosis of pancreatic neoplasms associated with cysts. Am J Surg 159:510–513
16. Sandy JT, Taylor RH, Christensen RM (1981) Pancreatic pseudocysts, changing concepts in management. Am J Surg 141:574–576
17. Siegelmannm SS, Copeland BE, Saba GP, Cameron IL, Sanders RC, Zerhouni EA (1980) CT of fluid collections associated with pancreatitis. AJR 134:1121
18. Sugawa C, Walt AJ (1979) Endoscopic retrograde pancreatography in the surgery of pancreatic pseudocysts. Surgery 86/4:639–647
19. Warshaw AL, Rattner DW (1980) Facts and fallacies of common bile duct obstruction by pancreatic pseudocysts. Ann Surg 192:33–37
20. Warshaw AL, Rutledge PL (1987) Cystic tumors mistaken for pancreatic pseudocysts. Ann Surg 205:393–398
21. Warshaw AL, Walt AJ, Lee KH (1980) Aging changes of pancreatic isoamylases and the appearance of "old amylase" in the serum of patients with pancreatic pseudocysts. Gastroenterology 79:1246–1251
22. Warshaw AL, David W, Rattner DW (1985) Timing of surgical drainage for pancreatic pseudocyst. Ann Surg 202/6:720–724

23. Warshaw AL, Compton CC, Lewandrowski K, Cardenosa G, Mueller PR (1990) Cystic tumors of the pancreas. New clinical, radiologic, and pathologic observations in 67 patients. Ann Surg 212:432–443
24. Yeo CJ, Bastidas JA, Lynchnyhan A, Fishman EK, Zinner MJ, Cameron JL (1990) The natural history of pancreatic pseudocysts documented by computed tomography. Surg Gynecol Obstet 170:411–417

Endoscopic Treatment of Pancreatic Cysts and Pseudocysts

J. SAHEL[1]

Introduction

Pancreatic cysts and pseudocysts are cavities containing pancreatic juice, either pure or mixed with necrosis debris or blood, contained or not within the pancreas from which they arise [1]. Anatomoclinical forms of pancreatic cysts are numerous. Besides cystic tumors such as cystadenomas and cystadenocarcinoma or parasitic cysts or congenital cysts, the most frequent varieties are observed during chronic pancreatitis and acute pancreatitis. In chronic pancreatitis, most cysts and pseudocysts are secondary to partial or complete ductal obstruction due to stenosis or intraductal stones or both phenomena. Distension of the ductal system results proximally to the obstacle. At the beginning, cysts are intrapancreatic collections, but when they grow, they can reach the capsule of the pancreas. If the capsule ruptures, cysts can sometimes migrate less far from the pancreas and are then limited by the neighboring organs or by a fibrous layer. These are called retention pseudocysts. Pseudocysts can also complicate acute pancreatitis, whatever the etiology (biliary acute panceatitis, acute attacks superimposed on chronic pancreatitis, for example). In this instance, necrotic pseudocysts result from the rupture of the ductal system.

Cysts and pseudocyts are observed in about 20% of cases of chronic pancreatitis [2] and in 25%–50% of cases of acute pancreatitis (Table 1). Although spontaneous resolution is possible and is observed in about 9% of cases [3], most cysts secondary to chronic pancreatitis persist and can lead to complications. Compression of the neighboring organs, viscera and vessels, haemorrhage, migration, infection, and fistulae are the most frequent complications.

The treatment of pancreatic cysts persisting more than 4–6 weeks is surgical. Presently two nonsurgical approaches are possible: percutaneous aspiration or drainage under ultrasonic or computed tomographic (CT) guidance and the endoscopic treatment.

[1] Service d'Hépato-Gastroentérologie, Hôpital Sainte-Marguerite, F-13009 Marseille Cedex, France

Beger/Büchler/Malfertheiner (Eds.)
Standards in Pancreatic Surgery

Table 1. Incidence of cysts in pancreatic diseases: personal series of 1200 consecutive ERCP examinations

Disease	Number of cases	Cysts	
		n	%
Chronic pancreatitis	198	40	20.2
Calcified	84	15	17.8
Precalcified	114	25	21.9
Acute pancreatitis	28	7	25.0
Pancreatic cancer	70	1	1.4
Cystadenoma and cyst-adenocarcinoma	3	3	
Islet cell carcinoma	1	1	
Senile pancreas	8	1	12.5
Total	308	53	17.2

Techniques for Endoscopic Drainage of Pancreatic Cysts

The aims of the endoscopic treatment are to drain correctly the collection and to postpone or avoid surgery.

Transductal Draining

Cysts communicating with the ductal system and located in the head or body of the pancreas can be efficiently drained by insertion through the papilla of Vater of a nasopancreatic catheter. The tip of the catheter should be placed either close to or into the cystic cavity. The catheter is permanently aspirated. The drawback of this method is discomfort to the patient because the external catheter is difficult to leave in the patient for longer than 1–2 weeks. Therefore, the nasopancreatic catheter can replaced by a prosthesis inserted through the main or minor papilla [4, 5]. The proximal tip of the prosthesis should be advanced either in the cystic cavity or in contact with the cyst. This method usually necessitates a previous pancreatic sphincterotomy. The size (7–10 F), length, and shape (straight or pigtailed) of the prosthesis should be adapted to the anatomy and diameter of the pancreatic duct as well as to the location of the cyst. The intraductal decompression results in drainage of the cysts into the duodenum. After disappearance or improvement of the symptoms and abnormal pancreatographic findings, the stent is removed after a period of 4–12 months.

The results obtained by this method are shown in Table 2. The complications reported were the formation of an abscess which was successfully treated by removal and exchange of the prosthesis [5] and in another case epigastric pain with hyperamylasemia due to obstruction of the prosthesis, which improved immediately after replacement of the tube [6].

Table 2. Morbidity and mortality associated with internal drainage by transpapillary prosthesis

Author	Year	No. of cases	Morbidity	Mortality
Grimm et al. [4]	1989	9	0	0
Huibregtse et al. [5]	1989	6	1	0
Dohmoto 1990 [6]	1990	9	1	0
Total		29	2	0

Direct Cystoenterostomy

The purpose of this technique is to create a communication between the cystic cavity and the digestive lumen. Two anatomical conditions should be observed before attempting this treatment. An obvious bulging due to the cyst should be observed during upper gastrointestinal endoscopy, and the distance between the cyst and gastric or duodenal wall should not exceed 1 cm. This distance can be measured either by percutaneous ultrasonography or by CT or endosonography. When a cyst leads to a visible compression of the upper digestive tract, the second is usually performed.

The successive steps of our personal procedure are the following [7]. ERCP may be performed but is not mandatory since it can be hazardous or complicated by infection of the cystic cavity when the endoscopic treatment fails [8]. After a careful observation of the gastric or duodenal compression, the first step consists in a diathermic puncture at the top of the bulge with a needle knife to create a fistula between the cyst cavity and the stomach or duodenum. The puncture should be performed perpendicular to the compression and is easier to perform when a lateral viewing endoscope is used. When the needle reaches the cyst cavity, which can be checked fluoroscopically, the needle is retracted, and a few milliliters of the cystic fluid are aspirated for biochemical and bacteriological assessment. Then the cyst is filled with a contrast agent to evaluate precisely its size and possible communication with the ductal system, if this has not been done previously by endoscopic pancreatography. The next stage is the cystostomy. A papillotome is inserted into the fistula tract either directly or guided by a metallic atraumatic wire; an opening is made using cutting and coagulation currents alternately. The length of the opening is 5–15 mm. The last and optional stage is the placement of a nasocystic catheter through the cystostomy for lavage of the cyst cavity with saline, either pure or with antibiotics selected according to the results of the cultures of the cyst fluid. The catheter is left for 2–7 days. Another option is to place a double pigtail prosthesis between the cyst cavity and the digestive tract lumen through the cystostomy to keep the cystostomy open in order to allow an adequate drainage of the cyst. Such prostheses are left in place for 1–2 months.

A new device called the cystoenterostome is now commercially available [9]. It consists in a coaxial system which has a 10-F sheath with a diathermic tip through the lumen of which the diathermic needle can be passed. With this instrument, the first step is similar to that previously described. When the needle knife has reached the cyst cavity, the large 10-F sheath is advanced in contact with the digestive wall, and the opening is made using only coagulation current.

Results of Endoscopic Treatment

The results are shown in Tables 2 and 3. The success rate is about 90%. After placement of the transpapillary prosthesis there was no mortality and a morbidity of 8.3%. Cystogastrostomy was successfully achieved in 88.8% of cases and cystoduodenostomy in 95.8%. The morbidity and mortality rates of cystoenterostomy were, respectively, 11.1% and 3.3%. Kozarek et al. [10] observed two cases of bleeding, one of which resulted in death in a patient with liver cirrhosis. In the Belgian series, three complications – one retroperitonitis, one infection of the cyst, and one arterial bleeding – occurred and were treated successfully medically. We observed three cases of retroperitoneal perforation, which were treated successfully by nasogastric suction, parental nutrition, and antibiotics for a few days, and two cases of bleeding, one of which led to death. This patient was a 30-year-old man presenting with alcoholic chronic pancreatitis complicated by a 10-cm cyst of the head of the pancreas and hemorrhagic pancreatic ascites. The bleeding was not due to the section of a vessel of the duodenal wall and occurred a few hours after completion of a cystoduodenostomy. Our explanation for this fatal complication is that the brutal decompression resulting from the cystoduodenostomy led to the reopening of preexisting cystovascular communications.

Table 3. Results of endoscopic cystoenterostomy

Author	Year	Cysto-gastrostomy		Cysto-duodenostomy		Morbidity	Mortality
		n	Successes	*n*	Successes		
Kozarek et al. [10]	1985	3	3	1	1	2[a]	1
Grimm et al. [4]	1987	1	1	8	8	0	1
Huibregtse et al. [5]	1989	–	–	1	1	0	0
Cremer et al. [11]	1989	11	11	22	21	3[b]	0
Sahel 1990	1990	3	1	40	38	5[c]	1
Total		18	16	72	69	10	3

[a] Two digestive bleedings.
[b] One retroperitoneal abscess, one cyst infection, one bleeding.
[c] Three retroperitoneal perforations, two bleedings.

Table 4. Results of endoscopic treatment of pancreatic cysts and pseudocysts (personal experience)

	Acute pancreatitis		Chronic pancreatitis	
	Cysto-enterostomy	Transpapillary drainage	Cysto-enterostomy	Transpapillary drainage
Number of patients	12	2	71	15
Number of procedures	12	2	78	15
Clinical success	10 (83%)	1 (50%)	62 (79.5%)	10 (66.7%)
Anatomical success	10 (83%)	1 (50%)	64 (82%)	10 (66.7%)
Recurrence	–	–	14 (17.9%)	5 (33.3%)
Morbidity	3 (25%)	0	12 (15.3%)	3 (20%)
Mortality	1 (8.3%)	0	1 (1.3%)	0

Our personal results of endoscopic cystoenterostomy in cases of cysts and pseudocysts complicating acute and chronic pancreatitis are shown in Table 4.

Discussion

The treatment of pancreatic cysts and pseudocysts should always be ecclectic. Abstention is recommended for small and asymptomatic cysts or in cases of cysts with a spontaneous tendency to resolution. However, in most cases surgery is necessary because of either pain or complications. According to the underlying disease (acute pancreatitis, chronic pancreatitis) and location of the cysts, cystogastrostomy, cystoduodenostomy, cystojejunostomy, or partial pancreatic resection can be performed [2].

Historically, the first endoscopic treatment was a transgastric needle aspiration of a pseudocyst: after temporary improvement the cyst recurred and surgery was indicated [12].

The insertion of a transpapillary prosthesis in the cyst cavity or in contact with the cyst is an interesting technique but can be limited or impossible because of the usual tortuosity of the Wirsung duct or the obstruction of the ductal system by stones in cases of chronic pancreatitis. Moreover, only cysts located close to the papilla are accessible to the treatment.

When successfully performed, cystogastrostomy or cystoenterostomy is probably the best method for drainage of pancreatic cysts in the stomach or duodenum. Our preliminary results with this method in chronic pancreatitis were encouraging [7] and prompted us to apply this technique in necrotic pseudocysts complicating acute pancreatitis [13] and in cystic tumors of the pancreas with untractable pain [14]. The morbidity and mortality rates compared favorably with those following surgery. The main risk of endoscopic cystoenterostomy seems to be uncontrolled bleeding. Therefore, the prior use of Doppler probes, CT, magnetic resonance imaging, or arteriography may be useful to check for potential bleeding into the cyst or for the vicinity of large vessels. Another precautionary measure is the simple aspiration of the cystic fluid using a needle catheter passed through the operating chanel of the endoscope: if blood is obtained, the endoscopic treatment should not be attempted (N. Sohendra, personal communication).

When successfully achieved, the results of the endoscopic drainage are immediate dramatic disappearance of pain or, in cases of infected cysts, improvement of sepsis. Usually we observed that when a good initial result was obtained, the drainage was sufficient to provide pain relief for a long period. Of course, the endoscopic treatment aims to drain the cystic cavity but has no influence on the evolution of the underlying disease, especially in cases of chronic pancreatitis. For this reason some authors complete the endoscopic drainage of pancreatic cyst by associated pancreatic ductal drainage achieved by pancreatic sphincterotomy and/or pancreatic stenting.

Conclusion

The following guidelines for the treatment of pancreatic cysts can be proposed. The persistence of a cystic collection of the pancreas after a period of 4–8 weeks is an indication for treatment. When imaging studies show that a pancreatic cyst has a gastric or paraduodenal location, the endoscopic treatment should be attempted and performed only when compression due to the cyst is obviously observed during upper GI endoscopy. In case of failure or technical impossibility of the endoscopic treatment, percutaneous drainage under ultrasonic or CT monitoring should be tried. When both instrumental invasive treatments failed or are followed by early recurrence, surgery is indicated.

References

1. Sarles H, Martin M, Camatte R, Sarles JC (1963) Le démembrement des pancréatites. Les pseudokystes des pancréatites aiguës et des pancréatites chroniques. Presse Med 5:237–240
2. Sarles JC, Sahel J, Sarles H (1979) Cysts and pseudocysts of the pancreas. In: Howat HT, Sarles H (eds) The exocrine pancreas. Saunders, Philadelphia, pp 463–483
3. Bourlière M, Sarles H (1989) Pancreatic cysts and pseudocysts associated with acute and chronic pancreatitis. Dig Dis Sci 34:343–348
4. Grimm H, Meyer WH, Nam C, Soehendra N (1989) New modalities for treating chronic pancreatitis. Endoscopy 21:70–74
5. Huigbregtse K, Schneider B, Vrij AA, Tytgat GNJ (1989) Endoscopic pancreatic drainage in chronic pancreatitis. Gastrointest Endosc 34:9–15
6. Dohmoto M (1990) Management of chronic pancreatitis with pseudocyst by endoscopic pancreatic prosthesis. Surg Endosc 4:83–87
7. Sahel J, Bastid C, Pellat B, Schurgers P, Sarles H (1987) Endoscopic cystoduodenostomy of cysts of chronic calcifying pancreatitis. A report of 20 cases. Pancreas 2:447–453
8. Cotton PB (1977) ERCP. Progress report. Gut 18:316–341

9. Cremer M, Deviere J, Baize M, Matos C (1990) New device for endoscopic cysto-enterostomy. Endoscopy 22:76–77
10. Kozarek RA, Brayko CM, Harlan J, Sanowski A, Cintora I, Kovac A (1985) Endoscopic drainage of pancreatic pseudocysts. Gastrointest Endosc 31:322–328
11. Cremer M, Deviere J, Engelholm L (1989) Endoscopic management of cysts and pseudocysts in chronic pancreatitis. Long-term results after 7 years of experience. Gastrointest Endosc 35:1–9
12. Rogers BH, Cicurel NJ, Seed RW (1975) Transgastric needle aspiration of pancreatic pseudocyst through an endoscope. Gastrointest Endosc 22:133 (letter)
13. Sahel J, Bastid C, Sarles H (1988) Dérivation endoscopique des pseudokystes et abcès au cours des pancréatites aiguës. Gastroenterol Clin Biol 12:431–435
14. Bastid C, Sahel J, Schurgers P, Sarles H (1987) Kystoduodénostomie endoscopique d'un cystadéno-carcinome du pancréas. Gastroenterol Clin Biol 11:258–259

Management of Pancreatic Pseudocysts

L.E. FLAUTNER[1]

Our knowledge of pancreatic pseudocysts has changed during the past few decades. Today it is unanimously agreed that acute and chronic pseudocysts are different. It is well known that the most frequent complication following acute pancreatitis is the development of a pseudocyst or pseudocyst-like fluid collection. With the help of computed tomography and ultrasound it is well documented that about 40% of pseudocysts resolve spontaneously. Therefore today our therapeutic tactics have changed accordingly. The application of interventional radiology – percutaneous drainage, combined endoscopic double pig-tail or endoscopically performed cysto-gastrostomy or cystoduodenostomy – has decreased the number of surgical operations.

A more significant development of surgical techniques can be observed in the field of chronic pancreatitis.

At the first Surgical Department of the Semmelweis Medical University of Budapest, 1698 operations were performed for the treatment of chronic pancreatitis and/or its complications from 1972 to 1990 (Table 1). Pseudocyst formation complicated the natural course of the disease in 70% of the patients.

In diagnosing a cystic lesion of the pancreas, we have to keep in mind that in 10%–15% of cases cystadenomas occur (Table 2).

Most frequently internal drainage procedures were used for pseudocysts (Table 3). Lately, instead of the transgastric Jurasz procedure, a posterior approach has been developed.

Frequently in the presence of pseudocyst we have to manage the morphologic alteration of the pancreatic duct at the same time. Upon follow-up, we found that subsequent operations were required more frequently after decompression and cyst drainage (Table 4). We found that in about 70% of the cases either a small unidentified pseudocyst or an unresolved obstruction of the pancreatic duct lay behind the symptoms. In order to overcome this drawback we developed cyst drainage with ductal decompression, the so called cystowirsungogastrostomy (Table 5, Fig. 1).

Pancreatoduodenectomy has become a standard procedure in the treatment of chronic pancreatitis localized mainly in the head of the pancreas. In

[1] Semmelweis University of Medicine, 1st Surgical Dept., H-1082 Budapest, Hungary

Beger/Büchler/Malfertheiner (Eds.)
Standards in Pancreatic Surgery

Table 1. Types of operations for chronic pancreatitis

Operation	No.	Deaths
Decompression	391	7 (1.79%)
Resection	350	21 (6.00%)
Cyst drainage	730	22 (3.01%)
Miscellaneous	227	9 (3.96%)
Total	1698	59 (3.47%)

Table 2. Frequency of cystic lesions of the pancreas

Lesion	Frequency
Pseudocyst	70%
Retention cyst	10%
Congenital cyst	2%–3%
Neoplastic cyst	10%–15%

Table 3. Types of operations for pseudocysts in chronic pancreatitis

Operation		No.	Deaths
Internal drainage		601	15 (2.50%)
Cystogastrostomy			
– transgastric	129		
– posterior	90		
Cystojejunostomy	38		
Cystoduodenostomy	146		
Blunt cystoduodenostomy	129		
External drainage		107	6 (5.61%)
Miscellaneous		22	1 (4.55%)
Total		730	22 (3.01%)

Table 4. Frequency of subsequent operations for recurrent symptoms

Primary operation	No.	Subsequent operation
Decompression	275	60 (21.8%)
Resection	238	30 (12.6%)
Cyst drainage	477	87 (18.2%)
Occlusion	15	7 (46.7%)
Miscellaneous	73	14 (19.2%)
Total	1078	198 (18.4%)

Table 5. Types of decompressions in chronic pancreatitis

Type of operation		No.	Deaths
Double plasty		182	4 (2.20%)
Distal decompression		209	3 (1.43%)
Wirsungojejunostoy	83		
Wirsungogastrostomy	51		
Cystowirsungogastrostomy	65		
Total		391	7 (1.79%)

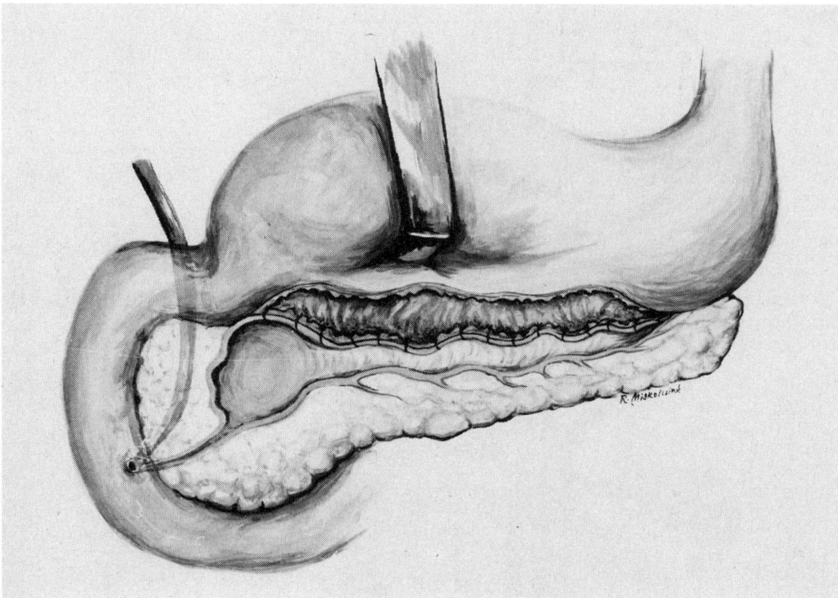

Fig. 1. Combined longitudinal cysto-Wirsungo-gastrostomy

our experience the pylorus-preserving method in combination with pancreatogastrostomy is the most valuable technique (Fig. 2).

On examination of the resected specimen we found that in nearly 60% of cases, small, cystic, necrotic cavities are the cause of head lesions. Longmire calls these cavities the pacemakers of the inflammatory process. Routine intraoperative ultrasonography localizes such cavities well, and with this method we are then able to drain them. This facilitates the regression of symptoms and of the inflammatory process. These cavities are situated deep in the pancreatic parenchyma, surrounded by fibrotic tissue, and are not palpable. They may cause the classic compression of the duodenum and the biliary and pancreatic ducts (Fig. 3).

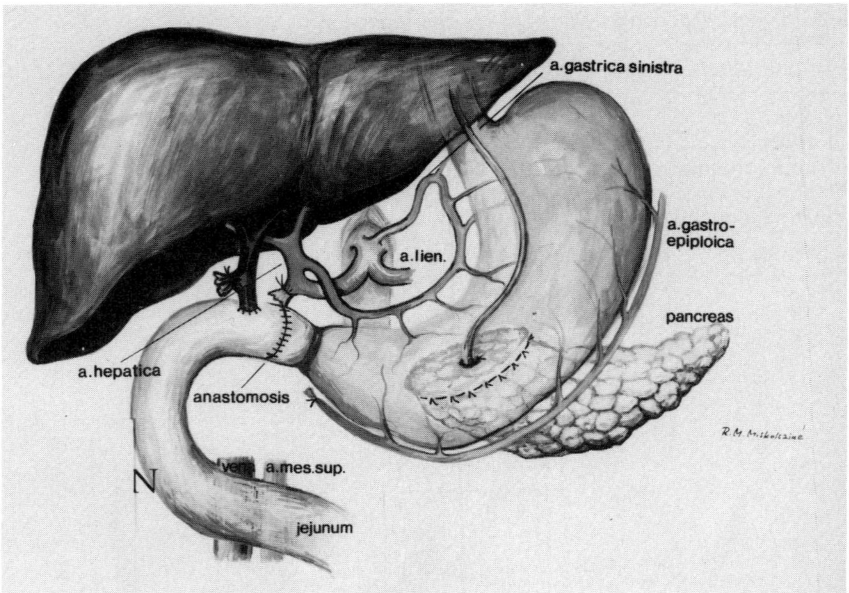

Fig. 2. Our modification of the pylorus preserving pancreatoduodenectomy. End-to-end duodenojejunostomy and pancreato-gastrostomy is performed

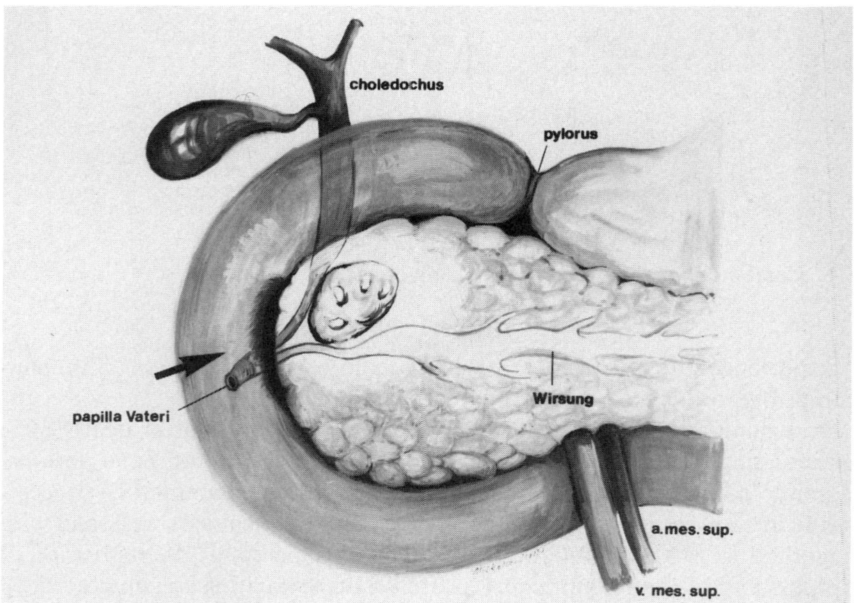

Fig. 3. The small cyst is situated deep in the parenchyma and usually cannot be palpated

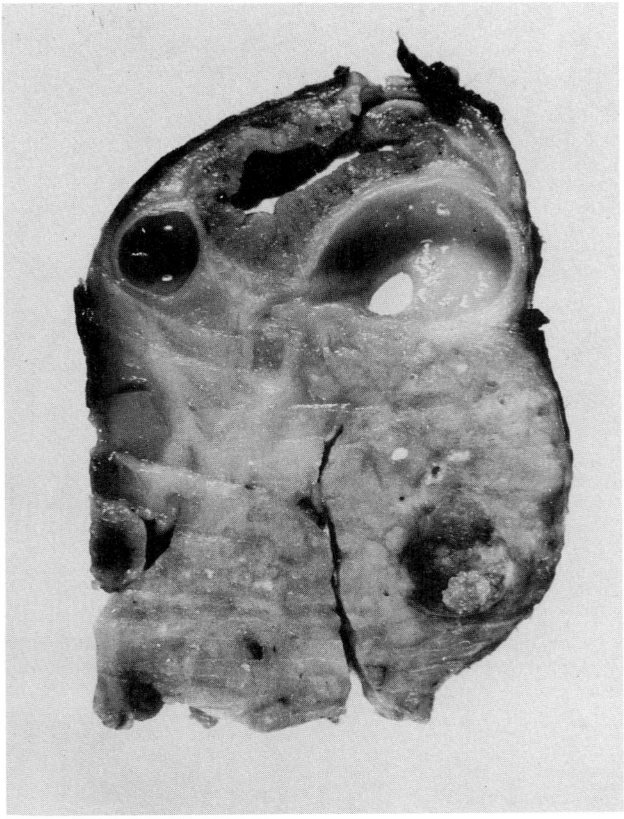

Fig. 4. Macroscopic picture of the resected specimen with multiple small cystic degenerations and pancreatic stone

On exploration, one can observe a large inflammatory mass in the head of the pancreas (Fig. 4).

When the cyst is localized, a duodenotomy is performed (Fig. 5). Through the medial wall of the duodenum, avoiding the papilla of Vater, a fine-tipped hemostatic clamp is forced through the pancreatic tissue, draining the cavity into the duodenum. In case of biliary or pancreatic obstruction a double plasty is also performed. To provide permanent drainage, the cut end of a T-tube is inserted in the cavity of the pseudocyst (Fig. 6).

Follow-up showed that after 1 year, the symptoms recurred in 9.3% of the patients (Table 6). Subsequent operations became necessary in only seven patients (5.4%).

With the availability of new techniques, and based upon our experience, our tactics in cases of pancreatic pseudocysts can be summarized as follows:

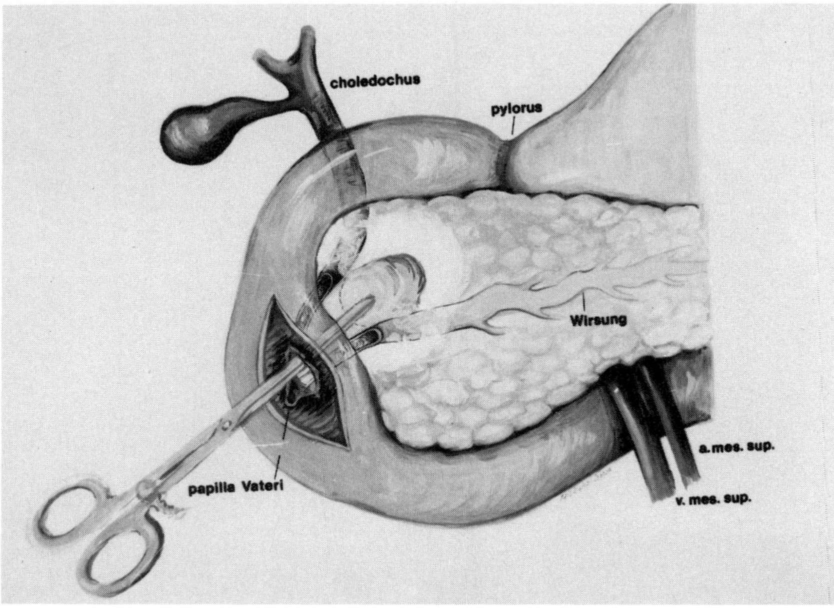

Fig. 5. After localisation by either intraoperativ sonography or by puncture it is drained by a blunt haemostatic clamp through the medial wall of the duodenum, avoiding the papilla of Váter

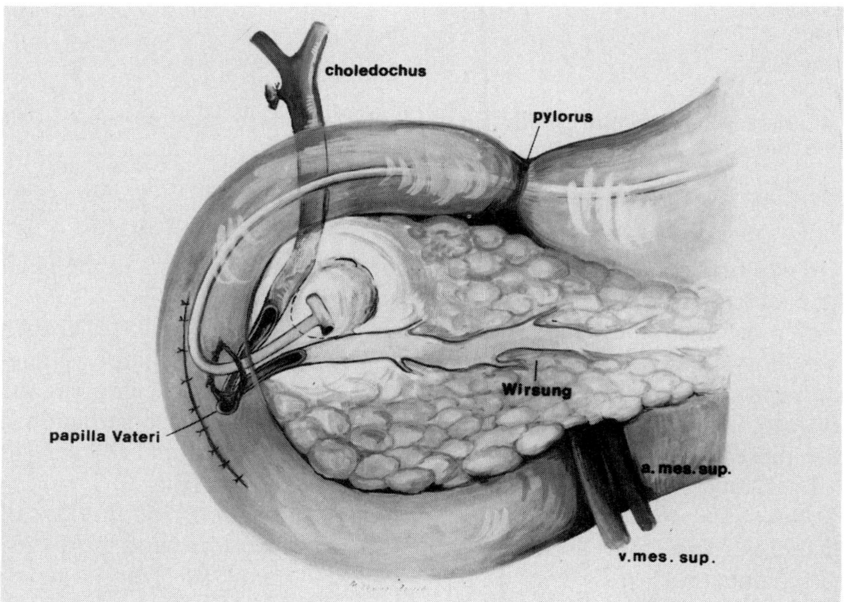

Fig. 6. Drainage is ensured by placing a short-cut T-tube into the cavity

Table 6. Treatment of recurrent complaints following blunt, forced cystoduodenostomy (n = 129)

Type of therapy	No. of patients
Medical Therapy	
Mild complaints	2
Delayed gastric emptying	2
Predelirium	1
Surgical Therapy	
Pancreatoduodenectomy	2 (4.2 months)
Cyst external drainage	1 (9 months)
Subphrenicabscess	2 (11.6 months)
Septic rupture of spleen: splenectomy, then adhesiolysis for intestinal obstruction	1 (11 months)
Fistula, peritonitis: laparotomy	1 (33 months)
Total	12 (9.3%)

- Without complications: wait (spontaneous regression)
- Depending upon Localization: US- or CT-guided drainage
- Clinical complaints or complications: surgical treatment (complications include exacerbations, compression, abscess, bleeding from erosion, and pleurisy or ascites)
- Relation with pancreatic duct: ERCP?

Conclusions

1. Instead of the transgastric approach a posterior cystogastrostomy is routinely performed.
2. The combined cysto-wirsungogastrostomy treats both the pseudocyst and chronic pancreatitis and also decreases the frequency of recurrences and the need for subsequent operations.
3. Blunt, forced, transparenchymal cysto-duodenostomy may take the place of pancreatic head resection in a significant number of cases.

Cystogastrostomy in the Treatment of Pancreatic Pseudocysts

T. Karavias,[1] P. Dollinger, and R. Häring

Introduction

The treatment of pancreatic pseudocysts today comprises the possibilities of internal and external drainage, and pancreas resection, as well as interventional procedures [8]. The drainage of pancreatic pseudocysts by anastomosis to the stomach is among the oldest internal drainage techniques. It was first described in 1921 by Jedlicka and later (1931) modified by Jurasz. Until the early 1960s, cystogastrostomy was the standard surgical procedure for internal drainage of pancreatic pseudocysts.

The following review of the literature investigates the current value of cystogastrostomy in the treatment of pancreatic pseudocysts. Older and more recent publications will be discussed, taking into account our own experiences.

Surgical Techniques

Concerning the different techniques, retrogastric or external cystogastrostomy and transgastric or transventricular cystogastrostomy are distinguished. The retrogastric technique involves mobilization of the free posterior gastric wall along the greater curvature and gastrotomy with subsequent anastomosis by suture to the incised cyst. In contrast, the transgastric procedure is started by opening the anterior gastric wall. A drainage opening between the cyst and the gastric lumen is created by incision in an area of the posterior gastric wall already adherent to the cyst through inflammation. The anastomosis is further secured by a continuous suture for hemostasis.

The described method is easy and fast to perform and especially suited for pseudocysts localized in the area of the head or corpus of the pancreas and already adherent to the stomach through inflammation.

[1] Chirurgische Klinik, Klinikum Steglitz der Freien Universität Berlin, W-1000 Berlin 45, FRG

Beger/Büchler/Malfertheiner (Eds.)
Standards in Pancreatic Surgery

Results

A comprehensive review of publications on surgical treatment of pancreatic pseudocysts was published by Warren et al. in 1958 [7]. His review included 481 patients. The number of internal and external drainage procedures was almost identical (43% and 47% respectively). At a rate of 10%, cystectomy was much less frequently performed. While mortality was almost equally low for both drainage procedures at 5% and 3%, reoperation was nearly twice as frequent after external than after internal drainage (24% vs 15%). In contrast, cystectomy was associated with a reoperation rate of 6% but with two- to fourfold higher mortality than drainage procedures (Table 1).

Twenty-five years later, Zirngibl et al. [9] discussed the findings of 16 authors and evaluated 1837 operations performed between 1968 and 1981, comparing internal and external drainage procedures. Statistical comparison of these studies taken together showed a twofold higher mortality and threefold higher recurrence rate of external than of internal drainage procedures, which confirms the superiority of the latter to external drainage procedures.

The further stratification of internal drainage procedures in Warren's statistic evaluation revealed cystogastrostomy at the most frequently applied method (Table 2). With regard to the passage of chyme from the stomach to the cyst pouch, Warren et al. [9] demonstrated that this was more frequently associated with the transgastric (eight of 25 cases) than with the retrogastric procedure (one of 25). In summary, a reoperation rate of 5% and mortality rate of 3% showed cystogastrostomy to be as efficient as anastomosis to the small intestine according to the method of Roux.

Table 1. Results of pancreatic pseudocyst treatment

Method	Number of cases	Reoperations (%)	Mortality (%)
Internal drainage	208	15	5
External drainage	225	24	3
Extirpation	48	6	12

Comprehensive statistical evaluation Warren et al. [9].

Table 2. Pancreatic pseudocysts: results of internal drainage

Type of anastomosis	Number of cases	Reoperation (%)	Mortality (%)
Jejunum	32	6	16
According to Braun	8	37	0
According to Roux	46	4	2
Stomach	107	5	3
Duodenum	15	20	7

Comprehensive statistical evaluation Warren et al. [9].

Nevertheless, this drainage procedure was not generally accepted during the following years [1]. A review of the literature by Kern et al. [5] revealed that drainage was insufficient after anastomosis to the stomach. Further shortcomings were the passage of gastric chyme to the cyst pouch with subsequent stagnation and inflammation, and finally erosion hemorrhage from the cyst wall as a feared complication.

Nielsen [6], who also reported on two cases of severe erosion hemorrhage in his review of the literature, found hemorrhage to be only slightly more frequent after cystogastrostomy than after cystojejunostomy. However, mortality was lower after anastomosis to the stomach than after anastomosis to the small intestine (Table 3). Zirngibl et al. [9] also reported a higher mortality associated with cystojejunostomy than with cystrogastrostomy (6% and 0% respectively). Both methods had an alarming late mortality rate, 23% and 43% respectively (Table 4). His review indicated the current trend towards less frequent application of external drainage procedures and cystogastrostomy and the preference of other, internal, draining methods.

Although in our patient collective (Table 5) internal drainage procedures were applied more frequently than external methods or resection – similar to other studies [2, 9] – anastomosis to the stomach was performed exceptionally seldom. The reason may be that the above-mentioned preconditions conducive to cystogastrostomy are seldom met with and that the percentage of resections and cystectomies followed by drainage has generally increased (34% in our patient collective).

On the other hand, there is a renaissance of cystogastrostomy as an interventional procedure. Current methods involve transcutaneous drainage

Table 3. Hemorrhage and mortality after cystojejunostomy and cystogastrostomy

	Cystogastrostomy	Cystojejunostomy
Number of cases	415	365
Mortality (%)	3.1	5.5
Hemorrhage (% of cases)	11	7.4

Comprehensive statistical evaluation Nielsen [6].

Table 4. Drainage of pancreatic pseudocysts – early and late mortality [9]

Procedure	Number of cases	Mortality (%)	
		Early	Late
Cystojejunostomy	120	5.8	23
Cystogastrostomy	7	0	43
Cystoduodenostomy	6	17	20
External drainage	20	10	50

Table 5. Pancreatic pseudocysts: surgical procedures

Surgical procedure	No.	%
Internal drainage	58	41
Resection	32	24
External drainage	14	10
Extirpation + drainage	14	10
Others	17	15

Surgical procedures performed on 135 patients (100 male, 35 female), mean age 45 (range 24–71), 1970–90. Mortality 4% (five patients).

of pancreatic pseudocysts in suitable locations into the stomach by means of special double-J catheters (assisted either by sonography or by endoscopy). A number of promising reports have been published [3, 4].

Conclusion

In summary, it can be said that cystogastrostomy remains a fast and easy internal drainage procedure. The transgastric method is particularly efficient and associated with very low intraoperative mortality when performed in carefully selected patients. Cystogastrostomy is carried out more rarely today (and largely replaced by anastomosis to the small intestine or pancreas resection). It is increasingly used as an interventional drainage method.

References

1. Andersson R, Janzon M, Sundberg I, Bengmark S (1989) Management of pancreatic pseudocysts. Br J Surg 76:550–552
2. Böttger T, Steegmüller K, Junginger T (1991) Ergebnisse der chirurgischen Therapie von Pankreaspseudozysten. Langenbecks Arch Chir 376:42–49
3. Grosso M, Gandini G, Cassinis C, Regge D, Righi D, Rossi P (1989) Percutaneous treatment (including pseudocystogastrostomy) of 74 pancreatic pseudocysts. Radiology 173:493–497
4. Heyder N, Flügel H, Domschke W (1988) Catheter drainage of pancreatic pseudocysts into the stomach. Endoscopy 20:75–77
5. Kern E, Kümmerle F, Hebell I (1960) Zur Differentialdiagnose und Therapie der Pankreaszysten. Chirurg 31:312–317
6. Nielsen OS (1979) Bleeding after pancreatic cystogastrostomy. Acta Chir Scand 145:247–249
7. Warren WD, Marsh W, Sandusky W (1958) An appraisal of surgical procedures for pancreatic pseudocyst. Ann Surg 147:903–920
8. Warshaw AL (1989) Pancreatic cysts and pseudocysts: new rules for a new game. Br J Surg 76:533–534
9. Zirngibl H, Gebhardt C, Faßbender D (1983) Drainagebehandlung von Pankreaspseudozysten. Langenbecks Arch Chir 360:29–41

Management of Pancreatic Pseudocysts: Pseudocystojejunostomy

H. Becker,[1] J.W. Heise,[1] and C. Niederau[2]

Introduction

Throughout the literature surgical procedures on pancreatic pseudocysts are usually dealt with as not much of a problem. The high percentage of reoperations required for recurrent disease – up to 10% [1, 2] – however, uncovers the fact that there might be uncertainty in terms of both indication to operate and the appropriate technique. The question of which treatment modality may be most beneficial cannot be definitively decided in favor of one or the other operation.

Once surgery has been chosen as the treatment of a pseudocyst, there are certain criteria for deciding on the kind of operation in each individual case (Table 1). One of the most important questions is that of the etiology of the pseudocyst [4]. Basically, pseudocysts may evolve following acute pancreatitis or as a complication of chronic pancreatitis. Morphologically, a retention cyst is often difficult to distinguish from a focal necrosis [13]. Although pseudocysts 2–5 cm in diameter may become symptomatic, there is general agreement that for cysts ⩾5 cm in diameter some kind of treatment has to be considered [17]. Others, however, do not see a critical diameter limit and advocate an aggressive aproach even in an asymptomatic situation, particularly because of the threat of bleeding complications [3, 7, 16]. The kind of surgical treatment also is influenced by the localization of the cyst, which can reach from the head of the gland towards the tail; it can occur in an atopical position, e.g., within the mediastinum, intrahepatically, or in the mesenteric root.

Regarding different treatment strategies, we have analyzed patients found to have pancreatic pseudocysts in our institution during the past 5 years. Reviews summarizing institutional experiences over two or even three decades are not very helpful, since the indication to operate on a pancreatic pseudocyst has changed tremendously by virtue of new interventional techniques developed within the past 10 years [6, 8, 15].

[1] Department of Surgery, General and Trauma Surgery
[2] Department of Medicine, Gastroenterology, Heinrich-Heine-Universität Düsseldorf, Moorenstraße 5, W-4000 Düsseldorf 1, FRG

Beger/Büchler/Malfertheiner (Eds.)
Standards in Pancreatic Surgery

Table 1. Criteria for deciding how to drain a pancreatic pseudocyst

Etiology	–	post-acute chronic
Morphology	–	focal necrosis retention cyst
Size	–	5 cm in diameter symptoms
Localization	–	cranial: tail or corpus caudal: head or uncinate process

Table 2. Distribution of treatment modalities among 72 patients with pancreatic pseudocysts from April 1986 to April 1991

Treatment	No.	Percentage
Conservative	24	33
Interventional	18	25
Surgical drainage	30	42

Patients

During the past 5 years, 72 patients with pancreatic pseudocysts were treated both in the surgical and in the medical department (Table 2). Some received only conservative treatment, which consisted in 6-week observation periods, but 25% of all patients underwent some kind of interventional procedure, mostly percutaneous catheterization. In five patients interventional measures were combined with surgical internal drainage, as illustrated by Fig. 1.

Looking at the patients treated exclusively with surgery (Table 3), 60% of them had post-acute pancreatitis cysts. Mostly, indication for the surgical approach was unquestionable, following necrotizing pancreatitis conservatively treated for at least 6 weeks (Fig. 2).

Particular attention should be paid to those patients in whom a pseudocyst is a sequela of chronic pancreatitis (Fig. 3a+b). Presented here are patients for whom the pseudocyst was the main indication for operative treatment, excluding those treated mainly for chronic pancreatitis with cysts found only incidentally. In the former group a meticulous diagnostic workup was be done preoperatively, in order to determine the entire morphology of the gland, particularly to assess whether large-duct disease is present. In five of our patients a hitherto unsuspected dilated main pancreatic duct was found (Fig. 4a+b), in addition to the pancreatic pseudocyst.

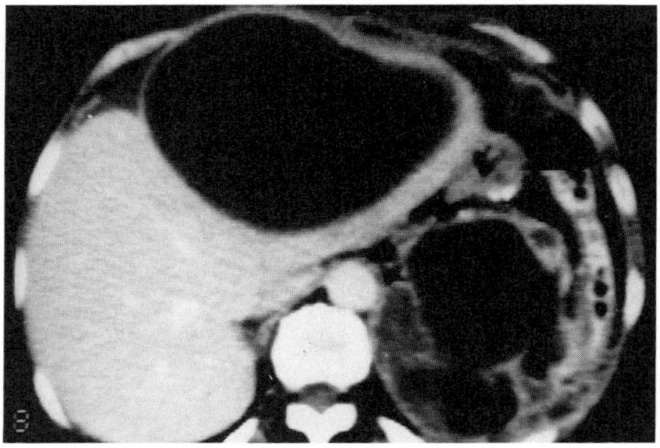

Fig. 1. CT scan of a 63-year-old woman in whom the larger cyst was first successfully treated by percutaneous catheterization. The smaller one was subsequently drained into a Roux-en-Y loop

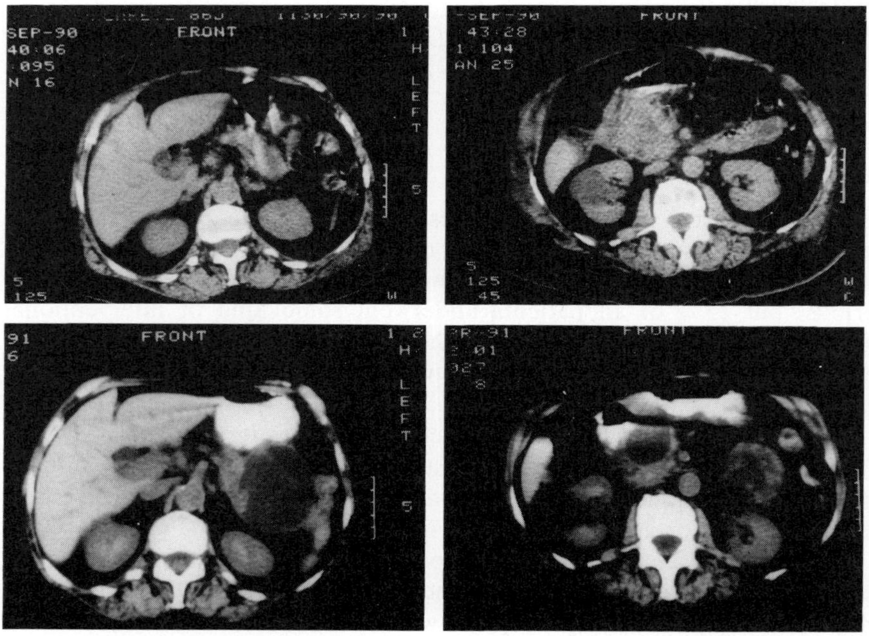

Fig. 2. Sequence of CT scans of an 85-year-old woman with acute pancreatitis. The *upper row* shows the acute state whereas the corresponding scans in the *lower row* represent the status 4 months later, with two mature thick-walled pseudocysts. Because of her age, she was treated interventionally by percutaneous catheterization

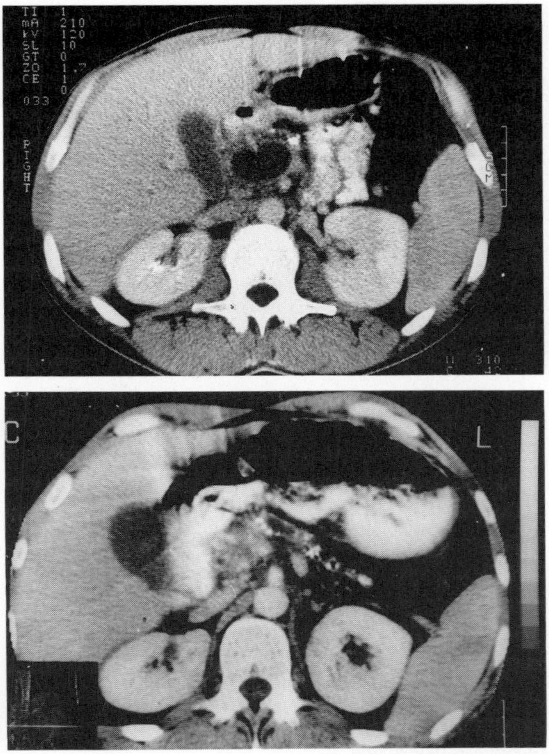

a

b

Fig. 3. **a** CT Scans of a 36-year-old man with long-lasting chronic pancreatitis who developed a pseudocyst within the head region. **b** Atrophic corpus and tail of the pancreas with large duct disease

Decision-Making on the Surgical Procedure

Pseudocysts After Acute Pancreatitis

In our patients who developed pseudocysts following acute pancreatitis, internal drainage employing cystojejunostomy was the treatment of choice. Usually, these were large cysts with an average diameter of 11 cm that developed within 3 months following the acute disease. Six patients who were thought to have a biliary etiology of the pancreatitis underwent simultaneously a standard cholecystectomy. In the literature persistent cholelithiasis is reported to increase the frequency of further complications in the pseudocyst patient.

a

b

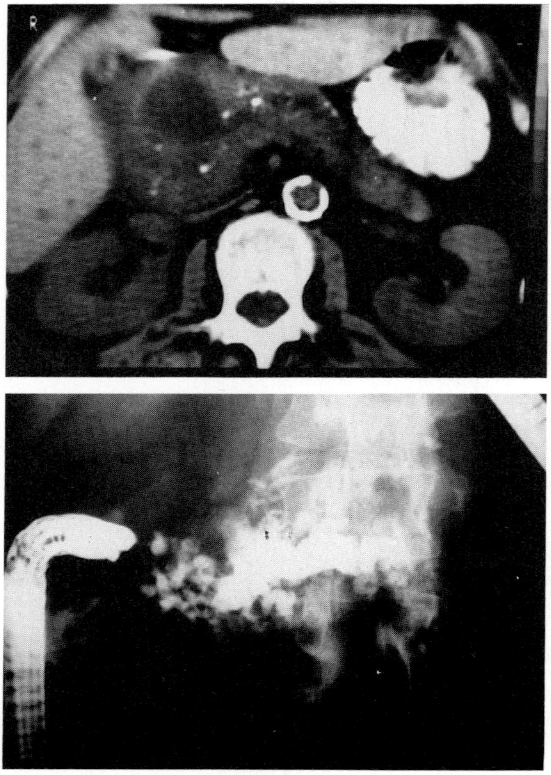

Fig. 4. **a** CT scan of a 41-year-old woman with a small pseudocyst in the head of the gland which became symptomatic with common bile duct obstruction; a dilated pancreatic duct was suspected. **b** Large duct disease confirmed by preoperative ERCP

Table 3. Etiology of pancreatic pseudocysts in 30 patients treated with surgical drainage

Etiology	No.	Percentage
Post-acute pancreatitis	18	60
Chronic pancreatitis	12	40
With large duct disease	5	
Without dilated duct	7	

Pseudocysts in Chronic Pancreatitis

In chronic pancreatitis patients the treatment plan must be highly individualized. A basic problem is whether pain or other symptoms are caused by the pseudocyst or by the chronic pancreatitis itself. It is therefore mandatory in this patient group that, besides the easily performed CT scan, a ductogram of the pancreatic system and if possible, of the biliary system should be obtained. It has been conclusively shown that the results of this type of investigation have a significant impact on the type of surgery performed in these patients [10, 14].

Some difficulties inherent in the process of decision-making may be illustrated by the following case report:

A 40-year-old man was admitted to our hospital because of symptomatic duodenal obstruction and signs of beginning cholestasis (Fig. 5a). CT scan of the upper abdomen revealed a pseudocyst only 4 cm in diameter within the head region (Fig. 5b). Scans of an upper level also raised the suspicion of a dilated pancreatic duct within the pancreatic body and tail (Fig. 5c). Pre-operative ERCP was impossible due to the duodenal obstruction. After exploration, a dilated duct was indentified and a pancreaticography was performed. It revealed a massively enlarged ductal system without communication of the cyst to the duct (Fig. 5d). The gland was totally exposed, the duct unroofed as far as possible towards the duodenum and towards the spleen, and the cyst was drained into it by excising some fibrotic parenchyma (Fig. 5e). Consecutively, a pancreaticojejunostomy covering the whole defect was undertaken in a standard fashion (Fig. 5f). Postoperatively, the duodenal and biliary obstruction resolved and chronic pain was also reduced drastically.

Based on our experience, a dilated duct always should be simultaneously drained in patients with large-duct chronic pancreatitis. The use of a jejunal Roux-en-Y loop as the organ to drain into is the technique of choice. In four of our patients with left-sided disease a resection of the pancreatic tail was considered appropriate.

Technical Aspects

In our hands a jejunal Roux loop is tailored to about 40 cm in length and in the post-acute type of cyst sewn to the deepest point, most commonly through the mesocolon. In large lesions with clear contents a limited cystostomy is sufficient. One should be very careful with débridement or even necrosectomy of more solid structures within the cavity of the cyst because hemorrhage might be induced, which is extremely difficult to deal with. The anastomosis is performed with an all-layer running suture of 3-0 Vicryl.

Advantages of Cystojejunostomy

If internal drainage into the small bowel is compared with other techniques, particularly cystogastrostomy, a major advantage is the ability to reach every part of the gland through the mobilized loop. Thus it is also possible to achieve drainage at the most dependent point of the cyst. There are several reports of an increased number of postoperative gastrointestinal hemorrhages following cystogastrostomy compared with cystojejunostomy [5, 11, 12]. However, the major benefit of employing the jejunum, in our view and that of other experienced centers [9, 15], is the possibility it provides of effectively treating the underlying chronic pancreatitis. The pseudocyst itself represents only a symptom or a complication of a different basic problem (Table 4). Prerequisite to successful use of the technique are a standardized preoperative diagnostic workup, including visualization of the pancreatic and common bile ducts, and being in control of every situation possible intraoperatively.

Summary

To decide whether surgery on a pancreatic pseudocyst is indicated, thorough knowledge of the natural history [3, 17] and alternative interventional

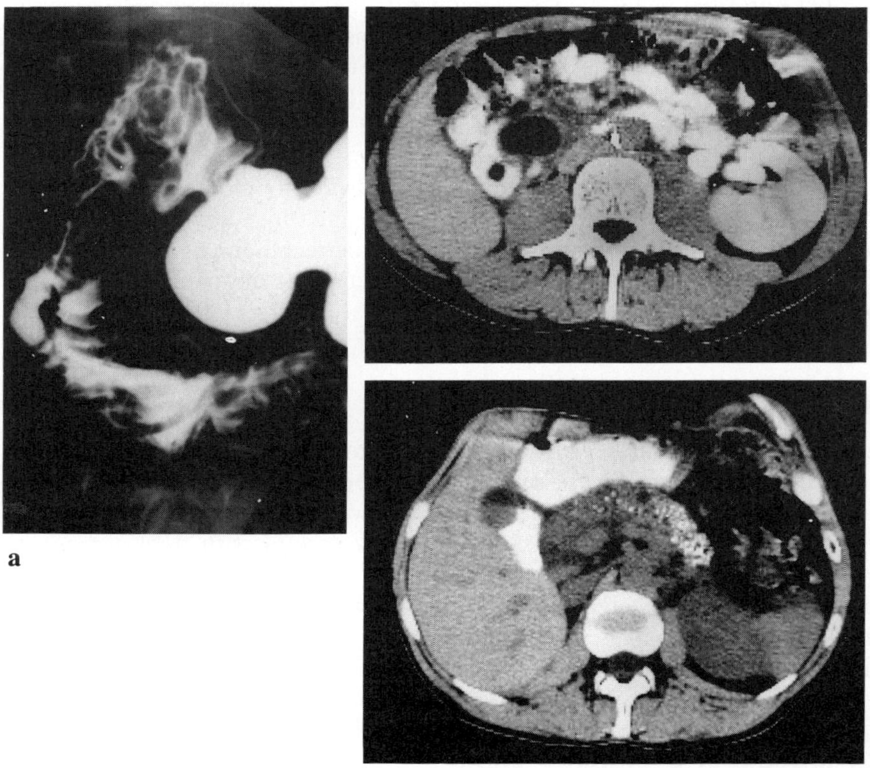

a b c

Fig. 5. a Highly symptomatic duodenal obstruction in a 40-year-old man. **b** CT scan showing a pseudocyst in the head region. **c** CT scan of the corpus/tail region with indication of duct dilatation. **d** Intraoperative pancreaticography. **e** The unroofed pancreatic duct and pseudocyst in the pancreatic head. **f** The pancreaticojejunostomy is performed in the typical fashion

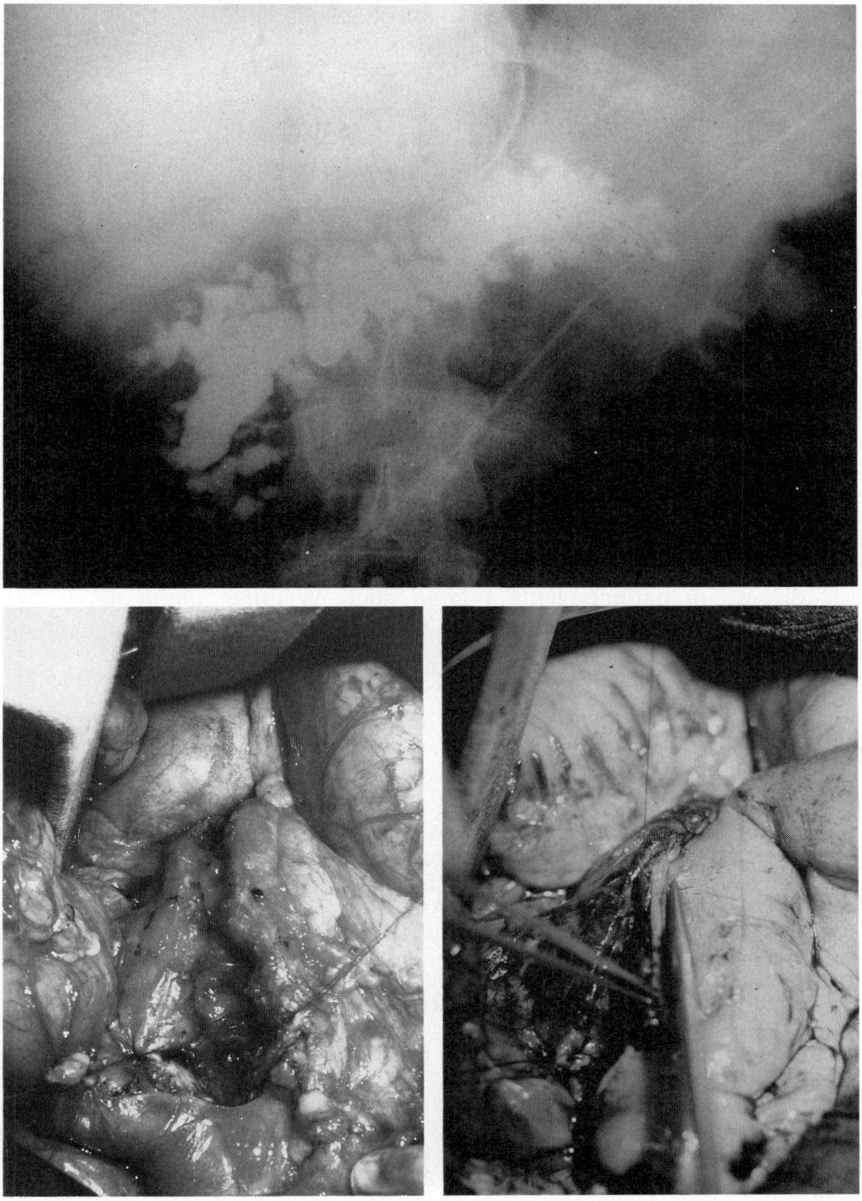

d

e

f

Fig. 5. *Continued*

Table 4. Diagnostic procedures essential for deciding on type of surgical drainage

1.	Ultrasonography
2.	Computed tomography
3.	ERCP
4.	Intraoperative pancreaticography[a]

[a] Intraoperative pancreaticography should be done only if ERCP is technically not feasible.

therapies [6, 8, 14] is necessary. A conclusive treatment strategy should be based on an interdisciplinary approach. The decision to operate at all, and when, and the choice of the surgical procedure are influenced mainly by the etiology. In case of pseudocysts following acute pancreatitis, treatment usually is not much of a problem and can be purely conservative, interventional, or surgical internal drainage. For us, cystojejunostomy is the gold standard. For pancreatic pseudocysts as a result of chronic pancreatitis, cystojejunostomy is by far the dominating alternative. Apart from some technical advantages, the most important point is the possibility to treat the basic disease in patients with a large duct. Whether simultaneous duct drainage as a prophylactic measure in the asymptomatic patient is justifiable is a matter of controversy.

References

1. Andersson R, Janzon M, Sundberg I, Bengmark S (1989) Management of pancreatic pseudocysts. Br J Surg 76:550–552
2. Böttger T, Steegmüller KW, Junginger T (1991) Ergebnisse der chirurgischen Therapie von Pankreaspseudozysten. Langenbecks Arch Chir 376:42–49
3. Bradley EL, Clements JL, Gonzales AC (1979) The natural history of pancreatic pseudocysts: a unified concept of management. Am J Surg 137:135–139
4. Crass RA, Way LW (1981) Acute and chronic pancreatic pseudocysts are different. Am J Surg 142:660–663
5. Frey CF (1978) Pancreatic pseudocyst – operative strategy. Ann Surg 188:652–662
6. Grewal HP, Carr-Locke D, Wood KF (1990) Endoscopic drainage of a recurrent pancreatic pseudocyst. Postgrad Med J 66:1081–1083
7. Kiviluoto T, Kivisaari L, Kivilaakso E, Lempinen M (1989) Pseudocysts in chronic pancreatitis – surgical results in 102 consecutive patients. Arch Surg 124:240–243
8. Lang EK, Paolini RM, Pottmeyer A (1991) The efficacy of palliative and definitive percutaneous versus surgical drainage of pancreatic abscesses and pseudocysts: a prospective study of 85 patients. South Med J 84:55–64
9. Munn JS, Aranha GV, Greenlee HB, Prinz RA (1987) Simultaneous treatment of chronic pancreatitis and pancreatic pseudocyst. Arch Surg 122:662–667
10. Nealon WH, Townsend CM, Thompson JC (1989) Preoperative endoscopic retrograde cholangiopancreatography (ERCP) in patients with pancreatic pseudocyst associated with resolving acute and chronic pancreatitis. Ann Surg 209:532–538

11. Newell KA, Liu T, Aranha GV, Prinz RA (1990) Are cystgastrostomy and cystjejunostomy equivalent operations for pancreatic pseudocysts? Surgery 108:635–640
12. Sankaran S, Walt AJ (1975) The natural and unnatural history of pancreatic pseudocysts. Br J Surg 62:37–44
13. Sarles H, Adler G, Dani R, Frey C, Gullo L, Harada H, Martin E, Norohna M, Scuro LA (1989) Classifications of pancreatitis and definition of pancreatic diseases. Digestion 43:234–236
14. Walt AJ, Bouwman DL, Weaver DW, Sachs RJ (1990) The impact of technology on the management of pancreatic pseudocyst. Arch Surg 125:759–763
15. Warshaw AL (1989) Pancreatic cysts and pseudocysts: new rules for a new game. Br J Surg 76:533–534
16. Warshaw AL, Rattner DW (1985) Timing of surgical drainage for pancreatic pseudocyst – clinical and chemical criteria. Ann Surg 202:720–724
17. Yeo CJ, Bastidas JA, Lynch-Nyhan A, Fishman EK, Zinner MJ, Cameron JL (1990) The natural history of pancreatic pseudocysts documented by computed tomography. Surg Gynecol Obstet 170:411–416

Pancreatic Pseudocysts: Late Results After Surgical Treatment

R.A. PRINZ[1]

Pancreatic pseudocysts are localized collections of pancreatic secretions often mixed with necrotic or hemorrhagic debris which results from inflammation or trauma. They are the most common cystic lesion of the pancreas and are characterized by their lack of an epithelial lining. The wall of a pseudocyst is composed of fibrotic or granulation tissue derived from the serosal surface or capsule of adjacent viscera, peritoneum, intestinal mesentery, or retroperitoneum. Pseudocysts are a well-recognized complication of both acute and chronic pancreatitis occurring in 1%–10% of patients with acute pancreatitis and as many as 35%–40% of patients with chronic pancreatitis [1]. However, not all fluid collections seen during the course of pancreatitis are pseudocysts or at least clinically significant pseudocysts. Noninvasive techniques such as ultrasound or computed tomography (CT) have shown that as many as 10%–50% of patients with moderately severe pancreatitis have an associated peripancreatic fluid collection [2]. However, these fluid collections resolve spontaneously in 30%–50% of patients [3, 4]. Factors indicating that resolution is unlikely include size greater than 5–6 cm, increase in size during observation, presence of chronic pancreatitis, and presence of multiple cysts.

Although pseudocysts smaller than 5–6 cm may be safely observed in asymptomatic patients [5], those that are greater than 6 cm or associated with symptoms should be treated surgically. Since pseudocysts may vary in etiology, size, location, age, number, anatomic relationships, and presence of infection, no one procedure is appropriate for every cyst and therapy must be individualized. Although CT and ultrasonographically guided percutaneous drainage and endoscopically guided internal drainage have proponents, pancreatic pseudocysts have been traditionally treated by surgery and this should still be considered the gold standard. Surgeons have three therapeutic options in dealing with pancreatic pseudocysts: external drainage, resection, or internal drainage of the cyst. Drainage procedures are usually preferred over resection because they preserve pancreatic function and have a lower mortality rate. External drainage carries a higher rate of recurrence and fistula formation and should be reserved for acute

[1] Department of Surgery, Loyola University Medical Center, 2160 South First Avenue, Maywood, Ill 60153, USA

Beger/Büchler/Malfertheiner (Eds.)
Standards in Pancreatic Surgery

cysts without a well defined wall and grossly infected cysts. Resection is an adequate alternative for small cysts in the tail, but safe removal is often not possible because of the size and/or location of the pseudocyst and its associated inflammation. This leaves internal drainage as the preferred approach in most cases.

Although external drainage has been recommended as the method of choice for treating pseudocysts by a few surgeons [6], most would reserve its use for acute problems. For those with gross infection, free rupture associated with peritonitis, and an immature wall that will not reliably hold sutures, external drainage is a necessary and life-saving operation. External drainage carries a higher rate of morbidity and mortality than other surgical options, but this is probably more a reflection of the severity of illness encountered than the inadequacies of the procedure itself. Mortality rates for external drainage are usually around 10% with a range of 2%–25% [7, 8]. Pancreatic fistula and recurrent pseudocyst formation as might be expected are also higher with external drainage. This is inherent in the procedure since underlying abnormalities in the pancreatic duct which may have caused the pseudocyst are unaltered. Persistent pancreatic fistulas occur in 10%–20% of patients with external drainage and recurrent pseudocysts in 8%–33%. Rates of fistula formation and recurrent pseudocysts are 11% and 33%, respectively, in our experience with external drainage [9]. These high rates are a reasonable price to get a patient over a life-threatening episode.

External drainage is performed by incising the cyst wall in an area with direct access to the abdominal wall (Fig. 1). Both the opening into the cyst and the abdominal wall incision should be placed for maximal dependent drainage. If an immature cyst wall is disrupted during the exploration, or it has spontaneously ruptured, this opening can be used for drain placement. All necrotic material and debris is removed, and internal loculations are broken. Care must be taken not to induce bleeding, and all hemorrhage must be controlled before wound closure. Specimens for gram stain and culture are obtained. However, it is not the mere presence of bacteria that dictates the need for external drainage. As many as a third of pseudocysts are contaminated by bacterial or fungal organisms. These may still be safely drained internally if there is no active inflammation or gross evidence of infection. Any suspicious areas of the wall of the pseudocyst are biopsied to rule out an underlying or associated malignancy. At least one large soft sump suction catheter is placed into the pseudocyst cavity and brought out to the abdominal wall. Care must be given to avoid proximity to blood vessels or the small or large intestine which can be eroded by the drains. The drains are kept in place until the pseudocyst has been completely decompressed and a well-formed track is present.

Resection is appropriate therapy for pseudocysts that are well localized to the tail of the gland and not widely adherent to adjacent structures. Pancreatico-duodenectomy or Whipple resection is almost never indicated

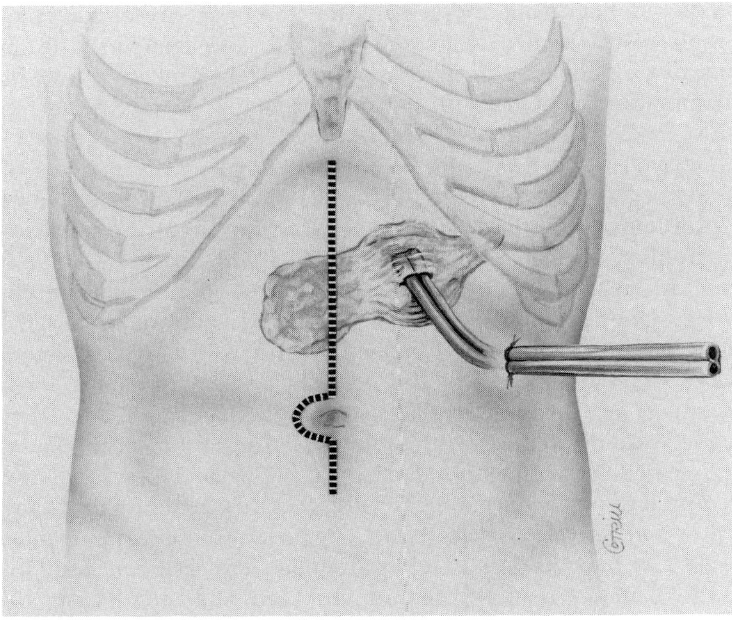

Fig. 1. External drainage is indicated for treatment of gross infection, free rupture, or cysts with immature walls. The cyst is evacuated of fluid, and debris and at least one large soft sump suction catheter is brought out through the abdominal wall

for pseudocyst disease. Likewise, extended or near total pancreatectomy should be avoided because of the high rate of postoperative diabetes. Frey reported that 32% of patients were diabetic on follow-up after 40%–80% distal pancreatectomy for pseudocyst disease [10]. This was not that dissimilar to the 26% rate with internal drainage procedures. However, 89% of patients were diabetic after 80%–95% resections and 15 of the 17 diabetic patients were insulin dependent.

Resection is usually technically more difficult than drainage because the inflammatory reaction associated with the pseudocyst and underlying pancreatitis may distort the anatomy and obliterate normal planes of dissection (Fig. 2). Mortality rates for pseudocyst resection range from 6–18%. The morbidity of resection can also be excessive if care is not given to patient selection. Endoscopic retrograde cholangiopancreatography (ERCP) can provide valuable information about the proximal pancreatic duct. This information is helpful in defining the extent of resection and the likelihood of success. Changes of chronic pancreatitis or a stricture of the more proximal duct indicate a greater chance for cyst recurrence and persistent pancreatic fistula formation. Kiviluto and coworkers noted recurrent pseudocyst development in 4 [13%] of 32 patients with chronic pancreatitis

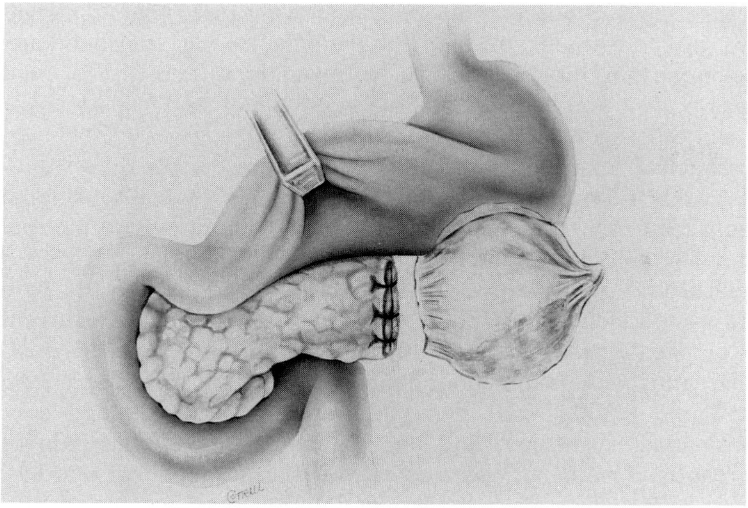

Fig. 2. Resection is appropriate management of pseudocysts that are well localized to the tail of the gland and not widely adherent to adjacent structures

treated primarily with distal pancreatectomy for pseudocyst disease [11]. Before using ERCP, two of the eleven patients treated by distal resection in our series of pseudocyst patients developed persistent pancreatic fistulas [9]. Both required reoperations and internal drainage.

Most studies support internal drainage as the preferred method of treating noninfected pseudocysts that have a mature wall. The stomach, duodenum or a Roux-en-Y loop of intestine can provide the site of drainage. Although the condition of the patient and anatomic considerations such as size, location, and adherence to surrounding structures may indicate one type of drainage rather than another, the decision is often dictated by the personal bias of the surgeon. Internal drainage of pseudocyts is most often accomplished by cystgastrostomy or Roux-en-Y cystenterostomy.

The infrequent use of cystduodenostomy cannot be explained on the basis of anatomic factors alone. Some surgeons have felt that an inordinate morbidity and mortality are associated with its use. Bradley has reviewed his own experience with cystduodenostomy and that reported in the literature to determine the origin of this controversy [12]. In 140 patients collected from the literature that had been treated with cystduodenostomy, the overall mortality rate was 7.8%; the complication rate was 18%; and the recurrence rate was 6.2%. However, in the 12 patients who had laterolateral cystduodenostomy, there were six deaths and eight complications. The most common complication and cause of death with laterolateral cystduodenostomy was suture line dehiscence and abscess formation. The morbidity and mortality of laterolateral cystduodenostomy far exceeded that of any other form of internal drainage, and Bradley concluded, and we agree, that it should rarely if ever be performed. In the 128 patients having transduodenal cystduodenostomy, mortality was 2.3%, complications were 7.8%, and recurrence was 6.2%. These results are as good if not better than those reported for any other form of internal drainage.

The location of recurrent cysts following transduodenal cystduodenostomy is rarely reported. It is altogether possible that a substantial number of these recurrences arise in an area remote from the site of internal drainage and are actually missed multiple cysts or are due to the progression of underlying chronic pancreatitis. In 11 patients we have reported with transduodenal cystduodenostomy, there were no deaths and no recurrent cysts [13]. Complications occurred in three patients and included postoperative pancreatitis, wound infection, pancreatic fistula, and intraoperative hemorrhage. Three patients had multiple cysts that were drained concomitantly with cystgastrostomy, and one patient had continued pain of chronic pancreatitis. This experience indicates that transduodenal cystduodenostomy is a safe and reliable method of internal drainage for mature cysts that are located in the head of the pancreas adjacent to the duodenum. Preoperative and intraoperative evaluation of the pancreas is necessary to rule out the presence of multiple pseudocysts or underlying chronic pancreatitis if optimal results are to be obtained.

Transduodenal cystduodenostomy is indicated for mature pseudocysts that are greater than 5–6 cm in diameter, that are located in a juxtaduodenal position, and that are not adherent to the stomach (Fig. 3). The operation begins with an extended Kocher maneuver so that the duodenum and pancreas are brought up into the wound where they can be thoroughly evaluated and safely dealt with. Ideally the cyst should be drained where it is closest to the medial wall of the duodenum. This point is identified grossly by the distortion or splaying of the duodenum by the cyst and can be confirmed by transduodenal needle aspiration. Intraoperative ultrasound can also help in defining the anatomic structures and how they are related in this area. The cyst can be drained into any portion of the duodenum although great care is needed to avoid common bile duct injury in the second portion. The lateral duodenal wall is opened longtitudinally directly opposite the area anticipated for cyst drainage. When the cyst is at all close to the common bile duct or ampulla of Vater, their location must be confirmed before proceeding. If there is any doubt, a Fogarty catheter can be positioned down the common bile duct and through the ampulla into the duodenum. This is usually placed through the cystic duct stump after cholecystectomy, but it can be placed directly into the common bile duct. An incision is made longtitudinally along the median plane of the medial wall of the duodenum to avoid injury to the anterior and posterior pancreaticoduodenal arteries. The incision must be at least 2 cm in length to insure adequate drainage. Fluid and debris are aspirated and loculations are broken. Bleeding is controlled with sutures between the medial duodenal

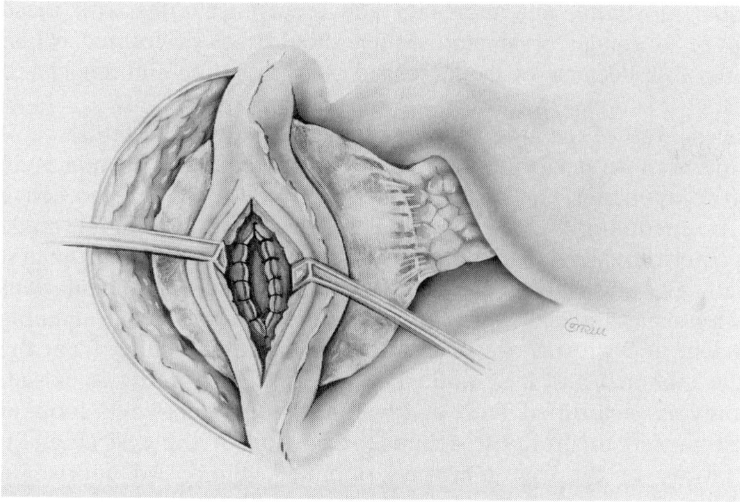

Fig. 3. Transduodenal cystduodenostomy is a safe, reliable method for mature pseudocysts that are in a juxtaduodenal position

wall and the cyst. One patient in our series had hemorrhage in the depths of the cyst that required placement of a Foley catheter through the stomach into the cystduodenostomy where tamponade by balloon inflation controlled the bleeding. With appropriate patient selection and care to avoid injury to the common bile duct and pancreatic vasculature, transduodenal cystduodenostomy can be performed with safety and success comparable to other forms of internal drainage.

Cystgastrostomy and Roux-en-Y cystenterostomy are the most common methods for elective drainage of pancreatic pseudocysts. We recently compared the efficacy of these operations in 39 patients treated with cystgastrostomy and 59 patients treated with cystenterostomy [14]. The groups were comparable in age, sex, cause of pancreatitis, pseudocyst location, symptoms, and preoperative serum amylase level. Cysts treated with cystgastrostomy were significantly larger than those treated with cystenterostomy with the mean diameters being 11.1 ± 0.9 versus 6.7 ± 0.7 cm ($p < 0.05$). The mean duration of operation of 148 ± 11 min for cystgastrostomy was significantly less than the 265 ± 15 min for cystenterostomy ($p < 0.05$). There was cyst recurrence in 10% with cystgastrostomy and 7% with cystenterostomy. Two patients died after cystgastrostomy for an operative mortality of 5%. Both deaths were related to upper gastrointestinal bleeding. There were two deaths after cystenterostomy for an operative mortality of 3%. Both deaths were related to intra-abdominal sepsis. The morbidity and mortality of these two drainage procedures were comparable although gastrointestinal bleeding was more common with cystgastrostomy and intra-abdominal abscess was more common with cystjejunostomy.

Given the equal morbidity and mortality and recurrence rates with these two methods of drainage, cystgastrostomy should be performed when anatomically feasible because of its decreased operative time and associated blood loss.

The posterior wall of the stomach must be adherent to the pseudocyst if cystgastrostomy is to be performed (Fig. 4). Only after this is certain is an anterior gastrotomy made. The cyst is needle aspirated to be sure no active hemorrhage is encountered. An opening greater than 2.5 cm is made through the posterior wall of the stomach into the cyst. A portion of the cyst wall is biopsied. The cyst is evacuated of all fluid and debris, and loculations are broken. Hemostasis is checked both within the cyst and at the opening into the stomach, and sutures are placed to control any bleeding from the opening of the stomach and cyst wall. The anterior gastrotomy is closed. Cystenterostomy is performed with a 40-cm isolated Roux-en-Y loop of intestine anastomosed to the most dependent portion of the cyst (Fig. 5). Once again biopsy of the cyst is always obtained. Fluid and debris are removed and loculations are broken. Gram stain and culture of the fluid is obtained.

All of the surgical options for pancreatic pseudocysts are relatively effective. Nevertheless, the choice of surgical intervention can affect the long-term outcome in pseudocyst disease. The effect of extended pancreatic resection on the development of diabetes has already been discussed. Two other long-term problems can be altered by our surgical decisions at the initial operation. Cyst recurrence and abdominal pain are the most frequent

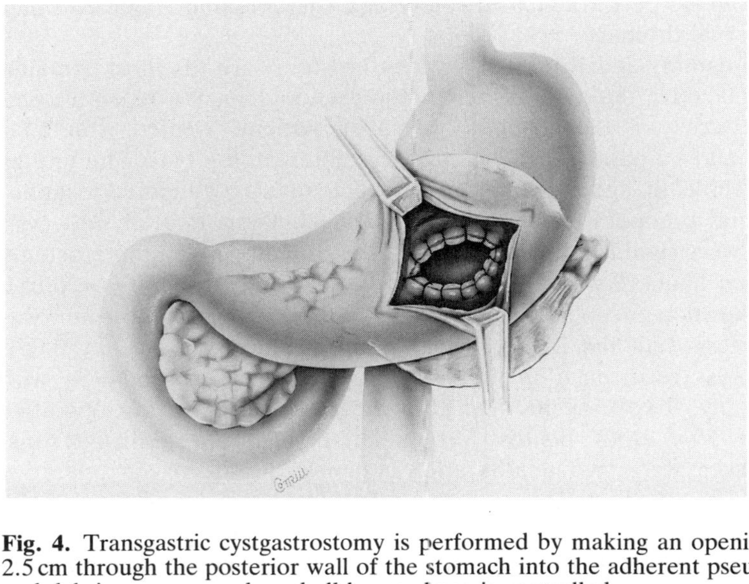

Fig. 4. Transgastric cystgastrostomy is performed by making an opening of at least 2.5 cm through the posterior wall of the stomach into the adherent pseudocyst. Fluid and debris are removed, and all hemorrhage is controlled

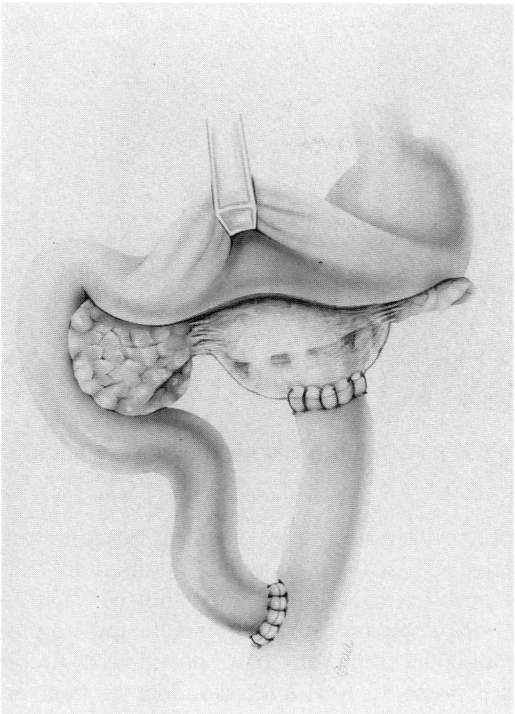

Fig. 5. Cystenterostomy is performed with a 40-cm isolated Roux-en-Y loop of intestine anastomosed to the most dependent portion of the pseudocyst

causes for reoperation in patients treated for pseudocysts. Frey reported that 40 of 120 patients undergoing operation for pseudocysts required reoperation [10]. Of these 40 patients, 26 had a second operation for a persistent or recurrent pseudocyst, and 11 were reoperated for persistent or recurrent abdominal pain. Fifteen of 81 patients operated on for pseudocyst that were reported from our center required reoperation [9]. Seven were for persistent or recurrent pseudocysts, and seven were for persistent or recurrent pain.

Cyst recurrence ranges from 5% to 20% in most series of surgically treated pseudocysts. Premature anastomotic closure is one possible cause for early recurrence. We believe this can be prevented by making a large anastomosis of at least 2.5 cm, evacuating all of the fluid and debris and breaking up the loculations within the cyst at the time of operation. A more likely cause for early recurrence in our opinion is missed multiple pseudocysts. Multiple pseudocysts occur in 3%–14% of patients with surgically treated pseudocysts [15]. If these are not recognized preoperatively or intraoperatively, they will not of course be treated appropriately. Con-

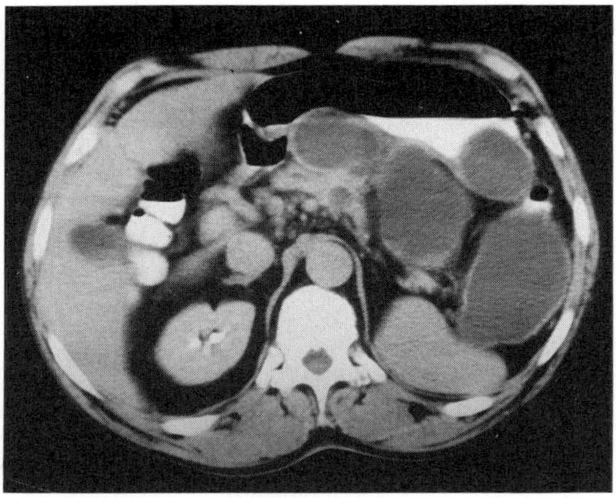

Fig. 6. Abdominal CT scan shows four separate pancreatic pseudocysts

sequently, we categorize cysts noted within 6 months of initial operation as persistent pseudocysts. Preoperative CT scans should be obtained to rule out multiple pseudocysts so this problem can be avoided (Fig. 6). Just as importantly, the pancreatic and peripancreatic areas should be thoroughly evaluated intraoperatively after elective treatment of a pseudocyst to be certain there are no other cysts present. Multiple pseudocysts can be dealt with by any combination of the various drainage procedures and/or resection. Bradley has also described internal cystocystostomy as a means to drain multiple pseudocysts that are relatively contiguous [16].

Cysts that are noted more than 6–12 months after operation are more likely new cysts. We would term these recurrent rather than persistent pseudocysts. Recurrent pseudocysts are more likely to develop in patients with chronic pancreatitis. This is true whether internal drainage or pancreatic resection is performed as the initial operation. Since neither method deals with the underlying chronic pancreatitis that precipitated the pseudocyst, neither can be expected to halt its progress. This problem can be rectified by a high index of suspicion for the presence of chronic pancreatitis. In patients with pancreatic calcifications, endocrine or exocrine insufficiency, a long history of alcohol abuse, or recurrent attacks of pain, we believe the pancreatic duct should be evaluated with ERCP prior to elective treatment of the pseudocyst. If a dilated pancreatic duct is identified, long-term success must take into account both the pseudocyst and the chronic pancreatitis. We have shown in patients with chronic pancreatitis and pseudocyst disease that lateral pancreaticojejunostomy can be used to drain both the pancreatic duct and the pseudocyst without an increase in morbidity and mortality. In 87 consecutive patients undergoing lateral pancreaticojejunostomy for chronic pancreatitis, 26 had combined pseudocyst and pancreatic duct drainage, and 61 had pancreatic duct drainage alone [17]. There was no difference in the operative morbidity or mortality, which was 19% and 8%, respectively, for combined drainage and 18% and 2% for ductal drainage alone. There were no recurrent pseudocysts noted with this approach of complete pancreatic duct drainage in either group.

The other long-term problem seen after pseudocyst drainage is persistent or recurrent abdominal pain. We believe this is also a reflection of the progression of chronic pancreatitis. Once again, if chronic pancreatitis is suspected, this problem can be anticipated and reoperation avoided by simultaneous pseudocyst and pancreatic duct drainage. Optimum treatment for pancreatic pseudocysts entails recognition of concomitant chronic pancreatitis. Combining pseudocyst drainage with lateropancreaticojejunostomy does not increase the morbidity or mortality, of either internal pseudocyst drainage or pancreatic duct drainage alone.

In conclusion, internal drainage is the preferred method of dealing with pancreatic pseudocysts. It does not hasten the development of diabetes as does pancreatic resection. If the problems of multiple pseudocysts and chronic pancreatitis are kept in mind and dealt with, the need for reoperation for persistent or recurrent pseudocyst and persistent or recurrent abdominal pain will be lessened.

Acknowledgements. I appreciate the assistance of Linda Wahrer in preparing the manuscript and Sue Cottrill, Pamela Wielgos, and Sharon Arizzi in preparing the illustrations.

References

1. Prinz RA (1990) Pseudocyst drainage in chronic pancreatitis. In: Beger HG, Büchler M, Ditschuneit H, Malfertheiner P (eds) Chronic pancreatitis. Springer, Berlin Heidelberg New York, pp 426–432
2. Siegelman SS, Copeland BE, Saba GP et al. (1980) CT of fluid collections associated with pancreatitis. AJR 134:1121–1132
3. Aranha GV, Prinz RA, Esguerra AC, Greenlee HB (1983) The nature and course of cystic pancreatic lesions diagnosed by ultrasound. Arch Surg 118:486–488
4. Bradley EL, Clements JL (1974) Implications of diagnostic ultrasound in the surgical management of pancreatic pseudocysts. Am J Surg 127:163–173
5. Yeo CJ, Bastidas JA, Lynch-Nyhan A et al. (1990) The natural history of pancreatic pseudocysts documented by computed tomography. Surg Gynecol Obstet 170:411–417
6. Elechi EN, Callender CO, Leffall LD et al. (1979) The treatment of pancreatic pseudocysts by external drainage. Surg Gynecol Obstet 148:707–710
7. Hunter JL, Ephgrave K (1987) Emergency surgery for pancreatic pseudocysts. South Med J 80:462–465
8. Walt AJ, Bouwman DL, Weaver DW, Sachs RJ (1990) The impact of technology on the management of pancreatic pseudocyst. Arch Surg 125:759–763
9. Aranha GV, Prinz RA, Freeark RJ et al. (1982) Evaluation of therapeutic options for pancreatic pseudocysts. Arch Surg 117:717–721
10. Frey CJ (1978) Pancreatic pseudocyst-operative strategy. Ann Surg 188:652–662

11. Kiviluoto T, Kivisaari L, Livilaakso E, Lempinen M (1989) Pseudocysts in chronic pancreatitis. Arch Surg 124:240–243
12. Bradley EL (1984) Cystoduodenostomy. Ann Surg 200:698–701
13. Altimari A, Aranha GV, Greenlee HB, Prinz RA (1986) Results of cystoduodenostomy for treatment of pancreatic pseudocysts. Am Surg 52:438–441
14. Newell KA, Liu T, Aranha GV, Prinz RA (1990) Are cystgastrostomy and cystjejunostomy equivalent operations for pancreatic pseudocysts? Surgery 108:635–640
15. Goulet RJ, Goodman J, Schaffer R et al. (1984) Multiple pancreatic pseudocyst disease. Ann Surg 199:6–13
16. Bradley EL, Austin H (1982) Multiple pancreatic pseudocysts: the principle of internal cystocystostomy in surgical management. Surgery 92:111–116
17. Munn JS, Aranha GV, Greenlee HB, Prinz RA (1989) Simultaneous treatment of chronic pancreatitis and pancreatic pseudocyst. Arch Surg 122:662–667

IV. Cancer of the Pancreas

Morphology of Pancreatic Exocrine Tumors

P.M. Pour,[1] J. Permerth,[2] and M. Mogaki

Classification of tumors is important for understanding the tumor histogenesis and prognosis. Since 1836, when pancreatic cancer was first described [1], progress has been made in pancreatic cancer morphology. However, there are still inconsistencies in the description and classification of pancreatic tumors, mostly because of the lack of information on the natural history of the disease. The silent course of the disease and its late clinical manifestation and diagnosis are contributing factors, as are the insufficient availability of tissues (biopsy, autopsy), the technique in preparation of the specimen, methods of histological examination (including the number of sections taken for evaluation), and personal experience. Therefore, some of the classifications have been either simplified, exaggerated by details or are incomplete [2–10]. For example, the classification by Cubilla and Fitzgerald [5] and Sommers and Meissner [10] include mixed duct-islet, duct-islet-acinar and acinar-islet tumors. In our experience and that of others [11–17], more than 70% of pancreatic carcinoma contains endocrine cells, some in a pattern consistent with the mixed-cell tumors of Cubilla and Fitzgerald (Figs. 1, 2). Therefore, Klöppel and Heitz [18] do not classify these tumors as separate entities, and rightly so. The same applies for the mixed acinar-islet and carcinoid-islet cell tumors that neither we nor other investigators have encountered in their material, except for rare tumors that contain both zymogen and endocrine granules [17]. Such tumors should not be regarded as mixed tumors but rather reflect altered differentiation.

The distinction between benign and malignant tumors has also not been worked out. Although previous classifications considered cystic serous tumors (microcystic adenoma) generally as benign, recent observations point to the malignant nature of some [19, 20].

There are no guidelines for preparation and processing of specimen for histological diagnosis. Because tumors may present different histological types in different regions, the number of tissues taken from each tumor determines the accuracy of classification. This has been shown experimentally to be one of the important considerations in such studies [21, 22].

[1] The Eppley Institute for Research in Cancer and Allied Diseases, University of Nebraska Medical Center, 600 S 42nd Street, Omaha, NE 68198-6805, USA
[2] Department of Surgery, University of Linköping, Sweden

Beger/Büchler/Malfertheiner (Eds.)
Standards in Pancreatic Surgery

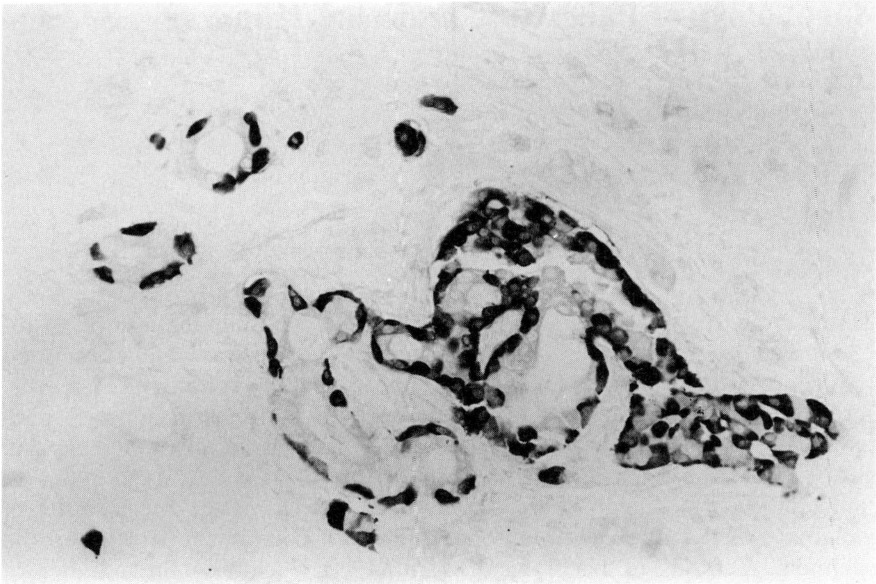

Fig. 1. A well-differentiated pancreatic ductal adenocarcinoma containing many cells immunoreactive with anti-glucagon antibody. (Peroxidase-antiperoxidase, ×210)

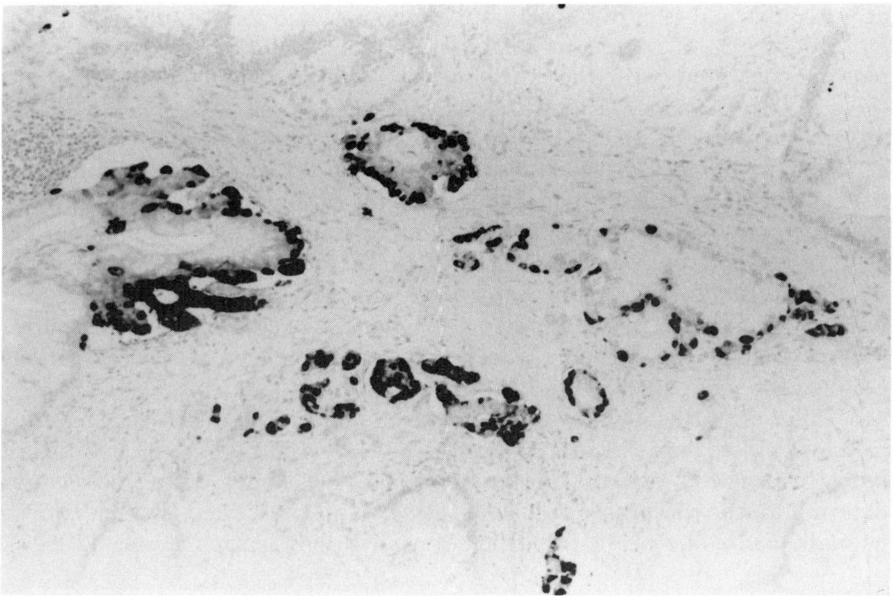

Fig. 2. A well-differentiated ductal adenocarcinoma with numerous cells immunoreactive with monoclonal anti-chromogranin A antibody. (ABC, ×100)

For example, many studies have shown that giant cell carcinoma, which was previously regarded as a separate entity [5, 10], represents a poorly differentiated variety of ductal adenocarcinoma.

The personal perception is another confounding factor in tumor diagnosis. Some consider small papillary projections occurring in some cystic tumors as papillary neoplasms, whereas others require dominant papillary structure as a prerequisite for lesions to be termed a papillary tumor.

Clearly, like tumors of other sites, some neoplasms cause problems in classification. The use of electron microscopy in tumor diagnosis has helped to solve some of the obstacles. For example, some of the "unclassified" or otherwise termed tumors, such as microadenocarcinoma of Cubilla and Fitzgerald [5], can now be categorized properly. Today, thanks to the development of many sophisticated methods, including diagnostic techniques for early tumor detection and examination, generation of antibodies for immunohistochemical studies, molecular biological studies, flow cytometry and DNA and proliferation index analysis [23], offers the possibility to advance significantly pancreatic cancer classification. The increasing collaboration between pathologists and clinicians is significant and fruitful in assessing tumor biology, therapeutic approaches, and prognosis.

Based on the above mentioned, a group of investigators realized the need for a new, more accurate, simple, and practical classification. For the first time in the history of pancreatic tumor classification, experts from different medical disciplines, including clinicians, pathologists, and basic researchers from around the world, gathered together to establish a universally accepted classification system [24]. Despite the initial scepticisms, this meeting, which took place August 1991 in Nagasaki, Japan, turned out to be a success. The experts worked out a new proposal for tumor classification and also recommended establishment of guidelines for tissue preparation and examination. The classification was based on reviewing a large number of histologic samples from different laboratories and a review of clinical data. Their recommendation will be published as an atlas: *Diagnostic Atlas for Exocrine Pancreatic Neoplasms. An International Guide to Classification*.

In this atlas, methods for tissue examination (sampling for routine and investigative purposes), intraoperative sampling diagnosis, staging and grading are recommended. To standardize the nomenclature of pancreatic and parapancreatic tissues, macroscopic and microscopic charactristics of the pancreas, including the terminology of ductal and vascular system, nerves, and lymphatic tissues will be given. Two classifications have been proposed. That according to morphological appearance is as follows:

Serous cystic tumors
  Serous cystadenoma (microcystic adenoma)
  Serous cystadenocarcinoma (microcystic carcinoma)
Intraductal tumors

Intraductal papillary tumors
- Noninvasive
- Invasive

Intraductal mucin hypersecreting tumors
- Noninvasive
- Invasive

Mucinous cystic tumors
- Noninvasive
- Invasive

Adenocarcinoma (ductal type)
- Well to moderately differentiated
- Poorly differentiated
- Mucinous carcinoma with or without signet ring cells
- Adenosquamous carcinoma

Acinar cell carcinoma
- Well differentiated
- Poorly differentiated

Anaplastic carcinoma

Miscellaneous
- Solid cystic tumor
- Pancreaticoblastoma
- Small cell carcinoma

Preneoplastic lesions

The classification according to biological behavior is as follows:

Benign
- Microcystic serous adenoma

Uncertain biological behavior
- Intraductal tumors
  - Mucinous cystic tumor
  - Solid-cystic tumor

Malignant
- Microcystic serous adenocarcinoma
- Mucinous cystadenocarcinoma
- Adenocarcinoma (variants)
- Acinar cell carcinoma
- Pancreaticoblastoma
- Small cell carcinoma
- Anaplastic tumor

Note that in this classification, some neoplasms are designated as "tumors" without assigning them to either benign (adenomas) or malignant lesions (carcinoma). This ambiguous designation reflects the unpredictable nature of such neoplasms. Additional morphologic phrases, such as "noninvasive" and "invasive," is to indicate their biological behavior. Such apparently "vague" terminology can help us to gather reliable information about such lesions.

This classification should not be considered as a Rosetta stone for pancreatic tumor classification, but it is an attempt to guide pathologists, clinicians and basic researchers in developing a clinically more useful classification system and in understanding the biology of pancreatic cancer.

References

1. Mondiére JT (1836) Recherches pour sevir á l'histoir pathologique du pancreás. Arch Gen Med 2e série 3:133–154
2. Ansari A, Burch GE (1968) A correlative study of proven carcinoma of the pancreas in 83 patients. Am J Gastroentrol 50:456–475
3. Arkin A, Weisberg SW (1949) Carcinoma of the pancreas. A clinical and pathologic studies of seventy-five cases. Gastroenterology 13:118–126
4. Becker V (1973) Bauchspeicheldrüse (Inselapparat ausgenommen). In: Doerr W, Seifert G, Uehlinger E (eds) Spezielle pathologische Anatomie, vol 6. Springer, Berlin Heidelberg New York
5. Cubilla AL, Fitzgerald PJ (1982) Tumors of the exocrine pancreas. Atlas of tumor pathology, 2nd series, fasc 19. Armed Forces Institute of Pathology, Washington DC
6. Frantz VK (1959) Tumors of the pancreas. In: Atlas of tumor pathology VII, fasc 27 and 28. Armed Forces Institute of Pathology, Washington DC
7. Gibson JB, Sobin LH (1978) Histological typing of tumors of the liver, biliary tract and pancreas. World Health Organization, Geneva (WHO, International histological classification of tumors, no 20)
8. Glenner G, Mallory GK (1956) The cystadenoma and related nonfunctional tumors of the pancreas. Pathogenesis, classification and significance. Cancer 9:980–996
9. Miller JR, Baggenstoss AH, Comfort MW (1951) Carcionoma of the pancreas. Effect of histological type and grade of malignancy on its behavior. Cancer 4:233–241
10. Sommers SC, Meissner WA (1954) Unusual carcinomas of the pancreas. Arch Pathol 58:101–111
11. Eusebi V, Capelle C, Bondi A, Sess F, Vezzandini P, Mancini AM (1901) Endocrine-paracrine cells in pancreatic exocrine carcinomas. Histopathology 5:599–613
12. Kamisawa T, Fukayama M, Koike M, Tabata I, Okamoto A (1987) So-called papillary and cystic neoplasm of the pancreas. An immunohistochemical and ultrastructural study. Acta Pathol Jpn 37:785–794
13. Kodama T, Mori W (1983) Morphological behaviour of carcinoma of the pancreas. 2. Argyrophil cells and Langerhans' islets in the carcinomatous tissues. Acta Pathol Jpn 33:483–493.
14. Ichijima K, Akaishi K, Toyoda N, Kobashi Y, Ueda Y, Matsuo S, Yamabe H (1985) Carcinoma of the pancreas with endocrine component in childhood. J Clin Pathol 83:95–100
15. Reid JD, Yuh S-L, Petrelli M, Jaffe R (1982) Ductuloinsular tumors of the pancreas: a light, electron microscopic and immunohistochemical study. Cancer 49:908–915
16. Schlossnagel DC, Campbell WG (1981) The papillary and solid neoplasm of the pancreas. A report of two cases with electron microscopy, one containing neurosecretory granules. Cancer 47:2603–2610

17. Ulich T, Cheng L, Lewin KL (1982) Acinar-endocrine cell tumor of the pancreas. Report of a pancreatic tumor containing both zymogen and neuroendocrine granulas. Cancer 50:2099–2105
18. Klöppel G, Heitz PU (1984) Pancreas pathology. Churchill Livingstone, Edinburgh
19. George DH, Murphy F, Michalski R, Ulmer BG (1989) Serous cystadenocarcinoma of the pancreas. A new entity? Am J Surg Pathol 13:61–66
20. Kamei●●
21. Pour PM, Wilson R (1981) Experimental pancreas tumor. In: Moossa AR (ed) Cancer of the pancreas. Williams and Wilkins, Baltimore, pp 37–158
22. Pour PM (1980) Experimental pancreatic ductal (ductular) tumors. In: Fitzgerald PJ, Morrison AB (eds) The pancreas. William and Wilkins, Baltimore, pp 111–139
23. Kamei K, Funabiki T, Orchial M, Amano H, Kasahara M, Sakamoto T (1991) Three cases of solid and cystic tumor of the pancreas. Analysis comparing the histopathological findings and DNA histograms. Int J Pancreatol (in press)
24. International Classification of Pancreatic Cancer (1991) The 3rd meeting of the International Pancreatic Cancer Study Group (IPCSG), Nagasaki, August 1991

The Molecular Pathology of Pancreatic Cancer

N.R. Lemoine[1]

Introduction

Our increased understanding of the molecular biology of oncogenes has allowed us to investigate the molecular events associated with pancreatic tumorigenesis. We are beginning to identify those oncogenic events that are necessary and sufficient to produce neoplasia and to determine their temporal sequence of activation. We can now reconstruct many of these events in vitro using gene transfer techniques to introduce activated cellular oncogenes into normal pancreatic epithelium in culture. These are exciting developments because we have the technology to detect oncogene activation for a molecular diagnosis of pancreatic cancer, and we have identified new targets for the design of therapeutic strategies.

Cellular oncogenes can be classified as components of signal transduction pathways, transmitting information from extracellular events through cytoplasmic cascades ending in the modulation of gene transcription within the nucleus. Here we will review recent advances in our understanding of these events in pancreatic cancer.

Growth Factors and Their Receptors

The EGF Receptor System

The epidermal growth factor (EGF) receptor (EGFR) is encoded by the c-*erbB1* proto-oncogene and is a transmembrane growth factor receptor with tyrosine kinase activity. Its known ligands include EGF, transforming growth factor-alpha, amphiregulin; other candidates include cripto and schwannoma-derived growth factor. We have found that transforming growth factor-alpha is expressed at low levels in normal ductal epithelium of the human pancreas and is expressed at higher levels in the reactive hyperplasia of chronic pancreatitis. In 95% of ductal adenocarcinomas of the pancreas this growth factor is highly overexpressed [1]. EGF is not expressed in the

[1] ICRF Oncology Group, RPMS, Hammersmith Hospital, Du Cane Road, London, W12 0NN, U.K.

Beger/Büchler/Malfertheiner (Eds.)
Standards in Pancreatic Surgery

normal pancreas but is expressed in an ulceration-associated cell lineage (UACL) that is involved in the repopulation of the epithelial lining of ducts involved in chronic pancreatitis. EGF is overexpressed in 12% of ductal adenocarcinomas of the pancreas [1]. EGFR is expressed only in the islets of the normal pancreas but in chronic pancreatitis is expressed at detectable levels by all cells of the ductal system including the centroacinar cells. Overexpression of EGFR occurs in 95% of ductal adenocarcinomas of the pancreas, and is the result of increased transcription since there is no evidence of gene amplification in these tumours. Therefore, there is the potential for autocrine growth stimulation of ductal epithelial cells both in reactive hyperplastic and neoplastic conditions of the human pancreas. We are now investigating the involvement of the other potential ligands for the EGFR in these conditions.

The c-*erbB2* Growth Factor Receptor

This receptor is closely related to the EGFR but has a separate class of ligands, identified recently as the heregulins and gp30 [9, 11, 12]. We have shown that the c-*erbB2* p185 protein is overexpressed in approximately 20% of ductal adenocarcinomas of the pancreas, and is sometimes associated with amplification of the c-*erbB2* gene.

Fibroblast Growth Factor Receptors

The dense stromal reaction often observed in pancreatic adenocarcinoma suggests the contribution of important epithelial-stromal interactions. An important category of growth factors involved in such interactions, responsible for the stimulation of angiogenesis and capable of mitogenic stimulation of both epithelial and stromal cells, is the family of fibroblast growth factors (FGF), also known as heparin-binding growth factors. This family currently comprises seven members namely acidic FGF (FGF1), basic FGF (FGF2), the product of the *int-2* oncogene (FGF3), the product of the *hst-1* oncogene (FGF4 or K-FGF), FGF5, FGF6 and keratinocyte growth factor (FGF7). The receptors for this family of growth factors are equally complicated, currently comprising at least four members, the product of the *flg* gene (FGFR1), the product of the *bek* oncogene (FGFR2), FGFR3 and FGFR4. We suspect that abnormalities of this system could contribute to the observed phenotype of pancreatic adenocarcinomas [7].

Cytoplasmic Oncogenes

Kirsten *ras* p21

This protein is a small (21 kDa) guanine nucleotide-binding protein associated with the inner surface of the plasma membrane which has been shown to be involved in the transduction of several growth factor signals including that of the insulin growth factor 1 (IGF1) receptor [3]. This oncogene is activated by specific point mutations at codon 12 in around 75% of pancreatic adenocarcinomas [6]. We have recently found that this activation is an early oncogenic event in pancreatic tumorigenesis, being present at high frequency in carcinoma in situ lesions [8]. The very high frequency of specific point mutations of this oncogene makes this a useful marker for early pancreatic malignancy which we are currently exploiting in the molecular diagnosis of cytological aspirates, and it also represents a potential target for anti-oncogene therapy using antisense oligonucleotide strategies to block transcription and translation of the mutant oncogenes.

Other Components of Signal Transduction Particles

Signal transduction involves the association of multiple cytoplasmic proteins in so-called signal transduction particles (STP). The components of STPs include *ras* p21 protein, the GTPase-activating proteins for *ras* p21 (p120 GAP and NF1 GAP), growth factor receptors with tyrosine kinase activity including the EGFR and the platelet-growth factor (PDGF) receptor, and the product of the c-*raf* oncogene which is a cytoplasmic protein with serine/threonine kinase activity.

Nuclear Oncogenes

The c-*myc* oncogene has been implicated in the regulation of cell proliferation and differentiation in a variety of tissues. It has been recently shown that overexpression of the c-*myc* oncogene under the control of the elastase gene promoter leads to exocrine pancreatic neoplasia in transgenic mice [10]. We do not yet know whether c-*myc* is directly involved in human ductal adenocarcinomas, and this is currently under investigation in several laboratories.

Tumour Suppressor Genes

p53

Inactivation of the p53 tumour suppressor gene by point mutation is now recognised as the most frequent genetic event in human malignancies, occurring in approximately 60% of tumours of the colon, lung, breast and liver. Using a combination of mutant-specific antibodies and gene sequence analysis we have found that point mutations of p53 occur in approximately 60% of ductal adenocarcinomas of the pancreas [2], and we are now investigating the spectrum of mutations that occur in larger tumour series. We are now using recombinant retroviruses expressing mutant p53 oncogene to immortalise primary cultures of human exocrine pancreas to develop models for oncogene cooperation.

Rb1 Retinoblastoma Gene

This was the first of the tumour suppressor genes to be identified, and it is inactivated by deletion of point mutation in all retinoblastomas as well as a proportion of other tumours including small cell lung cancer, breast cancer and melanoma. Such inactivation occurs in pancreatic cancer only at low frequency.

Other Candidate Tumour Suppressor Genes

The pioneering work of Vogelstein and his colleagues in the colon carcinoma model has identified other potential tumour suppressor genes including the DCC (delefed in colorectal carcinomas) gene on human chromosome 18q [4], and the MCC and APC genes on chromosome 5q21 [5]. We are investigating whether these genes might also be involved in pancreatic adenocarcinoma.

Future Directions

The depth and breadth of our understanding of the molecular basis of pancreatic cancer is rapidly increasing. We have already identified several new potential markers of malignancy for this tumour which can be used in modern objective diagnostic assays. The real excitement, however, lies in the potential for new therapeutic strategies for pancreatic cancer. Many groups are now working on inhibitors of growth factor receptors, some of which show promise in early trials, and our group is developing antisense strategies for the inhibition of the powerful *ras* oncogenes. The identification of several tumour suppressor genes may make it possible to replace their function by novel drug mechanisms, and possibly even by replacement of the defective genes by homologous recombination and gene therapy.

References

1. Barton CM, Hall PA, Hughes CM et al. (1991) Transforming growth factor alpha and epidermal growth factor in human pancreatic cancer. J Pathol 163: 111–116
2. Barton CM, Staddon SL, Hughes CM et al. (1991) Abnormalities of the p53 tumour suppressor gene in human pancreatic cancer. Br J Cancer 64:1076–1082
3. Bergering BMT, Medema RH, Maassen JA et al. (1991) Insulin stimulation of gene expression mediated by p21*ras* expression. EMBO J 10:1103–1109
4. Fearon ER, Cho KR, Nigro JM et al. (1990) Identification of a chromosome 18q gene that is altered in colorectal cancers. Science 247:49–56

5. Kinzler KW, Nilbert MC, Vogelstein B et al. (1991) Identification of a gene located on chromosome 5q21 that is mutated in colorectal cancers. Science 251:1366–1370
6. Lemoine NR, Hall PA (1990) Growth factors and oncogenes in pancreatic cancer. Bailliéres Clin Gastroenterol 4:815–832
7. Lemoine NR, Leung HT, Gullick WJ (1992) Growth factors and the gastrointestinal tract. Gut (in press)
8. Lemoine NR, Jain S, Hughes CM et al. (1991) Ki-*ras* activation in preinvasive pancreatic cancer. Gastroenterology 102:230–236
9. Lupu R, Colomer R, Zugmaier G et al. (1990) Direct interaction of a ligand for the c-*erbB-2* oncogene product with the EGF receptor and $p185^{neu}$. Science 249:1552–1555
10. Sandgren EP, Quaife CJ, Paulovitch AG, Palmiter RD, Brinster RL (1991) Pancreatic tumor pathogenesis reflects the causative genetic lesion. Proc Natl Acad Sci USA 88:93–97
11. Yarden Y, Peles E (1991) Biochemical analysis of the ligand for the *neu* oncogenic receptor. Biochemistry 30:3543–3550
12. Yarden Y, Weinberg RA (1989) Experimental approaches to hypothetical hormones: detection of a candidate ligand of the *neu* protooncogene. Proc Natl Acad Sci USA 86:3179–3183

Diagnosis of Pancreatic Cancer

J. Schölmerich[1]

Introduction

Textbooks of medicine from the first half of the century generally stated that the diagnosis of pancreatic cancer can only be made when it is palpable, and that this is too late for successful treatment. Very recently, Classen wrote in a current textbook of internal medicine [1]: "Diagnosis is easy using US, CT, ERCP and PTC. Treatment is by surgery but unfortunately impossible in the majority of cases. 1–4% of patients survive more than 5 years." Thus it seems that major progress has been made in the diagnostic approach, without change in the outcome, i.e., without real benefit to the patient. This short review deals with four problems in the diagnosis of pancreatic cancer: diagnosis in the symptomatic patient, differential diagnosis to other pancreatic diseases, the question of early diagnosis (screening), and staging before treatment.

Diagnosis in Symptomatic Patients

The list of symptoms that patients present at the time of diagnosis (Table 1) [2] shows that a high number of patients already have advanced disease, since hepatomegaly, ascites, and palpable mass can be taken as rather certain signs of extrapancreatic spread or extensive tumor.

When pancreatic cancer is suspected in such patients it is easy, as stated above, to make a diagnosis using endoscopic retrograde cholangiopancreatography (ERCP) or computed tomography (CT; Fig. 1). Ultrasound (US) can also give good results when visibility is sufficient [3, 4]. A pathological finding is obtained in most patients [5] (Table 2). However, when different techniques are compared, it becomes evident that CT is clearly superior to US (Fig. 2) [6]. Furthermore, several studies have shown that ERCP is even better in making the diagnosis of pancreatic abnormalities and tumors [4–10]. However, it must be noted that the positive and negative predictive values for carcinoma in contrast to "abnormal finding" are rarely better than 80% [11]. This is also true for

[1] Klinik und Poliklinik für Innere Medizin I, Universität Regensburg, Franz-Josef-Strauß-Allee, W-8400 Regensburg, FRG

Beger/Büchler/Malfertheiner (Eds.)
Standards in Pancreatic Surgery

Table 1. Symptoms and findings in pancreatic carcinoma at the time of diagnosis

Pain	72%–87%
Weight loss	92%–100%
Fatigue	35%–43%
Nausea	37%–45%
Icterus	
Head	82%
Body	7%
Palpable mass	13%–23%
Hepatomegaly	33%–83%
Ascites	14%–20%

Table 2. Comparison of several techniques in the diagnosis of pancreatic carcinoma (n = 32) (from [5])

	Pathological finding (%)	Tumor suspected (%)
US	67	59
CT	81	62
ERCP	100	87
Cytology	50	12
Serology	50	12

Table 3. Endosonography compared to other imaging techniques in 140 patients with suspected pancreatic tumor (from [11])

	Accuracy	
	Abnormal finding	Defined tumor
EUS	99	69
US	71	53
CT	82	61
ERCP	89	80
ERCP + CT	99	90

endosonography (Table 3) [11, 12]. A combination of techniques obviously improves accuracy, but even so definition or exclusion of malignancy is not possible in at least 10% of patients.

As an alternative to imaging, serological tests have been studied, i.e., tumor markers [13]. Several such markers have been proposed, and some have a rather good organ specificity but generally little diagnostic specificity for malignancy, such as pancreas elastase [14, 15], where a sensitivity of 72% and a specificity of 98% against healthy controls but only 72% and

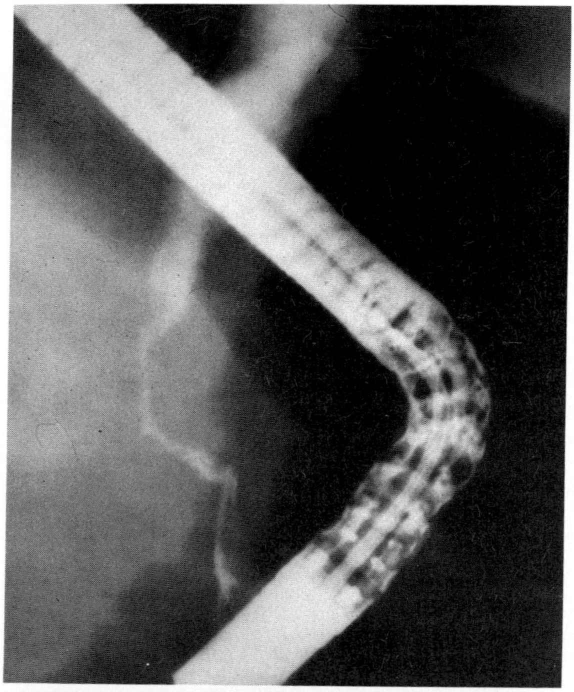

a

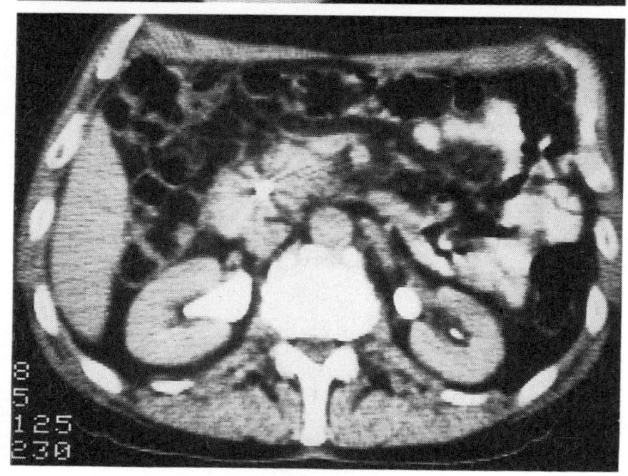

b

Fig. 1. a ERCP of a patient diagnosed as having pancreatic carcinoma. **b** CT of the same patient. Later, only chronic pancreatitis was found at surgery and at autopsy

60% against chronic pancreatitis was found [14]. Conversely, a number of oncofetal antigens exist that have high specificity for malignant change but little organ specificity. The best studied such antigen is the sialylated Lewis[a] antigen recognized by the Ca 19-9 antibody [16]. The sensitivity of this

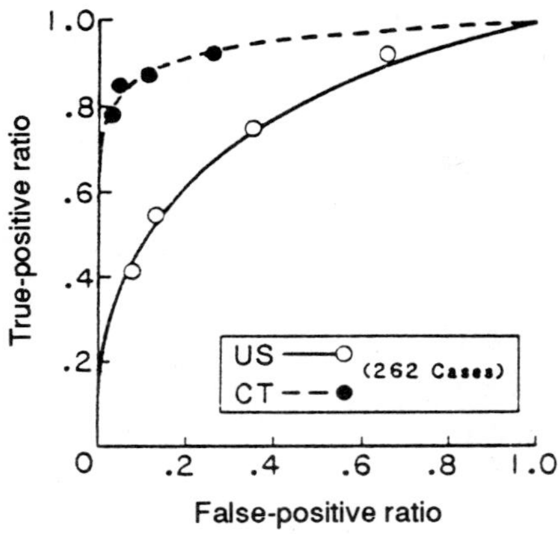

Fig. 2. Receiver operator characteristic curves comparing CT and US for diagnosis of pancreatic carcinoma. (From [6])

marker is 68%–93% and its specificity 72%–93% (for review see [13]). These figures are better than those for another marker, CEA, which has been evaluated to a significant degree (Table 4). Furthermore, combinations of CA 19-9 and elastase have been reported to have a sensitivity of 95% [17, 18]. Receiver operator characteristic analysis shows that specificity is the limiting factor rendering the positive predictive value too low (Fig. 3) [19]. Furthermore, the use of CA 19-9 is limited in patients with cholestasis and abnormal liver function, in particular cholestasis [13, 20]. Thus, overall these tests are probably useful in the evaluation of a nonjaundiced patient with unexplained abdominal pain or weight loss. However, there role is most probably only complementary to imaging techniques [21, 22].

Differential Diagnosis to Other Pancreatic Disorders

As stated above, differential diagnosis to other disorders, in particular to chronic pancreatitis, is difficult. Again, the value of tumor markers is limited, in particular for elastase-1 (Table 4) [14]. The analysis of pancreatic secretions for CA 19-9 has not proven to be helpful (Table 5) [21]. As seen

Table 4. Serological tests: a possible role

	Sensitivity (%)	Specificity (%)
CA 19-9	68–93	72–93
CEA	36–80	58–95
Elastase 1	35–70	(?)–82

Combinations reach sensitivity of 95%.

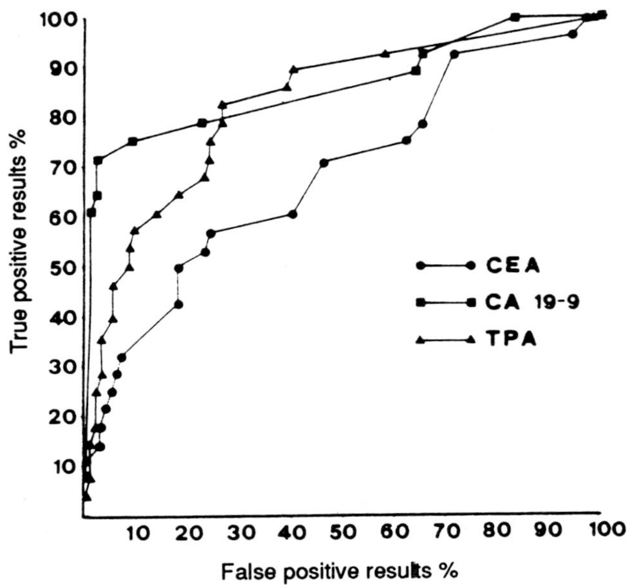

Fig. 3. Receiver operator characteristic curves comparing tumor markers for diagnosis of pancreatic carcinoma. (From [19])

Table 5. CA 19-9 in pancreatic secretions (from [21])

	Median (U/ml)	$>10^4$ U/ml (%)
Controls	0.80×10^4	30
Chronic pancreatitis	0.82×10^4	43
Carcinoma (ductal)	0.80×10^4	27

above, the imaging techniques, although detecting abnormal pancreatic morphology in a large number of patients, do not reliably enough provide a definitive diagnosis of a malignant lesion (Tables 2, 3). This is also true for endosonography (Table 3; for review see [23, 24]). Therefore, a large number of authors have proposed fine needle biopsy (FNB), either US- or CT-guided, as a major step in the diagnostic algorithm [25–32]. In our own institution sensitivity for malignant tumor was 87% and specificity 100% [33]. When comparing the reported data sensitivity ranges between 67% and 100%, and this does not depend on the number of patients studied (Fig. 4). In a recent study cytology was superior to histology (Table 6) [29], and a fine needle seems to be better than a coarse needle (Table 7) [34]. When the impact of FNB on patient management was studied, a significant reduction in surgery and hospital costs was obtained using this technique [35, 36]. However, a recent report indicated that in patients who underwent per-

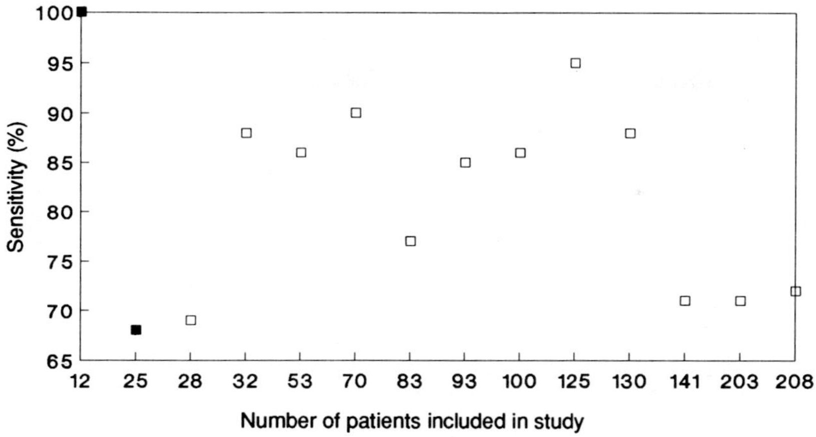

Fig. 4. Sensitivity for diagnosis of malignancy by percutaneous fine needle biopsy in different studies in relation to the number of patients included. ■, Before 1980; □, 1980 or later

Table 6. Cytology vs histology in pancreatic cancer (from [29])

Cytology	Histology		
	3 × M	Not 3 × M	Total
3 × M	31	20	51
Not 3 × M	8	41	49
Total	39	61	100

3 × M, Malignant in three examinations.

Table 7. Pancreatic cancer: fine-needle versus coarse-needle biopsy (from [34])

	Sensitivity (%)	Specificity (%)
Fine needle (22 g)	83	100
Coarse needle (18 g)	72	100

cutaneous needle biopsy a significantly higher number had a positive cytological finding in peritoneal washings during staging as compared to those without biopsy (Table 8) [37]. Thus, although FNB seems to be a helpful procedure in differentiating malignant lesions from other pancreatic diseases, it might be harmful. However, this must be further evaluated.

Table 8. The influence of certain factors on the proportion of patients with a positive cytological finding in peritoneal washings during staging (modified from [34])

	Positive finding (%)
Head	29
Body	40
Laparoscopy	33
Laparotomy	23
Ascites	50
No ascites	25
PNB	75
No PNB	19

Early Diagnosis: Screening

Up to now only 20%–30% of ductal carcinoma (95% of all pancreatic tumors) are resectable, but of these only 5% can be considered as cured [38]. If one uses available data for diagnostic tests and the prevalence of patients with pancreatic cancer in all patients having unspecific symptoms such as upper abdominal pain, a flow sheet indicates that even a test with 82% sensitivity and 95% specificity leeds to a high number of operated patients without cancer and results in the same number of deaths as compared to not performing this test (or test battery). Obviously this is an artificial system, but it high-lights the problem of screening (Fig. 5) [39]. When looking at the dependence of the posttest probability, it is seen that the CA 19-9 test has a good separating power only at a prevalence of approximately 20%, which requires a much better knowledge of risk factors than we have up to now (Fig. 6) [13]. As long as we do not know such risk factors increasing the a priori (pretest) probability of pancreatic cancer to 20% or more, a test would have to be 99.95% specific to allow for a reasonable screening (Table 9) [13, 40]. A recent study came to the conclusion that the use of CA 19-9 as a screening test is of no value [41] (Fig. 7). Thus, up to now screening seems not be possible, and we probably must search for better knowledge of risk factors and for better tests.

Staging of Pancreatic Cancer

Since surgery is the only potential curative treatment but causes some morbidity and mortality, it would be of great value and cost saving to have reliable staging techniques for defining resectable and/or curable cancer preoperatively. Unfortunately the imaging procedures do not fulfill these requirements (Table 10) [5, 42, 43]. Endosonography (EUS) seems to be

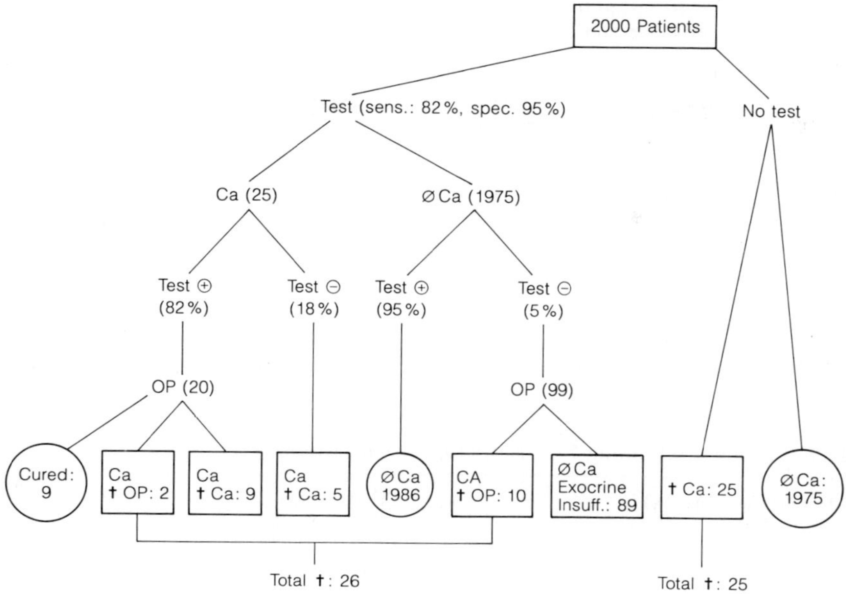

Fig. 5. Theoretical algorithm describing the outcome in 2000 patients having symptoms possibly related to pancreatic carcinoma – assuming a prevalence of 1.25%, sensitivity of a test of 82% and specificity of 95%, a curative operation in 50%, and a procedure-related mortality in 10% of those operated. Note that all assumptions are more or less optimistic. (From [39])

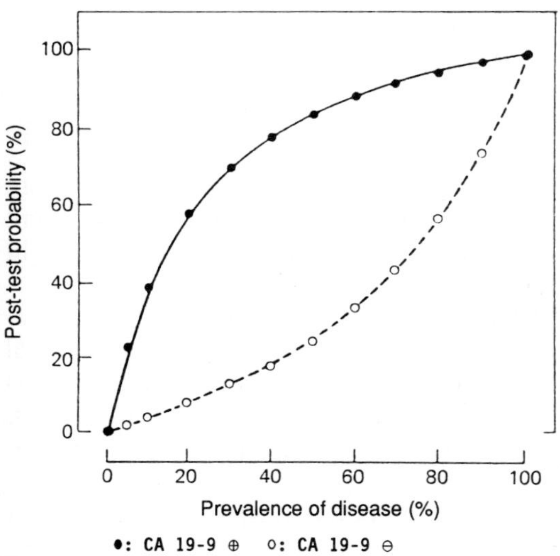

Fig. 6. Influence of the prevalence of the disease on the posttest probability for pancreatic carcinoma using Ca 19-9. (From [13])

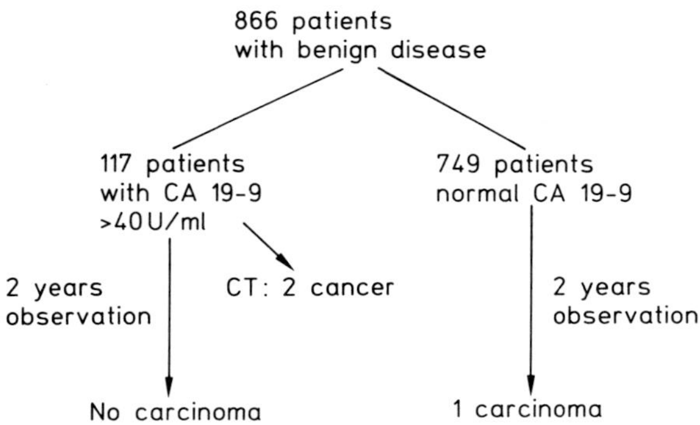

Fig. 7. Results of a prospective study of 866 patients using CA 19-9. (From [41])

Table 9. Problem: screening for pancreatic cancer (from [13])

Prevalence (>40 years)	≤20/100 000
Sensitivity 100% }	20 true positives
Specificity 99% }	1000 false positives

Table 10. Staging of pancreatic carcinoma: imaging (from [5])

	Liver metastases		
	1 or 2	Multiple	Total
US	2	2	4
CT	1	4	5
Angiography	1	–	1
Laparotomy	2	12	14

somewhat better, with about 75% accuracy for lymph node involvement [23], but it fails to detect distant metastasis. It is not clear to what extent magnetic resonance imaging or improved CT and US equipment might further increase preoperative staging with respect to metastasis.

A recent study analyzing 40 patients with pancreatic carcinoma considered potentially resectable by CT using salinic washing of the peritoneal cavity detected in 12 (30%) malignant cells in the peritoneal cavity (Fig. 8) [37]. As noted above, this was more often the case after FNB (Table 8). This technique has not been used widely and remains to be further evaluated.

Finally, radioimmunolocalization of tumors has raised hopes for better staging modalities [44–47]. However, the accuracy of this technique using antibodies against different antigens has not yet reached a level supporting its widespread application (Table 11).

Table 11. Radioimmunolocalization of pancreatic carcinoma (from [45, 46])

CEA antibody	
Staging correct	4/20
Neoplasia detected	13/20
False positive	9
CEA + CA19-9 antibody	
Patients correctly staged	15/21

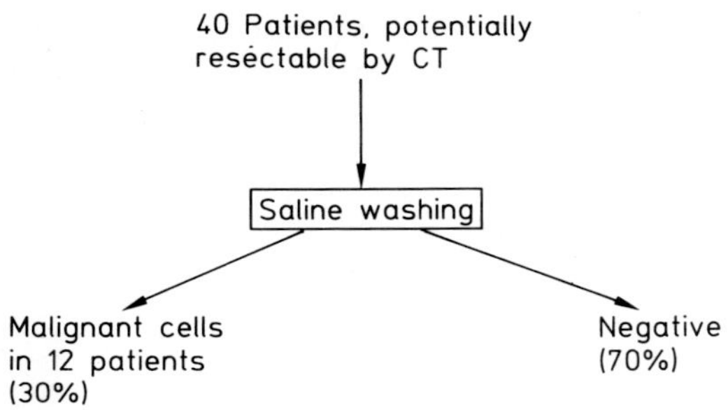

Fig. 8. Results of saline washing of the peritoneal cavity in 40 patients with pancreatic cancer. (From [37])

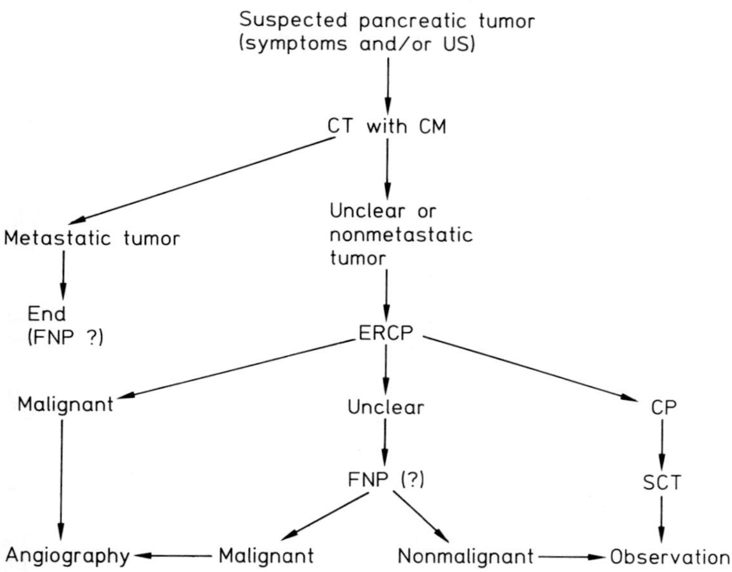

Fig. 9. Diagnostic algorithm for suspected pancreatic cancer

Summary

Up to now diagnosis in the symptomatic patient is by imaging, where ERCP, CT and EUS seem best. Combination may improve the accuracy and prediction of malignant lesions. Serological tests have a complementary character at best, and a combination of CA 19-9 and elastase-1 seems to be superior.

The differention to other pancreatic lesions is best by FNB, and cytological/histological evaluation after CT/ERCP has been performed. However, FNB may increase the spread of the disease. Due to the lack of adequate tests screening is not now possible. Risk factors must be found to increase pretest probability which allows for reasonable screening procedures.

Staging is carried out by CT and US. EUS for lymph node involvement and cytological examinations might be added in the routine in the future. Figure 9 gives an algorithm for the procedural steps used today where these new techniques might be implemented.

References

1. Classen M (1987) Erkrankungen des Pankreas. In: Siegenthaler W, Kaufmann W, Hornbostel H, Waller HD (eds) Lehrbuch der inneren Medizin. Thieme, Stuttgart, pp 1061–1072
2. Warshaw AL, Fernandez-Del Castillo C (1992) Pancreatic carcinoma. New Engl J Med 326:455–465
3. Campbell JP, Wilson SR (1988) Pancreatic neoplasms: how useful is evaluation with US? Radiology 167:341–344
4. Lindsell DRM (1990) Ultrasound imaging of pancreas and biliary tract. Lancet i:390–393
5. Soehendra N, Klapdor R, Lehmann U, Schmiegel WH, Brockman W-P, Vogel H, Klöppel G (1982) Moderne Diagnostik des Pankreaskarzinoms. Med Klin 77:289–293
6. Hessel SJ, Siegelman SS, McNeil BJ, Sanders R, Adams DF, Alderson PO, Finberg HJ, Abrams HL (1982) A prospective evaluation of computed tomography and ultrasound of the pancreas. Radiology 143:129–133
7. Foley WD, Stewart ET, Lawson TL, Geenan J, Loguiice J, Maher L, Unger GF (1980) Computed tomography, ultrasonography, and endoscopic retrograde cholangiopancreatography in the diagnosis of pancreatic disease: a comparative study. Gastrointest Radiol 5:29–35
8. Von Gmelin E, Weiss H-D, Fuchs H-D, Reiser M (1981) Vergleich der diagnostischen Treffsicherheit von Ultraschall, Computertomographie und ERPC bei der chronischen Pankreatitis und beim Pankreaskarzinom. Fortschr Röntgenstr 134(2):136–141
9. Smith KJ, Thurston DW, Strum WB (1989) Is ultrasound (US) equivalent to computerized tomography (CT) in the diagnosis of pancreatic cancer? Gastroenterology 96:A480
10. Gebel M, Stiehl M, Freise J (1985) Wert der sonographischen Pankreasgangdarstellung für die Diagnose der chronischen Pankreatitis und des Pankreaskarzinoms im Vergleich zur ERP. Ultraschall 6:127–130
11. Rösch T, Lorenz R, Braig C, Feuerbach S, Siewert JR, Classen M (1990) Endosonographische Diagnostik bei Pankreastumoren. Dtsch Med Wochenschr 115:1339–1347

12. Rösch T, Lorenz R, Braig C, Dancygier H, Classen M (1991) Endoskopischer Ultraschall bei kleinen Pankreastumoren. Z Gastroenterol 29:110–115
13. Rhodes JM, Ching CK (1990) Serum diagnostic tests for pancreatic cancer. Baillière's Clin Gastroenterol 4:833–852
14. Humano H, Hayakawa T, Kondo T (1987) Serum immunoreactive elastase in diagnosis of pancreatic diseases. Dig Dis Sci 32:50–56
15. Gullo L, Ventrucci M, Pezzilli R, Platé L, Naldoni P (1987) Diagnostic value of serum elastase 1 in pancreatic disease. Br J Surg 74:44–47
16. Koprowski H, Steplewski Z, Mitvhell K, Herlyn D, Fuhrer P (1979) Colorectal carcinoma antigens detected by hybridoma antibodies. Somat Cell Genet 5:957–972
17. Hayakawa T, Kondo T, Shibata T, Hamano H, Kitagawa M, Sakai Y, Ono H (1988) Sensitive serum markers for detecting pancreatic cancer. Cancer 61:1827–1831
18. Yamamura H, Tatsuta M, Ito M, Iishi H, Noguchi S, Okuda S, Yoshida M (1989) Effectiveness of discriminant analysis of serum CA 19-9 and elastase 1 in diagnosis of pancreatic carcinoma. Pancreas 4:401–405
19. Fabris C, Del Favero G, Basso D, Piccoli A, Meggiato T, Angonese C, Plebani M, Leandro G, Burlina A, Naccarato R (1988) Serum markers and clinical data in diagnosing pancreatic cancer: a contrastive approach. Am J Gastroenterol 83:549–553
20. Basso D, Fabris C, Del Favero G, Piccoli A, Angonese C, Pasquali C, Castoro C, Plebani M, Leandro G, Burlina A, Naccarato R (1990) How does liver dysfunction influence serum CA 19-9 in pancreatic cancer? Ital J Gastroenterol 22:1–6
21. Heptner G, Domschke S, Schneider MU, Domschke W (1985) Bedeutung des tumorassoziierten Antigens CA 19-9 in der Differentialdiagnose von Pankreaserkrankungen. Dtsch Med Wochenschr 110:624–628
22. Steinberg W (1990) The clinical utility of the CA 19-9 tumor-associated antigen. Am J Gastroenterol 85:350–354
23. Grimm H, Maydeo A, Soehendra N (1990) Endoluminal ultrasound for the diagnosis and staging of pancreatic cancer. Baillière's Clin Gastroenterol 4:869–888
24. Yasuda K, Nakajima M, Fujimoto S, Kiyoto K (1987) Detection of small tumors of the pancreas by endoscopic ultrasonography. In: Takemoto T, Kawai K (eds) Recent topics of digestive endoscopy. Excerpta Medica, Amsterdam, pp 87–95
25. Otto R, Deyhle P, Pedio L (1980) Sonographisch gesteuerte perkutane Feinnadelaspirationspunktion von Pankreastumoren unter permanenter Sicht. Dtsch Med Wochenschr 105:853–857
26. Søreide O, Skaarland E, Peersen OM, Larssen TB, Arnesjø B (1985) Fine-needle biopsy of the pancreas: results of 204 routinely performed biopsies in 190 patients. World J Surg 9:960–965
27. Yamamoto R, Tatsuta M, Noguchi S, Kasugai H, Okano Y, Okuda S, Wada A, Tamura H (1985) Histocytologic diagnosis of pancreatic cancer by percutaneous aspiration biopsy under ultrasonic guidance. Am J Clin Pathol 83:409–414
28. Celle G, Savarino V, Biggi E, Mansi C, Ceppa P, Cicio GR, Arcuri V (1986) Fine-needle aspiration cytodiagnosis: a simple and safe procedure for cancer of the pancreas. Gastroenterol Clin Biol 10:545–548
29. Glenthøj A, Sehested M, Torp-Pedersen S (1990) Ultrasonically guided histological and cytological fine needle biopsies of the pancreas. Reliability and reproducibility of diagnoses. Gut 31:930–933
30. Solmi L, Gandolfi L, Muratori R, Leo P, Bacchini P (1987) Echo-guided fine-needle biopsy of pancreatic masses. Am J Gastroenterol 82:744–748
31. Schwerk WB, Dürr H-K, Schmitz-Moormann P (1983) Ultrasound guided fine-needle biopsies in pancreatic and hepatic neoplasms. Gastrointest Radiol 8:219–225

32. Dickey JE, Haaga JR, Stellato TA, Schultz CL, Hau T (1986) Evaluation of computed tomography guided percutaneous biopsy of the pancreas. Surg Gynecol Obstet 163:497–503
33. Dinkel E, Helwig A, Jäger B, Rückauer K, Schölmerich J, Hauenstein KH, Wimmer B (1990) Computertomographisch gesteuerte Feinnadelbiopsie des Pankreas zur Histologiegewinnung. Radiologe 30:420–424
34. Swobodnik W, Janowitz P, Kratzer W, Wechsler JG, Hagel S, Eckert E, Binder T, Bültmann B, Kuhn K, Hagert N, Wenk H, Beck J, Ditschuneit H (1990) Vergleich ultraschallgezielter Feinnadel- und Grobnadelpunktionen bei umschriebenen Läsionen im Abdomen. Ultraschall 11:287–289
35. Mitty HA, Efremidis SC, Yeh H-C (1981) Impact of fine-needle biopsy on management of patients with carcinoma of the pancreas. AJR 137:1119–1121
36. Rapaccini GL, Grattagliano A, Pompili M, Rabitti C, Anti M, Aliotta A, Amadei E, Cedrone A, Gambassi G (1990) Clinical suspicion of pancreatic neoplasm: does echo-guided fine-needle biopsy modify patient management? Surg Endosc 4:206–208
37. Warshaw AL (1991) Implications of peritoneal cytology for staging of early pancreatic cancer. Am J Surg 161:26–30
38. Klapdor R (1989) Zum Stand der Früherkennung des Pankreaskarzinoms. Internist 30:752–758
39. Anschütz F (1982) Indikation zum ärztlichen Handeln. Springer, Berlin Heidelberg New York
40. Dahlmann N (1989) Alte und neue Tumormarker. Dtsch Med Wochenschr 114:1848–1853
41. Fredbourg T, Bercoff E, Manchon N, Senant J, Basuyau J-P, Breton P, Janvresse A, Brunelle P, Bourreille J (1988) The evaluation of CA 19-9 antigen level in the early detection of pancreatic cancer. Cancer 62:2287–2290
42. Schölmerich J, Groß V (1990) Unerwartete Befunde bei abdomineller Sonographie – Differentialdiagnose und Maßnahmen zur diagnostischen Klärung. In: Gerok W, Hartmann F, Mertelsmann R, Philipp T, Schuster HP, Sybrecht GW (eds) Klinik der Gegenwart, vol 4, pt 2. Urban and Schwarzenberg, Munich, pp 1–59
43. Schölmerich J, Volk BA, Neuner C, Fröhlich J, Gerok W (1984) Die Aussagefähigkeit der Sonographie bei Lebermetastasen unter besonderer Berücksichtigung des Primärtumors. Dtsch Med Wochenschr 109:326–329
44. Allum WH (1990) Radioimmunolocalization of tumours of the pancreas and biliary tree. Baillière's Clin Gastroenterol 4:853–868
45. Montz R, Klapdor R, Rothe B, Heller M (1986) Immunoscintigraphy and radioimmunotherapy in patients with pancreatic carcinoma. Nucl Med 25:239–244
46. Jewkes AJ, Macdonald F, Downing R, Drole Z, Allum WH (1991) Labelled antibody imaging in pancreatic cancer, cholangiocarcinoma, chronic pancreatitis and sclerosing cholangitis. Eur J Surg Oncol 17:354–357
47. Ballantyne KC, Perkins AC, Selby C, Wastie ML, Hardcastle JD (1988) Imaging of pancreatic and colorectal cancer using antibody fragments: a preliminary evaluation. Eur J Surg Oncol 14:393–398

Conventional Treatment of Pancreatic Cancer*

M. Korc[1]

Introduction

Carcinoma of the pancreas is the fourth leading cause of cancer death in the Western world [1]. Diabetes mellitus, high-fat diets, and tobacco smoking have been implicated as predisposing factors [2]. Ethanol consumption and pancreatitis may also be risk factors [2]. The 1-year overall survival rate in patients with pancreatic cancer is only 12% [3]. Three observations suggest that this malignancy will be an even more serious problem in the industrialized countries than it is today: (a) the incidence of pancreatic cancer increases dramatically after the fifth decade of life, and the general population in these countries is aging; (b) the incidence of diabetes in this population is increasing, and advances in the care of diabetic patients have led to an increase in their longevity; (c) the consumption of fat, alcohol, and tobacco is not abating. In view of the high mortality rate in patients with pancreatic cancer, there is an urgent need to improve the therapeutic options that are available for treating this disorder.

Conventional Therapeutic Modalities

In general, survival in pancreatic cancer is often limited to surgical cures in patients who were operated on during an early stage of their disease. Unfortunately, the diagnosis of pancreatic cancer is frequently established at a more advanced stage, which precludes the patients from having surgery. Furthermore, at the time of surgical exploration, as many as 50% of patients with pancreatic carcinomas are found to have either local spread or limited regional dissemination [4, 5]; theoretically, these patients may benefit from chemotherapy.

* This study was supported by Public Health Service Grant CA-40162, awarded by the National Cancer Institute.

[1] Division of Endocrinology and Metabolism, Departments of Medicine and Biological Chemistry, Medical Sciences I, C240, University of California, Irvine, CA 92717, USA

Beger/Büchler/Malfertheiner (Eds.)
Standards in Pancreatic Surgery

The current review is limited to a discussion of conventional nonsurgical treatment modalities for pancreatic cancer, which, with a few exceptions, have not produced encouraging results. This is due, in part, to the insidious onset of the disease and to the advanced stage at which many patients first develop symptoms. However, it is also due to the resistance of pancreatic cancer cells to chemotherapeutic agents, and to the tremendous growth advantage of these cells by comparison with noncancerous pancreatic cells. Although relatively little progress has been made in the areas of prevention, detection, and treatment in this disorder, we now have a better understanding of their unique tumor biology. Thus, we know that human pancreatic cancer cells exhibit a high frequency of mutations in the *ras* oncogene, overexpress the epidermal growth factor receptor, and produce large quantities of transforming growth factor-alpha [6–8]. In addition, these cells produce other growth factors [9, 10] that have been implicated in autocrine growth stimulation (e.g. insulin-like growth factor-I, fibroblast growth factors, platelet-derived growth factor), and most likely harbor mutated tumor supressor genes. However, to date, only the epidermal growth factor receptor and transforming growth factor-alpha have been found to be overexpressed in these cells.

There are several additional impediments to successful conventional therapy of pancreatic cancer. Even small primary tumors frequently have microscopic metastatic foci. The primary tumor often elicits an intense fibroblastic response within the contiguous pancreatic tissue, thereby creating a barrier to chemotherapeutic agents. The systemic administration of these drugs is also believed to result in inadequate levels within the tumor mass due to a relatively poor blood supply to the tumor. Furthermore, patients with pancreatic cancer are generally old and debilitated, and the toxicity of chemotherapeutic agents is greater in this population.

In spite of these difficulties, numerous attempts have been made to treat surgically inoperable pancreatic cancer. These attempts have included the use of single and combination chemotherapies, hormonal therapy, chemotherapy in conjunction with radiotherapy, and immunotherapy.

Single-agent chemotherapy has generally been unsuccessful [1]. Although intratumoral treatment with mitomycin-C adsorbed to activated charcoal particles resulted in a significant decrease in tumor-associated pain in 8 of 13 patients [11], it remains to be determined whether this type of therapy will be associated with increased survival. Combination therapy has produced somewhat better response rates than single-agent therapy. However, in randomized studies of combination therapy, the survival of patients has not been significantly prolonged [1]. Examples of combination regimen include 5-fluorouracil, doxorubicin, and mitomycin [12], and 5-fluorouracil, doxorubicin, and cisplatin [13].

Hormonal therapy is based on the premise that pancreatic cancer cell growth may be hormonally regulated. For example, the exocrine pancreas has low-affinity estrogen binding proteins [14]. Consequently, the anti-estrogen tamoxifen has been used in clinical trials. Similarly, the long-acting somatostatin analogue Sandostatin has been used in an effort to suppress the release of islet cell hormones and gastrointestinal hormones which are believed to enhance tumor growth. Unfortunately, the responses to tamoxifen [15] and to Sandostatin [16] have been disappointing.

Radiotherapy alone has been generally ineffective in the treatment of pancreatic cancer. However, when used in conjunction with chemotherapy, radiotherapy has shown some promise in terms of prolonging the median survival [17]. Furthermore, radiotherapy in combination with extensive pancreatic surgery and intraoperative infusion of mitomycin-C through either the hepatic artery or portal vein, has resulted in a 1-year survival rate of 86% [18]. An interesting approach which requires additional evaluation is the use of intraoperative radiation followed by the administration of intraoperative hyperthermia [19].

In view of the resistance of pancreatic cancer to conventional therapeutic modalities, it had been hoped that the use of immune-modifying agents would prove more successful. In culture, human pancreatic cancer cells bind the cytokines tumor necrosis factor and interferon-gamma, and are growth inhibited by these agents [20, 21]. Furthermore, in animal studies, adoptive immunotherapy with lymphokine-activated killer cells has yielded some success [22]. However, to date, clinical trials with immune-modifying agents have not been encouraging.

Conclusion

The prognosis of patients with pancreatic cancer is dismal, and current conventional therapeutic modalities are generally ineffective. As further advances are made in our knowledge of the basic pathophysiological processes that govern pancreatic tumor biology, every attempt should be made to devise new and novel therapies for this disease.

References

1. Wills JA (1989) Current status of chemotherapy in metastatic pancreatic cancer. Anticancer Res 9:1027–1032
2. Cubilla AL, Fitzgerald PJ (1985) Cancer of the exocrine pancreas: the pathological aspects. CA 35:2–35
3. Gudjonsson B, Livstone E, Spiro H (1978) Cancer of the pancreas: diagnostic accuracy and survival studies. Cancer 42:2494–2506
4. Tepper J, Nardi G, Suite H (1976) Carcinoma of the pancreas: review of MGH experience from 1963–1973. Cancer 37:1519–1524
5. Levine G, Remine WH, Hermann RE, Schein PS, Cohn I (1978) Cancer of the pancreas. Am J Surg 135:185–191
6. Almoguera C, Shibata D, Forrester K, Martin J, Arnheim N, Perucho M (1988) Most human carcinomas of the exocrine pancreas contain mutant c-K-ras genes. Cell 53:549–554

7. Korc M, Meltzer P, Trent J (1986) Enhanced expression of epidermal growth factor receptor correlates with alterations of chromosome 7 in human pancreatic cancer. Proc Natl Acad Sci USA 83:5141–5144
8. Smith JJ, Derynck R, Korc M (1987) Production of transforming growth factor α in human pancreatic cancer cells: evidence for a superagonist autocrine cycle. Proc Natl Acad Sci USA 84:7567–7570
9. Ohmura E, Okada M, Onoda N, Kamiya Y, Murakami H, Tsushima T, Shizume K (1990) Insulin-like growth factor I and transforming growth factor ∂ as autocrine growth factors in human pancreatic cancer cell growth. Cancer Res 50:103–107
10. Beauchamp RD, Lyons RM, Yang EY, Coffey RJ Jr, Moses HL (1990) Expression of and response to growth regulatory peptides by two human pancreatic carcinoma cell lines. Pancreas 5:369–380
11. Moriai T, Takebe T, Makino I, Ishii K (1989) Intratumoral treatment of pancreatic cancer with mitomycin-C adsorbed to activated carbon particles. Anticancer Res 9:1799–1804
12. Smith FP, Hoth DF, Levin BL et al. (1980) 5-Fluorouracil, Adriamycin and mitomycin-C (FAM) chemotherapy for advanced adenocarcinoma of the pancreas. Cancer 46:2014
13. Moertel CG, Rubin J, O'Connell MJ et al. (1986) A phase II study of combined 5-fluorouracil, doxorubicin and cisplatin in the treatment of advanced upper gastrointestinal adenocarcinoma. J Clin Oncol 4:1053
14. Pousetta A, Fernstad R, Haggmark A, Skoldefors H, Theve NO, Carlstrom K (1988) The estrogen binding protein in human pancreas: concentrations in subcellular fractions of normal pancreatic tissue, in duodenal juice during pancreatic stimulation and in peripheral serum in normal and pathological conditions. J Steroid Biochem 29:423–427
15. Bakkevold KE, Pettersen A, Arnesjo B, Espehaug B (1990) Tamoxifen therapy in unresectable adenocarcinoma of the pancreas and the papilla of Vater. Br J Surg 77:725–730
16. Klijn JGM, Hoff AM, Planting ASTh, Verweij J, Kok T, Lamberts SWJ, portengen H, Foekens JA (1990) Treatment of patients with metastatic pancreatic and gastrointestinal tumours with the somatostatin analogue Sandostatin: a phase II study including endocrine effects. Br J Cancer 62:627–630
17. The Gastrointestinal Tumor Study Group (1981) Therapy of locally unresectable pancreatic carcinoma: a randomized comparison of high dose (6000 rads) radiation alone, moderate dose radiation (4000 rads + 5-fluorouracil), and high dose radiation + 5-fluorouracil. Cancer 48:1705–1710
18. Ozaki H, Hojo K, Kato H, Kinoshita T, Egawa S, Kishi K (1988) Multidisciplinary treatment for resectable pancreatic cancer. Int J Pancreatol 3:249–260
19. Colacchio TA, Coughlin C, Taylor J, Douple E, Ryan T, Crichlow RW (1990) Intraoperative radiation therapy and hyperthermia. Arch Surg 125:370–375
20. Raitano AB, Scuderi P, Korc M (1990) Binding and biological effects of tumor necrosis factor and gamma interferon in human pancreatic carcinoma cells. Pancreas 5:267–277
21. Schmiegel WH, Caeser J, Kalthoff H, Greten H, Schreiber HW, Thiele HG (1988) Antiproliferative effects exerted by recombinant tumor necrosis factor-α (rTNF-α) and interferon-γ (rIFN-γ) on human pancreatic tumor cell lines. Pancreas 3:180–188
22. Marincola FM, Da Pozzo LF, Drucker BJ, Holder WD Jr (1990) Adoptive immunotherapy of human pancreatic cancer with lymphokine-activated killer cells and interleukin-2 in a nude mouse model. Surgery 108:919–929

Interventional Therapy for Pancreatic Cancer

N. SOEHENDRA,[1] K.F. BINMOELLER, and H. GRIMM

Introduction

Over the past two decades the incidence of pancreatic cancer has steadily increased. In the United States, pancreatic cancer ranks as the second most common gastrointestinal malignancy and ranks fifth among causes of cancer deaths [4, 35]. Despite tremendous progress in diagnostic technology including ERCP and ultrasound-guided needle aspiration, the prognosis continues to remain dismal. The main reason is delayed diagnosis. Pancreatic cancer is clinically silent during its initial growth phase, and by the time symptoms and signs such as weight loss, pain and jaundice appear, 85%–90% of cancers have already extended beyond the pancreas.

Palliative interventional therapy plays a major role in the management of patients with pancreatic carcinoma for several reasons. First, approximately 70% of pancreatic cancers are located in the pancreatic head, causing obstructive jaundice (Fig. 1). Second, the surgical resectability rate is only about 20% with a 5-year survival rate of less than 5% [5, 17]. Finally, patients tend to be poor surgical candidates to begin with. The average age at presentation is approximately 65 years. The peak incidence rate is, however, in the age group older than 75 years [37].

The main objective of palliative treatment is the relief of jaundice, which may be associated with debilitating pruritus, cholangitis, or pain. Pancreatic duct tumor obstruction rarely requires treatment and is generally not recommended. Pain of pancreatic cancer is multifactorial in etiology, and does not appear to be due to pancreatic duct obstruction alone.

Biliary Drainage: Percutaneous or Endoscopic Approach?

The bile duct can be decompressed either percutaneously or endoscopically. The endoscopic approach, introduced 42 years after the percutaneous [31, 38], is widely considered to be the procedure of choice because it is less invasive. In a review of the literature by Coene [9], endoscopic transpapil-

[1] Department of Endoscopic Surgery, University Hospital of Hamburg, Martinistraße 52, W-2000 Hamburg 20, FRG

Beger/Büchler/Malfertheiner (Eds.)
Standards in Pancreatic Surgery

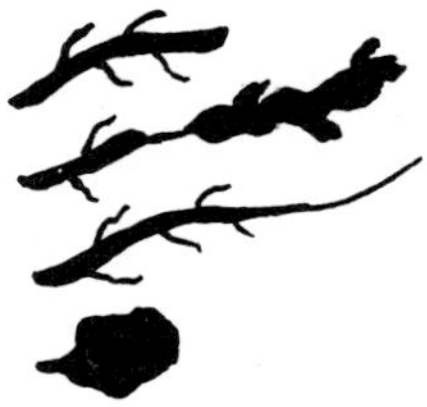
Type :
50 %
35 %
8 %
7 %
Location : Head 75 %
Body 20 %
Tail 5 %
Changings of common bile duct 80 %

Fig. 1. Frequency of type and location of pancreatic cancer on ERCP

lary drainage has lower rates of morbidity and 30-day mortality compared to percutaneous drainage (Table 1). A prospective study by Speer et al. [32] showed better success rates for endoscopic stent placement (89% versus 76%). In this study morbidity was 19% and 30-day mortality 15% in the endoscopic group compared to 67% and 33%, respectively, in the percutaneous group.

Recent progress achieved by the self-expandable metallic stents appears to reduce the risk of percutaneous-transhepatic drainage, since these stents can be inserted through a relatively thin catheter [1, 23]. However, the endoscopic procedure is still less invasive. The percutaneous method should therefore be reserved for endoscopic failures. In the case of Billroth-II gastrectomy or Roux-en-Y anastomosis, the percutaneous method can be combined with the endoscopic approach ("rendezvous" procedure) to enable implantation of a large diameter prosthesis with less trauma to the liver [22, 27].

Table 1. Endoscopic versus percutaneous-transhepatic biliary stent (from [8])

	Endoscopic (10)	Percutaneous (13)
Total no. of patients	2138	1160
Successful insertion	87%	90%
Successful drainage	85%	69%
30-day mortality	13%	23%
Early complications	19%	28%

In parentheses, number of published series.

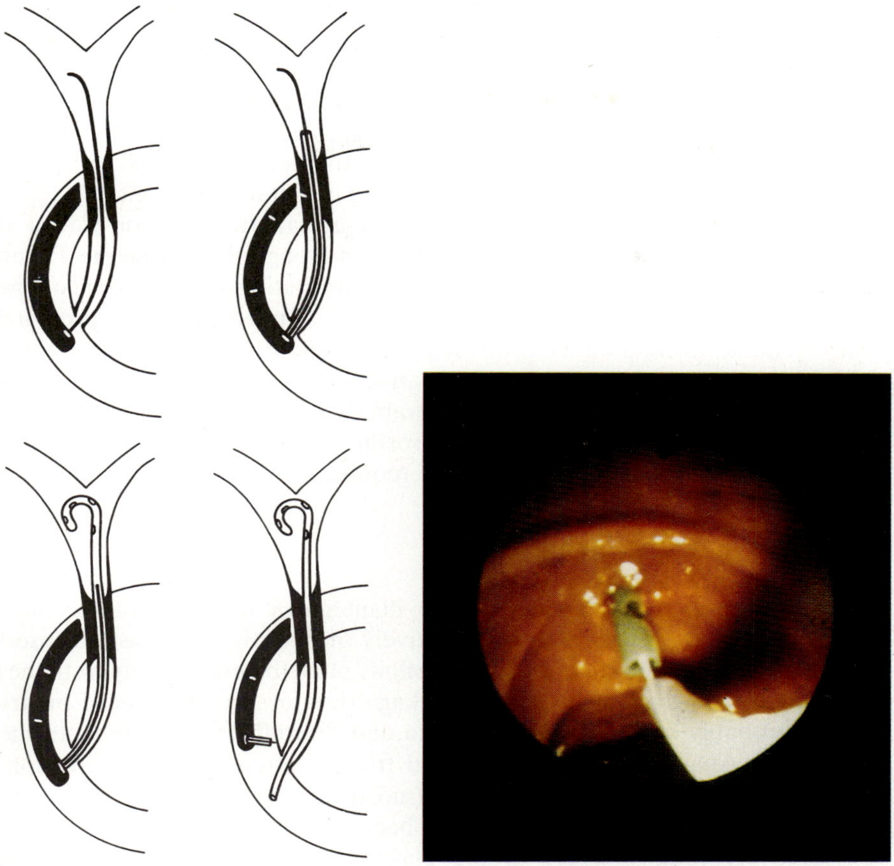

a b

Fig. 2. **a** Technique of endoscopic stent placement. **b** Endoscopic photo (Olympus TJF-1T 20) showing the insertion of a 10-F plastic prosthesis over a guidewire using a pusher catheter

Technique of Endoscopic Biliary Stenting

The method of endoscopic stent placement is based on the Seldinger technique. The prosthesis is pushed over a flexible guidewire into the bile duct using a pusher tube. To facilitate this, a small papillotomy is recommended (Fig. 2).

Two types of guidewires are recommended for endoscopic biliary stenting: (a) the hydrophilic polymer-coated steerable glidewire (Terumo, Tokyo, Japan or Wilson-Cook, Winston-Salem, USA); (b) the conventional Teflon-coated stainless steel guidewire. The Terumo glidewire is made of a titanium/nickel alloy which allows effective transmission of torque and is fairly kink-proof. Due to the polymer coating, the wire is very slippery when wet. Thus, it is a useful tool for negotiating complicated strictures. However, being very slippery, the Terumo wire is not suited for over-the-wire catheter or stent placement. For this purpose, the conventional 0.035″ 400-cm guidewire is still required. The new Tracer wire manufactured by Wilson-Cook combines the advantages of the Terumo and conventional guidewires by limiting the polymer coating to the distal 50–60 cm of the wire, leaving the remainder Teflon-coated for catheter placement.

To introduce the guidewire the universal catheter (Wilson-Cook) is recommended. This device is made of a 180-cm-long 6-F radiopaque Teflon catheter with a curved tip tapered to 4.5 F facilitating the insertion of the wire into the papillary orifice. A Y-adapter is connected to the proximal end to enable instillation of contrast media without having to remove the guidewire. A plastic pin vise handle is attached to the proximal end of the guidewire to improve grip and maneuverability of the wire.

Prior to insertion of larger plastic prostheses (10 or 12 F), dilation using catheter dilators (Wilson-Cook) may be required.

Stent Materials

Plastic prostheses, usually with an outer diameter of 10 F, are still the most widely employed because they are relatively inexpensive and easy to insert (Fig. 3). However, plastic materials (Teflon, polyethylene or polyurethane) are handicapped by a high rate of blockage due to accumulation of biliary sludge, probably encouraged by bacteria and the reflux of chyme from the duodenum. Analysis of sludge collected from occluded stents has demonstrated ample bacterial contamination (mostly *Escherichia coli*), and plant fibers [15, 24]. Presumably, a layer of bacterial bio-film initially forms on the relatively rough surface of the plastic prosthesis, which encourages adherence of sludge [33].

Antibacterial coating of stents has been proposed to solve this problem. An in vitro study showed that an impregnation with silver or chlorhexidine significantly reduced *E. coli* growth [16]. However, in our own clinical study [7] this result could not be reproduced. Silver-impregnated Teflon prostheses had almost the same duration of patency as the conventional Teflon prostheses (average 115 versus 111 days). Likewise, in another study using cephalosporin coating, no improvement was demonstrated [6].

In order to prevent duodeno-biliary reflux, we developed a stent which can be inserted above the papilla, leaving a tail-like "gutter" appendage extending into the duodenum for easy stent removal (Fig. 4). In a prospective clinical study, this stent model had a 20-day longer patency than the conventional one, provided that it did not dislodge.

Analyzing the sites of stent occlusion, sludge tends to accumulated along Side holes. One explanation for this might be the relatively rough edges of the holes, which are more prone to trap sludge and ascending chyme. In an

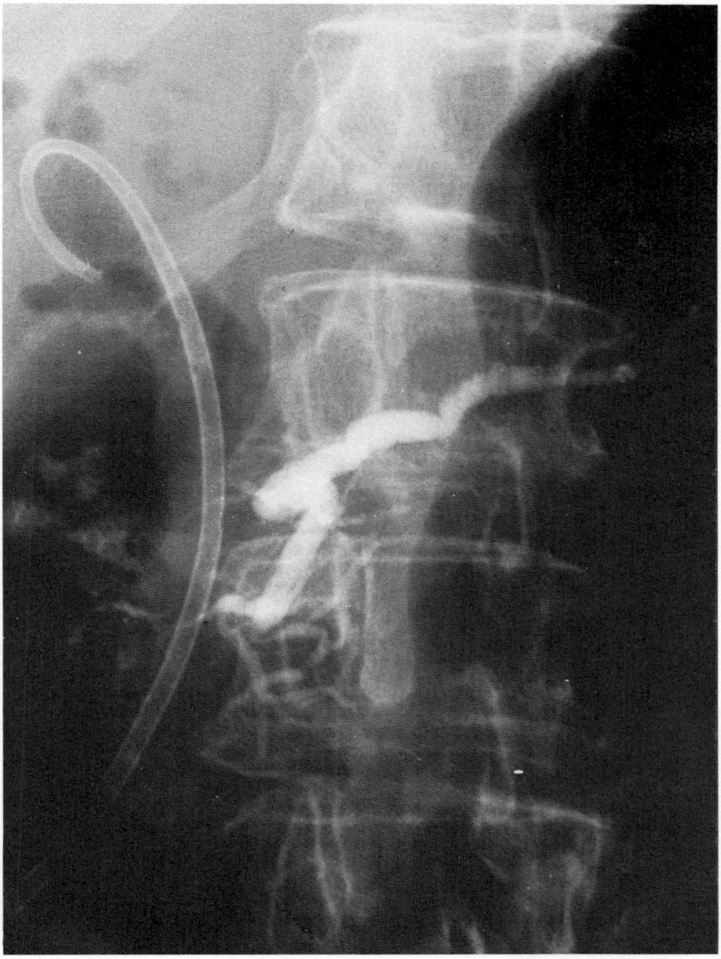

Fig. 3. Radiograph showing a 10-F "pigtail" plastic prosthesis in the bile duct. The patient had inoperable pancreatic head cancer. The main pancreatic duct is moderately dilated

experimental study, it could be demonstrated that Teflon prostheses without side holes have six times less sludge in the lumen than prostheses with side holes [8]. Side holes in conventional Amsterdam-type stents add little to drainage efficacy, so that these can be eliminated. Further clinical studies will show whether plastic prostheses without side holes offer significantly improved stent longevity.

Self-expandable metallic stents have been developed for placement in vessels and the urethra [28], and currently two are undergoing evaluation for use in the bile duct: the Wallstent and the Gianturco stent.

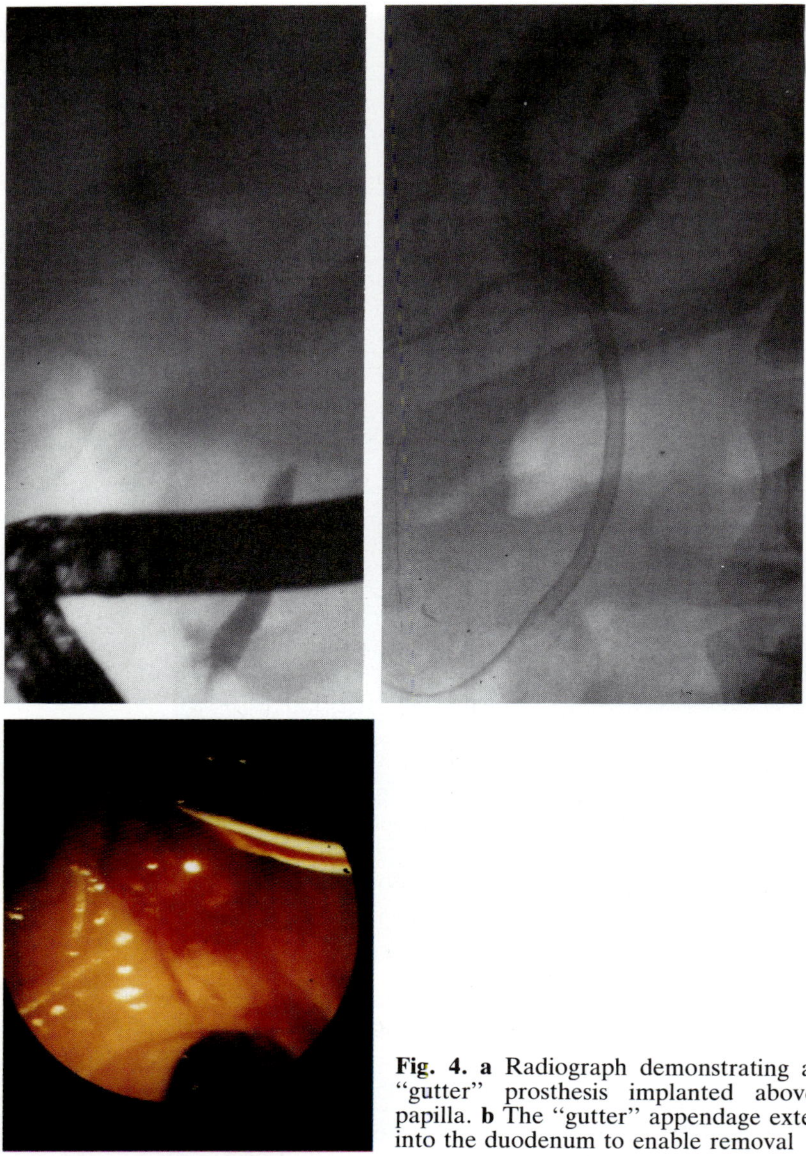

a

b

Fig. 4. a Radiograph demonstrating a 10-F "gutter" prosthesis implanted above the papilla. **b** The "gutter" appendage extending into the duodenum to enable removal

The Gianturco stent (Cook, Bloomington, USA) is made of stainless steel wire measuring 0.016″ or 0.018″ in diameter bent in a zig-zag pattern and soldered at the end to form a cylinder. The stent is introduced in a compressed state through a 12-F delivery catheter and expands to a diameter of 12 mm. The stent has been modified by adding monofilament nylon suture to connect the legs in order to limit stent expansion to a desired diameter. In addition, stents can be connected in an end-to-end fashion, increasingly the axial flexibility and making it easier to control stent placement [34]. In a European multicenter study comprising 11 patients with benign and 16 with malignant biliary strictures, initial relief of jaundice was achieved in all cases using the Gianturco stent. However, in a follow-up period of 6–21 months, two patients with benign and nine with malignant stricture developed recurrent jaundice and cholangitis [21]. In another study recurrent jaundice occurred in 22% of cases (5 of 23 patients) during a follow-up period of 2–59 weeks [36]. The Wallstent (Medinvent SA, Laussanne, Swiss) is woven in the form of tubular mesh from stainless steel alloy filaments measuring 0.09 mm in diameter. The stent is loaded onto a 7- or 9-F delivery catheter compressed in a double membrane. Upon release, the stent expands to a diameter of 7–10 mm. This stent has also shown relatively high rates of late recurrent jaundice, ranging from 18% to 42% in a mean/median follow-up period of 4–5 months [10, 13, 19, 26].

In conclusion, self-expandable metallic stents afford an attractive alternative to conventional plastic prostheses due to their larger luminal diameter. Clogging due to sludge formation is less likely to occur, but obstruction due to tumor ingrowth and overgrowth remains a problem. The rate of recurrent jaundice using the metallic stents has not decreased significantly compared to that of plastic prostheses. The occlusion rate of plastic prostheses is around 20% over the same length of observation [14, 18]. In view of their high cost at this time, metallic stents cannot be generally recommended. Whether membrane covering will improve results remains to be seen; a preliminary experimental study evaluating silicone and polyether-polyurethane coated metallic stents in dogs showed patency up to 24 weeks, but hyperplastic papillary mucosal proliferations resulting in different drgrees of luminal narrowing [2].

Results of Endoscopic Biliary Stenting

Endoscopic transpapillary stent placement is a well-standardized technique today. Success rates exceed 90% for the drainage of distal strictures secondary to pancreatic carcinoma. Failure is primarily due to inaccessibility of the papilla, as with extensive duodenal tumor invasion, or tumor infiltration of the papilla preventing cannulation (Fig. 5).

The overall procedure-related complication rate has been reported to be 3%–4% and the mortality rate less than 2% [14, 18, 30]. Complications are mainly related to papillotomy and include hemorrhage, pancreatitis and retroduodenal perforation. Cystic duct obstruction causing acute cholecystitis and risking perforation was seen in about 1% [14, 25].

In two studies comprising a total of 1035 patients with pancreatic cancer, the incidence of duodenal obstruction was 5%–10%. The 30-day mortality following endoscopic stenting was 11%–17%. Most early deaths were

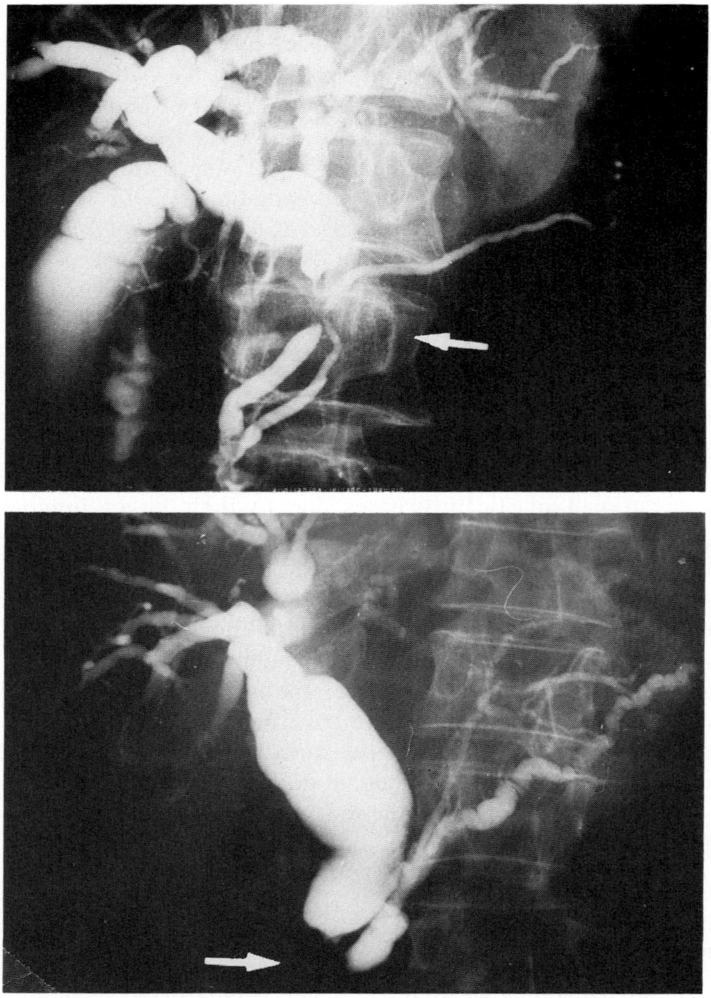

Fig. 5. ERCP showing two different sites of pancreatic head cancer causing obstructive jaundice. *Above*, typical so-called double duct sign due to tumor involvement of common bile duct and pancreatic main duct. *Below*, Pancreatic cancer located close to the papilla causing obstruction of the bile duct and main pancreatic duct. This type of obstruction is usually difficult to stent

related to the advanced disease or bacterial cholangitis secondary to inadequate drainage. Stent blockage occurred in 16%–29% of the cases [12, 20].

Of 180 patients with pancreatic head cancer that underwent successful stent placement, 175 could be followed until death. Following endoscopic biliary decompression, a total of 34 patients were considered suitable surgical candidates. Of these, 12 underwent curative resection, 19 palliative surgery, and three had only an exploratory procedure. The average survival was 12.7 months for resected patients, 12.5 months for palliatively bypassed patients and 7.7 months for endoscopically stented patients [14]. The shorter survival rate of endoscopically treated patients might be explained by the preselection poor surgical candidates.

Comparing results of endoscopic stenting and surgical bypass for unresectable pancreatic cancer, three prospective studies [3, 11, 29] have shown lower morbidity and 30-day mortality rates for endoscopic drainage. However, endoscopic treatment is burdened with late stent clogging, and surgery may ultimately be required for duodenal stenosis. Interestingly, the rate of duodenal stenosis after endoscopic drainage was 0%–14% compared to 0%–4% in the groups with surgical bypass, although prophylatic gastroenterostomies were not performed (Table 2).

Conclusion

Palliative nonsurgical biliary drainage plays an important role in the management of patients with pancreatic cancer. The majority of the cancers are located in the head of the pancreas and will eventually compress or invade the distal bile duct leading to obstructive jaundice. About 80% of the patients are either inoperable or incurable. Endoscopic drainage is generally preferable to the percutaneous approach because of easier accessibility to the distal bile duct and lower procedure risk. Endoscopic drainage has lower morbidity and 30-day mortality than surgical bypass, but recurrent jaundice is common due to stent clogging. Complications of stent clogging can be prevented by regular patient follow-up and serial laboratory checks for cholestasis. The average patency of plastic endoprostheses is 4–5 months, and approximately one-fifth of patients die of underlying disease before stent clogging occurs. Self-expandable metallic stents have larger luminal

Table 2. Palliative management of malignant obstructive jaundice – endoscopic stenting versus bypass surgery: comparison of three prospective studies

	Shepherd et al. [29]		Andersen et al. [3]		Dowsett et al. [11]	
	Stent	Bypass	Stent	Bypass	Stent	Bypass
No. of patients	23	25	25	25	65	62
Successful drainage	91%	92%	96%	76%	94%	94%
Complications	22%	40%	NA	NA	5%	11%
30-day mortality	9%	20%	NA	NA	6%	15%
Recurrent jaundice	43%	0%	28%	16%	17%	3%
Duodenal stenosis	9%	4%	0	0	14%	3%
Survival (weeks)	22	18	12	14	22	16

NA, Not available.

diameters and afford excellent initial drainage, but long-term stent patency is limited by tumor invasion and overgrowth.

Percutaneous drainage and surgical bypass should be reserved for endoscopic failures, which occur in approximately 10% of cases. Palliative surgery is indicated when duodenal stenosis is present. In patients with failed biliary cannulation or difficult anatomy, the percutaneous and endoscopic approaches can be combined in the "rendezvous" procedure.

Finally, the clinician should not always feel compelled to treat. Supportive treatment may be the best option for the terminally ill patient with a very short-life expectancy.

References

1. Adam A, Chetty N, Roddie M, Yeung E, Benjamin IS (1991) Self-expandable stainless steel endoprostheses for treatment of malignant bile duct obstruction. Am J Roentgenol 156:321–325
2. Alvarado R, Palmaz JC, Garcia OJ, Tio FO, Rees CR (1989) Evaluation of polymer-coated ballon-expandable stents in bile ducts. Radiology 170:975–978
3. Andersen JR, Sorensen SM, Kruse A, Rokkjaer M, Matzen P (1989) Randomised trial of endoscopic endoprosthesis versus operative bypass in malignant obstructive jaundice. Gut 30:1132–1135
4. Aoki K, Ogawa H (1978) Cancer of the pancreas, international mortality trends. World Health Stat Rep 31:2
5. Brooks JR (1987) Total pancreatectomy for pancreatic cancer. In: Howard JM, Jordan GL Jr, Reber HA (eds) Surgical diseases of the pancreas. Lea and Febiger, Philadelphia, p 715
6. Browne S, Schmalz M, Geenen J, Venu R, Johnson GK (1990) A comparison of biliary and pancreatic stent occlusion in antibiotic-coated vs. conventional stents. Gastrointest Endosc 36:206A
7. Brückner M, Seitz U, Mack D, Grimm H, Eckmann B, Soehendra N (1990) Vergleichende Untersuchung über Rinnen- und Silberprothesen bei der Drainage maligner Gallengangsstenosen. In: Henning H, Soehendra N (eds) Fortschritte der gastroenterologischen Endoskopie. Demeter, Gräfelfing, pp 17–21
8. Coene PPLO, Groen AK, Cheng J, Out MMJ, Tytgat GNJ, Huibregtse K (1990) Clogging of biliary endoprostheses: a new perspective. Gut 31:913–917
9. Coene PPLO (1990) Endoscopic biliary stenting. Mechanisms and possible solution of the clogging phenomenon. Krips Repro, Meppel, pp 13–50
10. Cremer M, Deviere J, Sugai B, Baize M (1990) Expandable biliary metal stents for malignancies: endoscopic insertion and diathermic cleaning for tumor ingrowth. Gastrointest Endosc 36:451–457
11. Dowsett JF, Russell RCG, Hatfield ARW, Cotton PB, Williams SJ, Speer AG, Houghton J, Lennon T, Macrae K (1989) Malignant obstructive jaundice: prospective randomized trial of by-pass surgery versus endoscopic stenting. Gastroenterology 96:A128
12. Dowsett JF, Williams SJ, Hatfield ARW, Vaira D, Ainley C, Polydorou AA, Cotton PB, Russell RCG (1989) Endoscopic management of low biliary obstruction due to unresectable primary pancreato-biliary malignancy – a review of 463 consecutive cases. Gastroenterology 96:A129
13. Gilliams A, Dick R, Dooley JS, Wallsten H, Eldin A (1990) Self-expandable stainless steel braided endoprosthesis for biliary stricture. Radiology 174:137–140

14. Grimm H, Sum PYS, Soehendra N (1988) Erfahrungen über die endoskopische biliäre Drainage. Verdauungskrankheiten 6:10–15
15. Groen AK, Huibregtse K, Delzenne B, Hoek FJ, Tytgat GNJ (1987) Characterization of the content of occluded biliary endoprostheses. Endoscopy 19:57–59
16. Haulk A, Danilewitz M (1989) Prevention of bacterial growth and colonization with antimicrobial impregnated stents – an in vitro study. Gastrointest Endosc 35:163A
17. Hirayama T, Waterhouse JAH, Fraumeni Jr JF (eds) (1980) Cancer risks by site. (UICC technical report series, vol 41) UICC. Geneva, pp 78–83
18. Huibregtse K, Katon RM, Coene PPLO, Tytgat GNJ (1986) Endoscopic palliative treatment in pancreatic cancer. Gastrointest Endosc 32:334–338
19. Huibregtse K, Cheng J, Coene PPLO, Fockens P, Tytgat GNJ (1989) Endoscopic placement of expandable metal stents for biliary stricures – a preliminary report on experience with 33 patients. Endoscopy 21:280–282
20. Huibregtse K (1990) Non-operative palliation of pancreatic cancer. In: Neoptolemos JP (ed) Clinical gastroenterology, vol 4. Bailliere Tindall, London, pp 995–1004
21. Irving JD, Adam A, Dick R, Dondelinger RF, Lunderquist A, Roche A (1989) Gianturco expandable metallic stens: results of a European clinical trial. Radiology 172:321–326
22. Kerlan RK, Ring EJ, Pogany AC, Jeffrey Jr RB (1984) Biliary endoprosthesis – insertion using a combined peroral-transhepatic method. Radiology 150:828–830
23. Lammer J, Klein GE, Kleinert R, Hausegger K, Einspieler R (1990) Obstructive jaundice: use of expandable metal endoprosthesis for biliary drainage. Work in progress. Radiology 177:789–792
24. Leung JWC, Ling TKW, Kung JLS, Vallance-Owen J (1988) The role of bacteria in the blockage of biliary stents. Gastrointest Endosc 34:19–22
25. Leung JWC, Chung SCS, Sung JY, Li MKW (1989) Acute cholecystitis after stenting of the commn bile duct for obstruction secondary to pancreatic cancer. Gastrointest Endosc 35:109–110
26. Neuhaus H, Hagenmüller F, Griebel M, Classen M (1991) Percutaneous cholangioscopic or transpapillary insertion in self-expanding biliary stents. Gastrointest Endosc 37:31–37
27. Robertson DAF, Hacking CN, Birch S, Ayres R, Shepherd H, Wright R (1987) Experience with a combined percutaneous and endoscopic approach to stent insertion in malignant obstructive jaundice. Lancet ii:1449–1452
28. Rösch J, Putnam JS, Uchida BT (1989) Expandable metallic stents in experimental and clinical use. In: Hiramatsu K, Zeitler E, Rossi P (eds) Recent advances in interventional radiology and new vascular imaging. Elsevier, Amsterdam, pp 9–15
29. Shepherd HA, Royle G, Ross APR, Diba A, Arthur M, Colin-Jones D (1988) Endoscopic biliary endoprosthesis in the palliation of malignant obstruction of the distal common bile duct: a randomized trial. Br J Surg 75:1166–1168
30. Siegel JH, Snady H (1986) The significance of endoscopically placed prostheses in the management of biliary obstruction due to carcinoma of the pancreas: results of nonoperative decompression in 277 patients. Am J Gastroenterol 81:634–641
31. Soehendra N, Rynders-Frederix V (1979) Palliative Gallengangdrainage: eine neue Methode zur endosopischen Einführung eines inneren Drains. Dtsch Med Wochenschr 104:206–207
32. Speer AG, Cotton PB, Russell RCG, Mason RR, Hatfield ARW, Leung JWC, MacRae KD, Houghton J, Lennon CA (1987) Randomised trial of endoscopic versus percutaneous stent insertion in malignant obstructive jaundice. Lancet ii:57–62

33. Speer AG,Cottopn PB, Rode J, Sedon AM, Neal CR, Holton J, Costerton JW (1988) Biliary stent blockage with bacterial biofilm. Ann Intern Med 108:546–553
34. Uchida BT, Putnam JS, Rösch J (1988) Modifications of Gianturco expandable wire stents. Am J Roentgenol 150:1185–1187
35. Young Jr JF, Aire AJ, Pollack ES (eds) (1978) SEER program. Cancer incidence and mortality in the United States 1973–1976. US Department of Health Education and Welfare, Bethesda
36. Yoshioka T, Sakaguchi H, Yoshimura H, Tamada T, Ohishi H, Uchida H, Wallace S (1990) Expandable metallic biliary endoprostheses: preliminary clinical evaluation. Radiology 177:253–257
37. Waterhouse J, Muir C, Correa P, Powell J (eds) (1976) Cancer incidence in five continents, vol 3. International agency for research on cancer, Lyon (IARC scientific publication no 15)
38. Wechsler RL, Wechsler L (1975) The first application of transhepatic cholangiography to the localization of liver or biliary tract pathology: Hanoi 1937. Am J Dig Dis 20:699–700

Indications for Surgery in Pancreatic Cancer

D.C. CARTER[1]

Introduction

Pancreatic cancer remains a devastating disease; despite advances in diagnostic imaging and surgical management, 90% of patients will die within a year of diagnosis, and survival beyond 5 years remains truly exceptional. This said, surgical resection does offer a prospect of cure to selected patients, and we have advanced from the situation in which review of the surgical literature revealed a mean operative mortality for the Whipple operation of 21% in almost 500 collected patients [14]. Nevertheless, in a more recent review, Gudjonsson [9] reported that from a total of 37 000 patients, 4100 of whom underwent resection, only 156 survived 5 years; this is an overall 5-year survival rate of only 0.4%. Accordingly, there are those who continue to doubt the value of resection in this disease, and even in specialist centres advocating extirpation whenever possible, representative resectability rates still range only from 14% to 22% [1, 10, 17]. Clearly, the majority of patients with this grim disease are not candidates for attempts at surgical cure, and the recent advent of percutaneous and endoscopic techniques to relieve biliary obstruction has brought into question the need for surgery as a means of palliation. It is against this background that the current indications for surgery in the management of pancreatic cancer will be reviewed. The discussion will be confined to the common problem of cancer arising in the head of the pancreas and will assume that tumours arising in the body and tail of the gland are rarely, if ever, resectable.

Patient Evaluation

It is now an article of faith that the clinical and radiological diagnosis of adenocarcinoma of the pancreas must be confirmed cytologically or histologically. The pitfalls of failing to obtain cytological or histological confirmation are well recognised but cannot be overemphasised. A variety of benign conditions can masquerade as cancer, and it is unforgivable to embark on potentially hazardous and inappropriate pancreatic resection for

[1] University of Edinburgh, The Royal Infirmary, Edinburgh EH3 9YW, U.K.

Beger/Büchler/Malfertheiner (Eds.)
Standards in Pancreatic Surgery

an impacted gallstone misdiagnosed as a "small, mobile, operative pancreatic cancer" solely on the basis of the findings at operation. Chronic pancreatitis is another potent source of diagnostic confirmation and in this particular context, doubt may remain despite every effort to exclude neoplasia by cytological and/or histological sampling. In my view, pancreatoduodenectomy using the Whipple resection or one of its variants is fully justified in this situation. The operation will present the pathologist with the biggest and best biopsy of the head of the pancreas that he is likely to receive, diagnostic doubt will be eliminated, and the operation offers effective treatment whether chronic pancreatitis is present alone or in conjunction with occult cancer. All surgeons with substantial experience of chronic pancreatitis will recall cases in which unsuspected, and in some cases curable pancreatic cancer was revealed in this way. Conversely, there are patients in whom a strong preoperative suspicion of co-existent cancer will prove to be groundless once the resection specimen has been examined fully.

It is also worth emphasising that a number of neoplasms can also masquerade as pancreatic adenocarcinoma, many of them carrying a much more optimistic outlook if appropriate treatment is instituted. For example, periampullary cancer and cholangiocarcinoma affecting the common bile duct are more frequently curable by resection; lymphoma obstructing the biliary system may respond dramatically to nonoperative therapy; and other primary pancreatic neoplasms such as cystadenoma, cystadenocarcinoma and APUDomas may carry superior survival prospects once the true nature of the condition is recognised.

Cytological/Histological Diagnosis

Preoperative diagnosis of pancreatic cancer can now be obtained safely by percutaneous fine-needle aspiration cytology or Trucut biopsy once a lesion has been targetted by ultrasonography or radiology. Such confirmation is also vitally important when the decision is taken to avoid surgery and relieve biliary obstruction by stenting, if inappropriate treatment is to be avoided. If diagnostic doubt remains in patients coming to operation, fine-needle sampling or Trucut biopsy (performed transduodenally wherever possible) should be employed, although sampling error is less likely when material is obtained under radiological/ultrasonographic control. Given a competent cytologist, false positivity is extremely rare but sampling error is still a potential source of false negativity. Although some groups have reported diagnostic accuracy rates of 100% [25], figures of 80%–90% may be more representative, and even in the best hands, an element of diagnostic doubt may remain in patients not undergoing resection. As already indicated, these sampling techniques have proved to be safe, with minimal risk of inducing acute pancreatitis, bleeding and fistula formation. The theoretical hazard of needle-track dissemination has not proved to be significant in practice, although multiple needle passes do carry a small but documented risk of needle-track dissemination and serosal spread, particularly when larger-calibre needles are employed [11].

Given cytological or histological confirmation of the diagnosis of pancreatic adenocarcinoma, which other factors are important in defining the indications for surgery? Patients presenting with pancreatic cancer occupy a spectrum ranging from relatively young, fit individuals with lesions which appear localised and eminently resectable, to elderly, unfit patients with significant intercurrent disease and with locally advanced or widely disseminated cancer. It is clear from the outset that the latter are not candidates for any form of surgery, let alone resection, and that they should be offered endoscopic stenting to relieve jaundice and pruritis. In some extreme cases, the kindest and correct decision may be to offer no intervention, accept the terminal nature of the condition, and simply ensure that unnecessary suffering is avoided.

Assessment of Resectability

Considerable clinical judgement is needed to determine which patients with pancreatic cancer should be offered which form of treatment. Patient age in itself is no longer a contra-indication to surgery, and specialist centres are now prepared to undertake resection in the elderly who have localised resectable cancer and who are otherwise deemed fit for major surgery. As discussed below, risk factors have been identified for use in patient evaluation. Preoperative demonstration of locally advanced or disseminated disease which would preclude resectional surgery remains problematic. Computerised tomography (CT) and ultrasonography are used widely to attempt to assess resectability. CT criteria for unresectability include evidence of hepatic and more distant metastasis and/or local signs of extension of cancer to contiguous structures, vascular encasement or invasion and local lymphadenopathy. However, recent reports indicate that CT is far from reliable in this regard and cannot be used as a basis for electing to manage pancreatic cancer nonoperatively [12]. It has also proved particularly disappointing in detecting metastatic lesions, with a reported sensitivity of 20%–38% [15]. Our own ongoing study of the use of CT scans following injection of iodised oil emulsion has confirmed the shortcomings of conventional CT scanning in detecting liver metastases. In this technique, the emulsion is taken up by the Kupffer cells of the hepatic reticuloendothelial system and metastases are revealed as filling defects. The technique carries a risk of sensitivity reaction and is unlikely to find a role in routine practice. However, in the context of colorectal cancer, intraoperative ultrasonography proved, in our hands, to be as accurate as iodised oil emulsion CT scanning in detecting hepatic metastases, and both techniques were superior to preoperative ultrasonography or conventional CT scanning (O.J. Garden, unpublished observations). Given the recent widespread adoption of laparoscopy in other areas of general surgical practice, laparoscopic ultrasonography may prove useful in evaluating resectability prior to laparotomy. Laparoscopy has also been advocated as a means of assessing resectability in its own right. Warshaw et al. [23] studied 40 patients with biopsy-proven pancreatic cancer who were thought to have curable lesions after conventional investigation; 14 showed evidence of hepatic or peritoneal spread that precluded cure, but laparoscopy failed to detect liver metastases in three patients found to have such lesions at subsequent laparotomy. Magnetic resonance imaging has also been evaluated as an alternative to CT scanning in assessing resectability, although to date the evidence in its favour is unimpressive [20].

Selective angiography is no longer used as a means of diagnosing the presence of pancreatic cancer, but its role as a routine preoperative means of defining significant vascular invasion and unresectability remains controversial. I still hold to the view that the investigation is of value in patients being considered for resection, accepting that this may be a minority view and that the technique can be misleading in the assessment of portal vein displacement or invasion. It is well recognised that such displacement does not necessarily mean unresectability, that venous invasion is not always revealed, and that such invasion does not necessarily preclude resection [17]. However, a comprehensive knowledge of vascular anatomy and overt vascular involvement is, in my view, valuable when one embarks on resection in pancreatic cancer.

Indications for Resection

As discussed earlier, it has been argued that there is no case for resection for carcinoma of the pancreas. The basis for this argument used to lie in the fact that the operative mortality was prohibitively high and the long-term survival rates were so poor [4, 9, 14]. However, it is now clear that the Whipple operation or its variants, such as pylorus-preserving pancreatoduodenectomy, can now be performed with mortalities that approximate to zero [5, 18, 19]. Recognition that a pancreaticojejunal anastomosis can be performed without high morbidity or mortality has greatly weakened the argument in favour of removing the entire pancreas, and in any event, total pancreatectomy does not appear to be a safer operation or to confer improved long-term survival [22]. There have been advocates of more radical or regional resection [7] and, more recently, of extended lymphadenectomy. These more radical procedures will be discussed elsewhere in this volume, but to date the case remains unproven. Actuarial 5-year survival rates of 18%–36% are now being reported following the Whipple operation [5, 19], and although survival for 5 years does not necessarily mean cure, it seems likely that this will remain the standard operative approach. When such surgery is undertaken while the primary cancer is small (i.e. less than 2 cm in diameter), 5-year survival rates of 30% have been recorded in a multicentre Japanese study, the figure rising to 44% in those with stage-I tumours [21]. Sadly, only 2% of Japanese patients with pancreatic cancer had such small tumours, and it remains clear that only a minority of patients will be candidates for resection. Nevertheless, it is evident that pancreatic cancer is not a contraindication to surgery and that worthwhile results will be achieved in some patients. Of recent interest, Griffen et al. [8] have analysed the pattern of failure after "curative" resection for pancreatic cancer. Of 36 patients, six remained free of disease and may have been cured, four died of intercurrent disease, and 26 manifested recurrence. Of the recurrences, 19% were local only, while 73% had a component of local failure. Peritoneal (42%) and hepatic (62%) recurrence were common, and while all patients had recurrent intra-adominal disease, only 27% had recurrence in an extra-abdominal site. The case for chemotherapy and/or radiotherapy as an adjunct to resection thus requires further evaluation as a means of improving survival prospects.

Indications for Palliative Surgery

The recent advent of stenting using an endoscopic, percutaneous or combined approach has resulted in a marked fall in the number of patients undergoing palliative surgery for pancreatic cancer. Prior to the availability of these techniques, surgery was the only means of relieving biliary obstruction with its attendant jaundice, pruritus, cholangitis and liver failure. While some surgeons advocated resection as a means of palliation, this has not been my practice, although I accept that in some operations commenced as curative resections it may become apparent in the later stages that the procedure will, in fact, be palliative. This consideration aside, palliative surgery in most hands consisted of biliary bypass (cholecyst-enterostomy or hepaticojejunostomy) with or without gastroenterostomy to treat or prevent duodenal obstruction. The recognition that such palliative surgery carried an overall operative mortality of almost 20% and was followed by a mean duration of survival of only 5.4 months [13], led to the ready abandonment of surgery as soon as nonoperative stenting became available. The results of early controlled comparisons certainly seemed to favour stenting, in that its technical success rate was just as good as that of surgical bypass, its mean survival rates were comparable, and its procedure-related mortality was less than 10% [3, 16]. It was clear from the outset that duodenal obstruction would be a problem in some patients (6%–14%) and that stent blockage might give rise to recurrent obstruction and biliary sepsis after some 3 months. However, it was argued that duodenal obstruction was never dealt with particularly well by surgery, in that the patients who needed gastro-enterostomy most appeared to benefit from it least [6, 24]. Furthermore, it was contended that stent blockage could be dealt with easily by changing of stent without the patient requiring long periods in hospital. In my view, the abandonment of surgical bypass in favour of stenting may have been too precipitate. While I accept that stenting is an effective method of relieving jaundice and that it has a lower procedure-related mortality when used nonselectively, I remain concerned about the problem of stent blockage and cholangitis, which may carry significant morbidity and erode the quality of life. Even with the combined percutaneous and endoscopic approach (the so-called rendevous technique) stents cannot be inserted in all patients, the procedure is not without problems (pancreatitis, bleeding and perforation), and there is a greater incidence of duodenal obstruction.

Our current approach to pancreatic cancer is as follows: Resection is undertaken whenever possible in eligible patients. When resection is not feasible, we divide the patients into two groups on the basis of risk assessment. A high-risk group of patients who, in the main, are elderly, profoundly jaundiced, and carry a large tumour burden are treated by stent insertion, using the endoscopic route whenever possible. The low-risk group of patients are then allocated on a random basis to have either surgical biliary bypass or stenting as part of a prospective controlled trial. The risk-factors assessment used is that defined earlier by our group, in which the serum bilirubin, albumin and creatinine are used in a discriminant function calculation [2]. It is our hypothesis that the quality of life following surgery will be superior to that which follows stenting, and analysis of data from our pilot study suggest that this will prove to be a reasonable contention.

Conclusions

Despite expressed views to the contrary, there are strong indications for surgery in some patients with pancreatic cancer. A minority (some 10%–20%) of patients may prove to be candidates for resection with the intention of cure, although realistically, survival rates in resected patients are liable to remain low in the absence of effective adjuvant treatment. Surgery may still be indicated as a method of palliation in selected patients who are not candidates for resection, accepting that there will be a large number of patients who are old, suffering from organ failure and/or burdened with extensive tumour who are at prohibitively high risk from operation and who will be best served by nonoperative relief of their biliary obstruction.

References

1. Andren-Sandberg A, Ihse I (1983) Factors influencing survival after total pancreatectomy in patients with pancreatic cancer. Ann Surg 198:605–610
2. Blamey SL, Fearon KCH, Gilmour WH et al. (1983) Prediction of risk in biliary surgery. Br J Surg 70:535–538
3. Bornman PC, Harries-Jones EP, Tobias R (1986) Prospective controlled trial of transhepatic biliary endoprosthesis versus bypass surgery for incurable carcinoma of head of pancreas. Lancet 1:69–71

4. Carter DC (1980) Surgery for pancreatic cancer. Br Med J 280:744–746
5. Crist DW, Sitzmann JV, Cameron JL (1987) Improved hospital morbidity, mortality and survival after the Whipple procedure. Ann Surg 206:358–365
6. Doberneck RC, Berndt GA (1987) Delayed gastric emptying after palliative gastrojejunostomy for carcinoma of the pancreas. Arch Surg 122:827–829
7. Fortner JG (1984) Regional pancreatectomy for cancer of the pancreas, ampulla and other related sites. Tumour staging and results. Ann Surg 199:418–425
8. Griffen JF, Smalley SR, Jewell W, Paradelo CJ, Reymond RD, Hassanein ESR, Evans RG (1990) Patterns of failure after curative resection of pancreatic carcinoma. Cancer 66:56–61
9. Gudjonsson B (1987) Cancer of the pancreas: 50 years of surgery. Cancer 60:2284–2303
10. Morrow M, Hilaris B, Brennan MF (1984) Comparison of conventional surgical resection, radioactive implantation and bypass procedures for exocrine carcinoma of the pancreas 1975–1980. Ann Surg 199:1–5
11. Rashleigh-Belcher HJC, Russell RCG, Lees WR (1986) Cutaneous seeding of pancreatic carcinoma by fine-needle aspiration biopsy. Br J Radiol 59:182–183
12. Ross CB, Sharp KW, Kaufman A et al. (1988) Efficacy of computerized tomography in the preoperative staging of pancreatic carcinoma. Am J Surg 54:221–225
13. Sarr MG, Cameron JL (1982) Surgical management of unresectable carcinoma of the pancreas. Surgery 91:123–133
14. Shapiro TM (1975) Adenocarcinoma of the pancreas: a statistical analysis of biliary bypass vs Whipple resection in good-risk patients. Ann Surg 182:715–721
15. Shimamoto K, Ishiguchi T, Sakuma S (1987) CT evaluation of pancreatic cancer – analysis of resected tumours. Eur J Radiol 7:37–41
16. Speer AG, Cotton PB, Russell RCG et al. (1987) Randomised trial of endoscopic versus percutaneous stent insertion in malignant obstructive jaundice. Lancet 1:57–62
17. Trede M (1985) The surgical treatment of pancreatic carcinoma. Surgery 97:28–35
18. Trede M, Schwall G (1988) The complication of pancreatectomy. Ann Surg 207:39–47
19. Trede M, Schwall G, Saeger H-D (1990) Survival after pancreatoduodenectomy. Ann Surg 211:447–458
20. Tscholakoff D, Hricak H, Thoeni R, Winkler ML, Margulis AR (1987) MR imaging in the diagnosis of pancreatic disease. Am J Radiol 148:703–709
21. Tsuchiya R, Noda T, Harada N (1986) Collective review of small carcinomas of the pancreas. Ann Surg 203:77–81
22. Warshaw AL, Swanson RS (1988) Pancreatic cancer in 1988 – possibilities and probabilities. Ann Surg 208:541–553
23. Warshaw AL, Tepper JE, Shipley WU (1986) Laparoscopy in the staging and planning of therapy for pancreatic cancer. Am J Surg 151:76–80
24. Weaver DW, Wieneck RG, Bouwman DL, Walt AJ (1987) Gastrojejunostomy – is it helpful for patients with pancreatic cancer? Surgery 102:608–613
25. Yamamoto R, Tatsuta M, Noguchi S (1985) Histocytologic diagnosis of pancreatic cancer by percutaneous aspiration biopsy under ultrasonic guidance. Am J Clin Pathol 83:409–414

Palliative Biliary Bypass for Pancreatic Cancer

J.P. NEOPTOLEMOS[1] and C. HENDRICKSE

Introduction

Pancreatic cancer affects 8–12 per 100000 population in Europe, North America and other industrialised countries and is the fourth or fifth commonest cause of death from cancer [26, 27]. The median age at presentation is 65–70 years. The long-term survival even with resection is exceptional and about 90% of patients are dead within 1 year of diagnosis [25, 26]. Resectability in specialist units is 10%–30% [47], but such data represent what may be possible rather than the general reality. Actual resectability may be as low as 2.6% as determined by a survey of nearly 10000 cases in the West Midlands, England (J.P. Neoptolemos et al., unpublished).

Because of the limited prognosis of the disease and the advanced age of the patients, palliation forms a major aspect of management. The most common complaints of patients with advanced pancreatic cancer are jaundice, weight loss, pain and vomiting. Obstructive jaundice is the presenting feature in 84%–90% of patients with cancer of the pancreatic head [31]. Modern imaging techniques now permit an accurate diagnosis; moreover they can determine not only whether the obstruction is correctable (multiple metastases vs a discrete lesion) but the exact level of biliary obstruction.

The important physiological benefits associated with the relief of obstructive jaundice are indicated in Table 1. The clinical benefits to the patient can be substantial and include improved digestion and energy utilisation; relief of pruritus; reduced peripheral oedema; improved clotting; and reduced risk of cholangitis.

The relief of obstructive jaundice is only one aspect of palliation and may need to be combined with measures for pain relief [51] and operative bypass for duodenal obstruction [32]. Many patients present with advanced disease (malignant ascites and multiple metastases) and in such cases tender loving care (TLC) is the only appropriate treatment; intervention (surgical or non-surgical) is best avoided. The mortality associated with laparotomy alone has usually been in the region of 20%–55% (Table 2). In nearly 10000 patients analysed in the West Midlands this represented 30% of cases and

[1] Academic Department of Surgery, Dudley Road Hospital, Birmingham, B18 7QH England

Beger/Büchler/Malfertheiner (Eds.)
Standards in Pancreatic Surgery

Table 1. Physiological benefits associated with the relief of obstructive jaundice

Improved hepatocyte metabolism – Carbohydrates – Fats – Hormones	Improved protein synthesis – Albumin and carrier proteins – Clotting factors – Increased oncotic pressure
Excretion – Waste products – Xenobiotics	Improved monocyte phagocytic system function – Decreased systemic endotoxaemia – Improved bacterial clearance
Bile salt enterohepatic circulation – Digestion of fats – Absorption of fats	

such a high figure is probably unjustified. The reason for not undertaking a bypass at laparotomy for pancreatic cancer was twofold: (a) carcinomatosis or advanced malignancy which can now usually be determined by non-operative means; (b) inability to effect a bypass due to incomplete pre-operative investigations.

Surgical Versus Non-Surgical Biliary Drainage

The investigative work-up must include an assessment of tumour burden and the fitness of the patient to undergo a surgical procedure, as such will determine the optimum approach (Fig. 1). There have been two prospective trials completed comparing surgical bypass with stenting [1, 52], and one trial based at the Middlesex Hospital, London is still in progress [19]. These trials suggest a reduced hospital mortality for endoscopic stenting compared to operative bypass (Table 3). Against this, is the greater risk of duodenal stenosis and recurrent jaundice associated with stenting (Tables 3, 4). A comparison of longterm survival rates between surgical series (Table 2) and endoscopic series (Tables 3, 4) suggests a survival advantage for operative bypass. This is supported by two recent retrospective studies comparing surgery with percutaneous stenting [35] or endoscopic stenting [30]. Indeed the most recent results of the Middlesex study suggest reduced long-term survival following hospital discharge in the stented group compared to the surgical group because of recurrent jaundice (C. Russell, personal communication).

Percutaneous transhepatic stenting is a useful alternative to endoscopic stenting but has similar long-term disadvantages [9]. Although one randomised trial has shown endoscopic stenting to be superior to percutaneous stenting [56], the choice depends largely upon local expertise.

A clear message seems to be emerging that stenting should be restricted to elderly, surgically unfit individuals with a life expectancy of 2–3 months. In contrast, younger patients with a low to moderate surgical risk are better palliated by surgical biliary decompression. A number of useful guidelines

Table 2. Mortality and survival associated with laparotomy alone and biliary bypass in obstructive jaundice for pancreatic cancer

Series	Year	Period	Number of patients	Hospital mortality (%)		Mean survival (months)	
				Laparotomy alone	Biliary-enteric bypass	Laparotomy alone	Biliary-enteric bypass
Sarr and Cameron [49][a]	1984	1945–1983	10814	27	18	3.4	5.5
Morrow et al. [36]	1984	1975–1980	122	20	14	3.0	4.0
Rosenberg et al. [45]	1985	1955–1978	341	30	16	2.9	6.3
Schouten [50]	1986	1968–1983	90	44	33	5.2	6.3
Dunn [21]	1987	1960–1982	126	30	25 (8)[b]	3.0	7.6
La Ferla and Murray [32]	1987	1974–1983	100	–	26	–	19%[c] (17%)[b]
Lea and Stahlgren [33]	1987	1980–1986	77	22	13	5.1	7.5
Singh et al. [54]	1990	1973–1988	221	–	8	3.9[d]–4.1[e]	8.0
Proctor and Mauro [42]	1990	1980 1987	70	–	0 (2)[h]	–	–
Potts et al. [41]	1990	1982–1987	147	0	2.5	<5.0	<8.0
Neoptolemos [37][f]	1991	1960–1984	6425	55	25	1.2	3.5

[a] Collected series ($n = 59$).
[b] With gastro-jejunostomy.
[c] 1-year survival (%).
[d] 1980.
[e] 1988.
[f] Single series, West Midlands, England (unpublished).

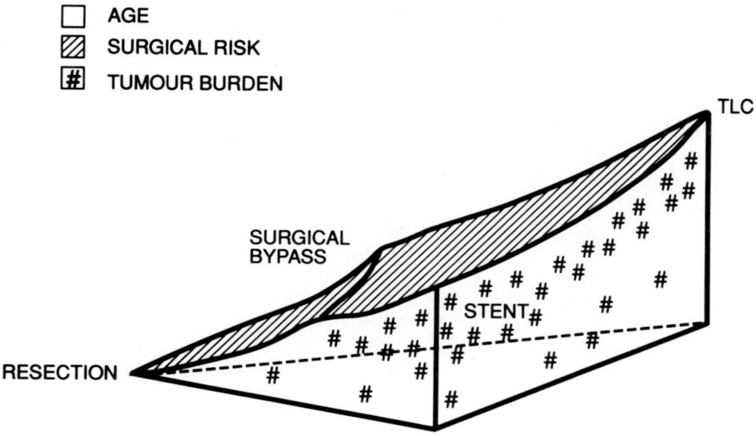

Fig. 1. Three-dimensional representation of the considerations that need to be taken into account before deciding the optimum approach for a patient with pancreatic cancer. *TLC*, "tender loving care"

Table 3. Randomised trials of endoscopic stenting vs operative biliary bypass for pancreatic cancer

Variable	Shepherd et al. [52] (1988)		Dowsett et al. [19] (1989)		Andersen et al. [1] (1989)	
	Stent	Surgery	Stent	Surgery	Stent	Surgery
Number of patients	23	25	101	103	25	19
Successful drainage	91%	92%	94%	91%	96%	84%
30-day mortality	9%	20%	7%[a]	17%	0%	0%
Recurrent jaundice	17%	2%	18%[a]	3%	28%	16%
Duodenal stenosis	0%	0%	6%[a]	1%	0%	0%
Survival	152 days[b]	125 days[b]	5 months[c]	5 months[c]	84 days[b]	100 days[b]

[a] Significantly different.
[b] Median.
[c] Mean.

have been proposed as to surgical risk in pancreatic cancer the most important of which seem to be concomitant medical problems and significant recent weight loss [6, 34, 35, 39, 40]. The suggestion that all patients with obstructive jaundice should be stented does not seem justified and most patients should have at least the benefit of a surgical consultation.

External biliary drainage as the only permanent means of relieving jaundice (performed surgically, endoscopically or radiologically) is not recommended [10]. It does not seem to prolong life, indeed it may shorten life because of sepsis and haemorrhage and above all, it seems to represent an intrusive indignity into the last few weeks of life.

Table 4. Results of endoscopic stenting for pancreatic cancer in three large consecutive series

Variable	St. Clare's and Doctors' Hospitals, New York [53] (1986)	Middlesex Hospital, London [20] (1989)	University of Amsterdam [14] (1990)
Number of patients	311	463	632
Mean age	73 years	NA	71 years
Successful drainage	89%	85%	87%
30-day mortality	18%	17%	11%
Survival	4.3 months[a]	4.5 months[b]	5 months[b]
Stent blockage	70%[c]	16%	29%
Duodenal stenosis	NA	5%	9%

NA, Not available.
[a] Median.
[b] Mean.
[c] At 6 months.

Choice of Surgical Procedures

The survival of patients following biliary operative bypass is around 13% (Fig. 2). The choice of which procedure to undertake may influence hospital mortality, length of survival and the quality of survival.

The mortality from surgical bypass remains high, averaging up to 15% in specialist teaching units & even higher in unselected series (Tables 2, 5). Mortality is affected by those risk factors already discussed, by the effect of the surgical procedure, and by whether the bypass is being undertaken as a primary procedure or because non-operative means of bypass have failed. In the latter case, mortality is higher because of greater risk factors and the problems of biliary tract sepsis associated with non-surgical biliary instrumentation. In order to minimise operative morbidity and mortality, it is, important to undertake adequate pre-operative preparation along the same lines as would be undertaken if resection were being planned.

Such precautions include the following: (a) clear pre-operative identification of the level of obstruction and likely sites of biliary bypass; (b) correction of anaemia by blood transfusion (>11 g/dl) and hypoalbuminaemia by albumin infusion (>30 g/l); (c) treatment of pre-existent infection as far as possible and routine intravenous prophylactic antibiotics; (d) correction of clotting abnormalities with parenteral vitamin K and, if need be, fresh frozen plasma; (e) oral lactulose 20 ml twice daily for 3–5 days before surgery to increase gut luminal endotoxin binding, thereby reducing protal and systemic endotoxaemia and the risk of renal failure [38]; (f) use of intravenous H_2 blockade during and immediately following surgery may help to reduce the small but significant incidence of upper gastrointestinal haemorrhage [18]; (g) adequate rehydration with intravenous fluids is im-

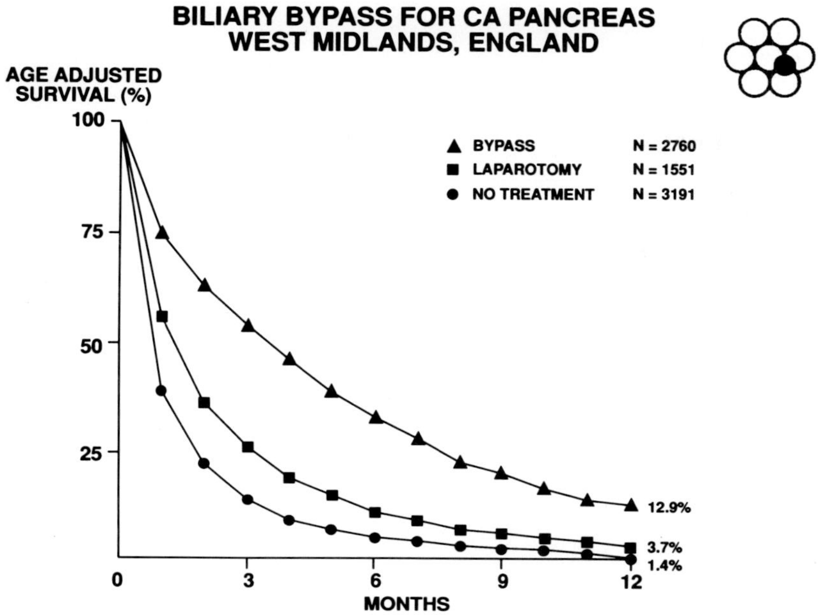

Fig. 2. Survival in a large complete cohort of patients from the West Midlands, England, with pancreatic cancer – comparing biliary bypass with laparotomy alone and no treatment

portant output (60 ml/h) during and after surgery. Intravenous mannitol (100 ml of 20%) is recommended for maintaining a good urinary output although a loop diuretic may be preferable in the presence of congestive cardiac failure.

Controversies continue regarding the optimum surgical approach. The gallbladder may be used for bypass with anastomosis to the stomach, duodenum or small bowel. Alternatively, the main bile ducts may be used as the upstream site of bypass. In general, the stomach has been abandoned as the downstream site of bypass because of troublesome biliary gastritis and oesophageal reflux. Although anastomosis between the gallbladder and small bowel are technically much easier (Fig. 3) than between the main bile duct and small bowel (Fig. 4) mortality does not seem to be any higher for choledocho-enterostomy (Table 5). In our personal experience of 33 patients (median age 68 years; range 33–84) that had a side-to-side choledocho-enterostomy, there were four post-operative deaths (12%). Although perhaps technically more demanding, choledocho-enterostomy does seem to provide a longer survival time than cholecysto-enterostomy (Table 5). In our experience, side-to-side choledocho-enterostomy produced a median survival rate of 8 months (range 1–22 months) in these 33 consecutive cases.

Table 5. Hospital mortality and mean survival following biliary bypass by cholecysto-enterostomy or choledocho-enterostomy for pancreatic cancer

Series	Year	Period	Number of patients	Cholecysto-enterostomy		Choledocho-enterostomy	
				Hospital mortality	Mean survival (months)	Hospital mortality	Mean survival (months)
Sarr and Cameron [49]	1984[a]	1945–1983	1850	16%	5.3	20%	6.5
Gough and Mumme [24]	1984	1970–1983	66	–	5.0	–	5.0
Rosenberg et al. [45]	1985	1955–1978	341	14%	6.0	12.5%	10.5
Ubhi and Doran [58]	1986	1978–1981	88	–	7.2[b]	–	10.9[b]
Schouten [50]	1986	1968–1983	55	39%	5.6	30%	6.6
La Ferla and Murray [32]	1987	1974–1983	100	26%	17[c]–19 1-year	–	–
Condie et al. [15]	1989	1975–1985	71	10%	–	3%	–
Hyoty and Nordback [30]	1990	1980–1987	63	0%	–	2.9%	–
Potts et al. [41]	1990	1982–1987	122	9.4%	5–8	0%	5–8
Singh et al. [54]	1990	1973–1988	154	5.4%	8.6–9.6[c]	11.7%	6.1–6.8[c]

[a] Collected series ($n = 19$).
[b] Median.
[c] With gastro-enterostomy.

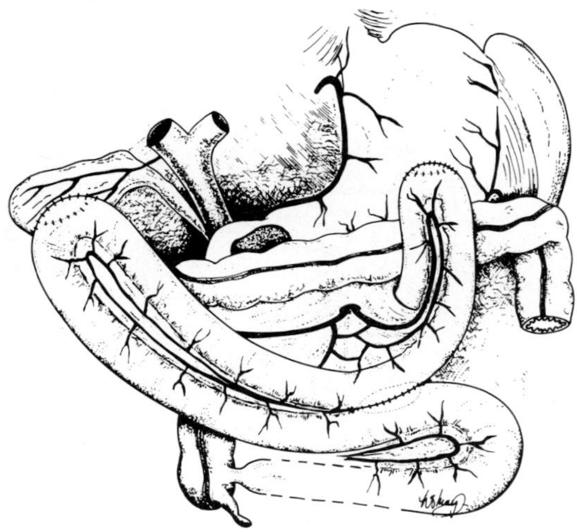

Fig. 3. Cholocysto-enterostomy with side-to-side entero-enterostomy for pancreatic cancer. An ante-colic gastro-jejunostomy is also shown

The difficulties that may encountered using the gallbladder are several: (a) there may be gallstones, chronic cholecystitis and a relatively narrow cystic duct thereby compromising retrograde bile drainage; (b) the gallbladder wall may show areas of patchy necrosis secondary to over-distension; (c) the cystic duct may be involved in the pancreatic tumour mass because of low entry into the bile duct, which occurs in about 18%; (d) the cystic duct is liable to early obstruction because of its position, relatively small size and the tendency for metastases to occur preferentially in the cystic duct lymph node. Based on four studies with a total of 298 patients, cholecysto-enterostomy did not produce clinical resolution of jaundice in 18% of cases (Table 6). It is of interest, however, that Singh et al. [54] also reported that clinical jaundice failed to resolve in 14/60 (23%) patients who had undergone choledocho-enterostomy. This is difficult to explain and may suggest problems with patient selection or the choice of sites for bypass in that series. Moreover, the incidence of recurrent jaundice in patients who have had cholecysto-enterostomy is generally greater than in those who have had choledocho-enterostomy (Table 7). This is presumably because of early encroachment by the cancer on the cystic duct.

A Roux-en-Y reconstruction for choledocho-enterostomy has the important advantage of reducing the risk of subsequent acute cholangitis from reflux of intestinal contents. This can also be achieved by a side-to-side entero-enterostomy if a loop reconstruction is used, but this has the disadvantage of removing a large part of the small bowel from contact with luminal contents. This may compound existing problems associated with maldigestion, malabsorption and cancer-induced cachexia. Acute cholangitis

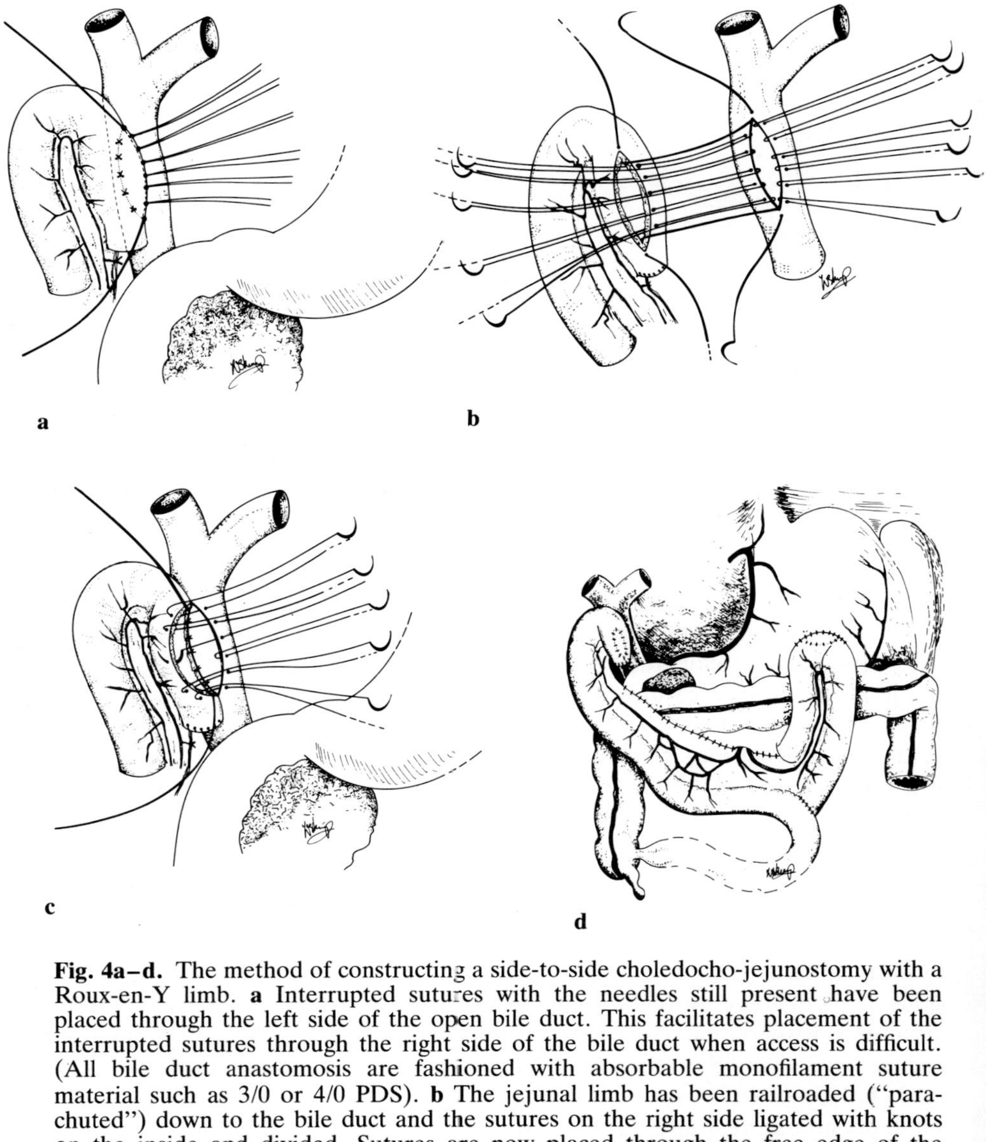

Fig. 4a–d. The method of constructing a side-to-side choledocho-jejunostomy with a Roux-en-Y limb. **a** Interrupted sutures with the needles still present have been placed through the left side of the open bile duct. This facilitates placement of the interrupted sutures through the right side of the bile duct when access is difficult. (All bile duct anastomosis are fashioned with absorbable monofilament suture material such as 3/0 or 4/0 PDS). **b** The jejunal limb has been railroaded ("parachuted") down to the bile duct and the sutures on the right side ligated with knots on the inside and divided. Sutures are now placed through the free edge of the jenunostomy. **c** The sutures on the left side of the anastomosis have been ligated and are about to be divided. **d** The completed Roux-en-Y side-to-side choledocho-jejunostomy with an ante-colic gastro-jejunostomy

Table 6. Incidence of incomplete resolution of clinical jaundice following cholecysto-enterostomy for pancreatic cancer

Series	Year	Number of patients	Failure to resolve clinical jaundice
Bufkin et al. [13]	1967	141	25 (18%)
Eastman and Kune [22]	1980	30	3 (10%)
Gough and Mumme [24]	1984	53	7 (13%)
Singh et al. [54]	1990[a]	74	19 (26%)
Total		298	54 (18%)

[a] In this series choledocho-enterostomy also resulted in incomplete resolution of clinical jaundice in 14/60 patients (23%).

Table 7. Incidence of recurrent jaundice following cholecysto-enterostomy (CCE) or choledocho-enterostomy (CDE) for palliative biliary bypass in pancreatic cancer

Series	Year	Number of patients	Recurrent jaundice (%)	
			CCE	CDE
Vijaynagar and Tolins [60]	1970	23	11 (10)[a]	0
Stuart et al. [57]	1971	46[b]	–	0
Elmslie and Slavotinek [23]	1972	27	6	0
Richards and Sosin [43]	1973	74	6 (4)[a]	0
Blievernicht et al. [7]	1980	108	8	0
Eastman and Kune [22]	1980	38	43 (10)[c]	0
Ross and Jonas [46]	1980	55	8	0
Brooks et al. [11]	1981	38	0	7
Gough and Mumme [24]	1984	66	26 (13)[c]	0
Ubhi and Doran [58]	1986	88	64	17
Schouten [50]	1986	34	27	4
Sarfeh et al. [48]	1988[d]	19	50	22
Condie et al. [15]	1989	66	24	7
Potts et al. [41]	1990	117	19	4
Hyoty and Nordback [30]	1990	63	0	0
Singh et al. [54]	1990	154	14	13

[a] Acute cholangitis.
[b] All had choledocho-duodenostomy.
[c] Failure of jaundice to resolve initially.
[d] Prospective randomized trial.

seems to be more frequent following cholecysto-enterostomy [44] but not always [30], suggesting that case selection and precise operative technique are perhaps more important.

An important alternative operative option is side-to-side choledocho-duodenostomy (Fig. 5). This is an operation that can be performed quickly through a relatively small incision. It seems particularly suitable for the older patient at moderate to high surgical risk and would be the operation of

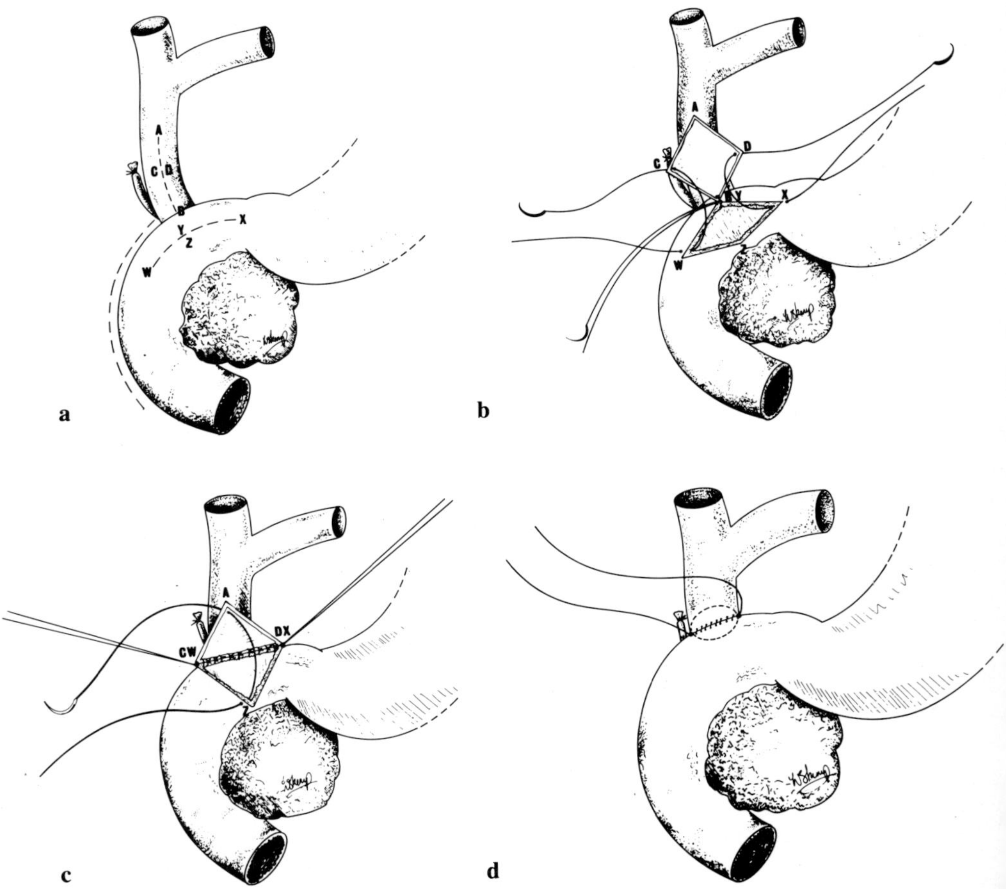

Fig. 5. a Sites of incision into the main bile duct and proximal duodenum for performing a side-to-side choledocho-duodenostomy. **b** The anastomosis is commenced by placing lateral sutures as shown and then a central suture for the posterior anastomotic layer. **c** The posterior anastomotic layer has been completed with interrupted sutures, ligated with knots on the inside and divided. The anterior anastomotic layer is being commenced with a central suture having been placed. **d** The completed choledocho-duodenostomy

choice following failure of non-operative stenting. Although a choledocho-duodenostomy may have the theoretical disadvantage that the anastomosis may become involved with tumour enlarging within the duodenum (as well as proximally into the bile duct) this cannot be substantiated by the literature. Indeed, a detailed analysis of several studies would suggest that this provides an excellent form of biliary drainage and seems superior to types of bypass utilising the gallbladder (Table 8).

Table 8. Mean survival rates (months) associated with different types of biliary bypass involving either the gallbladder or main bile duct

Series	Year	Number of patients	CCJ[a]	CCJ (Loop)	CCJ (Roux-en-Y)	CCD	CDE[a]	CDJ (Loop)	CDJ (Roux-en-Y)	CDD
Bowers [10]	1964	58	6.4	–	–	–	6.0	–	–	–
Buckwalter et al. [12]	1965	179	–	5.4	4.0	4.4	–	6.6	11.8	7.7
Bufkin et al. [13]	1967	141	–	4.4	5.3	–	–	–	–	–
Vijaynagar and Tolins [60]	1970	28	–	4.0	3.3	–	–	–	–	–
Stuart et al. [57]	1971	46	–	–	–	–	–	–	–	7.0
Aston and Longmire [3]	1973	75	5.0	–	–	6.4	10.3	–	–	10.7
Richards and Sosin [43]	1973	111	6.9	–	–	5.5	5.6	–	–	5.7
Hertzberg [28]	1974	113	–	7.1	–	–	–	–	–	–
Anderson and Bergdahl [2]	1976	83	5.5	–	–	7.5	2.5	–	–	5.0
Hines and Burns [29]	1976	65	–	4.5	–	–	(10.0)[b]	–	–	(10.0)[b]
Bergstrand et al. [4]	1978	201	3.6	–	–	5.7	5.3	–	–	7.4
Brooks et al. [11]	1981	34	6.0	–	–	–	6.0	–	–	–
Van Heerden [59]	1984	27	6.0	–	–	–	–	–	–	6.0
Gough and Mumme [24]	1984	66	5.0[c]	–	–	–	6.0[c]	–	–	–
Sonnenfield et al. [55]	1986	24	7.0	–	–	–	–	–	–	7.0
Schouten [50]	1986	55	5.6	–	–	–	5.6	–	–	12.0
La Ferla and Murray [32]	1987	100	17%[d]–19% 1-year	–	–	–	–	–	–	–
Singh et al. [54]	1990	154	8.6–9.6[d]	–	–	–	6.1–6.8[d]	–	–	–
Potts et al. [41]	1990	61	–	–	–	–	–	–	–	8.0

CCJ, Cholecysto-jejunostomy; CCD, cholecysto-duodenostomy; CDE, choledocho-enterostomy; CDJ, choledocho-jejunostomy; CDD, choledocho-duodenostomy.

[a] Not specified.

[b] Types not separated.

[c] Median.

[d] With gastro-jejunostomy.

The lower part of the bile duct may not be suitable for bypass in many cases because of primary tumour extension or involvement of cancer by retrograde lymphatic spread in the hepatoduodenal ligament. In this situation, it is necessary to use the common hepatic or the left hepatic duct. The latter follows an extrahepatic course for the first 3–5 cm and can usually be easily located by dissection and lowering of the hepatic hilar plate and its left extension [8, 17]. Occasionally this may not be possible but alternative approaches are available. These include location of the segment III bile duct though the round ligament and very occasionally it is justified to approach the segment V duct following excision of a V-shaped segment of liver to the right of the gallbladder [5]. By careful pre-operative planning it should therefore be possible to obtain adequate surgical biliary bypass in the vast majority of patients with extrahepatic biliary obstruction [37].

Whether or not to undertake a selective gastro-jejunostomy because of duodenal obstruction by the primary cancer or to perform this routinely is also controversial. The evidence indicates the following: (a) adding a routine gastro-jejunostomy does not increase the hospital mortality; (b) in unselected cases which have not had gastro-jejunostomy, a second operation is required in around 15% because of duodenal obstruction [32, 49]; (c) although there is no strict evidence that adding a routine gastro-jejunostomy improves long-term survival, there is a tendency in this direction [49, 54]. Certainly, it is psychologically disturbing for the patient to undergo a second palliative procedure. Indeed, the vomiting and weight loss which occurs can easily be misconstrued as being due to terminally advanced cancer when such is not the case.

The gastro-jejunostomy may be sited retro-colically at the site of maximum dependence in the hope of achieving more reliable drainage. In preference the antecolic approach can be taken because at this site there is less risk of subsequent blockage by local tumour extension.

Conclusions

Palliation of obstructive jaundice in patients with pancreatic cancer is by far and away the commonest indication for operation. Careful pre-operative investigation, not only with regards to diagnosis but also with regards to the level of obstruction is required in order to achieve a pleasing result.

The proposal that decompression of the biliary tree falls entirely into the territory of the endoscopist or interventional radiologist is now considered incorrect. For relatively younger patients, surgery seems to provide the best and kindest form of treatment. One approach to the problem is shown in Fig. 6. Finally it is important to obtain a histological diagnosis of pancreatic adenocarcinoma as occasionally both the surgeon and radiologist can be deceived with potentially distressing consequences for the patient, his friends and relatives.

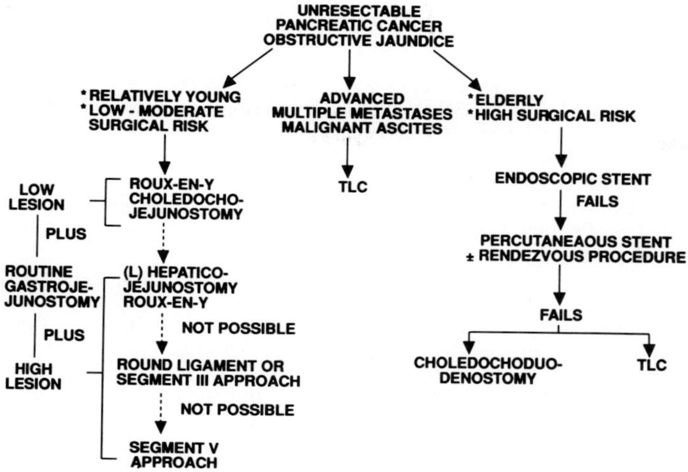

Fig. 6. A suggested algorithm for the palliative treatment of a patient with obstructive jaundice

Acknowledgements. We are grateful to Jean Powell for her assistance with the pancreatic cancer data from the West Midlands; to Wendy Kemp for the excellent art work; to the Medical Photography Department, Dudley Road Hospital, for preparing the illustrations; and to Fay Cox and Dilys Thomas for preparing the manuscript.

References

1. Andersen JR, Sorenson SM, Kruse A, Rokkjaer, Matzen P (1989) Randomised trial of endoscopic endoprosthesis versus operative bypass in malignant obstructive jaundice. Gut 30:1132–1135
2. Anderson A, Bergdahl L (1976) Carcinoma of the pancreas. Ann Surg 42:173
3. Aston SJ, Longmire WP (1973) Pancreatico-duodenal resection. Arch Surg 106:813–817
4. Bergstrand D, Ahlberg J, Ewerth S, Hellers G, Holmstrom B (1978) A retrospective study of carcinoma of the pancreas with special reference to results of surgical treatment. Acta Chir Scand Suppl 482:26–28
5. Bismuth H, Corlette MB (1975) Intrahepatic cholangioenteric anastomosis in carcinoma of the hilus of the liver. Surg Gynecol Obstet 140:170–178
6. Blamey SL, Fearon KCH, Gilmour WH, Osborne DH, Carter DC (1983) Prediction of risk in biliary surgery. Br J Surg 70:535–538
7. Blievernicht SW, Neifeld JL, Terz JJ, Lawrence KW (1980) The role of prophylactic gastrojejunostomy for unresectable periampullary carcinoma. Surg Gynecol Obstet 151:794–796
8. Blumgart LH, Kelley CJ (1984) Hepaticojejunostomy in benign and malignant high bile duct stricture: approaches to the left hepatic ducts. Br J Surg 71:257–261
9. Bornman PC, Harries-Jones EP, Tobias R, Van Stiegmann G, Terblanche J (1986) Prospective controlled trial of transhepatic biliary endoprostheis versus bypass surgery for incurable carcinoma of head of pancreas. Lancet i:69–71

10. Bowers RF (1964) What can be done for carcinoma of the pancreas? Clin Med 71:59
11. Brooks DC, Ostreen RT, Gray EB, Steele GD, Wilson RE (1981) Evaluation of palliative procedures for pancreatic cancer. Am J Surg 141:430–433
12. Buckwalter JA, Lawton RL, Tidrick RT (1965) Bypass operations for neoplastic biliary tract obstruction. Am J Surg 109:100–106
13. Bufkin WJ, Smith PE, Krementz FT (1967) Evaluation of palliative operations for carcinoma of the pancreas. Arch Surg 94:240
14. Coene PLO (1990) Endoscopic biliary stenting. Krips Repro, Meppel
15. Condie JD, Nagpal S, Peebles SA (1989) Surgical treatment for ductal adenocarcinoma of the pancreas. Surg Gynecol Obstet 168:437–445
16. Cotton PB (1990) Management of malignant bile duct obstruction. J Gastroenterol Hepatol Suppl 1:63–67
17. Couinaud C (1989) Exposure of the left hepatic ducts through the hilum or in the umbilicus of the liver: anatomic considerations. Surgery 105:21–27
18. Dixon JM, Armstrong CP, Duffy SW, Elton RA, Davies GC (1984) Upper gastrointestinal bleeding. A significant complication after surgery for relief of obstructive jaundice. Ann Surg 199:271–275
19. Dowsett JR, Williams SJ, Hatfield ARW et al. (1989) Endoscopic management of low biliary obstruction due to unresectable primary pancreato-biliary malignancy: a review of 463 consecutive cases. Gastroenterology 96:A129
20. Dowsett JR, Russell RCG, Hatfield ARW et al. (1989) Malignant obstructive jaundice: a prospective randomized trial of surgery versus endoscopic stenting. Gastroenterology 96:A128
21. Dunn E (1987) The impact of technology and improved perioperative management upon survival from carcinoma of the pancreas. Surg Gynecol Obstet 164:237–244
22. Eastman MC, Kune GA (1980) The objectives of palliative surgery in pancreas cancer, a retrospective study of 73 cases. Aust NZ J Surg 50:462–464
23. Elmslie RG, Slavotinek AH (1972) Surgical objectives in unresected cancer of the head of the pancreas. Br J Surg 59:508–512
24. Gough IR, Mumme G (1984) Biliary and duodenal bypass for carcinoma of the head of the pancreas. J Surg Oncol 26:282–284
25. Gudjonsson B, Livstone EM, Spiro HM (1978) Cancer of the pancreas. Diagnostic accuracy and survival statistics. Cancer 42:2494–2506
26. Gudjonsson B (1987) Cancer of the pancreas. Fifty years of surgery. Cancer 60: 2284–2303
27. Haddock G, Carter DC (1990) Aetiology of pancreatic cancer. Br J Surg 77:1159–166
28. Hertzberg J (1974) Pancreatico-duodenal resection and bypass operation in patients with carcinoma of the head of the pancreas, ampulla and distal end of the common duct. Ann Surg 42:441
29. Hines LH, Burns RP (1976) Ten years experience treating pancreatic and periampullary cancer. Acta Chir Scand 156:391–396
30. Hyoty MK, Nordback IH (1990) Biliary stent or surgical bypass in unresectable pancreatic cancer with obstructive jaundice. Acta Chir Scand 156:391–396
31. Kalser MH, Barkin J, MacIntyre JM (1985) Pancreatic cancer: assessment of prognosis by clinical presentation. Cancer 56:397–402
32. La Ferla G, Murray WR (1987) Carcinoma of the head of the pancreas: bypass surgery in unresectable disease. Br J Surg 74:212–213
33. Lea MS, Stahlgren LRH (1987) Is resection appropriate for adenocarcinoma of the pancreas? Am J Surg 154:651–654
34. Little JM (1987) A prospective evaluation of computerized estimates of risk in the management of obstructive jaundice. Surgery 473–476
35. Malangoni MA, McCoy DM, Richardson JD, Flint LM (1985) Effective palliation of malignant biliary obstruction. Ann Surg 201:554–557

36. Morrow M, Hilaris B, Brennan MF (1984) Comparison of conventional surgical resection, radioactive implantation, and bypass procedures for exocrine carcinoma of the pancreas 1975–1980. Ann Surg 199:1–5
37. Neoptolemos JP (1992) Cancer of the pancreas and gallbladder. In: Burn I, Wellwood J (eds). Farrand, London (in press)
38. Pain JA, Cahill CJ, Gilbert JM, Johnson CD, Trapnell JE, Bailey ME (1991) Prevention of postoperative renal dysfunction in patients with obstructive jaundice: a multicentre study of bile salts and lactulose. Br J Surg 78:467–469
39. Pedrazzoli S, Bonadimani B, Spert C et al. (1987) Forecast of surgical risk in pancreatic cancer. Am J Surg 153:374–377
40. Pitt HA, Cameron JL, Postier RG, Gadacz TR (1981) Factors affecting mortality in biliary tract surgery. Am J Surg 141:66–71
41. Potts JR, Broughton TA, Hermann RE (1990) Palliative operations for pancreatic carcinoma. Ann J Surg 159:72–78
42. Proctor HJ, Hauro M (1990) Biliary diversion for pancreatic carcinoma: matching the methods and the patient. Am J Surg 159:67–71
43. Richards AB, Sosin H (1973) Cancer of the pancreas: the value of radical and palliative surgery. Ann Surg 177:325–331
44. Rosemurgy AS, Burnett CM, Wasselle JA (1989) A comparison of choledochoenteric bypass and cholecystoenteric bypass in patients with biliary obstruction due to pancreatic cancer. Am Surg 55:55–60
45. Rosenberg JM, Welch JP, Macaulay WP (1985) Cancer of the head of the pancreas: an instutional review with emphasis on surgical therapy. J Surg Oncol 28:217–221
46. Ross H, Jonas RA (1980) The results of surgery for carcinoma of the pancreas. Aust NZ J Surg 50:454–458
47. Russell RCG (1990) Surgical resection for cancer of the pancreas. Clin Gastroenterol 4:889–916
48. Sarfeh IJ, Rypins EB, Jakowatz JG, Juler GL (1988) A prospective, randomised clinical investigation of cholecystenterostomy and choledochoenterostomy. Am J Surg 155:411–414
49. Sarr MG, Cameron JL (1984) Surgical palliation of unresectable carcinoma of the pancreas. World J Surg 8:906–918
50. Schouten JT (1986) Operative therapy for pancreatic carcinoma. Am J Surg 151:626–630
51. Sharfman WH, Walsh TD (1990) Has the analgesic efficacy of neurolytic celiac plexus block been demonstrated in pancreatic cancer pain? Pain 41:267–271
52. Shepherd HA, Royle G, Ross APR, Diba A, Arthur M, Colin-Jones D (1988) Endoscopic biliary endoprostheis in the palliation of malignant obstruction of the distal common bile duct: a randomised trial. Br J Surg 75:1166–1168
53. Siegel JH, Snady H (1986) The significance of endoscopiically placed prostheses in the management of biliary obstruction due to carcinoma of the pancreas: results of non operative decompression in 277 patients. Am J Gastroenterol 81:634–641
54. Singh SM, Longmire WP, Reber HA (1990) Surgical palliation for pancreatic cancer. Ann Surg 212:132–139
55. Sonnenfield Y, Nyberg B, Perbeck L (1986) The effect of palliation bilodigestive operation for unresectable pancreatic cancer. Acta Chir Scand 530:47–50
56. Speer AG, Cotton PB, Russell RG et al. (1987) Randomised trial of endoscopic versus percutaneous stent inversion in malignant obstructive jaundice. Lancet ii:52–62
57. Stuart M, Keo T, Hermann RE, Hoerr SO (1971) Palliation of malignant obstruction of the common bile duct by side-to-side choledochoduodenostomy. Am J Surg 121:505–509
58. Ubhi CS, Doran J (1986) Palliation for carcinoma of head of pancreas. Ann R Coll Surg Engl 68:159–162

59. Van Heerden JA (1984) Pancreatic resection for carcinoma of the pancreas. Whipple versus total pancreatectomy – an institutional perspective. World J Surg 8:880–888
60. Vijayanagar R, Tolins SH (1970) Evaluation of palliative operations for carcinoma of the head of the pancreas: a ten year study. Mt Sinai J Med (NY) 37:115

Palliative Treatment of Gastric Outlet Obstruction in Advanced Pancreatic Carcinoma

Å. ANDRÉN-SANDBERG[1] and I. IHSE[1]

There is controversy concerning the optimal surgical palliation for patients with pancreatic cancer. One issue debated is whether to add gastroenterostomy routinely in patients undergoing palliative biliary bypass for obstructive jaundice and, lately, also whether gastroenterostomy is helpful in any patients with pancreatic cancer. According to the literature, gastroenterostomy produces variable and often disappointing results in duodenal obstruction due to pancreatic carcinoma [1, 2]. Opponents and proponents abound on both sides. Data on the effectiveness of biliary decompression and the incidence of recurrent biliary obstruction in pancreatic cancer are easily found; in contrast, surprisingly little has been reported on the efficacy of gastrojejunostomy in alleviating nausea and vomiting or enabling the patient to eat once pancreatic carcinoma obstructs the gastric outlet. Despite this lack of data, some surgeons by tradition routinely add gastrojejunostomy as a palliative procedure, whatever the state of the duodenum or the size and situation of the tumor, when operating on a patient with pancreatic carcinoma. We have compiled the experience of gastroenterostomy in pancreatic cancer in our hospital, with special reference to the changing policy of using gastroenterostomy over time.

Material and Methods

The charts of 404 patients treated at the Department of Surgery at Lund University Hospital for adenocarcinoma of the pancreas from 1969 to 1986 were reviewed. Only patients with the diagnosis verified by cytologic or histologic examination – either by biopsy or by postmortem examination – were accepted for analysis. Patients with tumors of the duodenum, distal bile duct, papilla of Vater, or the endocrine pancreas were excluded. Seventy-seven percent of the patients were treated entirely at our hospital, whereas 23% had part of their diagnostic workup and therapy at referring hospitals.

Of the 404 patients, 96% died of their disease. Three percent died with the disease, but of causes most likely unrelated to pancreatic cancer, and

[1] Department of Surgery, Lund University, S-221 85 Lund, Sweden

Beger/Büchler/Malfertheiner (Eds.)
Standards in Pancreatic Surgery

five patients (1%) were alive at least 8 years after laparotomy (i.e., without signs of recurrent disease at the end of 1991).

Results

The number of patients with pancreatic cancer has increased over the years. However, the absolute number of laparotomies for this disease has remained unchanged, which means a decreased relative frequency of laparotomies (Table 1). Biliary bypass with concomitant gastroenterostomy has decreased in number, whereas the use of isolated gastroenterostomy has remained constant. During the 18-year-period in question only 12 such procedures, all but three without the use of a Roux loop, were done at the time of diagnosis. In nine patients a gastrojejunostomy was needed when gastric stasis later became a problem. The 30-day mortality did not differ statistically between early and delayed isolated gastroenterostomy, or between the first and the second 9-year period (Table 2).

At the time of diagnosis, gastric outlet obstruction was present in only 21 of the 404 patients (Table 3). Eighteen of these 21 patients had an early gastroenterostomy. These 21 patients had a considerably shorter median survival than most of the other patients; only patients presenting with gastrointestinal bleeding had a worse outcome. The functional results of gastroenterostomy were good in nine, fair in six, and bad in three of the 18 patients. However, only 11 of the 21 patients were discharged from the hospital alive after the diagnosis had been settled. During the 18 years regastroenterostomy was performed in three patients only. None of these operations were of any clinical benefit to the patients.

Discussion

In the comprehensive collective review by Sarr and Cameron [2] the benefits of palliative surgery for carcinoma of the pancreas were scrutinized in over 8000 patients described in the English-language literature from 1965 to 1980. Their results suggested that biliary bypass prolongs survival, relieves the sequelae of extrahepatic biliary obstruction, and improves the quality of life. They recommended a concomitant gastroenterostomy in all patients undergoing surgery when prolonged survival was expected. The authors claimed that the addition of a gastroenterostomy did not increase the operative mortality risk, and that 13% of patients could be expected to develop subsequent duodenal obstruction if gastroenterostomy was not performed. Overall, they advocated surgical intervention, which, as well as providing a diagnosis and indicating feasibility of resection, also offers chances of considerable palliative benefit for the patient with nonresectable pancreatic cancer.

Table 1. Surgical management of patients with pancreatic cancer in Lund 1969–1986

Year	No. of patients treated	No. of patients operated on	No. of patients with biliary (single) bypass	No. of patients with biliary bypass + GE	No. of patients with "early" (single) GE	No. of patients with "delayed" (single) GE
1969	16	13	3	7	1	1
1970	20	17	3	8		
1971	19	15	3	8		
1972	21	15	4	6	1	
1973	18	15	2	5		2
1974	19	16	4	6	1	
1975	23	20	10	5	1	1
1976	18	16	8	4		1
1977	19	15	7	4		
1978	22	15	6	3	2	1
1979	20	14	7	2		
1980	24	16	3	5	1	
1981	27	17	3	6		
1982	22	13	2	3	2	1
1983	28	14	4	3	1	2
1984	30	14	3	4	1	
1985	27	12	3	2		
1986	31	13	3	2	1	
Total	404	270 (62%)	78 (19%)	83 (21%)	12 (3%)	9 (2%)

Table 2. Thirty-day mortality after isolated palliative gastroenterostomy for pancreatic carcinoma

	First 9-year period	Second 9-year period	Total
"Early" gastroenterostomy	1/4	3/8	4/12
"Delayed" gastroenterostomy	3/5	2/4	5/9

Table 3. Symptoms and signs at the time of diagnosis

Symptom/sign	*n*	Median survival (days)
Jaundice	311	152
Pain (regular use of analgetics)	282	106
Weight loss >8 kg	212	93
Nausea/vomiting	162	109
Changed bowel habits	161	121
Palpable tumor	83	68
Diabetes (regular use of antidiabetic drugs)	41	93
Gastrointestinal bleeding	23	26
Steatorrhea	22	72
Gastric outlet obstruction	21	54
History of acute or chronic pancreatitis	12	178
Venous thrombosis	9	156

Because some patients eventually develop duodenal obstruction, many surgeons believe that a gastrojejunostomy should be performed prophylactically along with biliary bypass. Indeed, in a collective series of 900 patients who underwent biliary bypass only (i.e., no evidence at operation of duodenal obstruction), 23% subsequently developed duodenal obstruction as early as 1 month later. Because the addition of gastrojejunostomy to biliary bypass did not increase the operative morbidity or mortality (17% vs. 18%), the authors recommended that it be used prophylactically in all patients with a calculated survival of more than 1 or 2 months [3].

In Lund, gastroenterostomy was a common procedure (38% of all cases) when laparotomy was done for pancreatic carcinoma during the first 6 years of the study period, but it was less common during the second (18%) and the third 6-year periods (15%). After the introduction of percutaneous transhepatic, and later endoscopically placed biliary stents for relief of jaundice the frequency of laparotomies decreased, as did the number of "early" gastroenterostomies, but "delayed" gastroenterostomies were done equally infrequently (2%–3% of all patients in both groups). Thus, it is reasonable to assume that prophylactic gastroenterostomy was done too often during the first 6-year period.

The 30-day mortality after palliative operations for pancreatic carcinoma was high. The patients operated on for gastric outlet obstruction had a hospital mortality of 42% and a short median survival. It is probably not a consequence of a hazardous operation per se, but it indicates that the gastric outlet obstruction was part of the terminal course of the disease.

In a recent series reviewed by Geoghegan et al. [1] comprising 51 patients who had palliative surgery for carcinoma of the pancreas, only five required early gastroenterostomy. Three patients subsequently had signs of delayed gastric emptying. It is not uncommon in our practice that patients with advanced pancreatic cancer and severe and prolonged vomiting show unimpeded passage of food at a barium meal. In such cases antiemetics and neuroleptics may help to some degree. However, the overall survival is short and the quality of life poor.

Our observations are supported by the data of Weaver et al. [4] indicating that effective palliation rarely is achieved in patients with significant nausea and vomiting associated with pancreatic carcinoma with or without impingement on the duodenum; 90% of their patients had a poor outcome. Even patients with nausea and vomiting before placement of a gastrojejunostomy and no evidence of duodenal impingement had a poor outcome. The small subset of patients with nonadvanced disease and symptoms of nausea and vomiting fared every bit as poorly as those with advanced disease and the same symptoms. The authors therefore suggested that the problem of vomiting is independent of advanced disease and in itself a harbinger of outcome failure. They conclude by claiming that "it is a frustrating observation that those who stand to gain the most from gastrojejunostomy for pancreatic cancer seem to benefit the least."

The reason for the poor outcome of gastroenterostomy is probably that nausea and vomiting seldom are due to a morphological obstruction of the gastric outlet, but rather to a functional intestinal disturbance or an endocrine dysfunction causing CNS-induced vomiting. Therefore, the diagnosis of clear-cut duodenal obstruction should always be made preoperatively by upper gastrointestinal roentgenograms or perhaps gastroduodenoscopy before surgery should be contemplated.

Our results are in accordance with those of another series of 55 patients with carcinoma of the pancreas who underwent gastrojejunostomy alone or in conjunction with biliary bypass. The mortality for gastrojejunostomy alone was 18%, although the corresponding figure for the combined biliary and duodenal bypass operation was 5%. Fifteen patients (26%) had delayed gastric emptying postoperatively for periods extending from 9 to 31 days. Five patients (33%) died. Eight (57%) of 14 patients with preoperative duodenal obstruction and five (42%) of 12 patients with retrocolic gastroendostomy experienced delayed gastric emptying postoperatively. The authors concluded that delayed gastric emptying is a frequent and serious problem in patients with unresectable pancreatic cancer even after gastrojejunostomy [5].

In conclusion, we feel that gastrojejunostomy is an easy and appropriate operation to be done in advanced cases of exocrine pancreatic cancer with verified gastric outlet obstruction. However, the indication for surgery is seldom present, as most cases of nausea and vomiting are not caused by morphological duodenal obstruction, but rather by functional disturbance during the terminal part of the disease, and are not to be treated surgically.

References

1. Geoghegan J, Delaney PV, Egan TJ (1990) Duodenal obstruction in advanced pancreatic carcinoma: how effective is gastroenterostomy in palliation? Ir J Med Sci 159:213–214
2. Sarr MG, Cameron JL (1982) Surgical management of unresectable carcinoma of the pancreas. Surgery 91:123–133
3. Reber HA (1987) Palliative operations for pancreatic cancer. In: Howard JM, Jordan GL, Reber HA (eds) Surgical diseases of the pancreas. Leo and Febiger, Philadelphia, pp 725–733
4. Weaver DW, Wiencek RG, Bouwman DL, Walt AJ (1987) Gastrojejunostomy: is it helpful for patients with pancreatic cancer? Surgery 102:608–612
5. Dobernech RC, Berndt GA (1987) Delayed gastric emptying after palliative gastrojejunostomy for carcinoma of the pancreas. Arch Surg 122:827–829

The Whipple Pancreaticoduodenectomy for Pancreatic Cancer

H.A. Reber[1]

Whipple first described pancreaticoduodenal resection in 1935, for a cancer of the ampulla of Vater [1]. Within a short time, the operation was being performed for carcinoma of the head of the pancreas, although it underwent a number of modifications before the one-stage operation that we know today was developed [2, 3]. By 1953, Cattell and Warren reported that they had performed 102 Whipple procedures at the Lahey Clinic [4]. Of these, 88 were for malignant disease of the periampullary area, and 46 of the 88 were for carcinoma of the head of the pancreas. Nineteen of the 46 were done as one stage resections, the others had some form of biliary decompression performed as an initial procedure. The mortality rate in this early series of 46 patients was 17.3% (eight deaths).

Today the operation continues to be a major surgical undertaking, with such technical complexity that the best results are obtained only by those who perform it frequently. Indeed it is only in the last decade that the mortality rate reported by Cattell and Warren has been significantly and widely improved upon. Today experienced pancreatic surgeons around the world perform the operation with mortality rates around 5% [5, 6]. In a number of major centers, the operative mortality rate is about 2% [7].

A recent survey of pancreatic surgeons in the United States revealed that the Whipple procedure is still the preferred operation for carcinoma of the head of the pancreas [8]. Although the pylorus preserving modification has a number of proponents, the standard Whipple is done in about two thirds of cases. The pylorus is preserved in most of the rest. Total pancreatectomy and other more radical operations are almost never done.

About 28000 new cases of pancreatic cancer are diagnosed yearly in the United States. How many of these patients undergo Whipple resections? The statistics are not available, but if all of them were operated upon (they are not), there would be about 4200 instances of resectable cancers, assuming a resectability rate of 15%. (This may be a conservative estimate, since recent data suggests that about 20%–25% now undergo resection in major centers.) If two thirds of them had a Whipple resection, there would be 2800 such resections performed yearly.

[1] UCLA Medical Center, Division of General Surgery, 10833 Le Conte Avenue, Los Angeles, CA 90024, USA

Beger/Büchler/Malfertheiner (Eds.)
Standards in Pancreatic Surgery

The United States experience suggests that about 9% of all patients with pancreatic cancer who undergo the Whipple resection are alive 5 years later [8]. Even in this group, about 40% eventually die with recurrent disease. When the tumor has not metastasized to any lymph nodes, there is evidence that the 5-year survival is significantly greater than that, perhaps 20%–30%. Nevertheless little information is available on this point because the majority of surgeons in the United States do not routinely perform a lymphadenectomy as part of the Whipple resection [8]. Moreover the pathologists do not always examine all of the lymph nodes.

Although the major technical details of the operation have been agreed upon, a number of areas of controversy remain. One of these is the need for a positive tissue diagnosis of cancer before undertaking the resection. This was much more of an issue some years ago, when the mortality rate of the operation was higher than it is today. Many surgeons were understandably reluctant to perform the Whipple procedure when the operative mortality rate was 15% or 20%, especially when the chance for cure was less than 10%. The desire for diagnostic proof of malignancy is influenced as well by the experience of the surgeon. Many feel that they are able to make the diagnosis on clinical grounds alone based on the findings at operation. This is particularly true for the small cancer where tissue for diagnosis may be very difficult to obtain. Moreover the Whipple operation is an effective treatment for other nonmalignant lesions (e.g., chronic pancreatitis) that can produce similar findings. The surgical risk of the patient is also a factor. I often resect the pancreas without obtaining tissue proof of malignancy in patients who are good operative candidates. In higher risk patients, I am more likely to insist on proof of cancer. Although a number of techniques for obtaining a sample of the tumor tissue are available, the various needle biopsy methods that provide an actual core of tissue are being used less often. Instead a fine needle aspiration for cytologic examination is preferred. It is just as sensitive and specific as the biopsy methods, and it is safer.

As mentioned previously, the extent of nodal dissection in the Whipple resection as performed in the United States is variable. Some surgeons remove the soft tissue and lymph nodes along the major vessels and up into the porta hepatis routinely; others do not. Since the Japanese experience with extensive soft tissue and node dissection suggests some value to this approach [9], this question needs to be resolved by an appropriately designed study.

Other areas of debate among pancreatic surgeons include the best technique for the pancreatic anastomosis, the need for a stent for the pancreatic duct, and whether to perform a vagotomy [10]. My personal approach to these questions (and many others) has been based on a two-part philosophy: (a) if one approach were clearly superior to any other, we would know it by now, and (b) the simplest technique that works for you is the one to use. Thus, although I have tried a number of methods over the years, I prefer an end-to-end pancreaticojejunostomy in which the pancreas is "dunked" into the end of the jejunum [11]. A specific duct-to-mucosa anastomosis is not performed. I do not use a pancreatic duct stent, even when the duct is small. I do not perform a vagotomy, but generally maintain the patient indefinitely on acid antisecretory medication. I have no objection to many of the other approaches in common use, however.

In the United States, the criteria for resectability in patients who are candidates for the Whipple resection have changed little over the more than 50 years that the procedure has been done [8]. In the opinion of most surgeons, distant metastases, major vascular invasion, and direct growth of the tumor into adjacent structures such as the stomach or colon preclude resection. Extension of the tumor into the duodenum or common bile duct is not generally considered a contraindication. Neither is involvement of regional lymph nodes that would normally be removed with the Whipple specimen. Thus the teaching and practice have been that the Whipple operation is only done in circumstances where cure is possible. The Whipple procedure is not done (intentionally) for palliation. In retrospect, of course, we know that at least 90% of patients who undergo the procedure are only palliated by it. With the low operative mortality rates now being achieved for the Whipple resection, however, it may be time for a new look at this issue. Would the mortality rate for the operation be higher in patients with more extensive disease? Again, from the experience of the Japanese, there is evidence that patients with stage II disease tolerate the so-called extended Whipple procedure with an operative mortality rate similar to that of patients with stage I tumors (about 5%) [12]. Stage II disease implies extension of the cancer into the stomach, colon, or spleen, and/or the major vessels, but without distant metastases. These observations raise the question of whether a standard Whipple resection, done deliberately for palliation in selected patients, might be indicated. The answer would require a prospective study in which patients would be randomized between Whipple operation and the usual biliary and gastric bypass that is done commonly for palliation. Since the mean survival for the latter group is only about 7 months, the answer should be apparent in a short time.

In summary, the Whipple pancreaticoduodenectomy is still the standard operation for the treatment of potentially curable cancer of the head of the pancreas. The mortality rate of the operation is less than 5% in the hands of experienced surgeons. In the United States, the overall 5-year survival rate is about 9%, but some of those patients still die with recurrent disease. In lymph node negative patients, 5-year survival is 20%–30%. Issues that might be addressed in the future include: (a) a definition of the importance of a lymph node dissection as part of the procedure, (b) a rigorous comparison between the standard Whipple operation and other operations now being done (e.g., pylorus-preserving Whipple, extended Whipple with lymph node, and soft tissue dissection), and (c) a determination of the safety and efficacy of the Whipple operation performed for palliation in selected patients with more advanced disease.

References

1. Whipple AO, Parsons, Mullins CR (1935) Treatment of carcinoma of ampulla of Vater. Ann Surg 102:763–779
2. Whipple AO (1941) Rationale of radical surgery for cancer of the pancreas and periampullary region. Ann Surg 114:612–615
3. Cattell RB (1948) A technique for pancreatoduodenal resection. Surg Clin North Am 28:761–775
4. Cattell RB, Warren KW (1953) Surgery of the pancreas. Saunders, Philadelphia, p 374
5. Trede M, Schwall G, Saeger HD (1990) Survival after pancreatoduodenectomy. 118 consecutive resections without an operative mortality. Ann Surg 211:447–458
6. Tsuchiya R, Noda T, Harada N et al. (1986) Collective review of small carcinomas of the pancreas. Ann Surg 203:77–81
7. Singh SM, Longmire WP Jr, Reber HA (1986) Surgical palliation for pancreatic cancer. Ann Surg 212:132–139
8. Livingston EH, Welton ML, Reber HA (1991) The United States experience with surgery for pancreatic cancer. Int J Pancreatol (in press)
9. Tsuchiya R, Harada N, Tsunoda T et al. (1988) Long term survivors after operation on carcinoma of the pancreas. Int J Pancreatol 3:491–496
10. Jordan GL Jr (1989) Pancreatic resection for pancreatic cancer. In: Reber HA (ed) Surg Clin North Am 69:569–597 Saunders, Philadelphia
11. Jordan GL Jr (1987) Pancreatic resection for pancreatic cancer. In: Howard JM, Jordan GL Jr, Reber HA (eds) Surgical diseases of the pancreas. Lea and Febiger, Philadelphia, pp 666–689
12. Tsuchiya R, Tsunoda T, Yamaguchi T (1990) Operation of choice for resectable carcinoma of the head of the pancreas. Int J Pancreatol 6:295–306

Early Results of Subtotal Pancreatectomy for Cancer: An Interim Report

I. Ihse,[1] Å. Andrén-Sandberg, J. Permerth, and J. Larsson

In several institutions, including our own, total pancreatectomy for many years was the operation of choice for attempted radical pancreatic cancer surgery [1]. Although initial reports were promising [2, 3], the operation did not meet expectations when enough experience was collected. The mortality and morbidity rates were not convincingly advantageous, and long-term survival was dismal [4–6]. Furthermore, troublesome nutritional and metabolic sequelae were frequent [4]. Therefore, we decided to give up the operation as our routine procedure and instead adopted subtotal pancreatectomy as described by Gall and coworkers [7]. This paper gives a preliminary report of our early operative results with subtotal pancreatectomy for cancer and analyzes the importance of surgical experience for postoperative mortality and morbidity.

Patients and Methods

The study comprised 100 patients operated on at the Departments of Surgery in Lund and Linköping, Sweden, between 1985 and 1990. There were 59 men and 41 women, and the median age was 67 years.

As the aim was to report early surgical results and *not* the long-term survival of a specific disease, all diagnoses giving rise to a subtotal pancreatectomy were included (Table 1).

Ninety-two of the operations (92%) were done by four surgeons with a special interest in pancreatic surgery, and these surgeons were generally operating together, two and two. Eight operations were done by surgeons with a main interest in other areas of gastrointestinal surgery.

The operation included removal of at least 50% of the distal stomach, 60%–80% of the duodenum, distal bile duct (transected above the entrance of the cystic duct), gallbladder, and pancreas with the exception of 5 cm of the tail. No vagotomy was performed, and the spleen was preserved. The specimen was removed en bloc, and regional lymph nodes were exstirpated. The bile flow was in all cases secured by an end-to-side hepatico-jejunostomy. In about half the patients the gastroenteroanastomosis (GE) was

[1] Department of Surgery, Lund University, S-221 85 Lund, Sweden

Beger/Büchler/Malfertheiner (Eds.)
Standards in Pancreatic Surgery

Table 1. Diagnoses in 100 patients operated on with subtotal pancreatectomy

	Number of patients
Pancreatic cancer	59
Ampullary cancer	20
Bile duct cancer	10
Duodenal cancer	5
Cystadenocarcinoma	2
Endocrine tumor	2
Metastasis of hypernephroma	1
Metastasis of malignant melanoma	1
Total	100

carried out using a Roux-en-Y loop and in the other half by an end-to-side GE with an additional enteroanastomosis. The main pancreatic duct of the tail was doubly ligated, and in about half the patients the pancreatic resection surface was closed by staplers and in the other half by a continuous suture line. Thus, no pancreatico-jejunostomy was performed.

Results

To study the effect that the factor of practice in a specific kind of surgery has on the results, the first 50 operations were compared with the next 50. As different diagnoses were included, appropriate and uniform tumor staging was not feasible. Therefore, we simply used tumor size as an approximation of what can be called the surgical stage of the disease. As shown in Table 2, there was no difference in tumor size when the first 50 and the next 50 patients were compared. Still, however, there was a statistically significant reduction in perioperative blood loss, operative time, and the length of hospital stay (Table 2).

The 30-day mortality was 2% and the hospital mortality 5%. There was no obvious association between operative mortality and age of the patient, tumor size, diagnosis, perioperative blood loss, or operative time. It seemed, however, that operative mortality was operator related, even if the low number of fatalities did not allow statistical calculations. Four of the five operative deaths were among the first 50 operations.

Postoperative complications are listed in Table 3. Altogether 31% of patients had a clinically relevant complication, and these tended to be more common in the first 50 operations, although a statistically significant difference was not reached. Reoperations were needed in 10% of patients: in three cases of abdominal bleeding, three cases of abdominal abscess, two cases of delayed gastric emptying, one case of persistent pancreatic fistula,

Table 2. Tumor size, peroperative blood loss, operative time, and duration of hospital stay in 100 patients operated on with subtotal pancreatectomy

	First 50 operations	Second 50 operations	*p*
Tumor size (cm)			
Median	3.00	3.00	
Mean ± SEM	3.5 ± 0.2	3.2 ± 0.2	NS
Blood loss (ml)			
Median	2000	1450	
Mean ± SEM	2333 ± 167	1656 ± 143	<0.005
Operative time (h)			
Median	7	6	
Mean ± SEM	6.7 ± 0.2	5.6 ± 0.2	<0.005
Hospital stay (days)			
Median	24	18	
Mean ± SEM	32 ± 4	22 ± 2	<0.001

NS, Not significant.

Table 3. Postoperative complications in 100 patients operated on with subtotal pancreatectomy

	Number of patients
Intraabdominal bleeding	4
Intraabdominal abscess	4
Delayed gastric emptying	8
Persistent pancreatic fistula	1
Transient pancreatic fistula	19
Venous thrombosis	4

and one case of intraductal tumor growth needing removal of the pancreatic tail at a second laparotomy.

As only 5 cm of the pancreatic tail was saved and the main duct closed, the pre- and postoperative frequency of diabetes was of special interest. Before the operation 16% of patients had manifest diabetes and immediately postoperatively the figure had increased to 34%, including the patient who underwent exstirpation of the pancreatic tail at a second laparotomy. Thus, the subtotal pancreatectomy per se caused diabetes in 17 of the preoperatively nondiabetic 84 patients (20%).

Discussion

The results of this preliminary study indicate that subtotal pancreatectomy can be regarded as a safe procedure. With increasing experience of the surgeons in the particular surgical procedure, the operative mortality and morbidity decreased, as did the intraoperative blood loss, operative time, and hospital stay. Although there may be covariation by other factors, we feel that the findings are strongly supportive for the opinion that "practice makes perfect." Furthermore, they are in agreement with what previously has been reported by Crist and coworkers [8]. To us, it goes without saying that a surgical procedure should be carried out only in units in which it is practised often enough to make reliable follow-up possible.

The complication rate of the present series compares favorably with the results of other groups [6–9]. It may be of interest to call attention to the absence of stomal ulcerations in our patients, although none of them had a vagotomy. Thus, the relatively high frequency of delayed gastric emptying (8%) was not a consequence of ulcer formation. It is intriguing that all instances of delayed gastric emptying occurred in patients with stapled GE and stapled pancreatic remnant. It may be speculated that localized leak from the pancreatic remnant or the nonacidic stomach causes dysfunction of the proximal gastrointestinal tract. However, in all cases but two the gastric emptying normalized on conservative treatment. Today we think that the two reoperations were done too early, and that a spontaneous resolution could have occurred as well. Blind closure of the pancreatic remnant led to pure pancreatic fistula in 20% of the patients. One fistula needed surgical repair whereas 19 healed spontaneously. In did not matter for the fistula formation whether the pancreatic resection surface was stapled or hand-sewn. Although pancreatic fistulas if adequately drained do not cause additional morbidity, the high frequency in our series questions the surgical technique used for closure of the tail remnant.

As surgery is fundamental for cure of malignancies of the pancreas, distal bile duct, ampulla, and duodenum, it is gratifying that clearly improved operative results after pancreaticoduodenectomy are reported by several groups including our own [8–10]. For improved long-term survival, however, surgery needs to be complemented with adjunctive treatment modalities. The challenge for the future will therefore be to develop such useful methods based on radiotherapy, chemotherapy, immunotherapy, hormonal therapy, or other treatment principles.

References

1. Ihse I, Isaksson G (1984) Pancreatic cancer: diagnosis and treatment. Clin Gastroenterol 13:961–984
2. Brooks JR, Culebras JM (1976) Cancer of the pancreas: palliative operation, Whipple procedure of total pancreatectomy? Am J Surg 131:516–520
3. Ihse I, Lilja P, Arnesjö B, Bengmark S (1977) Total pancreatectomy for cancer. Ann Surg 186:675–680
4. Andrén-Sandberg Å, Ihse I (1983) Factors influencing survival after total pancreatectomy in patients with pancreatic cancer. Ann Surg 198:605–610
5. Edis AJ, Kierman PD, Taylor WF (1980) Attempted curative resection of ductal carcinoma of the pancreas. Mayo Clin Proc SS:531–536
6. Commoly MM, Dawson PJ, Michelassi F, Moossa AR, Lowenstein F (1987) Survival in 1001 patients with carcinoma of the pancreas. Ann Surg 206:366–373

7. Gall FP, Hermanek P, Gebhardt CH, Meier H (1981) Erweiterte Resektion der Pankreas- und periampullären Karzinome. Regionale, totale und partielle Duodenopankreatektomie. Leber Magen Darm 11:179–184
8. Crist DW, Sitzmann JV, Cameron JL (1987) Improved hospital morbidity, mortality, and survival after the Whipple procedure. Ann Surg 206:358–365
9. Grace PA, Pitt HA, Tompkins RK, DenBesten L, Longmire WP (1986) Decreased morbidity and mortality after pancreaticoduodenectomy. Ann Surg 151:141–149
10. Trede M (1985) The surgical treatment of pancreatic carcinoma. Surgery 97:28–35

Whipple Operation for Pancreatic Carcinoma: Japanese Experience

F. Hanyu,[1] M. Suzuki, and T. Imaizumi

Introduction

Whipple operation for carcinoma of the periampullary malignant disease has become a safe operation with less than 5% postoperative mortality [1, 2]. Whipple operation results in fairly good survival in patients with carcinoma of the ampulla of Vater or carcinoma of the distal bile duct. Five-year survival rates in such patients have been reported to be between 30% and 50% [3, 4]. However, Whipple operation does not produce survival benefits in patients with carcinoma of the pancreas, for whom the 5-year survival rate is less than 10% [5]. Although complete removal of the tumor by surgery is the only curative treatment and provides a chance of long-term survival for patients with carcinoma of the pancreas, the majority of surgeons do not choose extended radical Whipple operation. The present study was done to determine the effectiveness of surgical treatment of extended radical Whipple operation for pancreatic cancer.

Materials and Methods

From 1968 to December 1990, 566 patients with carcinoma of the pancreas were admitted to our institution. Of the 566 patients, 224 received Whipple operation for ductal adenocarcinoma of the head of the pancreas. Ductal adenocarcinoma of the pancreas was classified as follows: (1) the tumor had to demonstrate both epithelial and glandular differentiation, and (2) cystadenocarcinomas and mucin-producing intraductal adenocarcinomas were excluded. Of the 224 ductal adenocarcinomas, tubular adenocarcinomas comprised 87.5%, papillary adenocarcinoma 11.6%, adenosquamous carcinoma 1.3%, and signet ring cell carcinoma 0.4% (Table 1). All 224 patients had complete reports of preoperative or postoperative histopathological evaluation of the tumor. Four patients (2%) were classified as stage 1; the tumor was less than 2 cm in size and was located within the pancreatic parenchyma without lymph node involvement. Twenty-seven patients (12%) were classified as stage 2; the tumor was less than 4 cm in

[1] Department of Gastroenterological Surgery, Tokyo Women's Medical College, Tokyo, Japan

Beger/Büchler/Malfertheiner (Eds.)
Standards in Pancreatic Surgery

Table 1. Histopathology in 224 patients receiving Whipple operation for ductal adenocarcinoma of the pancreas

Histological findings	Patients	
	(*n*)	(%)
Tubular adenocarcinoma	196	87.5
Papillary adenocarcinoma	26	11.6
Adenosquamous carcinoma	3	1.3
Signet ring cell carcinoma	1	0.4

Table 2. Clinicopathological staging in 198 patients with ductal adenocarcinoma of the pancreas who received Whipple operation

Stage	Description	Patients	
		(*n*)	(%)
1	Tumor size <2 cm, tumor located within pancreas, no lymph node involvement	4	2
2	Tumor size 2–4 cm, tumor located within pancreas, parapancreatic lymph node involvement	27	12
3	Tumor size 4–6 cm, tumor exposed on surface of pancreas, positive lymph node involvement (distant)	139	62
4	Tumor size >6 cm, tumor invading extrapancreatic tissue, positive lymph node metastasis (distant)	54	24

size and was located within the pancreatic parenchyma with parapancreatic lymph node involvement. One hundred and thirty-nine patients (62%) were classified as stage 3; the tumor size was between 4 and 6 cm with the tumor exposed on the surface of the pancreas, with positive lymph node metastasis. The remaining 54 patients (24%) were classified as stage 4; the size of the tumor was greater than 6 cm with the tumor exposed on the surface of the pancreas, with positive lymph node metastasis (Table 2).

Of the 224 patients, 17 received a standard Whipple operation between 1968 and 1977. This operation included resection of the head of the pancreas, duodenectomy, antrectomy, and cholecystectomy, but regional lymphadenectomy was not carried out. Between 1978 and 1990, 167 patients received extended radical Whipple operation. Of these patients 145 (87%) had regional lymphadenectomy, 124 (74%) had perineural dissection, 103 (62%) had portal vein resection and reconstruction, and eight patients had resection and reconstruction of the hepatic or the superior mesenteric artery (Table 3).

Table 3. Procedures carried out in extended radical Whipple operation on 167 patients for ductal adenocarcinoma of the pancreas

Procedures	Patients	
	(*n*)	(%)
Regional lymphadenectomy	145	87
Perineural dissection	124	74
Portal vein resection	103	62
Arterial resection	8	5

Results

The resectability and curability in patients receiving standard Whipple operation were 14% and 2% respectively. After the introduction of extended radical Whipple operation, the resectability increased from 14% by standard Whipple operation to 58%. The curability also increased from 2% by standard Whipple operation to 23% by extended radical Whipple operations. The overall postoperative mortality rate among the 224 patients receiving Whipple operation for ductal adenocarcinoma of the head of the pancreas was 5.3%, but it has been 1% in the last 5 years. Mortality after standard Whipple operation performed from 1968 to 1977 was 13%; it was 3% after extended radical Whipple operation performed from 1978 to 1990. Morbidity rates did not differ between the patients who received the standard Whipple operation and the patients received the extended radical Whipple operation (Table 4).

The survival rate after standard Whipple operation was 35% at 1 year, but 0% at 3 years and 5 years. Survival rates in the patients who received extended radical Whipple operation were 44%, 9%, and 8% at 1 year, 3 years, and 5 years respectively (Table 5). Of the 167 patients receiving extended radical Whipple operation, 94 had curative resection of the tumor, which was confirmed by histological study postoperatively. In the 94 patients

Table 4. Mortality, morbidity, resectability, and curability in standard Whipple operation and extended radical Whipple operation

	Standard Whipple operation (%)	Extended radical Whipple operation (%)
Mortality	13	3
Morbidity	23	25
Resectability	14	58
Curability	2	23

Table 5. Survival rates (%) after standard Whipple operation and extended radical Whipple operation

Survival rate at	Standard Whipple operation (%)	Extended radical Whipple operation
1 year	35	44
3 years	0	9
5 years	0	8

Table 6. Survival rates (%) in patients with curative resection and with noncurative resection after extended radical Whipple operation

Survival rate at	Extended radical Whipple operation	
	Curative	Noncurative
1 year	62	35
2 years	38	7
3 years	29	2
5 years	27	0

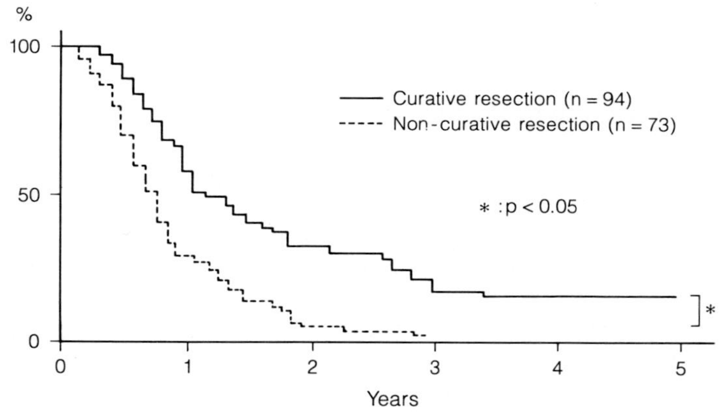

Fig. 1. Survival curves after extended radical Whipple-operation for ductal adenocarcinoma of the pancreas

with curative resection, the survival rate was 62% at 1 year, 38% at 2 years, and 27% at 5 years. Among the 73 patients with noncurative resection, however, the 1-year and 2-year survival rates were 35% and 7%; no patients survived more than 3 years after the operation (Table 6, Fig. 1). Seven patients survived more than 5 years after extended radical Whipple operation. The seven long-term survivors were all male. The tumor size was

1.8–8.0 cm. Five out of the seven survivors had lymph node involvement in the retroperitoneum. Four patients had tumor invasion to the portal vein and they received portal resection and vascular reconstruction by end-to-end anastomosis. All the seven patients had curative resection by extended radical Whipple operation (Table 7).

Discussion

Modern advances in diagnostic techniques such as ultra-sonography or computed tomography (CT) can provide earlier diagnosis in some patients with carcinoma of the pancreas. However, the majority of patients with carcinoma of the pancreas still have advanced tumor, including wide lymph node metastasis, and massive tumor invasion to the surrounding organs. Ductal adenocarcinoma of the pancreas is known as having wide tumor invasion to the perineural and the perivascular connective tissues as well as lymph nodes in the retroperitoneum.

The survival rate in patients with carcinoma of the pancreas is extremely poor. Very few patients with ductal adenocarcinoma of the head of the pancreas can obtain long-term survival following the treatments, usually less than 5% at 5 years. As surgical treatments did not provide survival benefits in the majority of patients with ductal adenocarcinoma of the pancreas, many surgeons have chosen not to perform radical pancreatic resection for patients with ductal adenocarcinoma of the pancreas.

Some surgeons prefer a biliary by-pass operation for patients with pancreatic carcinoma because of the high mortality rate and the poor postoperative prognosis associated with radical pancreatic resection. However, improvements in operative and perioperative management have lessened the postoperative mortality and morbidity in patients receiving radical pancreatic resection. Crist et al. [1] found that among 41 patients operated on from 1969 to 1980 hospital mortality and morbidity were 24% and 59% respectively, compared with 2% and 36% among 47 patients operated on from 1981 to 1986. In 1986, Grace et al. [2] reported that the mortality rate after pancreatoduodenectomy decreased from 10% to 2% between the two 5-year periods 1975–1979 and 1980–1984. Fortner [6] in 1984 reported 35 patients receiving regional pancreatectomy with a postoperative mortality rate of 25%. In our series, the postoperative mortality rate after extended radical Whipple operation was 3%. The Whipple procedure for peripancreatic malignant disease is not an easy operation, but postoperative mortality and morbidity rates have become acceptably low. Surgeons no longer avoid the Whipple operation for periampullary malignancies.

Traditionally, the Whipple procedure has been utilized to resect localized disease in patients with periampullary malignancies. The standard Whipple operation does not include regional lymphadenectomy or wide dissection of the perivascular connective tissues. Expected 5-year survival

Table 7. Long-term survivors after extended radical Whipple operation for ductal adenocarcinoma of the pancreas

Case	Age (years)	Sex	Pathology/prognosis	Tumor size (cm)	Lymph node involvement	Portal invasion	Survival (years)	Outcome
1	67	Male	Tubular adenocarcinoma	1.8	Yes	No	11.4	Alive
2	67	Male	poor	2.5	Yes	No	10.8	Alive
3	50	Male	Tubular adenocarcinoma	4.5	No	Yes	7.5	Alive
4	51	Male	Papillary adenocarcinoma	8.0	Yes	Yes	6.7	Alive
5	70	Male	Tubular adenocarcinoma	2.3	Yes	No	5.8	Alive
6	54	Male	Tubular adenocarcinoma	4.1	No	Yes	5.1	Alive
7	72	Male	Tubular adenocarcinoma	2.0	Yes	Yes	5.0	Died

rates after the operation range from 30% to 50% in patients with carcinoma of the ampulla of Vater or the distal bile duct [3, 4]. Some patients survived for 10 or 20 years after the operation. However, in patients with carcinoma of the pancreas, the expected 5-year survival rate is under 10%, and about 50% of patients who undergo resection have local recurrences within the tumor bed [7]. Whipple operation without regional lymphadenectomy and wide dissection of the perivascular connective tissue is not appropriate for patients with ductal adenocarcinoma of the pancreas. The survival rates of patients in Fortner's series were 50% at 1 year and 10% at 3 years. Similar survival rates were reported by Sindelar [7] in 1989. In our series the overall survival rate in patients who had extended radical Whipple operation for ductal adenocarcinoma of the pancreas was 10% at 5 years. Among the patients who had extended radical Whipple operation but had a noncurative operation conformed by postoperative histological study, the 1-year survival rate was 35%, but no patients survived more than 5 years after the operation. In the patients with curative resection, the survival rate was 62% at 1 year, 38% at 2 years, and 27% at 5 years.

Using modern imaging techniques such as CT or selective abdominal angiography, it has been possible to determine preoperatively whether a patient has massive tumor invasion to the major vascular and retroperitoneal tissue or whether a patient has a chance of curative operation. If a patient has massive tumor invasion to the celiac artery or the superior mesenteric artery, even extended radical Whipple operation cannot provide any survival benefits. The criteria for extended radical Whipple operation for ductal adenocarcinoma of the pancreas in our series are as follows: (1) no hepatic metastasis or peritoneal dissemination, (2) no evidence of tumor invasion to the major arteries, and (3) no massive tumor invasion to the retroperitoneal connective tissues. In Fortner's series and Sindelar's series, there were no substantial differences in the expected survival of patients who underwent regional pancreatectomy as compared with standard Whipple resections. They did not select patients for regional pancreatectomy. In our series, 27% of the patients who had extended radical Whipple operation for ductal adenocarcinoma of the pancreas survived 5 years.

Extended radical Whipple operation can be performed with an acceptably low risk that does not exceed that of standard Whipple operation. Extended radical Whipple operation should be considered as a choice of treatment in selected patients, determined by using preoperative imaging techniques.

References

1. Crist DW, Sitzmann JV, Cameron JL (1987) Improved hospital morbidity, mortality, and survival after the Whipple procedure. Ann Surg 206:358–365
2. Grace PA, Pitt HA, Tompkins RK et al. (1986) Decreased morbidity and mortality after pancreatoduodenectomy. Am J Surg 151:141–149

3. Tarazi RY, Hermann RE, Vogt DP et al. (1986) Results of surgical treatment of periampullary tumors: a thirty-five-year experience. Surgery 100:716–723
4. Monson JR, Donohue JH, McEntee GP et al. (1991) Radical resection for carcinoma of the ampulla of Vater. Arch Surg 126:353–357
5. Cameron JL, Crist DW, Sitzmann JV et al. (1991) Factors influencing survival after pancreatoduodenectomy for pancreatic cancer. Am J Surg 161:120–125
6. Fortner JG (1984) Regional pancreatectomy for cancer of the pancreas, ampulla and other related site: tumor staging and results. Ann Surg 199:418–425
7. Sindelar WF (1989) Clinical experience with regional pancreatectomy for adenocarcinoma of the pancreas. Arch Surg 124:127–132

Cancer of the Pancreas – Extensive Lymph Node Dissection

F.P. GALL[1] and H. ZIRNGIBL

Introduction

Ductal carcinoma of the pancreas is a malignant tumour with one of the most dismal prognoses. A recent literature review quotes a 5-year survival rate of 5%–6% [5]. Long-term results have not improved despite the introduction of imaging techniques in early diagnosis. The results of adjuvant radio- and chemotherapy have been equally unsuccessful [16]. The only chance for cure remains radical surgical resection, however, few patients benefit from this.

This begs the question why operative treatment of pancreatic carcinoma has reached a standstill whereas great surgical advances have been achieved in other gastrointestinal tumours, notably in gastric and colorectal carcinomas. The successes in treatment of the latter can be attributed to radical tumour excision with adequate margins of clearance and extended lymph node dissection. Efforts to transfer these principles to pancreatic carcinoma were made in the 1970s by Fortner [4], who was unable to improve results despite the introduction of his so-called regional duodenopancreatectomy. Consequently the value of extended lymph node dissection in pancreatic carcinoma remained controversial. The main argument against radical dissection remained the fact that only patients without positive lymph nodes in the resection specimen had a reasonable chance of survival.

New studies, notably those by Japanese authors [6, 9, 11], report a markedly improved 5-year survival rate following tumour resection with extended lymph node dissection. Our goal was to adopt this concept and to test on our patient population whether extensive lymph node dissection improved the prognosis for ductal pancreatic carcinoma.

Methods

Extended lymph node dissection was applied in combination with pancreatic resection since 1978. Prospective data collection was undertaken by the clinical Tumour Registry of the Department of Surgery. Numerous clinical

[1] Chirurgische Universitätsklinik und Poliklinik Maximiliausplatz, W-8520 Erlangen, FRG

Beger/Büchler/Malfertheiner (Eds.)
Standards in Pancreatic Surgery

and histopathological data were collected. The 1987 UICC TNM/pTNM classification and staging were retrospectively applied to already collected prospective data. The survival curves were calculated using the Kaplan-Meier method and corrected for age, and postoperative mortality was not excluded. The 95% confidence interval was given for the 5-year survival rate. Differences between survival curves were tested using the log-rank test, differences in the incidences in the χ^2 test were tested for statistical significance.

Results

Operability and Resectability

The extremely poor prognosis of ductal carcinoma of the pancreas is mainly due to the large number of inoperable cases at the time of diagnosis. Even in recent times, more than two-thirds of patients in our study group were primarily inoperable. Out of these patients only 117, representing 19.8–23% of the entire group, could be curatively resected (R0; Table 1).

Contraindication for resection was the presence of distant metastases in 67%. Thirty-three percent of all tumours which could not be resected had already infiltrated the retroperitoneum, sometimes with invasion of large vessels. The remaining patients were not operated on because of their poor physical condition.

The reason for a non-curative (R1, 2) resection was residual tumour in the retroperitoneum dorsal to the head of the pancreas in 83% of cases. In the remaining cases tumour remained in the pancreatic or choledochal resection lines.

These figures emphasize the need for an adequate margin of clearance not only from the tumour to the pancreatic resection line, but especially also to the retroperitoneal space.

Complication Rate and Operative Mortality

Extended lymph node dissection did not increase the complication rate in our study group. Following extended lymph node dissection, we observed a complication rate of 33.3% vs 31.9% where there was no dissection. As far

Table 1. Resectability and curability in ductal carcinoma of the pancreas 1969–1990 (n = 687)

Time period	Patients	Resections		R0 resection	
	(n)	(n)	(%)	(n)	(%)
1969–1977	153	14	9.2	10	6.5
1978–1982	182	53	29.1	36	19.8
1983–1990	352	125	35.5	81	23.0
Total	687	192	27.9	127	18.5

Table 2. Postoperative complications and mortality following 192 surgical resections for ductal carcinoma of the pancreas with and without extended lymph node dissection

	Extended lymph node dissection	
	Yes (n = 139)	No (n = 53)
Complications		
No complications	66.7%	68.1%
Surgical complications pancreas specific	9.0%	4.3%
Other surgical complications	18.0%	14.9%
General complications	6.3%	12.8%
Mortality		
1967–1977	–	1/14 (7%)
1978–1982	4/45 (9%)	1/8 (13%)
1983–1990	6/94 (6%)	4/31 (13%)
Total	10/139 (7%)	6/53 (11%)

as pancreas-specific complications were concerned, after lymph node dissection there was an increase in the incidence of pancreatic fistulae; in non-pancreas-specific complications, there was an increase in seromas. These complications could be treated conservatively without surgical intervention and did not contribute to operative mortality. From 1969 to 1990, the operative mortality for the entire study group and for all operations (partial, subtotal, total duodenopancreatectomy and left-sided resection) was 7% with extended lymph node resection and 11% without (Table 2).

Lymph Node Metastases: Incidence and Site

All operative specimens were carefully prepared and histopathologically examined and, especially, the number and site of all lymph nodes with and without metastases were recorded.

If an extended dissection was performed, we found lymph node metastases in 75% (76 out of 101) of all resections, in contrast, only in 62% (16 out of 26) without dissection. This emphasizes the importance of complete lymph node dissection not only for the patient's prognosis, but also for the comparability of staging. Of special note is the difference in the incidence of lymph node metastases depending on the number of examined lymph nodes. If up to 20 lymph nodes were examined, lymph node metastases were found in 47%; if 21–30 lymph nodes were examined, then 67%; and if 30 or more lymph nodes were examined, then 80%.

In the majority of cases metastasis of pancreatic carcinoma is an orderly process, the peripancreatic nodes near the tumour are affected first, followed by more distant lymph nodes (Table 3). Lymph node skipping is

Table 3. Site of lymph node metastases in curative lymph node positive resection specimens (R0) compared with noncurative resection of ductal carcinoma of the pancreas (R1, 2)

Localisation of the lymph node metastases	R0 pN1 (n = 92)		R1, 2 pN1 (n = 49)	
	n	%	n	%
Peripancreatic only	59	64	30	61
Also distant[a]	31	34	17	35
Only farther away	2	2	2	4

[a] Lymph nodes on the gastroepiploic artery, hepatoduodenal ligament, coeliac trunk, superior mesenteric artery, superior para-aortal lymph nodes.

seldom, and out of all R0 resections (n = 127), we found only two skips. Within the resection specimens with positive lymph nodes, the incidence was 2%.

In the group of lymph nodes close to the carcinoma of the pancreas head, the pancreaticoduodenal lymph nodes were the most frequently invaded, followed by the suprapancreatic and infrapancreatic nodes. In tumours of the body of the pancreas, in 29% of cases suprapancreatic node metastases were discovered, in 10% infrapancreatic. Lymphatic spread to the splenic hilum in pancreatic carcinoma could not be found in six total duodenopancreatectomy resection specimens. This underlined the adequate resectability of subtotal duodenopancreatectomy as treatment for carcinoma of the pancreatic head.

Even more distant lymph node stations are already affected in a high percentage of curatively resected carcinomas of the pancreatic head. Lymph node metastases were found at the hepatoduodenal ligament in 33% of cases, at the superior mesenteric artery in 24%, and in the region of the superior para-aortal lymph node groups in 12% (Table 4).

Late Results

A relevant 5-year survival rate can be achieved only in patients where the pancreatic carcinoma can be operatively removed. A 5-year survival rate of 8% was achieved for all resected patients. If the tumour was curatively (R0) resected, then the age-corrected 5-year survival rate is 10%, in case of a non-curative (R1, 2) resection no patient survived 5 years (Table 5).

A decisive step towards improved prognosis can be found in curatively-resected patients in stages I and II, in other words, patients without node invasion. A 5-year survival rate of 28% with a median survival time of 28 months was achieved in these stages, compared with a 5% rate and 10 months in stage III. If only one lymph node is infiltrated, then the 5-year survival rate is 9%, compared to 7% in the group where more than one lymph node is affected. The difference is also evident in the median survival

Table 4. Site of lymph node metastases in curative lymph node positive resections of ductal carcinoma of the head of the pancreas (pN1, R0, $n = 83$)

Site of lymph node metastases	Patients	
	n	%
Peripancreatic		
anterior pancreaticoduodenal	24/58	41
posterior pancreaticoduodenal	40/62	65
pancreaticoduodenal (not further specified)	18/29	62
suprapancreatic head	28/78	36
suprapancreatic body	17/59	29
intrapancreatic head	23/72	32
intrapancreatic body	5/51	10
splenic hilus	0/6	0
Distant		
right gastroepiploic	2/67	3
hepatoduodenal ligament	23/70	33
coelicac trunk	5/51	10
superior mesenteric artery	12/51	24
superior para-aortal	5/43	12

times of 13.2 vs 8.8 months. This difference is not statistically significant, but shows that prognosis is worse in more advanced disease.

A slight, also not statistically significant difference was found in R0 patients in stage III when only peripancreatic nodes were affected. The 5-year survival rate was 6%. If nodes of the second stage were involved, then no patient survived for five years (Table 5).

The benefits of extended lymph node dissection did not extend to patients in stage III following lymph node resection, in other words, in positive lymph node cases, there is no improvement of prognosis compared to non-resected patients. The median survival times were the same for both groups – 9.5 months (Table 5, Fig. 1). Even when we could not find a statistically significant improvement in survival rates following extended lymph node dissection in our entire study group, we found a clear difference in prognosis in the small number of patients in whom no lymph node metastases were found according to histopathological criteria. Accordingly, when only one lymph node was infiltrated, prognosis was slightly better.

In order to justify radical tumour surgery, it is not sufficient to simply extend the margin of clearance to the left. Cubilla and Fitzgerald [3] observed a perineural and lymphatic infiltration in more than 90% of all pancreatic carcinomas. Nagai et al. [12] could demonstrate a microinvasion in the surrounding soft tissue even in small T1 tumours with a diameter of less than 1 cm. Miyazaki et al. [10] emphasize the necessity of retroperitoneal dissection; they showed that retroperitoneal infiltration behind the pancreas (rP factor) also represents the most important factor for T1 tumours. In his

Table 5. Observed cumulative survival rates (Kaplan-Meier) in resected ductal carcinoma of the pancreas (postoperative mortality not excluded), 1978–1989/1990 6 patients were in R0, stage IV

Tumor resection	Patients	Age corrected		Median survival rate
		2 years survival rate	5 years survival rate	(months)
R0*	107	31 ± 10	10 ± 8	11.1 }*
R1, 2	58	7 ± 9	0	7.8
R0, 1, 2	165	25 ± 8	8 ± 5	10.3
R0, stage I/II	25	63 ± 23	28 ± 24	28.1 }*
R0, stage III	76	22 ± 11	5 ± 7	9.8
R0, stage III, 1 lymph node	13	40 ± 28	9 ± 17	13.2
R0, stage III >1 lymph node	63	19 ± 11	7 ± 9	8.8
R0, stage III				
Only peripancreatic	52	11 ± 14	6 ± 8	10.0
Second station	24	22 ± 17	0	7.6
R0, stage III extended dissection				
No	9	23 ± 41	25 ± 44	9.5
Yes	67	21 ± 11	3 ± 6	9.5
R0, stage/I/II extended dissection				
No	6	48/50	0	22.3
Yes	19	67 ± 26	35 ± 29	31.8

* $p < 0.05$

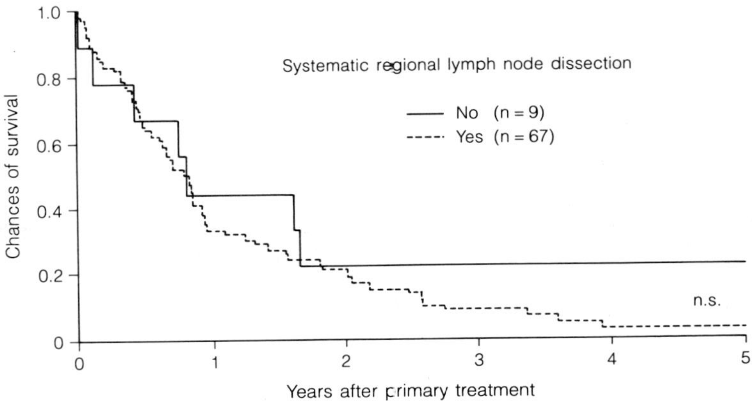

Fig. 1. Observed cumulative survival rates (Kaplan-Meier) following R0 resected stage III, ductal carcinoma of the pancreas with and without extended lymph node dissection (postoperative mortality not excluded), 1978–1989/1990

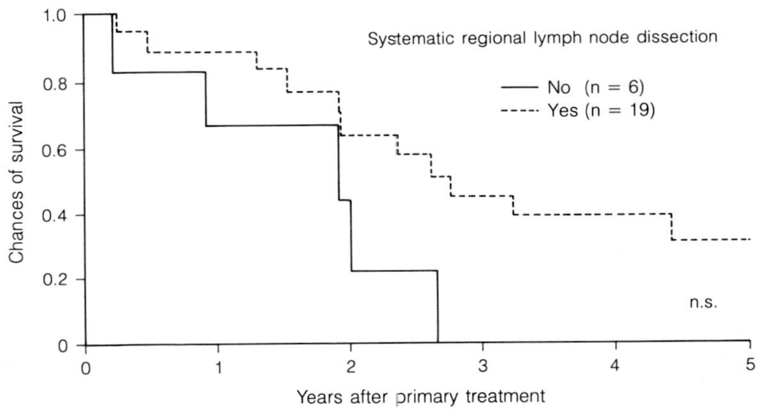

Fig. 2. Observed cumulative survival rates (Kaplan-Meier) following R0 resected stage I and II ductal carcinoma of the pancreas with and without extended lymph node dissection (postoperative mortality not excluded), 1979–1989/1990

anatomical and pathological studies, Nagai [13] found a close relationship between pancreatic lymphatics (peripancreatic lymph nodes) and the para-aortal lymph nodes on the bilateral and anterior regions of the aorta from the coeliac trunk up to the inferior mesenteric artery. Out of ten autopsy cases with relatively small pancreatic carcinomas, four had microscopic metastases in a few para-aortal lymph nodes. He concluded that there is a need for the lymph node disection of the para-aortal region in apparently resectable tumours to include en bloc removal of the lymph nodes and the surrounding soft tissue from the coeliac trunk to the inferior mesenteric artery.

Since Ulrich's report [15] that perineural infiltration can serve as a path for the lymphatic spread of tumour cells, it can be assumed that the perineural and lymphatic infiltration may represent completed lymphatic spread prior to tumour cell invasion of lymph nodes. From this one might conclude that a microinvasion of the second lymph node station has already occurred, even when histologically, the lymph node invasion is limited to the peripancreatic lymph nodes (first station). The simultaneous removal of already present microinvasion of peripancreatic lymphatics and lymph nodes may explain the improvement of prognosis for our lymph node negative patients following extended dissection.

Ishikawa et al. [6] differentiate between a limited lymph node dissection of the region of the pancreatic head (R1) from an extended dissection (R2) which includes complete removal of more distant lymph node stations along the large vessels including para-aortal regions as well as renal vessels. He was able to observe a 3-year survival rate of 38% for the extended dissection vs 13% following limited resection. This difference was statistically significant. The 5-year survival rate was also clearly different: 28% vs 9%. Furthermore, he was able to show that through extended dissection, the cumulative death rate of 16% at 3 years postoperatively attributed to local recurrence was considerably lower than that of limited resection (67%). The death rate as a consequence of distant metastases was not affected by extension of dissection.

We are of the opinion that it is those patients with small tumours and early tumour stages who profit from an extended lymph node dissection. In advanced pancreatic carcinoma, radical tumour surgery alone cannot control disease and these patients must be offered adjuvant therapy [14]. As long as there is no way to improve early diagnosis and as long as there is no effective adjuvant treatment in sight, surgical removal of the tumour with adequate margins of clearance on all sides, as practised in extended lymph node dissection, is the method with the best results.

References

1. Bittner R, Roscher R, Sati F, Dopfer H-P, Schölzel E, Beger HG (1989) Der Einfluß von Tumorgröße und Lymphknotenstatus auf die Prognose des Pankreaskarzinoms. Chirurg 60:240–245
2. Böttger T, Zech J, Weber W, Sorger K, Junginger T (1989) Prognostisch relevante Faktoren beim duktalen Pankreascarcinom. Chirurg 60:521–528
3. Cubilla AL, Fitzgerald PJ (1980) Surgical pathology of tumors of the exocrine pancreas. In: Moosser AR (ed) Tumors of the pancreas. Williams and Wilking, Baltimore, pp 159–193
4. Fortner JG (1984) Regional pancreatectomy for cancer of the pancreas, ampulla and other related sites. Tumor staging and results. Ann Surg 199:418–425

5. Hohenberger W, Zirngibl H, Gall FP (1989) Pancreatic and periampullary carcinoma. In: Veronesi U (ed) Surgical oncology. A European handbook. Springer, Berlin Heidelberg New York, pp 578–621
6. Ishikawa O, Ohhigashi H, Sasaki Y, Kabuto T, Fukuda I, Furukawa H, Imaoka S, Iwanga T (1988) Practical usefulness of lymphatic and connective tissue clearance for the carcinoma of the pancreas head. Ann Surg 208:215–220
7. Kümmerle F, Rückert K (1984) Surgical treatment of pancreatic cancer. World J Surg 8:889–894
8. Manabe T, Naitoh A, Suzuki T, Tobe T (1985) An appraisal of the surgical management of stage I and II cancers of the pancreas. Nippon Geka Gakkai Zasshi 86:1089–1092
9. Manabe T, Hoshio G, Baba N, Miyshita T, Asano N, Tamura K, Yamaki K, Nonaka A, Tobe T (1989) Radical pancreatectomy for ductal cell carcinoma of the head of the pancreas. Cancer 64:1132–1137
10. Miyazaki I, Nagakawa T, Higashino Y (1985) Surgical results and problems of pancreatic cancer. Gan To Kagaku Ryoho 12:220–226
11. Miyazaki I (1989) Significance of extensive surgery in pancreatic cancer. Gan To Kagaku Ryoho 16:1064–1069
12. Nagai H, Kuroda A, Morioka Y (1986) Lymphatic and local spread of T_1 and T_2 pancreas cancer: a study of autopsy material. Ann Surg 204:65–71
13. Nagai H (1987) An anatomical and pathological study of autopsy material on the metastasis of pancreatic cancer to para-aortic lymph nodes. Nippon Geka Gakkai Zasshi 88:308–317
14. Trede M (1987) Treatment of pancreatic carcinoma: the surgeon's dilemma. Br J Surg 74:78–80
15. Urich H (1976) Disease of peripheral nerves. In: Blackwood W, Corsellis JAN (eds) Greenfield's neuropathology, 3rd edn. Arnold, London, pp 688–770
16. Warshaw AL, Swanson RS (1988) Pancreatic cancer in 1988. Possibilities and probabilities. Ann Surg 208:541–553

Pancreaticogastrostomy After Resection of the Pancreatic Head

C.D. JOHNSON[1]

Resection of the pancreatic head is a major surgical undertaking which can only be accomplished safely if all parts of the reconstruction heal satisfactorily. Historically, the most feared step in the reconstruction has been the anastomosis between the pancreatic remnant and the small bowel. Most surgeons report a high incidence of leakage from this anastomosis which overall runs at 13.6% (Table 1). This serious complication carries a mortality of 19%, which makes it one of the major causes of postoperative death. Some authors have noted a falling mortality from pancreaticoduodectomy, but they found no corresponding reduction in pancreatic fistula rates when pancreaticojejunostomy was used [3, 7].

A possible reason for the frequency and severity of leakage from the pancreaticojejunal anastomosis is that pancreatic proteolytic enzymes, which are secreted in an inactive form, are activated by enterokinase in the lumen of the small bowel. These activated enzymes may digest the healing anastomosis, and after leakage through the anastomosis will attack and destroy surrounding tissue. The harmful effects of activated enzymes are well illustrated by the excoriation that occurs around a duodenal fistula, in contrast with the absence of skin reaction to a fistula of pure pancreatic juice.

Various technical modifications of pancreaticojejunostomy have been described in an attempt to minimise leakage (Table 2). An alternative approach is to anastomose the pancreatic remnant to the stomach. This has several practical and theoretical advantages. The stomach lies immediately anterior to the pancreas and the anastomosis can be made without extensive intestinal or pancreatic mobilisation. The anastomosis is tension free as the organs are naturally apposed. There is no enterokinase in the gastric lumen, so pancreatic enzymes are not activated at the anastomosis. Indeed, a low intragastric pH totally inhibits the activity of these enzymes, and may permanently denature them [31]. Thus the anastomosis can heal without enzymatic attack, and if leakage should occur the resulting fistula is easy to manage and heals rapidly.

[1] University Surgical Unit, F Level, Centre Block, Southampton General Hospital, Southampton SO9 4XY, U.K.

Beger/Büchler/Malfertheiner (Eds.)
Standards in Pancreatic Surgery

Table 1. Pancreatic fistula and operative mortality after pancreaticoduodenectomy with pancreaticojejunostomy

Author(s)	Number of patients	No. with pancreatic fistula	Fistula-related deaths (*n*)	Operative mortality (*n*)
Wise et al. [45]	39	4	NS	6
Sato et al. [34]	66	8	2	5
Van Heerden et al. [43]	146	17	2	6
Obertop et al. [26]	24	3[a]	3	3
Herter et al. [10]	102	9	1	15
Piorkowski et al. [30]	39	3	0	6
Lerut et al. [19]	96	15	3	8
Jones et al. [14]	87	13	2	4
Grace et al. [7]	74	18	1	3
Tarazi et al. [36]	94	26[b]	NS	9
Braasch et al. [1]	71	7	0	2
Dunn [4]	22	2	NS	3
Funovics et al. [6]	112	16	NS	8
Kairaluoma et al. [15]	51	13	2	6
Tashiro et al. [37]	112	14	10	11
Crist et al. [3]	88	12	0	11
Neoptolemos et al. [25]	24	6	NS	3
Trede and Schwal [40][c]	233	14[d]	4	6
Pellegrini et al. [28]	51	9	0	11
Lygidakis et al. [20]	55	1[a]	1	3
Hall et al. [9]	14	2	0	0
Trede et al. [41][c]	118	9	0	0
Roder et al. [32]	110	27	0	2
Total	1828	248 (13.6%)	31 (1.7%)	31 (7.1%)

NS, Not stated.
[a] At least. Only reoperations and deaths were reported.
[b] Also acute pancreatitis.
[c] Some overlap of series.
[d] Also included 11 acute pancreatitis with one death.

Table 2. Techniques described for dealing with the pancreas after resection of the head

Pancreaticojejunostomy
end-to-end
"dunking" end-to-end
invaginating end-to-side
mucosa-to-mucosa end-to-side
Duct ligation
Duct occlusion
Total pancreatectomy
Pancreaticogastrostomy

Pancreaticogastrostomy was described in experimental animals in the 1930s [29, 42]. The technique has been applied clinically after resection of the pancreatic head, initally in relatively few patients, but recently in increasing numbers (Table 3).

Pancreaticogastrostomy was initially carried out by simple implantation of the transected pancreas into the posterior wall of the stomach [5, 12, 23, 33, 35, 44]. This technique was followed by scarring and fibrosis of the pancreatic stump, with subsequent occlusion of the duct and pancreatic insufficiency. Some authors [16, 21] deliberately ligated the pancreatic duct before the insertion of the pancreas into the stomach. Wells et al. [44] were the first to describe direct duct-to-mucosa anastomosis. Telford et al. [39] examined the various options in an experimental study, and demonstrated that long-term patency of the anastomosis could be achieved by direct suture of pancreatic duct to gastric mucosa, whereas other forms of pancreaticogastric anastomosis were usually followed by fibrotic stricture and obstruction. The importance of duct-to-mucosa anastomosis has been confirmed recently in an experimental study of pancreaticojejunostomy [8]. Telford and Mason [38] subsequently reported excellent clinical results with the technique of duct-to-mucosa anastomosis.

Surgical Technique

After resection of the pancreatic head and division of the neck of the pancreas, 1–2 cm of pancreas is mobilised to allow the placement of sutures. A stay suture is placed at the superior and inferior border of the pancreas to permit traction and to incorporate any bleeding points at these sites (Fig. 1). The stomach is retracted superiorly to expose its posterior surface and the pancreas and stomach are approximated. After Whipple resection with distal gastrectomy it is advisable to make the pancreatic anastomosis at least

Table 3. Pancreatic fistula and operative mortality after pancreaticoduodenectomy with end-to-side pancreaticogastric anastomosis

Author(s)	Number of patients	No. with pancreatic fistula	Fistula-related deaths (*n*)	Operative mortality (*n*)
Park et al. [27][a]	19	0	0	2
Mackie et al. [21]	25	1	0	2[b]
Telford and Mason [38]	9	0	0	0
Flautner et al. [5]	27	0	0	0
Kapur [16]	31	0	0	2
Icard and Dubois [11]	17	0	0	0
Total	128	1	0	6

[a] Reviews previous experience.
[b] One death from acute pancreatitis.

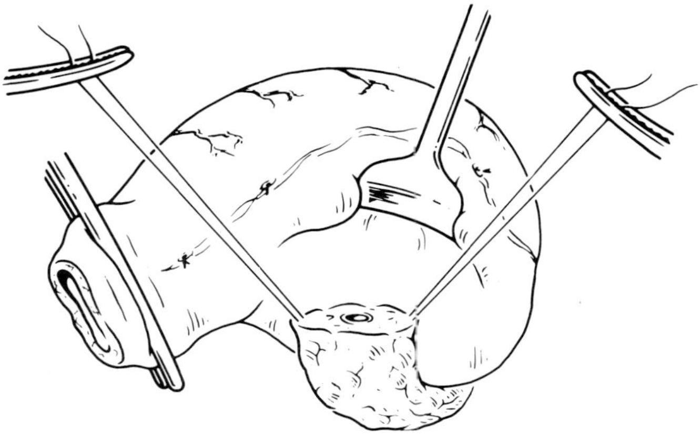

Fig. 1. The stomach is retracted superiorly and the pancreatic neck is secured with two sutures at the superior and inferior border. (From [2])

3 cm from the gastric closure line. At a convenient point, without tension, the pancreatic capsule is sutured to the serosa of the stomach with a continuous suture. This should not be of rapidly absorbable material. My own preference is to use 3/0 polyglactin (Vicryl, Ethicon) for this stitch (Fig. 2). After completion of the first continuous suture, an incision is made in the posterior wall of the stomach to match the pancreatic duct. This is most easily achieved with a pointed scalpel. Sometimes the gastric mucosa is thick and mobile, and is not easily penetrated from without by the scalpel. In these cases the clamp is removed from the distal gastric resection line and a curved forceps (such as Lahey's) is passed into the lumen of the stomach to push the gastric mucosa out through the serosal incision. This mucosa is then incised and picked up with full thickness sutures before the Lahey's forceps is withdrawn. A short length of polypropylene tubing (4 F gauge) can then be inserted into the pancreatic duct. The purpose of this tube is to avoid occlusion of the duct by the duct-to-mucosa sutures. One or two sutures are inserted to appose the gastric mucosa to pancreatic duct epithelium posteriorly (Fig. 3), and the tube stent is then passed into the gastric lumen before completion of the anastomosis with interrupted 3/0 sutures of polydioxanone (PDS, Ethicon) (Fig. 4). The number of sutures required depends upon the diameter of the pancreatic duct. For a normal duct of 2–3 mm, only three or four sutures are used. A stent is not necessary for pancreatic ducts larger than 4 mm.

After completion of the duct-to-mucosa anastomosis, the serosa-to-pancreatic capsule continuous suture is carried across the front of the anastomosis (Fig. 5).

When the pancreaticogastric anastomosis has been constructed, intestinal continuity is restored by end-to-end gastrojejunostomy and end-to-side

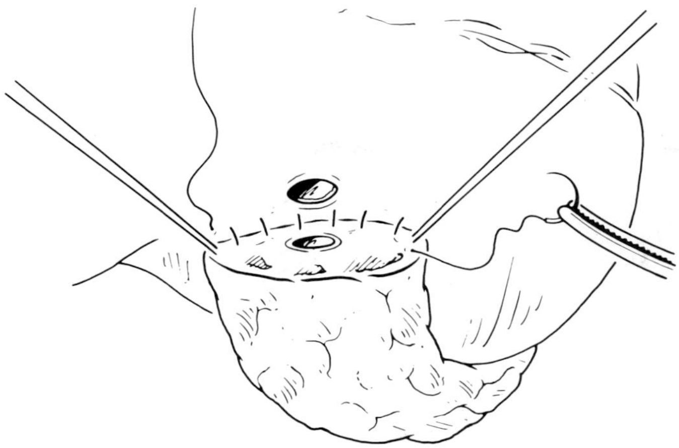

Fig. 2. The anterior surface of the pancreatic capsule is sutured to the serosa of the posterior wall of the stomach with a continuous stitch. An incision is made in the posterior wall of the stomach to correspond to the pancreatic duct. (From [2])

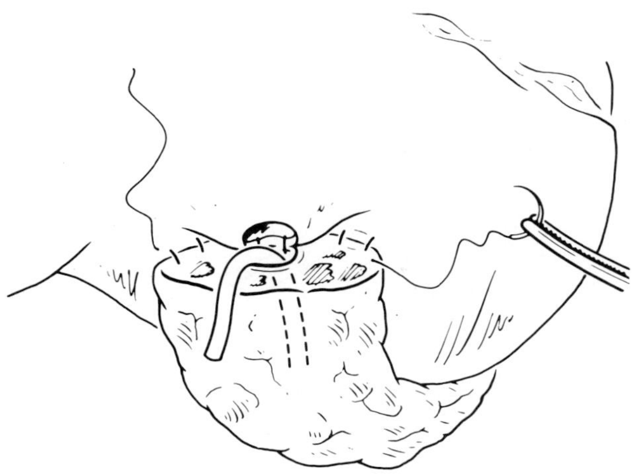

Fig. 3. The duct mucosa and gastric mucosa are approximated with interrupted sutures. A fine polyethylene tube has been placed in the pancreatic duct to prevent occlusion of the duct by the suture. (From [2])

choledochojejunostomy (Fig. 6). The choledochojejunostomy is placed 45 cm from the gastrojejunostomy after standard Whipple resection, to prevent bile reflux (Fig. 7). After pylorus-preserving resection, the duodenojejunostomy is made end to end and the biliary anastomosis is made at a convenient short distance from this.

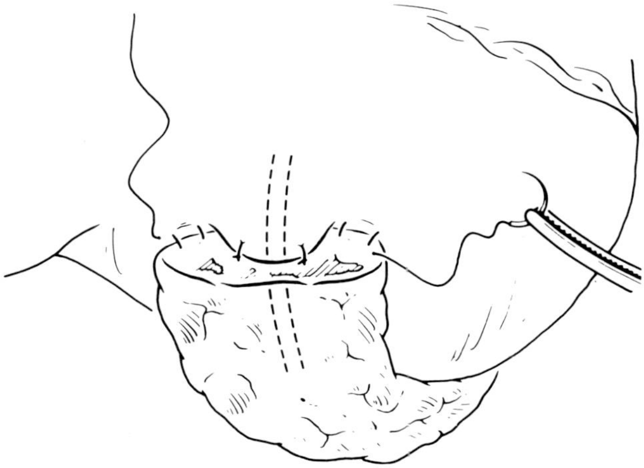

Fig. 4. The polyethylene tube is passed through the gastric incision into the lumen and the duct-to-mucosa anastomosis is completed with interrupted sutures. (From [2])

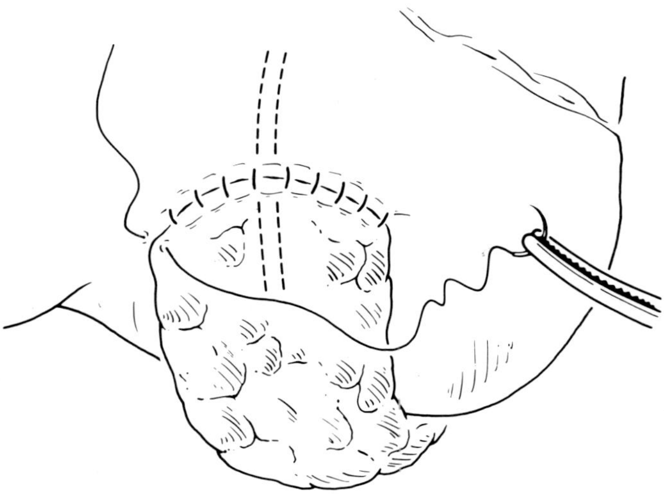

Fig. 5. The posterior wall of the stomach and posterior capsule of the pancreas are approximated with he the continuous suture to complete the anastomosis. (From [2])

A tube drain is placed behind the stomach, in the region of the pancreaticogastric anastomosis. This is led past the biliary anastomosis to the right flank. No external anastomotic stents are used. If the pancreaticogastric anastomosis is stented, the tubing will pass spontaneously. This is occasionally aspirated in the nasogastric tube or may be passed in the first bowel action.

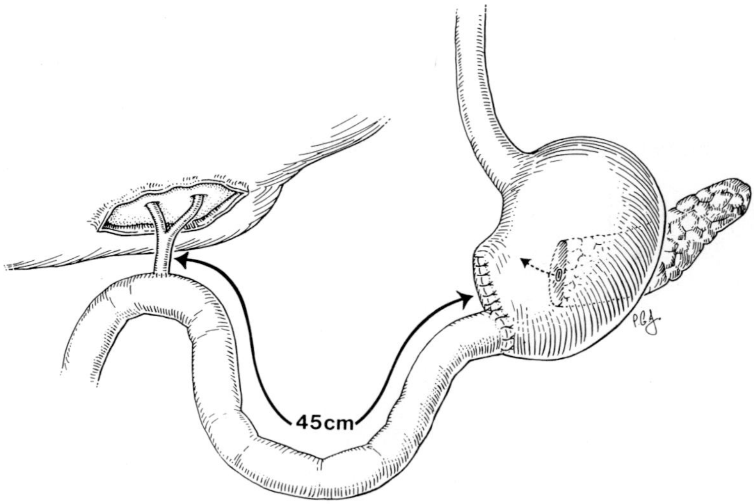

Fig. 6. Reconstruction after standard Whipple resection with distal gastrectomy. After formation of the pancreaticogastric anastomosis, and partial closure of the gastric resection line, an end-to-end gastrojejunostomy is made in the manner of a Billroth I gastrectomy. An end-to-side choledochojejunostomy is made 45 cm distal to the gastrojejunostomy

Surgical Results

We have used this technique in 50 patients suffering from periampullary malignancy and chronic pancreatitis (Table 4). Anastomotic complications were few. There were two pancreatic fistulas diagnosed by drainage of clear fluid rich in amylase. One fistula closed spontaneously after 5 days; the other closed after parenteral nutrition for 21 days. In neither case was there evidence of intra-abdominal sepsis. One patient developed a peripancreatic fluid collection and fever, 7 days after operation. Percutaneous drainage of the fluid collection produced a resolution of the fever within 24 h, and ileus resolved at 48 h. The drainage fluid was dark brown and rich in amylase but within 24 h had reduced to a negligible volume. This case probably represents postoperative pancreatitis rather than anastomotic leakage. One patient developed a biliary anastomotic leak which closed after 6 days of conservative management.

There were two deaths within 30 days of operation. One patient died from septicaemia secondary to cholangitis. Preoperative biliary drainage had been unsuccessful and uncontrolled cholangitis was present at the time of operation. One patient died from perioperative haemorrhage. There was no death related to anastomotic leakage.

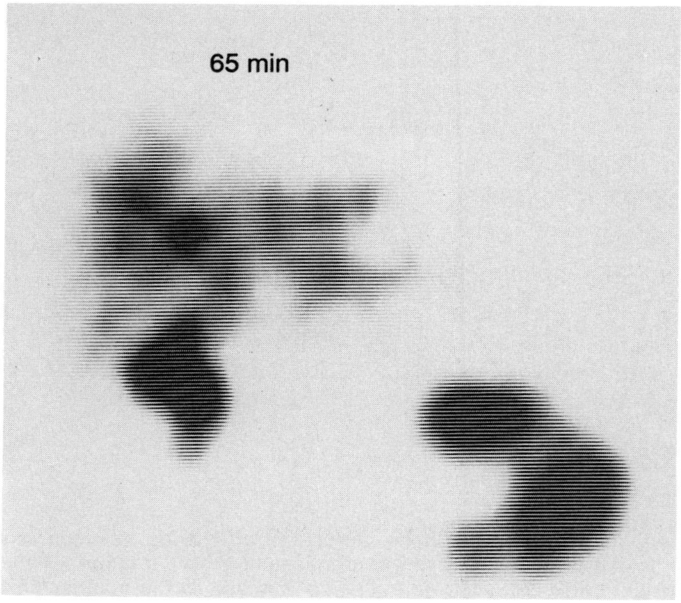

a

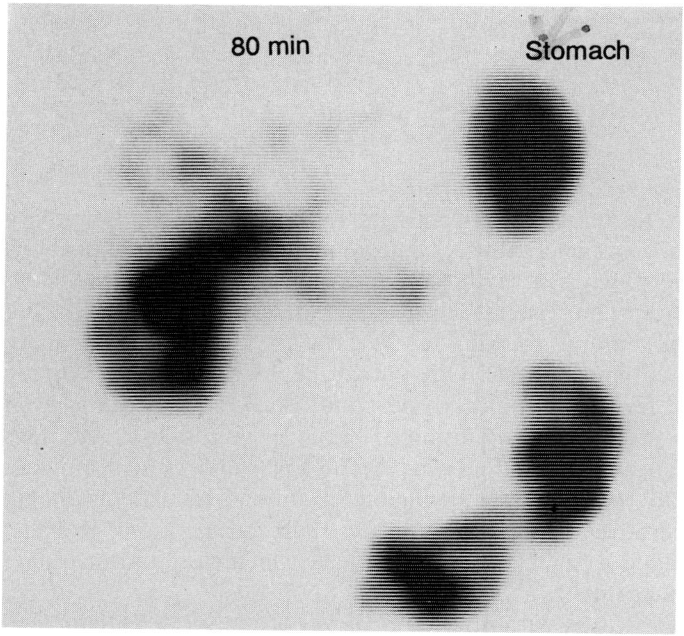

b

Fig. 7a,b HIDA biliary excretion scan from a patient with a reconstruction as shown in Fig. 6. Activity has passed from the liver into the small bowel (**a**) but there is no activity in the area corresponding to the gastric remnant, outlined by isotope swallow (**b**). (Courtesy of Dr. R.J. Jewkes)

Table 4. Diagnosis of 50 cases of pancreatic resection with end-to-side pancreaticogastric anastomosis

Diagnosis	Number of patients
Pancreatic adenocarcinoma	21
Ampullary adenocarcinoma	13
Bile duct tumours	10
Chronic pancreatitis	4
Islet cell tumour	1
Duodenal adenocarcinoma	1

Late Results

Two patients who had not been diabetic preoperatively developed diabetes mellitus after operation.

One patient developed postanastomotic ulceration. He had undergone a pylorus-preserving pancreatectomy for an apparently localised small carcinoma of the pancreas. Subsequent histological examination revealed involvement of pancreatic resection margins. He received postoperative radiotherapy (40 Gy in two fractions, with 5-FU as a radiosensitiser) and was started on monthly treatment with 5-FU. He was unable to tolerate this treatment and it was discontinued. Six months after operation he developed symptoms of gastric outlet obstruction. Barium examination showed ulceration and stricturing in the proximal jejunum, which was shown to be benign on endoscopic biopsy. His symptoms were relieved and the radiographic appearances improved during continuous therapy with omeprazole, which he continues to take. He is well 30 months after operation, although he requires pancreatic enzyme supplements.

Functional Results

Long-term functional results were assessed in 16 patients who had operations for malignancy more than 6 months previously. Patients with chronic pancreatitis were not studied because all had evidence of impaired pancreatic function prior to operation.

All but one patient had gained weight (median 6 kg, range 0–22 kg) after operation. Two patients reported clinical evidence of steatorrhoea despite enzyme supplements. Five of the 16 patients were taking pancreatic enzyme supplements to control their bowel habit. Six patients agreed to attend for investigation by endoscopy, HIDA biliary excretion scintigraphy and a gastric intubation test for assessment of gastric and pancreatic function.

Endoscopy

Two patients showed evidence of gastric mucosal erythema, and in two patients there was histological evidence of gastritis. In none of the six patients could the pancreatic duct anastomosis be identified. The erythema and gastritis was seen in patients operated on early in the series who had the biliary anastomosis close to the gastric remnant. The two patients with normal mucosal appearances and normal histology had a distal biliary anastomosis.

Biliary Scintigraphy

Biliary excretion scintigraphy confirmed the absence of bile reflux to the stomach in patients with a distal choledochojejunostomy (Fig. 7).

Combined Function Test

Six patients underwent a combined gastric and pancreatic function study. A nasogastric tube was passed and the gastric content was aspirated. Resting secretion was then collected for 30 min prior to an injection of pentagastrin 6 μg/kg. Secretion was collected for 1 h in 15 min aliquots. An intravenous bolus injection of secretin 75 units and cholecystokinin (CCK) 75 units was then given, and secretion was aspirated for a further hour. The results are shown in Table 5.

All patients had normal gastric secretion. Of the six patients in whom pancreatic enzyme secretory capacity was assessed, all but one patient had demonstrable enzyme activity in the gastric aspirate. The patient with no detectable enzymes had no clinical evidence of pancreatic insufficiency, and he had very high basal values for gastric secretion and a peak acid output of 22 mmol/h. It is likely that this patient was producing pancreatic enzymes, but that in the conditions of the test the enzymes were inactivated by the high gastric acidity.

Table 5. Secretory outputs of stomach and pancreas in response to pentagastrin 6 μg/kg and secretin 1 U/kg with CCK 1 U/kg respectively

	Basal		Peak	
	Median	Range	Median	Range
Gastric acid (mmol/h)	1.2	0–9	12.7	6.2–22
	Total		Peak	
	Median	Range	Median	Range
Pancreatic enzymes				
Amylase (U/h)	1660	0–14 200	2450	0–36 800
Lipase (U/h)	500	0–1315	750	0–1750

None of the patients showed normal pancreatic enzyme outputs, which is not surprising in view of the prior resection of a large part of the gland. Nevertheless, two thirds of these patients were able to maintain a normal diet without pancreatic enzyme supplements and without evidence of malabsorption. Although pancreatic enzymes are inactivated at low pH, the conditions found in the gastric lumen immediately after a meal will be favourable for normal activity of the pancreatic enzymes. Intragastric pH rises rapidly to levels above pH 5.5 during ingestion of a meal, and remains elevated for some time until gastric emptying nears completion. This buffering capacity of the food presumably protects the pancreatic enzymes from denaturation at the time when they are required. The enzymes will then pass with the chyme into the small bowel where activation by enterokinase can proceed.

Conclusions

The pancreatic anastomosis is a critical part of the reconstruction following resection of the pancreatic head. Pancreaticojejunostomy is troublesome, and leakage from this anastomosis is a serious complication. In contrast, pancreaticogastrostomy with duct-to-mucosa suture is a simple anastomosis to perform, and has a very low leak rate. If leakage occurs its consequences are usually minor. Pancreaticogastrostomy has been used in several series with very low rates of leakage and low rates of operative mortality. Some of these series are all the more remarkable in that they were reported before the recent dramatic reductions in mortality following pancreaticoduodenal resection [13].

Late function after pancreaticogastrostomy is good, with normal gastric function and demonstrable pancreatic enzyme secretion in most patients several years after operation. These figures are similar or better than the long-term functional results of pancreaticojejunostomy [9, 18, 24].

Pancreaticogastric anastomosis is a useful, safe technique for pancreatic reconstruction after pancreatic head resection. It simplifies reconstruction and allows "in line" gastrojejunal anastomosis. There appear to be no long-term complications. Pancreaticogastrostomy with duct-to-mucosa anastomosis is recommended as the procedure in the reconstruction after resection of the pancreatic head.

References

1. Braasch JW, Rossi RL, Watkins E, Deziel DJ, Winter PF (1986) Pyloric and gastric preserving pancreatic resection. Ann Surg 204:411–418
2. Bradbeer JW, Johnson CD (1990) Ann R Coll Surg Engl 72:266–269
3. Crist DW, Sitzman JV, Cameron JL (1987) Improved hospital morbidity and survival after the Whipple procedure. Ann Surg 206:358–373

4. Dunn E (1987) The impact of technology and improved perioperative management upon survival from carcinoma of the pancreas. Surg Gynecol Obstet 1164:237–244
5. Flautner L, Tihanyi T, Szecseny A (1985) Pancreatogastrostomy: an ideal complement to pancreatic head resection with preservation of the pylorus in the treatment of chronic pancreatitis. Am J Surg 150:608–611
6. Funovics JM, Zoch G, Wenzl E, Schulz F (1987) Progress in reconstruction after resection of the head of the pancreas. Surg Gynecol Obstet 164:545–548
7. Grace PA, Pitt HA, Tomkins PK, Longmire WP (1986) Decreased morbidity and mortality after pancreaticoduodencetomy. Am J Surg 161:120–125
8. Greene BS, Loubeau JM, Peoples JB, Elliot DW (1991) Are pancreaticoenteric anastomoses improved by duct-to-mucosa sutures? Am J Surg 161:45–50
9. Hall RI, Rhodes M, Isabel-Martinez L, Kelleber J, Venables CW (1990) Pancreaticendocrine function after a sutureless pancreaticojejunostomy following pancreaticoduodenectomy. Br J Surg 77:83–85
10. Herter FP, Cooperman AM, Allborn TN, Antinori C (1982) Surgical experience with pancreatic and periampullary cancer. Ann Surg 195:274–281
11. Icard P, Dubois F (1988) Pancreaticogastrostomy following pancreaticogastrostomy 207:253–256
12. Ingebritsen R, Langfeldt E (1952) Pancreaticogastrostomy. Lancet 263:270
13. Johnson CD (1991) Why resect pancreatic cancer? In: Johnson CD, Imrie CW (eds) Pancreatic disease: progress and prospects. Springer, Berlin Heidelberg New York, pp 97–102
14. Jones BA, Langer B, Taylor BR, Girotti M (1985) Periampullary tumours. Which ones should be resected? Am J Surg 149:46–52
15. Kairaluoma MI, Kiviniemi H, Stahlberg M (1987) Pancretic resection for carcinoma of the pancreas and the periampullary region in patients over 70 years of age. Br J Surg 74:116–118
16. Kapur BML (1986) Pancreaticogastrostomy in pancreaticoduodenal resection for ampullary carcinoma. Surgery 100:489–493
17. Kümmerle F, Duckert K (1984) Surgical treatment of pancreatic cancer. World J Surg 8:889–894 (not cited in text)
18. Lai ECS, King W, Longmire WP, Tompkin RK (1987) Pancreaticojejunostomy after Whipple's operation. In vivo examination of long term patency: a preliminary report. Surgery 101:544–548
19. Lerut JP, Gionello PR, Otte JB, Kestens MD (1984) Pancreaticoduodenal resection. Ann Surg 199:432–437
20. Lygidakis NS, vander Hyde MN, Houthoff HJ, Schipper MEI, Huibregste K et al. (1989) Resectional surgical procedures for carcinoma of the head of the pancreas. Surg Gynecol Obstet 168:157–165
21. Mackie JA, Rhoads JE, Park CD (1975) Pancreaticogastrostomy: a further evaluation. Ann Surg 181:541–545
22. Millbourn E (1958) Pancreaticogastrostomy in pancreaticoduodenal resection for carcinoma of the head of the pancreas or papilla of Vater. Acta Chir Scand 116:12–27
23. Nanson EM (1954) An unusual case of carcinoma of the head of the pancreas. Br J Surg 41:439–441
24. Niebel W, Hotz J, Dostal G, Goebtell H, Eigler FW (1980) Pancreatic function in the early and late postoperative period after surgical treatment of chronic pancreatitis. Eur Surg Res 12 Suppl 2:36
25. Neoptolemos JP, Talbot IC, Carr-Locke DL (1987) Treatment and outcome in 52 consecutive cases of ampullary carcinoma. Br J Surg 74:957–961
26. Obertop H, Bruining HA, Geftink Schattenkerk M, Eggink WF, Jeekel J, von Houten H (1982) Operative approach to cancer of the head of the pancreas and periampullary region. Br J Surg 69:573–576
27. Park CD, Mackie JA, Rhoads JE (1967) Pancreaticogastrostomy. Am J Surg 113:85–89

28. Pellegrini CA, Heck CF, Roper S et al. (1989) Analysis of the reduced morbidity and mortality rates after pancreaticoduodenectomy. Arch Surg 124:778–781
29. Person EC, Glenn F (1939) Pancreaticogastrostomy. Experimental transplantation of the pancreas into the stomach. Arch Surg 39:530–550
30. Piorkowski RJ, Blievernicht SW, Lawrence W et al. (1982) Pancreatic and periampullary carcinoma. Am J Surg 143:189–193
31. Rinderknecht H (1986) Pancreatic secretory enzymes. In: Go VLW, Gardner JD, Brooks FP et al. (eds) The exocrine pancreas. Raven, New York, pp 163–183
32. Roder JD, Stein HJ, Huttl W, Siewert JR (1992) Pylorus preserving versus standard pancreaticoduodenectomy. Br J Surg 79:152–154
33. Sames CP (1952) Pancreaticogastrostomy. Lancet 262:718
34. Sato T, Noto N, Matsumo S, Miyakawa K (1981) Follow-up results of surgical treatment for chronic pancreatitis. Am J Surg 142:317–323
35. Silverstone M (1956) Pancreaticoduodenectomy and pancreaticogastrostomy. Br J Surg 44:299–302
36. Tarazi RY, Hermann RE, Vogt DP, Hoerr SO, Esselstyn CB et al. (1986) Results of surgical treatment of periampullary tumors: a thirty-five year experience. Surgery 100:716–723
37. Tashiro S, Murata E, Hiracka T, Nakakuma K, Watanabe E, Miyauchi Y (1987) New technique for pancreaticojejunostomy using a biological adhesive. Br J Surg 74:392–394
38. Telford GL, Mason GR (1984) Pancreatico-gastrostomy. Clinical experience with a direct pancreatic duct to gastric mucosa anastomosis. Am J Surg 147:832–837
39. Telford GL, Ormsbee HS, Mason GR (1980) Pancreaticogastrostomy improved by a pancreatic duct-to-gatric mucosa anastomosis. Curr Surg 37:140–142
40. Trede M, Schwal G (1988) The complications of pancreatectomy. Ann Surg 207:39–47
41. Trede M, Schwall G, Saeger HD (1990) Survival after pancreaticoduodenectomy. 118 consecutive cases without operative mortality. Ann Surg 211:447–458
42. Tripodi AM, Sherwin CF (1934) Experimental transplantation of the pancreas into the stomach. Arch Surg 28:345–356
43. Van Heerden JA, McIlrath DC, Dozois RR, Adson MA (1981) Radical pancreatectomy – a procedure to be abandoned? Mayo Clin Proc 56:601–606
44. Wells C, Shepherd JA, Gibbon N (1952) Pancreaticogastrostomy. Lancet 262: 588–589
45. Wise L, Pizzimbono C, Dehner LP (1976) Periampullary cancer. Am J Surg 131:141–148

Adjuvant Intraoperative Radiation Therapy During Duodenopancreatectomy

K. Glaser,[1] E. Bodner,[1] and A. Klingler[2]

Introduction

Intraoperative radiation therapy (IORT) is a modern oncological treatment, utilizing radiotherapy and surgery at the same time. The idea to administer radiation to internal structures was first published by Carl Beck, a Berlin surgeon, in 1908 in a paper entitled "*On external Roentgen treatment of internal structures (eventration treatment)*" [1].

The modern development of IORT was mainly perpetuated by Prof. Abe of Kyoto during the mid-1960s. Following the Japanese publications [2], IORT was enthusiastically adopted and investigated in the United States and Europe. The principle of administering a large single dose of irradiation to a surgically exposed tumor volume is very intriguing, and many surgical oncologists have shown interest in the method. To date about 4000 patients have been treated with IORT in over 50 centers throughout the world. Nevertheless, due to the absence of a sufficient number of controlled prospective randomized trials, the possible benefits of IORT have never been proven, and attitudes towards IORT remain controversial [3, 4].

According to the scientific and clinical interests of our department, we have used IORT mainly in treating pancreatic cancer [5, 6] and since December 1984 also as an adjuvant measure during Whipple's resection. At the same time in our operative strategy we have adopted a more aggressive approach including extended regional lymphadenectomy.

The incidence of pancreatic cancer in Austria is about 10 per 100000 inhabitants, approximately 700 patients per year [7]. As in the rest of the world, the results of our therapeutic endeavours are poor. Remarkable developments in diagnostic procedures and the reduction of operative risks have not improved the outlook. Resectability rates remain low at 10%–30%. More than half of the patients who undergo radical resections develop local recurrences [8]. Median survival following radical resection is 12–14 months; less than 5% of patients with ductal pancreatic cancer survive more than 5 years after resection.

[1] Second Department of Surgery, University of Innsbruck, Anichstraße 35, A-6020 Innsbruck, Austria
[2] Division of Theoretical Surgery, Second Department of Surgery, University of Innsbruck, Anichstraße 35, A-6020 Innsbruck, Austria

Beger/Büchler/Malfertheiner (Eds.)
Standards in Pancreatic Surgery

Indication Criteria and Rationale for IORT

According to our approach, IORT is indicated in resectable pancreatic cancer without detectable tumor spread to the liver, distant lymph nodes, and the peritoneum. After exposure, the tumor is irradiated in situ immediately before resection for the following reasons:

1. Since the operation is started in the radiation therapy unit (three floors away from the operating theater) it is only necessary to transport the patient once, thus considerably reducing the expenditure of time and manpower.
2. IORT is performed with the intention to limit growth of malignant cells, which may be spread during surgical manipulations, and to eliminate microscopic residual disease which may be left behind after curative resection.
3. The use of electron beams also allows sufficient radiation doses to the tumor bed and lymphatic drainage system with the tumor still in situ.

Method and Material

Preoperative Diagnosis

To avoid unnecessary occupation of the radiation therapy unit, an attempt must be made to assess the tumor stage exactly preoperatively. Ultrasound and computed tomography are used to judge local resectability and metastases. Laparoscopy is most helpful in the detection of small metastases (<5 mm) and peritoneal spread.

Intraoperative Diagnosis and Exposure

The abdomen is opened in the radiotherapy unit. The liver, peritoneal cavity, and lymphatic nodes are examined for extrapancreatic tumor spread. Fine-needle aspiration biopsy is carried out for cytological confirmation of the diagnosis. Liver and pancreatic tumor are examined by means of intraoperative ultrasound to further rule out small liver metastases and confirm local resectability. Afterwards the tumor is exposed utilizing the "no-touch method" as far as possible.

Radiotherapeutic Intervention

High-velocity electrons from a linear accelerator (Philips SL75/20) are used in a single dose of 15–20 Gy. Eight electron energy stages can be selected between 5 and 20 meV in order to adapt the maximum dose to the particular topographic situation. In correlation to the diameter and depth of the tumor, the electron energy is chosen so that the tumor bed is positioned within the 80% isodose curve. Additionally, the distal hepatoduodenal ligament, superior mesenteric root, and celiac trunk are included in the IORT field. Surrounding tissue (hollow viscera and abdominal organs) are pushed aside by the treatment cone which is placed over the tumor. The IORT dose administered is 15 Gy in the case of a soft pancreatic remnant and 20 Gy in patients with congestive pancreatic induration. During IORT, which usually lasts 4–6 min, the patient, respirator, and ECG are observed via television monitors. After temporary closure of the wound, the patient is transported to the operating theater for resection and reconstruction.

Surgical Intervention

In all cases an extensive lymph node resection, classified as a regional pancreatectomy type 0 according to Fortner [9], was undertaken. Reconstruction was carried out with end-to-end pancreatojejunostomy (telescope type anastomosis without pancreatic duct occlusion), end-to-side hepaticojejunostomy, Billroth II gastroenterostomy and Braun anastomosis (side-to-side jejunojejunostomy). With a few exceptions, patients did not receive any postoperative therapy such as chemotherapy or external beam irradiation.

Patients

Since 1984, 38 patients with a median age of 67 years (range 45–82) suffering from ductal cancer of the head of the pancreas underwent adjuvant IORT during resection. According to the UICC classification 17 patients (45%) had stage I and II disease, and 21 patients (55%) had stage III tumors. In two cases, partial resection of the portal vein was necessary.

Results

There were no intraoperative mishaps during irradiation or operation. Three patients developed leakage of the pancreatojejunostomy, and reoperation was unavoidable in one case. The leakage could be drained by means of percutaneous ultrasound-guided pig-tail drainage in one other case and subsided spontaneously in the third patient. One patient had to be reoperated on because of hemorrhage from the gastric anastomosis. We observed two perioperative deaths, both from unrelated causes (hepatorenal syndrome and cardiopulmonary failure).

As a late complication one patient developed a peptic ulcer of the jejunum necessitating gastric stump resection, and one patient was reported to have died from a massive intestinal hemorrhage of unknown origin.

Nine (24%) patients developed local recurrences at the superior mesenteric artery and celiac trunk (Table 1). Median survival is presently

Table 1. Type of recurrence of pancratic cancer in 38 patients who underwent Whipple resection plus IORT between 1984 and 1990

Stage	Local recurrence rate (*n*)	%	Liver metastasis (*n*)	Peritoneal carcinoma (*n*)
I	2	5	1	1
II	1	3	–	–
III	6	16	3	1

18 months (Fig. 1). As compared to a historical control group without extensive lymphadenectomy and IORT (median survival 14 months), the survival improvement is encouraging, but not statistically significant (Fig. 2). Furthermore the rate of early and late complications did not differ between the two groups.

Conclusion

Our experience demonstrates that IORT can be administered in an adjuvant setting without an increase in perioperative morbidity and lethality. IORT may help to reduce local recurrences and improve overall survival. Never-

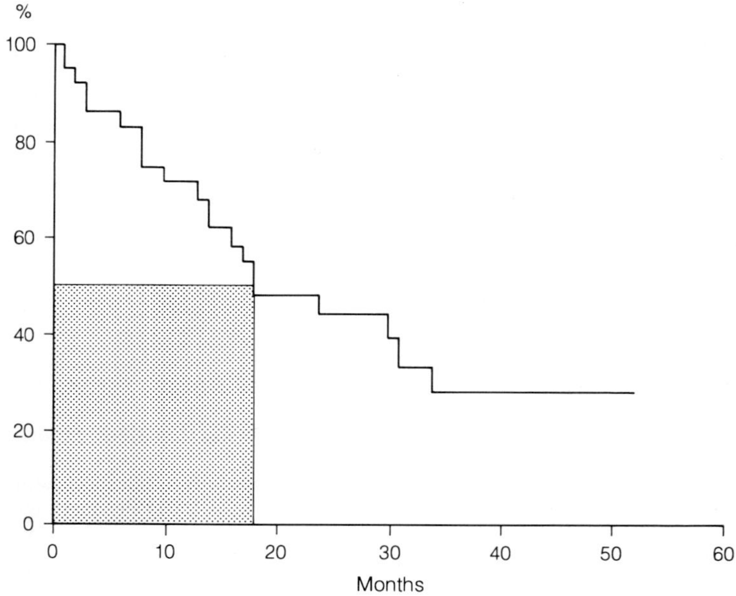

Fig. 1. Survival analysis of 38 patients with pancreatic cancer following IORT and whipple resection (1984–1991)

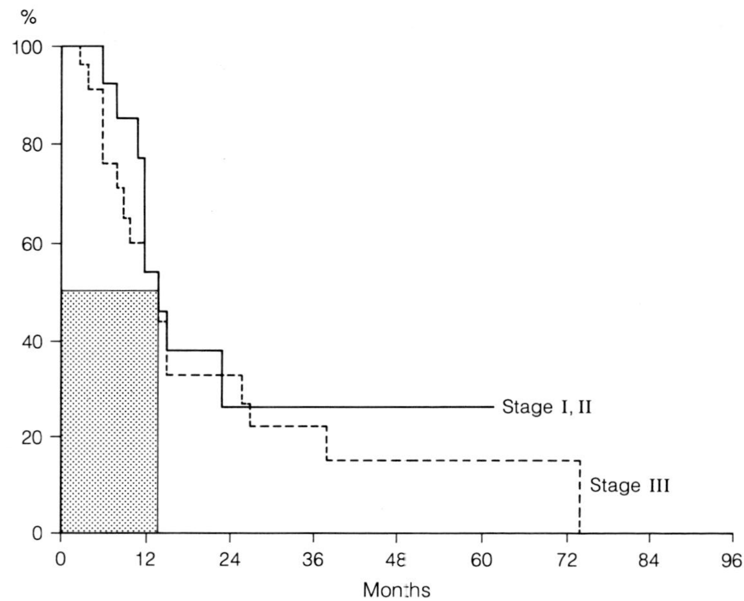

Fig. 2. Survival analysis of the historical control group of pancreatic cancer patients (1976–1983). Fourteen patients had stage I or stage II disease; 24 patients had stage III disease

theless, from our results it remains unclear whether a possible improvement can be ascribed to IORT or to the more extended resectional technique or both. In spite of the use of IORT surgeons are required to perform an adequate resection, preferably a regional subtotal pancreatectomy type O or I according to Fortner. There is definitively a need for a prospective randomized trial to further evaluate and confirm the results which can be achieved by adjuvant IORT in pancreatic cancer.

References

1. Beck C (1909) On external Roentgen treatment of internal structures (Eventration treatment). NY Med J 11:27
2. Abe M, Takahashi M (1981) Intraoperative radiotherapy: the Japanese experience. Int J Radiat Oncol Biol Phys 7:869
3. Hiraoka T, Tashiro S, et al. (1991) Combination of intraoperative radiation with resection for cancer of the pancreas. In: Abe M, Takahashi M (eds) Proceedings of the Third International Symposium on Intraoperative Radiation Therapy. Pergamon, New York, pp 239–241
4. Hanyu F, Hatori T et al. (1991) Intraoperative radiation therapy for patients with carcinoma of the head of the pancreas. In: Abe M, Takahashi M (eds) Proceedings of the Third International Symposium on Intraoperative Radiation Therapy. Pergamon, New York, pp 242–243

5. Bodner E, Glaser K et al. (1986) Intraoperative Strahlenbehandlung beim Pankreaskarzinom, erste klinische Erfahrungen. Dtsch Med Wochenschr 111: 892–896
6. Glaser K, Bodner E et al. (1989) Intraoperative radiation therapy in Austria. In: Dobelbower RR, Abe M (eds) Intraoperative radiation therapy. CRC, Boca Raton, pp 363–376
7. Österreichische Krebsstatistik (1984) Statistische Nachrichten 3:172
8. Tepper J, Nardi G et al. (1981) Carcinoma of the pancreas – review of MGH experience from 1963–1973. Analysis of surgical failure and implications for radiation therapy. Cancer 47:1456
9. Fortner JG (1984) Regional pancreatectomy for cancer of the pancreas, ampulla, and other related sites. Ann Surg 199:418

Surgical Management of Endocrine Pancreatic Tumors

H.J. Peiper[1]

Functionally active pancreatic tumors (FATs) are generally uncommon. They do, however, exhibit a typical clinical picture and can be diagnosed with considerable certainty thanks to the advances made in diagnosis. Endocrine pancreatic tumors are not only those which originate from the islets, but also those which arise from cells that are not present in this region. The former include insulinomas (producing insulin), somatostatinomas (somatostatin), glucagonomas (glucagon), and PPomas (pancreatic polypeptide). The latter group comprises non-secreting tumors: VIPomas (vasoactive intestinal polypeptide), neurotensinomas (neurotensin), GRFomas (growth hormone releasing factor), gastrinomas (gastrin), corticotropinomas (corticotropin), and calcitoninomas (calcitonin).

Insulinomas account for 70%–75% of all endocrine pancreatic tumors. Gastrinomas make up about 20%, VIPomas only 3%–4%, glucagonomas roughly 1%. The other types of endocrine tumors (PPomas, somatostatinomas) are rare. According to the literature 5%–10% of all insulinomas, 35% of the VIPomas, 50%–80% of the glucagonomas, 55%–70% of the somatostatinomas, and over 60% of gastrinomas are malignant.

The diagnosis and classification of endocrine tumors of the pancreas are based on:

1. Symptoms
2. Analysis of the stomach secretion
3. Radioimmunoassay for the serum hormone level
4. Provocation tests
5. Suppression tests
6. Localizing methods
   - Selective celiacography
   - Computed tomography (CT)
   - Ultrasound
   - Endoscopy
   - Percutaneous, transhepatic portovenous collection of serum for hormone measurement
   - Intraoperative findings

[1] Abt, Allgemeinchirurgie, Klinik und Poliklinik, Georg-August-Universität, Robert-Koch-Straße 40, W-3400 Göttingen, FRG

Beger/Büchler/Malfertheiner (Eds.)
Standards in Pancreatic Surgery

In addition, the tumor type is determined by morphological and biochemical analyses of the tumor tissue, immunohistological tests, immunocytochemical tests, and electron microscopy. Results of preoperative localizing techniques naturally must be viewed in relation to the time in which they were evaluated. Recent data have been published by Rothmund et al. which stem from their international study conducted in 1990 and from another large international review on insulinomas. Norton et al. recently published data for gastrinomas. The figures show positive results for – in ascending order – ultrasound, CT, and angiography. Some authors have reported good results for PTP; however, we consider this technique to be too complicated and time-consuming and our gastroentologists have abandoned it completely.

The main problems associated with endocrine pancreatic tumors are their exact diagnosis and localization. Therapy is aimed at treating the effects of hypersecretion and excessive hormone incretion, as well as the tumor itself under oncological aspects. Surgical management includes the following techniques:

- Enucleation of the adenoma
- Pancreatic tail resection
- Stepwise resection (in some cases as "blind" resection)
- Subtotal pancreatic tail resection
- Partial duodenopancreatectomy or a duodenum-preserving head resection
- Total duodenopancreatectomy
- Reduction of tumor mass by lymph node extirpation
- Total gastrectomy
- Selective proximal vagotomy (in combination with H_2-blockers or omeprazole)
- Arterial occlusion of liver metastases

Extensive surgical exploration is important to localize the tumor. Besides the pancreas, the entire abdominal cavity must be inspected because of the possible presence of ectopic tumors. The importance of the surgeon's experience cannot be stressed enough and, as Jaffe put it, "The surgeon's hand is the best localizing instrument, but it must be an experienced hand!."

This hand should also palpate areas of the pancreas that are not easily accessible, such as the uncinate process. In addition, a major improvement has been made in intraoperative diagnosis: intraoperative ultrasound (IOUS). The new diagnostic technique proves to be extremely valuable when the adenoma has not been localized preoperatively and when there are no reliable intraoperative palpatory findings. IOUS is particularly beneficial in determining the rare occurrence of multiple adenomas (10%). One of our patients had an 8-mm insulinoma, which only ultrasound was able to localize, between the superior mesenteric vein and the isthmus of the pancreas. I was able to enucleate the mass by severing the isthmus and I closed the two sutured areas without anastomosis.

First I should like to address *organic hyperinsulinism*. The following morphological changes must be considered:

- Insulinoma (solitary or multiple)
- Polyhormonal tumor
- Diffuse islet hyperplasia? (occurs only in childhood)
- Focal adenomatosis (very rare)
- Multiple endocrine adenomatosis
- Islet cell carcinoma

The insulinomas found in our patients (n = 52) are distributed evenly throughout the entire pancreas, a phenomenon known from the literature. In addition to the 45 benign lesions, we treated six malignant B cell tumors, one of which was an ectopic adenoma. For insulinomas we proceed as follows. If the adenoma has been localized, it is enucleated or removed by means of pancreatectomy. If the tumor cannot be localized, a "blind" resection is carried out in the form of a distal pancreatectomy or stepwise resection, or by taking portal blood intraoperatively to determine the plasma level of immunoreactive insulin intraoperatively and to measure the radio-immunological insulin level postoperatively. If the tumor can then be found, it is removed. Otherwise, treatment with diazoxide is given and finally a secondary exploratory procedure is performed.

Enucleation should be aimed for whenever possible. This applies particularly to the head of the pancreas, where small and concealed adenomas can be located by means of IOUS with the aid of needle markings after the parenchyma has been incised. Larger adenomas in the tail region usually require a more or less extensive left resection. Blind resection, sometimes in the form of a so-called stepwise resection, which used to be very common in the case of occult adenoma, today no longer seems justified. It would seem better to interrupt the operation after blood samples have been taken from the various segments of the portal system and to repeat it at a later date if necessary. The blind left resection can bring about undesirable results. As an example, in one of our patients in whom a blind distal 80% resection turned out to be unsuccessful, arteriography later revealed a pea-size adenoma at the duodenal wall. This called for a duodenopancreatectomy, which in this particular case meant total pancreatectomy. Such extensive treatment for benign disease is not warranted and today can largely be avoided. A further example shows that the adenoma was found during a second operation in the mesentery after an unsuccessful blind distal pancreas resection.

Thus, a partial duodenopancreatectomy today is reserved for very rare cases. Many years ago, I performed a duodenum-preserving subtotal resection of the head of the pancreas in such a case and found a small insulinoma that was depicted by angiography. This is a technique that Beger reported for chronic pancreatitis.

Two large collective reviews of the literature deal with tumor localization.

We compiled statistics from the literature comprising 2687 cases from 1926 to 1982, which reflect the changes that took place over various time periods and shows that tumor localization improved considerably. The figures also show the ratio of localized tumors to those that were not found until further surgery or were not found at all. The most recent review by Rothmund et al. from 1990, which includes my data, reveals that no tumor was found in only 5.1% of 394 primary operations, while the error rate rose to 28.6% in 44 reoperations.

Our collective review also shows that the surgical techniques used have changed over the years. Left resections have been performed more often than enucleation, while partial duodenopancreatectomy and total pancreatectomy have been reserved for isolated cases. Rothmund's collective review showed a similar trend among their 383 cases. Most of the adenomas located in the head region were removed by enucleation. One out of 10 patients underwent Whipple's operation to remove the insulinoma in the head region. About one-third of these patients could be managed by enucleation. In repeat operations Whipple's resection was done just as often as enucleation to remove insulinomas in the head region. These reoperations ended in total pancreatectomy in five patients, because in the previous operations a portion of the gland had already been removed.

The results reported in the literature show that the percentage of patients cured of organic hyperinsulinism has constantly grown, while the number of cases with persisting hyperglycemia has continuously decreased. Rothmund's latest collective review published in an international report in 1990 shows that in the course of 419 operations on 396 patients only 2.5% could not be classified as cured.

Our own statistics disclose the frequency of the various operations (Table 1) with a total mortality of 4%. In only one of the patients followed-

Table 1. Surgical procedures in insulinomas (Department of Surgery, University of Göttingen, 1969–91)

Insulinomas	55
Benign	49
Malignant	6
Treatment	
Enucleation	18
Pancreatic tail resection	18
50% – subtotal resection	9
Duodenum-preserving head resection	1
Partial duodenopancreatectomy	1
Total pancreatectomy	1
Extirpation of ectopic insulinoma	1
Laparotomy without tumor finding	3
Extirpation of metastases	2
Arterial occlusion or embolisation	3
Removal of insulinoma (total)	49
Operative mortality	2 (4%)

up for years was a persisting hypoglycemia detected, which, however, could be successfully treated with diazoxide. In this case part of an insulinoma located in the head region had remained after enucleation.

Our results are included in the above-mentioned international review published by Rothmund et al. in 1990.

Gastrinoma is the second most common endocrine tumor of the pancreas, which has unique pathophysiological features. This tumor, which is most often cancerous, often metastasizes to the liver. The therapeutic principles described by Zollinger and Ellison in 1955 have changed considerably in the last decade. Today, we know that duodenal tumors are relatively common and that they can be detected by endoscopy and intraoperative duodenotomy. The development of H_2-blockers and especially omeprazole has made it possible to reduce the secretion of gastric acid. The tumor can be localized by means of radiographic techniques, ultrasound, and selective venous catheterization for hormone determination. We know that a relatively high percentage of patients can be cured by removal of the primary tumor if no metastases have arisen. When the gastrinoma cannot be found or when metastasis is suspected, selective proximal vagotomy is performed, which allows the amount of medication necessary to reduce the acid secretion to be decreased. Total gastrectomy, which used to be a common procedure, today is indicated only when the drugs available cannot adequately control the ulceration.

The so-called gastrinoma triangle in the duodenopancreatic region plays a major role in localizing gastrinomas. Furthermore, the entire pancreas, the duodenal wall, the regional lymph nodes, the liver, and the extrapancreatic region must be carefully inspected. Gastrinomas are characteristically small, located outside the pancreas, and occult, as reported by Howard and Passaro in 1989. Kaplan et al., in a recent report, showed in 29 cases that this tumor most often arises in the duodenum, so that this is where a careful search should be undertaken. The authors found 38% of the gastrinomas in the duodenum, 34% in the pancreas (sporadically in 24%, MEN I in 10%), 10% outside the pancreas and duodenum; 17% were not localized. This shows that the tumor could be localized in as many as 82% of the patients.

During the first 10 years of our experience, total gastrectomy was the most common surgical procedure. In subseqent years, tumor removal was preferred, since the hyperacidity could be treated better with drugs or by additional vagotomy. Today, the surgical management of Zollinger-Ellison syndrome offers the following prospects:

- A definitive cure for more patients.
- A potential cure for patients with extrapancreatic and extraintestinal gastrinomas.
- Death from liver or distant metastases is not expected for a period of 25 years, even in patients with lymph node involvement, and the survival rate is the same as in patients without residual tumor.

This favorable prognosis for malignant disease can be demonstrated by a case example: 20 years ago, a 47-year-old woman with a duodenal gastrinoma had been treated by Billroth II gastrectomy prior to diagnosis. After the duodenal gastrinoma had been detected, I performed a partial duodenopancreatectomy and removed a regional lymph-node metastasis along with the primary tumor. The patient has been followed up regularly since then. Her general condition is good and the serum gastrin levels are normal. We can thus expect a permanent cure.

So-called microgastrinomas in the duodenal wall deserve mention. The improved prognosis of duodenal gastrinomas is important because of the frequency of the tumor alone. An occult duodenal gastrinoma can be concealed behind microgastrinomas. According to figures published by Kaplan et al., gastrinomas in this location are apparently less commonly malignant (36%) than the sporadic pancreatic gastrinomas (71%). Malignancy is confirmed by the presence of lymph-node metastases, and even then the prognosis and the resectability are better. Our experience shows that the chances of achieving normal gastrin levels in serum postoperatively are greater after the tumors have been removed. The modern strategy in treating Zollinger-Ellison syndrome entails the possibility of removing the gastrinoma with the prospect of a definitive cure. In addition, it is a matter of discussion whether a selectively proximal vagotomy can reduce the H_2-blocker dosage, which would be relevant in the case of malignant gastrinoma. Total gastrectomy today is indicated only for emergency cases, when compliance is poor, and when severe side effects are caused by the drugs being taken. The rate of cure expected today is derived from a review of the recent literature. A total of 92 patients were evaluated by Norton, Malagelada, Vogel and Ellis and their colleagues. In 32% of them a cure was achieved. Thus, the goal must be to remove the tumor when there is no metastasis and to apply drug therapy in the case of a metastasizing gastrinoma.

Many of the relatively large number of patients seen in Göttingen were treated in the initial era, in which 17 out of 45 patients underwent gastrectomy, some along with tumor removal. In the last few years, conservative treatment modalities have become employed for metastasizing gastrinomas, while partial duodenopancreatectomies were performed in four cases with duodenal gastrinomas (Table 2).

Less common endocrine tumors such as glucagonomas and VIPomas are treated with the same measures.

The metastases of malignant endocrine pancreatic tumors require special drug and surgical measures:

- Palliative tumor enucleation or reduction of the metastasis mass
- Resection of metastases (liver resection or enucleation of isolated metastases)
- Ligation of the hepatic artery

Table 2. Treatment of patients with Zollinger-Ellison syndrome ($n = 45$) at the University of Göttingen, 1969–1991

	Number of patients
Surgical therapy	
Total gastrectomy	17
Partial duodenopancreatectomy	4
Laparotomy	24
Vagotomy	7
Antrectomy + selective gastric vagotomy	1
Postoperative conservative therapy	
(H_2 – blockers, omeprazole)	22

- Embolization of the right or left hepatic artery (with cholecystectomy)
- Drug therapy (diazoxide, propranolol, streptozotocin plus 5-fluorouracil, octreotide)

The effectiveness of these measures can be proven, for example, by the reduction of serum insulin levels after embolization of a hepatic artery. The effect of streptozotocin in the presence of metastasizing VIPomas is demonstrated by the decrease in VIP levels in the serum, reduction of offensive-smelling stools, and regression of liver metastases in CT.

The variable prognosis of metastasizing endocrine pancreatic tumors is illustrated by the case of a woman with a metastasizing insulinoma: 20 years ago, we removed multiple lymph-node metastases from the peripancreatic region and a plum-size tumor from the tail of the pancreas. At the time the liver already showed diffuse metastasis. By repeated treatment with streptozotocin, which was partially administered intraarterially, along with intraoperative embolization of the hepatic artery, the growth of the liver metastases could be checked so that today the patient is alive and in good general condition. Such developments are known from malignant gastrinomas. On the other hand, such tumor may cause death within a very short time.

V. Prevention and Treatment of Complications Following Pancreatic Surgery

Effects of Somatostatin and Octreotide on Pancreatic Function

T.P. Kemmer, M. Büchler, and P. Malfertheiner[1]

Introduction

The tetradecapeptide hormone somatostatin was first detected in the ovine hypothalamus and was described as growth hormone release inhibitor by Brazeau et al. [13]. Numerous studies have been performed to elucidate effects and possible therapeutic uses of this hormone. More recently analogs of somatostatin were synthesized and investigated with different aims in various animal and human studies.

Historical Aspects

In 1973, Brazeau et al. described the structure and de novo synthesis of a peptide extracted from the ovine hypothalamus which inhibited growth hormone release in vitro and named the substance "somatotropin release-inhibiting factor" (SRIF) or somatostatin. Ten years later, a synthesized analog of somatostatin, octreotide, became available for investigational use [5]. Based on the structure of native somatostatin, this compound possessed greater potency and an increased resistance to degradation, resulting in a longer biologic half-life.

Pharmacological Aspects of Somatostatin and Octreotide

Native somatostatin occurs in two biologically active forms, as tetradecapeptide (somatostatin-14) and as a 28-residue peptide (somatostatin-28) containing the somatostatin-14 at its carboxyl terminus [74]. Both are derived from a larger polypeptide precursor, prosomatostatin [71]. More recently, a larger precursor of somatostatin with more than 100 amino acids has been described and called preprosomatostatin [88].

Somatostatin has a widespread tissue distribution, including the central and peripheral nervous system [13, 29, 70], pancreas and gastrointestinal tract [4, 57, 69], thyroid [14], and body fluids, suggesting a mainly paracrine

[1] Universität Ulm, Abteilung Innere Medizin II, Robert-Koch-Straße 8, W-7900 Ulm, FRG

Beger/Büchler/Malfertheiner (Eds.)
Standards in Pancreatic Surgery

rather than endocrine function for the peptide [67]. The greatest amount of somatostatin is contained in the gastrointestinal tract (mucosal and neural cells) and pancreas, with a predominating amount of somatostatin-14 in the upper tract and pancreas and a progressive increase distally in the proportion of somatostatin-28 [4, 69].

Exogenous somatostatin has a very short half-life (0.5–3.0 min) and, therefore, it has to be administered as a continuous intravenous infusion [66]. Liver, pancreas, lungs, and kidneys have been proposed for the clearance site of somatostatin [19, 72, 78, 97].

In the gastrointestinal tract, somatostatin is released from the stomach and duodenum to systemic circulation in response to the presence of luminal nutrients [68, 73]. The stimulation for the release of somatostatin may be carried out through a cyclic adenosine monophosphate (cAMP)-dependent system, activated by epinephrine and beta-adrenergic agonists [104], and through a cAMP-independent system, activated by gastrin and cholecystokinin (CCK) [92]. Pancreatic somatostatin release is stimulated by gastrointestinal peptides like gastric inhibitory polypeptide (GIP) and vasoactive intestinal polypeptide (VIP), glucagon, glucose, and arginine [38, 82].

Octreotide is a synthetic cyclic octapeptide with a 4-amino acid sequence (Phe-Trp-Lys-Thr) in common with somatostatin-14, which is responsible for biologic activity (Fig. 1). In the design of somatostatin analogs it became evident that incorporation of structural elements of natural somatostatin, namely Phe at the NH_2 terminal and especially D-Phe, was very advantageous. By the same consideration, COOH-terminal elongation of the cyclic lead by Ser or Thr further improved activity. The corresponding amino alcohol Thr-ol finally gave the best results, showing that D-Phe and Thr-ol protect the sensitive ends of the molecule in an ideal manner against degrading enzymes [5] (Fig. 1). Octreotide is administered parenterally (intravenously or subcutaneously) because of poor oral absorption, and has an elimination half-life of approximately 90 min [48].

Biologic Functions of Somatostatin and Octreotide

Somatostatin, present in the brain, gut, and pancreas, exerts an inhibitory effect on the release of several pituitary and gut peptides [13, 77, 90] as well as on nutrient absorption and gastrointestinal motility [40, 47, 85]. Somatostatin has also been shown to be a potent inhibitor of gastric and pancreatic secretion [27, 28, 44, 96]. Because of its potent inhibitory action somatostatin was thought to be of benefit in acute pancreatitis (Table 1).

Since the first descriptions of an inhibition of exogenously stimulated gastric and pancreatic secretion and gallbladder contraction by somatostatin in 1975 [9, 21, 49], numerous studies have been conducted into the effect of somatostatin on gastrointestinal functions [3, 60], and the following biologic effects could be determined:

Natural somatostatin-14

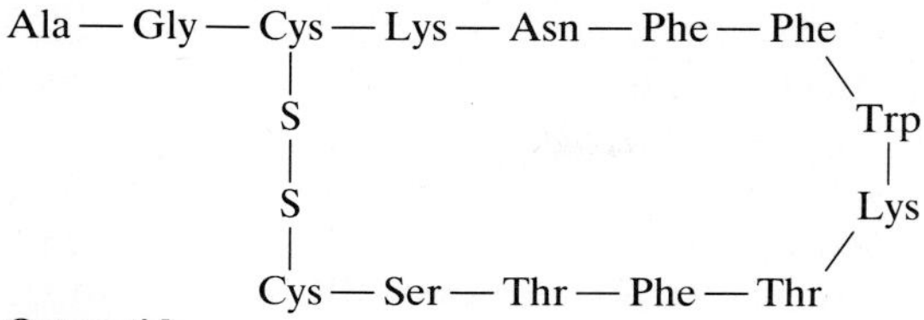

Octreotide

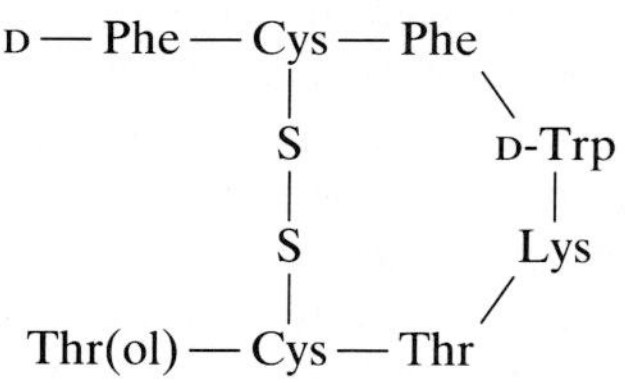

Fig. 1. Amino acid sequence of natural somatostatin-14 and octreotide

Table 1. Somatostatin in the therapy of human acute pancreatitis

Authors [Reference]	Study type	Patients (*n*)	Controls (*n*)	Deaths		Significance
				Patients (*n*)	Controls (*n*)	
Usadel et al. [98]	con/db	36	41	4	7	ns
Schöndube et al. [84]	con	20	23	3	8	ns
Sanchez et al. [80]	con/db	27	20	1	4	ns
Choi et al. [16]	con	35	36	1	2	ns
D'Amico et al. [23]	con	82	82	2	7	ns

(con, controlled study; db, double blind study; ns, not significant.)

- Reduction of gastric acid secretion
- Inhibition of gastric release
- Delay of gastric emptying
- Inhibition of exocrine pancreatic secretion
- Decrease in insulin and glucagon release
- Inhibition of amino acid absorption
- Prolongation of intestinal transit time

Pharamacological dosages of somatostatin have a dual mechanism of action: suppression of the release of regulatory peptides and direct inhibition of target organs.

Somatostatin has a strong effect on various gastrointestinal hormones and on the function of the digestive system. It inhibits exocrine secretion (such as secretion of gastric acid and pepsinogen, pancreatic secretion, bile flow, and ductular hepatic secretion) [31, 68, 89], and neuroendocrine secretion (such as secretion of gastrin, CCK, secretin, VIP, GIP, motilin, acetylcholine, insulin, glucagon, and pancreatic polypeptide) [1, 9–11, 43, 53, 64]. Regarding the effects of somatostatin on the exocrine pancreas, there is general agreement that exogenous administration of the peptide causes marked, dose-dependent inhibition of interdigestive pancreatic enzyme outputs in animals [15, 91, 95], whereas reports of its effects on unstimulated water and bicarbonate secretion are more conflicting [21, 76]. Somatostatin also inhibits stimulated pancreatic enzyme output in animals [15, 45, 91, 95, 99] and humans [34, 35, 51, 65, 76] irrespective of the mode of stimulation [15, 45, 91]. However, volume and bicarbonate secretion are markedly reduced in response to intravenous somatostatin only after endogenous stimulation, but not after exogenous stimulation [15, 35, 45, 91], suggesting an indirect mechanism of action by inhibition of several mediators (e.g., CCK, secretin, and neurotransmitters). This hypothesis is supported by the observation that somatostatin lacks any effect on the exocrine pancreas in vitro [62].

Reports of the effect of somatostatin on pancreatic bicarbonate and fluid secretion have been conflicting, with both an inhibitory effect and no effect being reported [32]. The effects on pancreatic output may be mediated by the inhibition of CCK release [52, 93] or by the inhibition of nervous transmission, since somatostatin has been shown to inhibit carbachol-induced pancreatic secretion [49]. A recent study [33] also showed that the effect of somatostatin was due to inhibition of amino acid uptake by acinar cells. Other gastrointestinal effects are the reduction of gastric emptying, duodenal motility, and gallbladder contraction [11, 21]. Splanchnic blood flow is reduced during continuous intravenous somatostatin infusion [79]. A cytoprotective, systemic organoprotection and vasculoprotection by somatostatin has also been described [101].

In recent years, several analogs of somatostatin tested in animal studies [46] have been shown to exert more specific effects with regard to the potency and pattern of activity on different target organs than the naturally occurring hormone [5, 54, 100, 102]. Such an analog which has recently become available for clinical use is octreotide (SMS 201-995). Octreotide can be administered by subcutaneous injection [59] and is a potent inhibitor of endocrine and exocrine pancreatic secretion.

Therapeutic Studies with Somatostatin and Octreotide

Somatostatin has been used in the treatment of variceal hemorrhage [39], diarrhea due to carcinoid syndrome and VIP-secreting tumors [18], and enterocutaneous fistula [36].

In 1975, Creutzfeldt et al. [21] reported that in man somatostatin inhibits the pancreatic juice and enzyme secretion and gallbladder contraction induced by secretin and CCK-pancreozymin administration. Dollinger et al. [27] showed that somatostatin did not inhibit secretin-stimulated volume and bicarbonate secretion. Somatostatin, however, reduced pancreatic enzyme secretion stimulated by CCK-pancreozymin. Because of its additional ability to inhibit circulating plasma gastrin and gastric secretion [2, 9] as well as to reduce requirements for exogenous insulin [8, 61] it has been suggested as a useful therapeutic adjunct in the treatment of acute pancreatitis [27, 56] and in the prevention of post endoscopic retrograde cholangiopancreatography (ERCP) pancreatitis [12].

The potential usefulness of somatostatin in acute pancreatitis is based on its inhibitory effect on exocrine pancreatic function by suppressing glandular secretion and the release of CCK and gastrin. Several studies have been published on the effects of somatostatin in experimentally induced acute pancreatitis and their results are conflicting [6, 24, 26, 50, 58, 83, 86].

Although the use of somatostatin in the treatment of human acute pancreatitis was introduced more than 10 years ago, not many controlled clinical trials have been carried out with the aim of evaluating the efficacy of this therapy. Therapeutic trials with somatostatin in acute pancreatitis, however, have failed to confirm a significant benefit (Table 1).

The somatostatin analog octreotide has proven to be therapeutically useful in the closure of pancreatic and high-output small-bowel fistulas [20, 25, 87]. Several other indications for possible treatment with octreotide such as gastrointestinal hemorrhage, pancreatitis, short-bowel syndrome, gastroenteropancreatic tumors, and diarrhea syndromes have been or are currently being evaluated in clinical studies [17, 30, 75, 81, 94, 103].

Octreotide was shown to exert a significant inhibitory effect on exocrine pancreatic function in animals [46]. Human studies [7, 21, 22, 37, 41, 42, 52, 103] indicate that octreotide inhibits basal and stimulated pancreatic enzyme secretion, and this effect diminishes with time [37, 52]. Octreotide also inhibits the release of pancreatic polypeptide, a hormone that is known to decrease pancreatic enzyme and bicarbonate secretion.

Studies in man have shown a significant inhibition of pancreatic secretion by octreotide, but the experimental conditions and doses as well as the route of administration were different (Table 2). Köhler et al. [42] found the lowest effective dose of octreotide to be 27 ng/kg per hour to inhibit secretin (250 ng/kg per hour) plus cerulein (25 ng/kg per hour) stimulated pancreatic secretion. This finding was confirmed and extended in a recent study by Kemmer et al. [41] who found that 5 μg/h octreotide

Table 2. Inhibition of exocrine pancreatic secretion by octreotide

Authors [Reference]	Species	Dosage	Percentage of enzyme inhibition of secretion
Köhler et al. [42]	man	27 ng/kg per hour i.v.	80
Creutzfeldt et al. [22]	man	2 × 25 μg/day s.c.	80
Lembcke et al. [52]	man	2 × 25 μg/day s.c.	80
Baxter et al. [7]	pig man	200 μg/h i.v. 100 μg s.c.	100 75
Konturek et al. [46]	dog	2 μg/kg per hour i.v.	80
Kemmer et al. [41]	man	5 μg/h i.v.	80

Table 3. Long-term effects of octreotide treatment in man

Authors [Reference]	Dosage	Duration	Inhibition (%)
Creutzfeldt et al. [22]	2 × 25 μg s.c.	7 days	50
Lembcke et al. [52]	2 × 25 μg s.c.	7 days	50

was the lowest effective dose to inhibit maximally stimulated pancreatic secretion by secretin (290 ng/kg per hour) plus cerulein (120 ng/kg per hour). The knowledge of the lowest effective dose of octreotide is of practical value if one considers the tachyphylaxis after long-term treatment with octreotide reported in several studies [22, 37, 52] (Table 3).

References

1. Alberti KG, Christensen NJ, Christensen SE et al. (1973) Inhibition of insulin secretion by somatostatin. Lancet 2:1299–1301
2. Arnold R, Creutzfeldt W (1975) Hemmung der Pentagastrin-induzierten Säuresekretion des Magens beim Menschen durch Somatostatin. Dtsch Med Wschr 100:1014–1016
3. Arnold R, Lankisch PG (1980) Somatostatin and the gastrointestinal tract. Clin Gastroenterol 9:733–753
4. Baldissera FGA, Holst JJ, Jensen SL, Krarup T (1985) Distribution and molecular forms of peptides containing somatostatin immunodeterminants in extracts from the entire gastrointestinal tract of man and pig. Biochim Biophys Acta 838:132–143
5. Bauer W, Briner U, Doepfner W, Haller R, Huguenin R, Marbach P, Petcher TJ, Pless J (1982) SMS 201-995: A very potent and selective octapeptide analogue of somatostatin with prolonged action. Life Sci 31:1133–1140

6. Baxter JN, Jenkins SA, Day DW et al. (1985) Effects of somatostatin and a long-acting somatostatin analogue on the prevention and treatment of experimentally-induced acute pancreatitis in the rat. Br J Surg 72:382–385
7. Baxter JN, Ellenbogen S, Roberts N, Mackie CR, Jenkins SA (1988) The effects of a somatostatin analogue, SMS 201-995, on pancreatic secretion in the pig and in man. Surg Res Comm 4:215–228
8. Besser GM, Mortimer CH, McNeilly AS, Thorner MO, Batistoni GA, Bloom SR, Kastrup KW, Hanssen KF, Hall R, Coy DH, Kastin AJ, Schally AV (1974) Long-term infusion of growth hormone release inhibiting hormone in acromegaly: effects on pituitary and pancreatic hormones. Br Med J 4:622–627
9. Bloom SR, Mortimer CH, Thorner MO, Besser GM, Hall R, Gomez-Pan A, Roy M, Russell RCG, Coy DH, Kastin AJ, Schally AV (1974) Inhibition of gastrin and gastric acid secretion by growth-hormone release-inhibiting hormone. Lancet 2:1106–1109
10. Bloom SR, Ralphs KN, Besser GM et al. (1975) Effect of somatostatin on motilin levels and gastric emptying. Gut 16:834
11. Boden G, Sivitz MC, Owen OE, Essa-Koumar N, Landor JH (1975) Somatostatin suppresses secretin and pancreatic exocrine secretion. Science 190:163–165
12. Bordas JM, Toledo V, Mondelo F, Rodes J (1988) Prevention of pancreatic reactions by bolus somatostatin administration in patients undergoing endoscopic retrograde cholangiopancreatography. Horm Res 29:106–108
13. Brazeau P, Vale W, Burgus R, Ling N, Butcher M, Rivier J, Guillemin R (1973) Hypothalamic polypeptide that inhibits the secretion of immunoreactive growth hormone. Science 179:77–79
14. Buffa R, Chayvialle JA, Fontana P, Usellini L, Capella C, Solcia E (1979) Parafollicular cells of rabbit thyroid store both calcitonin and somatostatin and resemble gut D cells ultrastructurally. Histochemistry 62:281–288
15. Chariot J, Roze C, Vaille C, Debray C (1978) Effects of somatostatin on the external secretion of the pancreas of the rat. Gastroenterology 75:832–837
16. Choi TK, Mok F, Zhan WH, Fan ST, Lai ECS, Wong J (1989) Somatostatin in the treatment of acute pancreatitis: a prospective randomised controlled trial. Gut 30:223–227
17. Christiansen J, Yotis A (1986) The role of somatostatin and a long-acting analogue, SMS 201-995, in acute bleeding due to peptic ulceration. Scand J Gastroenterol 21[Suppl 119]:109–114
18. Comi RJ, Maton PN, Go VLW (1989) Somaostatin and somatostatin analogue (SMS 201-995) in treatment of hormonesecreting tumors of the pituitary and gastrointestinal tract and non-neoplastic diseases of the gut. Ann Intern Med 110:35–50
19. Conlon JM, Whittaker J, Hammond V, Alberti K (1981) Metabolism of somatostatin and its analogues by the liver. Biochim Biophys Acta 677:234–242
20. Cooper MM, Wright FH, Smith JL, Corry RJ (1989) Successful treatment of a high-output fistula with a somatostatin analogue following pancreas transplantation. Transplant Proc 21:3738–3741
21. Creutzfeldt W, Lankisch PG, Fölsch UR (1975) Hemmung der Sekretin- und Cholecystokinin-Pankreozymin-induzierten Saft- und Enzymsekretion des Pankreas und der Gallenblasenkontraktion beim Menschen durch Somatostatin. Dtsch Med Wochenschr 100:1135–1138
22. Creutzfeldt W, Lembcke B, Fölsch UR, Schlieser S, Koop I (1987) Effect of somatostatin analogue (SMS 201-995, Sandostatin) on pancreatic secretion in humans. Am J Med 82[Suppl 5B]:49–54
23. D'Amico D, Favia G, Biasiato R, Casaccia M, Falcone F, Fersini M, Marrano D, Napolitano F, Oliviero S, Rodolico A (1990) The use of somatostatin in acute pancreatitis – results of a multicenter trial. Hepatogastroenterol 37:92–98
24. Degertekin H, Ertan A, Akdamar K et al. (1985) Effects of somatostatin and a somatostatin agonist on diet-induced pancreatitis in mice. Peptides 6:1245–1247

25. Delbert Kwan BA, Aufses AH (1989) Short-term administration of SMS 201-995 in the management of an external pancreatic fistula. Am J Gastroenterol 84:326–328
26. De Rai P, Franciosi C, Confalonieri GM et al. (1988) Effects of somatostatin on acute pancreatitis induced in rats by injection of taurocholate and trypsin into a temporarily closed duodenal loop. Int J Pancreatol 3:367–374
27. Dollinger HC, Raptis S, Pfeiffer EF (1976) Effects of somatostatin on exocrine and endocrine pancreatic function stimulated by intestinal hormones in man. Horm Metab Res 8:74–78
28. Domschke S, Domschke W, Rosch W (1977) Inhibition by somatostatin of secretin-stimulated pancreatic secretion in man: a study with pure pancreatic juice. Scand J Gastroenterol 12:59–63
29. Elde R, Hökfelt T, Johansson O, Schultzberg M, Efendic S, Luft R (1978) Cellular localization of somatostatin. Metabolism 27[Suppl 1]:1151–1159
30. Fedorak RN (1989) Long acting somatostatin analogue: Clinical potential for gastrointestinal disease. Can J Gastroenterol 3:77–81
31. Gomez-Pan A, Reed JD, Albinus M et al. (1975) Direct inhibition of gastric acid and pepsin secretion by growth-hormone release-inhibiting hormone in cats. Lancet 1:888–890
32. Gullo L, Priori P, Scorpignato C et al. (1987) Effect of somatostatin-14 on pure human pancreatic secretion. Dig Dis Sci 32:1065–1070
33. Gullo L, Pezzelli R, Barbara L (1989) Effect of somatostatin in plasma amino acids uptake by human pancreas. Gastroenterology 97:732–736
34. Gyr K, Beglinger C, Köhler E, Tratzl U, Keller U, Bloom SR (1987) Circulating somatostatin – a physiological regulator of pancreatic function? J Clin Invest 79:1595–1600
35. Hanssen LE, Hanssen F, Myren J (1977) Inhibition of secretin release and pancreatic bicarbonate secretion by somatostatin infusion in man. Scand J Gastroenterol 12:391–394
36. Hild P, Dobroschke J, Henneking K et al. (1986) Treatment of enterocutaneous fistulas with somatostatin. Lancet 2:626
37. Hopman WPM, van Liessum PA, Pieters GFFM, Smals AGH, Tangerman A, Jansen JBMJ, Rosenbusch G, Lamers CBHW, Kloppenborg PWC (1990) Pancreatic exocrine and gallbladder function during long-term treatment with octreotide (SMS 201-995). Digestion 45[Suppl 1]:72–76
38. Ipp E, Dobbs RE, Arimura A, Vale W, Harris V, Unger RH (1977) Release of immunoreactive somatostatin from the pancreas in response to glucose, amino acids, pancreozymin-cholecystokinin, and tolbutamide. J Clin Invest 60:760–765
39. Jenkins SA, Baxter JN, Corbett W et al. (1985) A prospective randomised controlled clinical trial comparing somatostatin and vasopressin in controlling acute variceal hemorrhage. Br Med J 290:275–278
40. Johansson C, Wisen O, Efendic S, Uvnas-Wallensten K (1981) Effects of somatostatin on gastrointestinal propagation and absorption of oral glucose in man. Digestion 22:126–137
41. Kemmer TP, Malfertheiner P, Büchler M, Frieß H, Meschenmoser L, Ditschuneit H (1992) Inhibition of human exocrine pancreatic secretion by the long-acting somatostatin analogue octreotide (SMS 201-995). Aliment Pharmacol Ther 6:41–50
42. Köhler E, Beglinger C, Dettwiler S, Whitehouse I, Gyr K (1986) Effect of a new somatostatin analogue on pancreatic function in healthy volunteers. Pancreas 1:154–159
43. Koerker DJ, Ruch W, Chideckel E et al. (1974) Somatostatin: hypothalamic inhibitor of the endocrine pancreas. Science 184:482–484
44. Konturek SJ, Tasler J, Obtulowiew W (1976) Effect of growth hormone release inhibiting hormone on hormones stimulating exocrine panceatic secretion. J Clin Invest 58:1–6

45. Konturek SJ, Cieszkowski M, Bilski J, Konturek J, Bielanski W, Schally AV (1985) Effects of cyclic hexapeptide analogue of somatostatin on pancreatic secretion in dogs. Proc Soc Exp Biol Med 178:68–72
46. Konturek SJ, Bilski J, Jaworek J, Tasler J, Schally AV (1988) Comparison of somatostatin and its highly potent hexa- and octapeptide analogues on exocrine and endocrine pancreatic secretion. Proc Soc Exp Biol Med 187:241–249
47. Krejs GJ, Browne R, Raskin P (1980) Effect of intravenous somatostatin on jejunal absorption of glucose, amino acids, water and electrolytes. Gastroenterology 78:26–31
48. Kutz K, Nuesch E, Rosenthaler J (1986) Pharmacokinetics of SMS 201-995 in healthy subjects. Scand J Gastroenterol 21[Suppl 119]:65–72
49. Lankisch PG, Arnold R, Creutzfeldt W (1975) Wirkung von Somatostatin auf die Betazol-stimulierte Magensekretion und die Carbachol-stimulierte Pankreassekretion und die Gallenblasenkontraktion des Menschen. Dtsch Med Wochenschr 100:1797–1800
50. Lankisch PG, Koop H, Winckler K, Fölsch UR, Creutzfeldt W (1977) Somatostatin therapy of acute experimental pancreatitis. Gut 18:713–716
51. Layer P, Boekstegers A, Müller MK, Lötte A, Goebell H (1987) Cyclical interdigestive pancreatic secretion in response to physiologic doses of somatostatin-14 in humans. Gastroenterology 92:1495
52. Lembcke B, Creutzfeldt W, Schlieser S, Ebert R, Shaw C, Koop I (1987) Effect of the somatostatin analogue Sandostatin (SMS 201-995) on gastrointestinal, pancreatic and biliary function and hormone release in normal men. Digestion 36:108–124
53. Lennon JR, Sircos W, Bloom SR et al. (1975) Investigation and treatment of a recurrent vipoma. Gut 16:821–822
54. Lightman SL, Fox P, Dunne MJ (1986) The effect of SMS 201-995, a long-acting somatostatin analogue, on anterior pituitary function in healthy male volunteers. Scand J Gastroenterol 21[Suppl 119]:84–95
55. Lin TM, Evans DC, Shaar CJ, Root MA (1983) Action of somatostatin on stomach, pancreas, gastric mucosal blood flow and hormones. Am J Physiol 244:G40–G45
56. Limberg B, Kommerell B (1980) Treatment of acute pancreatitis with somatostatin. N Engl J Med 303:284
57. Luft R, Efendic S, Hökfelt T, Johansson O, Arimura A (1974) Immunohistochemical evidence for the localization of somatostatin-like immunoreactivity in a cell population of the pancreatic islets. Med Biol 52:428–430
58. Mann NS, Mauch MJ (1981) Inhibitory effect of cycloheximide, somatostatin and 5-aza cytidine on acute experimental pancreatitis. Am J Proctology 32:24–32
59. Maton PN, O'Dorisio TM, Howe BA, McArthur KE, Howard JM, Cherner JA, Malarkey TB, Collen MJ, Gardner JD, Jensen RT (1985) Effect of a long-acting somatostatin analogue (SMS 201-995) in a patient with pancreatic cholera. N Engl J Med 312:17–21
60. McIntosh CHS (1985) Gastrointestinal somatostatin: distribution, secretion and physiological significance. Life Sci 37:2043–2058
61. Meissner C, Thum C, Beischer W, Winkler G, Schröder KE, Pfeiffer EF (1975) The antidiabetic action of somatostatin – assessed by artificial pancreas. Diabetes 24:988–996
62. Müller MK, Kessel B, Hütt T, Layer P, Goebell H (1988) Effects of somatostatin-14 on gastric and pancreatic responses to hormonal and neural stimulation using an isolated perfused stomach and pancreas preparation. Pancreas 3:303–310
63. Ohe M, Layer P, Wollny C, Beglinger C, Goebell H (1989) Effects of physiological doses of somatostatin-28 on cyclical interdigestive pancreatic secretion and upper gastrointestinal motility in humans. Gastroenterology 96:A374

64. Orci L, Baetens D, Ravazzola M, Stefan Y, Malaisse-Lagae F (1976) Pancreatic polypiptide and glucagon: non-random distribution in pancreatic islets. Life Sci 19:1811–1815
65. O'Shaughnessy DJ, Long RG, Adrian TE et al. (1985) Somatostatin-14 modulates postprandial glucose levels and release of gastrointestinal and pancreatic hormones. Digestion 31:234–242
66. Patel YC, Wheatley T (1983) In vivo and in vitro plasma disappearance and metabolism of somatostatin-28 and somatostatin-14 in the rat. Endocrinology 112:220–225
67. Pearse AG (1980) The APUD concept and hormone production. Clin Endocrinol Metab 9:211–222
68. Penman E, Wass JAH, Medback S et al. (1981) Response of circulating immunoreative somatostatin to nutritional stimuli in normal subjects. Gastroenterology 81:692–699
69. Penman E, Wass JAH, Butler MG et al. (1983) The distribution and characterization of immunoreactive somatostatin in human gastrointestinal tract. Regulatory Peptides 7:53–65
70. Pevet P, Ebels I, Swaab DF, Mud MT, Arimura A (1980) Presence of AVT-alpha-MSH- LHRH- and somatostatin-like compounds in the rat pineal gland and their relationship with the UMO5R pineal fraction. An immunochemical study. Cell Tissue Res 206:341–353
71. Pless J, Bauer W, Briner U, Doepfner W, Marbach P, Maurer R, Petcher TJ, Reubi J-C, Vonderscher J (1986) Chemistry and pharmacology of SMS 201-995, a long-acting octapeptide analogue of somatostatin. Scand J Gastroenterol 21[Suppl 119]:54–64
72. Polonsky KS, Jaspan JB, Berelowitz M, Emmanouel DS, Dhorajiwala J (1981) Hepatic and renal metabolism of somatostatin-like immunoreactivity. J Clin Invest 68:1149–1157
73. Polonsky KS, Shoelson SE, Docherty HM (1983) Plasma somatostatin-28 increases in response to feeding in man. J Clin Invest 71:1514–1518
74. Pradayrol L, Jornvall J, Mutt V, Ribet A (1980) N-terminally extended somatostatin: The primary structure of somatostatin-28. FEBS Lett 109:55–58
75. Primrose JN (1990) Octreotide in the treatment of the dumping syndrome. Digestion 45[Suppl 1]:49–59
76. Regal H, Fink M, Luger T, Ogris E, Irsigler K (1977) Suppression der endokrinen und exokrinen Pankreasfunktion durch Somatostatin beim Menschen unter Stimulation durch Sekretin und Cholecystokinin-Pankreozymin. Wien Klin Wochenschr 89:580–586
77. Reichlin S (1983) Somatostatin. N Engl J Med 309:1556–1563
78. Ruggere MD, Patel Y (1985) Somatostatin metabolism by the isolated rat lung. Endocrinology 117:1870–1873
79. Samnegard H, Tyden G, Thulin L, Friman L, Uden R (1980) Effect of somatostatin on regional splanchnic blood flows in man. Angiographic studies. Acta Chir Scand [Suppl] 500:71–73
80. Sanchez D, Sanchez A, Zurdo JR, Arriaza R, Chimpen V, Portugal J (1988) Pancreatitis aguda: Estudio clinico y terapeutico. Valoracion de la eficacia de Somatostatina. Ann Med Intern 3:40
81. Schally AV, Cai R-Z, Torres-Aleman I, Redding TW, Szoke B, Fu D, Hierowski MT, Colaluca J, Konturek SJ (1986) Endocrine, gastrointestinal and antitumor acitivity of somatostatin analogues. In: Moody TW (ed) Neural and endocrine peptides and receptors. Plenum, New York, pp 73–88
82. Schauder P, McIntosh C, Arends J, Arnold R, Frerichs H, Creutzfeldt W (1977) Somatostatin and insulin release from isolated rat pancreatic islets in response to D-glucose, 1-leucine, alpha-ketoisocaproic acid or D-glyceraldehyde: evidence for a regulatory role of adenosine-3′,5′-cyclic monophosphate. Biochem Biophys Res Commun 75:630–635

83. Schlarman DE, Beinfeld MC, Andrus C, Kaminski DL (1987) Effects of somatostatin on acute canine experimental pancreatitis. Intern J Pancreatol 2:247–255
84. Schöndube S, Klempa I, Baca I, Menzel J (1987) Nekrotisierende Pankreatitis – ein Beitrag zur studiengerechten operativen Therapie (abstract). Österreichische Gesellschaft für Chirurgie, Lanz
85. Schusdziarra V (1980) Somatostatin – a regulatory modulator connecting nutrient entry and metabolism. Horm Metab Res 12:563–577
86. Schwedes U, Althoff PH, Klempa I et al. (1979) Effect of somatostatin on bile-induced acute hemorrhagic pancreatitis in the dog. Horm Metab Res 11:655–661
87. Scott NA, Finnegan S, Irving MH (1990) Octreotide and gastrointestinal fistulae. Digestion 45[Suppl 1]:66–71
88. Shen LP, Pictet R, Rutter W (1982) Human somatostatin I: Sequence of the cDNA. Proc Natl Acad Sci USA 79:4575–4579
89. Seal A, Yamada T, Debas H et al. (1982) Somatostatin-14 and -28: Clearance and potency on gastric function in dogs. Am J Physiol 243:G97–102
90. Siler TM, Yen SSC, Vale W, Guillemin R (1974) Inhibition by somatostatin on the release of TSH induced in man by thyrotropin-releasing factor. J Clin Endocr Metab 38:742–745
91. Singh M (1986) Effect of somatostatin on amylase secretion from in vivo and in vitro rat pancreas. Dig Dis Sci 31:506–512
92. Soll AH, Amirian DA, Park J, Elashoff JD, Yamada T (1985) Cholecystokinin potently releases somatostatin from canine fundic mucosal cells in short-term culture. Am J Physiol 248:G569–573
93. Stöckmann F, Richter G, Lembcke B, Conlon JM, Creutzfeldt W (1986) Long-term treatment of patients with endocrine gastrointestinal tumours with the somatostatin analogue SMS 201-995. Scand J Gastroenterol 21[Suppl 119]:230–237
94. Stöckmann F, Creutzfeldt W (1988) Behandlung gastrointestinaler neuroendokriner Tumoren mit dem Somatostatin-Analog Octreotide (Sandostatin). Z Gastroenterol 26:665–675
95. Susini C, Esteve JP, Bommelaer G, Vaysse N, Ribet A (1978) Inhibition of exocrine pancreatic secretion by somatostatin in dogs. Digestion 18:384–393
96. Susini C, Esteve JP, Vaysse N, Pradayrol L, Ribet A (1980) Somatostatin 28: Effects on exocrine pancreatic secretion in conscious dogs. Gastroenterology 79:720–724
97. Taborsky G, Ensinck J (1983) Extraction of somatostatin by the pancreas. Endocrinology 112:303–307
98. Usadel KH, Überla KK, Leuschner U (1985) Treatment of acute pancreatitis with somatostatin: Results of the multicenter double-blind trial (APTS-Study). Dig Dis Sci 30:992
99. Vaysse N, Chayvialle A, Pradayrol L et al. (1981) Somatostatin-28: comparison with somatostatin-14 for plasma kinetics and low-dose effects on the exocrine pancreas in dogs. Gastroenterology 81:700–706
100. Veber DF, Freidinger RM, Perlow S, Paleveda WJ, Holly FW, Strachan RG, Nutt RF, Arison BH, Homnick C, Randall WC, Glitzer MS, Saperstein R, Hirschmann R (1981) A potent cyclic hexapeptide analogue of somatostatin. Nature 292:55–58
101. Wdowinski JM, Schwedes U, Faulstich H et al. (1981) Beneficial effect of somatostatin in phalloidin-intoxicated rats. Influence on survival rate, biochemical and morphological data, and ^{3}H-demethyl-phalloin absorption rate by the liver. Res Exp Med 178:155–163
102. Whitehouse I, Beglinger C, Fried M, Gyr K (1984) The effect of an octapeptide somatostatin analogue (SMS 201-995) and somatostatin-14 (SST-14) on pentagastrin-stimulated gastric acid secretion: A comparative study in man. Hepatogastroenterol 31:227–229

103. Williams ST, Woltering EA, O'Dorisio TM, Fletcher WS (1989) Effect of octreotide acetate on pancreatic exocrine function. Am J Surg 157:459–462
104. Yamada T, Soll AH, Park J, Elashoff J (1984) Autonomic regulation of somatostatin release. Studies with primary cultures of canine fundic mucosal cells. Am J Physiol 247:G567–573

Exocrine and Endocrine Pancreatic Secretion Following Pancreatic Resection

I. Klempa,[1] I. Baca,[1] J. Menzel,[1] H. Morr,[1] and V. Schuszdiarra[2]

Introduction

The Whipple procedure, i.e. a partial duodeno-pancreatectomy, is the gold standard in the operative treatment of cancer of the pancreatic head aiming at cure [15, 17]. In spite of recent advances in operative techniques and postoperative intensive care, perioperative morbidity and mortality remain high [17]. Tryptic activity of the pancreatic remnant may lead to postoperative pancreatitis or breakdown of the anastomosis with fistula formation. It is therefore necessary to look for a therapeutic principle which inhibits the exocrine pancreatic secretion before, during, and after surgery. Atropin, aprotinin, glucagon, somatostatin, and calcitonin have been under investigation, but results have not been very satisfactory and remain under discussion [7, 8, 13]. Numerous studies report on the effects of somatostatin on the endocrine and exocrine pancreatic function [2, 3, 14]. With respect to the clinical course after pancreatic surgery, positive results have been reported with the administration of somatostatin [7, 8]. However, almost nothing is known about the exocrine and endocrine function of the pancreatic remnant after a Whipple procedure under somatostatin.

We present here the results of our study on these topics. The metabolic effects of somatostatin in the postoperative course were studied because somatostatin is an inhibitor of the release of insulin and glucagon, which act in protein metabolism. In addition, we studied the excretory function of the pancreatic remnant after stimulation and its reaction to a somatostatin bolus, after surgery, and after continuous postoperative somatostatin administration.

Patients and Methods

Thirty patients entered this prospective, randomized trial, suffering either from carcinoma of the head of the pancreas or of the papilla of Vater. After

[1] Klinik für Allgemein- und Gefäßchirurgie (Direktor: Prof. Dr. med. I. Klempa), Zentralkrankenhaus St.-Jürgen-Straße, W-2800 Bremen, FRG

[2] II. Medizinische Klinik (Direktor: Prof. Dr. med. M. Classen) der Technischen Universität München, W-8000 München, FRG

Beger/Büchler/Malfertheiner (Eds.)
Standards in Pancreatic Surgery

laparotomy the decision was made whether partial duodenopancreatectomy with curative intent was feasible or not. This was followed by randomization to receiving or not receiving somatostatin prior to the gross dissection of the gland; 15 patients received somatostatin and 15 did not. (The hormone was administered continuously at 250 μg/h until the end of the 6th postoperative day.) As the Table 1 shows, there were no significant differences between the groups as to indication for resection, mean age, sex, type of operation, duration of the operation, or mean intraoperative blood loss. Six of the 30 patients dropped out of the study, three from each group. In four patients we noted a dislocation or occlusion of the small silicone catheter which was placed in the pancreatic duct; this made collection of pancreatic fluid impossible. Two patients suffered from severe chronic fibrosing pancreatitis and were therefore excluded.

The operative procedure is described elsewhere. We estimate that about 50% of the gland was resected. In all cases reconstruction was carried out with an end-to-end pancreatico-jejunostomy. Before this, a small silicone catheter (inner diameter 2 mm) with multiple perforations at the end was put into the duct of the pancreatic rest. This catheter was brought out through the jejunum and through the abdominal wall by a stab incision (Fig. 1).

Postoperatively, total parenteral nutrition was instituted. Fluids and electrolytes were given according to individual needs, while administration of carbohydrates and amino acids was standardized: 30 g/kg body weight carbohydrates and 1 g/kg amino acids per day.

Table 1. Patient characteristics

	Group A (n = 12)	Group B (n = 12)
Operative indication		
Pancreatic cancer	10	9
Ampullary cancer	2	3
Mean age	54 ± 7	59 ± 8
Sex		
Men	8	7
Women	4	5
Symptoms		
Jaundice	8	7
Weight loss	9	7
Palpable gallbladder	6	5
Diabetes mellitus	2	3
Operative procedure		
Partial pancreatectomy/gastrectomy	12	12
Operative data		
Operative time (h)	2.7 ± 0.5	2.9 ± 0.9
Intraoperative blood transfusion (ml)	2000 ± 800	1800 ± 700

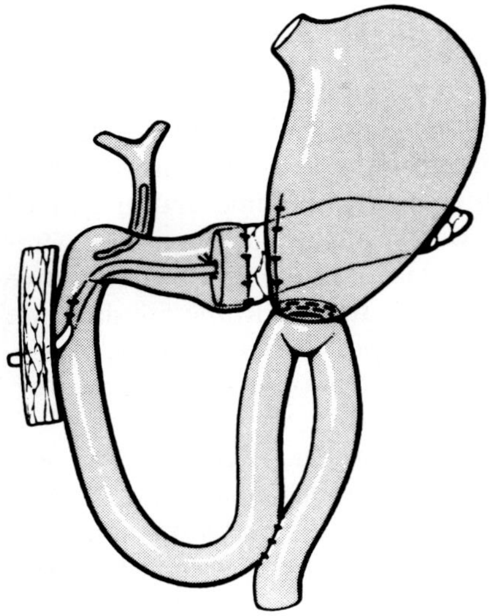

Fig. 1. Reconstruction of the upper abdomen after a partial duodeno-pancreatectomy. A small silicone catheter is put into the duct of the pancreatic remnant and brought out through the abdominal wall

Pancreatic juice was collected at intervals of 24 h and frozen until analysis. Amylase, lipase, bicarbonate, and protein contents were measured. Bicarbonate was measured in only five patients of each group. All analyses were done with commercially available kits. The pancreatic fluid collected over the period of the first 4 postoperative days was taken as basal because oral intake was not allowed before the 5th postoperative day.

To examine the effect of somatostatin on the stimulated secretion of the pancreatic remnant, we injected secretin (1 IU/kg per hour) and cerulein (25 μg/kg per hour) over a total period of 150 min on the 7th postoperative day. After 60 min we gave somatostatin, for a first period of 30 min at 4 μg/h and for a second period of a further 30 min at 8 μg/h. During the complete time of testing, pancreatic juice was collected every 15 min for analysis of amylase, lipase, bicarbonate, and protein. Daily routine laboratory tests included insulin, glucagon, cortisol, electrolytes, amylase, lipase, serum d-aspartat aminotranspherase (AST), serum alanin-aminotranspherase (ALT), cholinesterase, and serum protein. Urine was collected at 24-h samples. Analysis was carried out for amylase, lipase, epinephrine, norepinephrine, glucose, and blood urea nitrogen. The daily nitrogen balance was calculated.

The secretion of the pancreas was calculated from the 24-h samples after stimulation from two 15-min samples, following one after the other. Means and standard deviations were calculated from these individual values. For testing of significance a two-tailed t test for unpaired samples was used. Significance was taken as $p < 0.05$.

Results

Somatostatin inhibited baseline pancreatic secretion during the postoperative period. Secretory volume and content of amylase and, more so, that of lipase and protein were inhibited after somatostatin. A significant reduction was observed during the first 2 days with respect to volume and enzymatic content. Obviously, the inhibitory effect was strongest at that time. After somatostatin, bicarbonate production was reduced on the 2nd postoperative day (3.6 ± 1.1 versus 5.2 ± 1.2 mmol/day). From the 3rd to the 5th days, we observed a continuous increase in the total output in both groups. A significant reduction in output over the complete time of observation, however, was found only for lipase (Fig. 2).

After stimulation with cerulein and secretin pancreas secretion was inhibited by somatostatin as well. Secretory volume and lipase and amylase activities were inhibited after 60–90 min with 4 μg/kg per hour and after 90–120 min with 8 μg/kg per hour somatostatin. There was a tendency toward a dose-dependent inhibitory effect (Fig. 3).

A marked increase in serum amylase levels was seen on the 1st and 2nd postoperative days. However, this change was not significant either in serum or in urine. The same was true for lipase. This may point to the fact that no postoperative pancreatitis occurred in either group. Transaminase levels were lower in the somatostatin group, with significant results for AST on the 1st and 2nd, for ALT from the 3rd to the 5th postoperative days (Fig. 4). In summary, we saw an early normalization for AST, ALT, and cholinesterase.

No differences were found in glucose levels between the two groups, although two patients in the somatostatin group needed continuous infusion of insulin during total parenteral nutrition. Measuring epinephrine norepinephrine, and glucose in urine did not reveal any differences between the two groups.

The releasing of insulin and glucagon was inhibited most strongly in the early postoperative period up to the 5th day after operation. Glucagon was more strongly inhibited, leading to a shift in the insulin-glucagon ratio. This was also significant after the 3rd postoperative day with 5 ± 2 versus 9 ± 4 mol/mol (Fig. 5).

The nitrogen balance was positive as early as on the 2nd postoperative day in the group with somatostatin. Without somatostatin this did not occur before the 4th day. Over all, the nitrogen balance was definitely better with somatostatin, with a significant difference on the 3rd and 4th postoperative days (Fig. 6).

No patient died in the somatostatin-treated group. Among those without somatostatin there was one death from a bleeding complication and a second-look procedure of the pancreaticojejunal anastomosis.

The rate of perioperative complications was higher without somatostatin. The incidence of pancreatic fistula formation was twice as high and that of

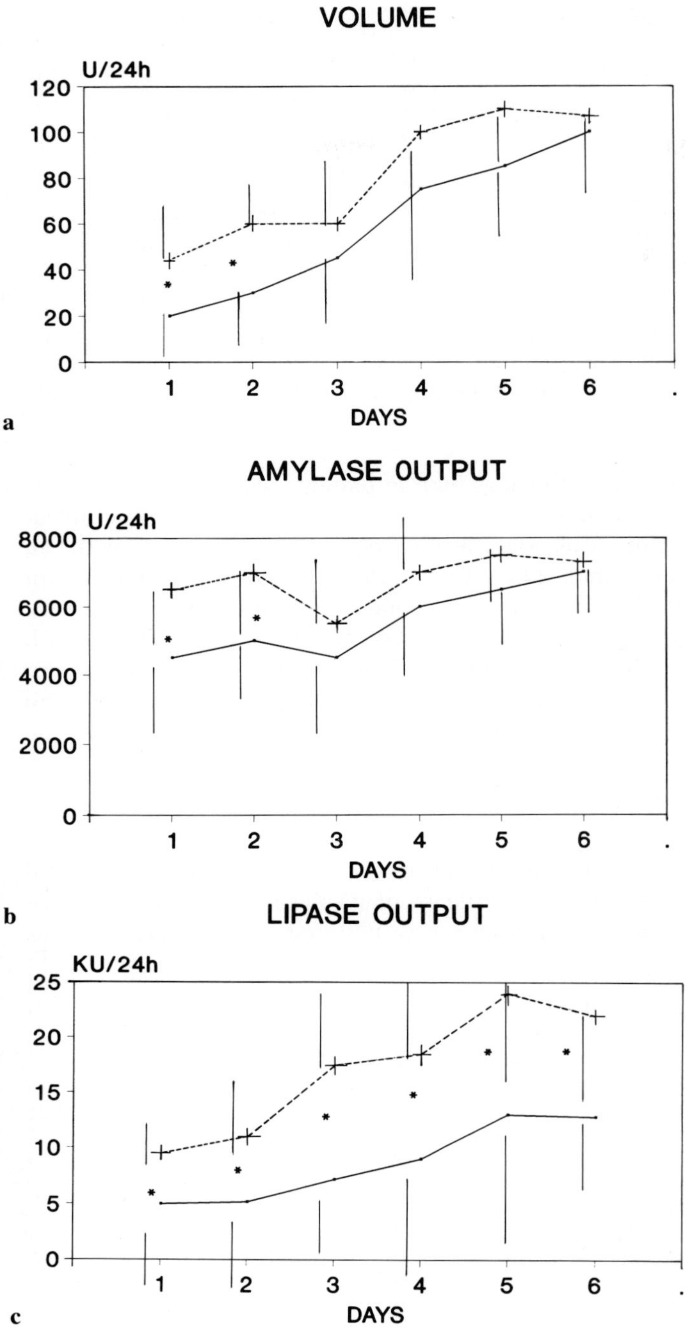

Fig. 2. Postoperative secretory volume (**a**), amylase (**b**), and lipase output (**c**) of the exocrine pancreatic remnant with (*solid line*) and without (*broken line*) somatostatin. *, $p < 0.05$ between groups

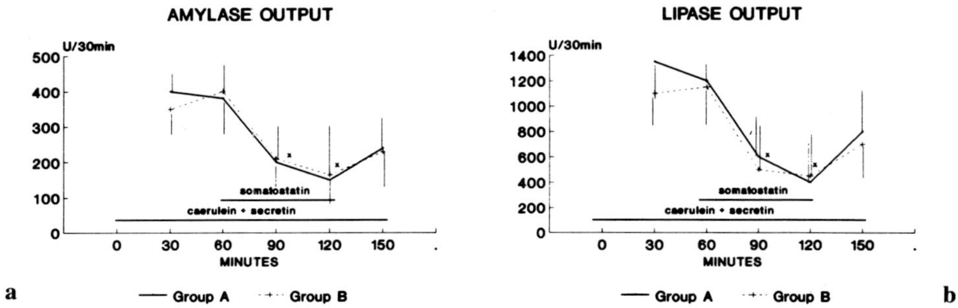

Fig. 3. Amylase (**a**) and lipase output (**b**) after stimulation with cerulein and secretin without (*broken line*) and with (*solid line*) somatostatin administration in different concentrations (after 60–90 min 4 μg/kg per hour and after 90–120 min 8 μg/kg per hour). *, $p < 0.05$ between groups

bleeding complications three times as high in patients without somatostatin. Of the bleeding complications two were gastrointestinal and one intra-abdominal. Two second-look operations were necessary, one with an unfavorable outcome, as mentioned above. In the group with somatostatin we observed one bleeding complication from the superior mesenteric vein with subsequent reoperation. Total morbidity was 8.3% in the group with somatostatin and 33.3% in that without. Nonspecific complications were pneumonia, urinary tract infections, and wound infections. There was no difference between the two groups of patients (Table 2).

Discussion

Somatostatin inhibits the release of probably all of the gastrointestinal hormones [2, 10]. In our study the release of insulin and glucagon was not inhibited to the same degree. Glucagon was inhibited more effectively, thus

Table 2. Mortality and morbidity

	Group A	Group B
Overall morbidity	3	6
Individual complications		
Pancreatic fistula	1	2
Wound infection	2	3
Upper gastrointestinal bleeding	–	2
Intra-abdominal hemorrhage	1	1
Gastric outlet obstruction	3	2
Pneumonia	3	4
Urinary tract infection	3	4
Overall mortality	–	1
Hospitality (days)	26 ± 8	29 ± 6

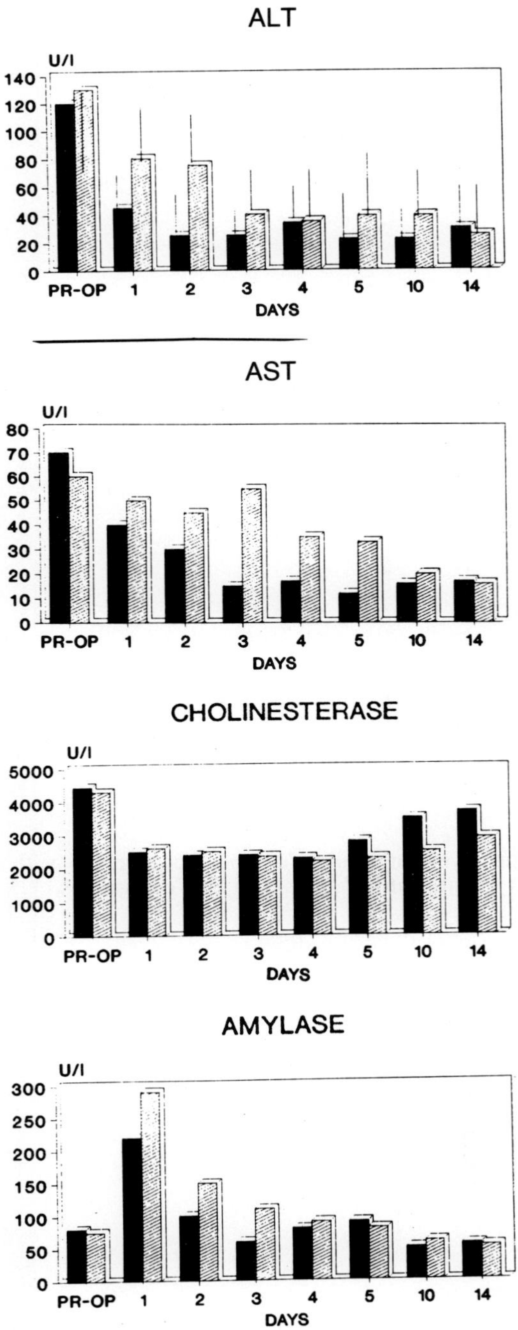

Fig. 4. Pre- and postoperative serum levels of ALT (**a**), AST (**b**), cholinesterase (**c**), and amylase (**d**) with (*dark columns*) and without (*hatched columns*) somatostatin. *, $p < 0.05$ between groups

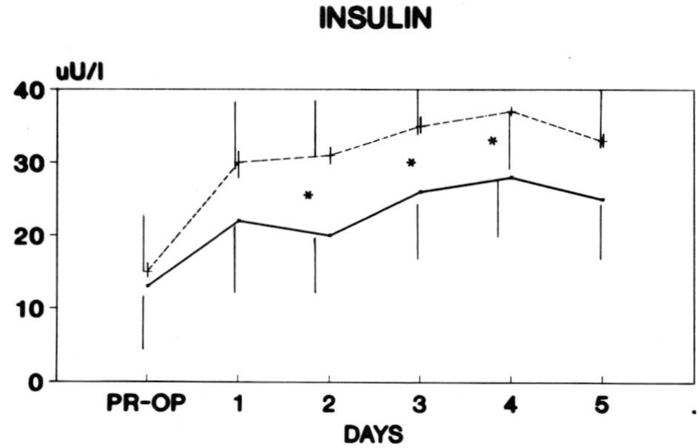

a

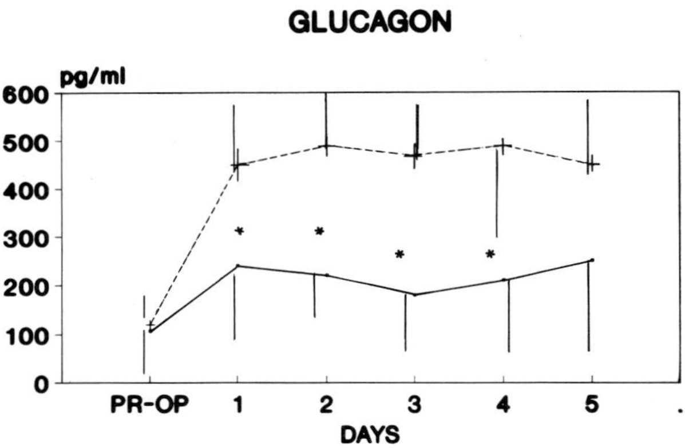

b

Fig. 5. Pre- and postoperative serum levels of insulin (**a**) and glucagon (**b**) with (*solid line*) and without (*broken line*) somatostatin. *, $p < 0.05$ between groups

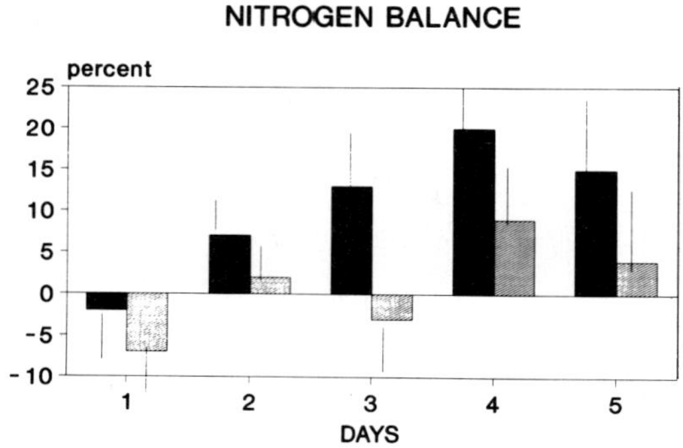

Fig. 6. Nitrogen balance (in percentage) from the 1st to the 5th postoperative days with (*dark columns*) and without (*hatched columns*) somatostatin. *, $p < 0.05$ between groups

leading to a shift in the insulin-glucagon ratio. There was no difference in the values of cortisol or catecholamines between the two groups. Therefore somatostatin is probably responsible for the early positive nitrogen balance. There is reason to believe that this effect is a consequence of the shift in the insulin-glucagon ratio in favor of insulin. Similar results were presented by Shaw and coworkers in 1988 [12]. In spite of these very interesting findings, we focus on the exocrine pancreas function. Pancreatic fistula and anastomotic breakdown are complications of major importance after duodenopancreatectomy, causing morbidity and mortality [1, 6].

By means of pancreatic duct catheterization we demonstrated a considerable amount of pancreatic fluid being secreted postoperatively. Total volume output and the amount of amylase, lipase, bicarbonate, and total protein on the secretion of the pancreatic remnant are physiologically relevant. Furthermore, we must take into consideration the different amount of secretion at the baseline and stimulated status. The inhibitory effect of somatostatin on the pancreatic secretion is a rational basis for the administration of this hormone in procedures involving pancreatic resection [10, 14]. In clinical studies published until now, a more favorable outcome after duodeno-pancreatectomy was demonstrated with the administration of somatostatin [7, 8]. In our own prospective, randomized trial we showed a significant inhibition of volume output and amylase activity by somatostatin in the early postoperative period. The inhibitory effect on lipase lasted for as long as 7 days. The decline in the inhibitory effect was found for the somatostatin analogue SMS. Creutzfeldt and coworkers found similar results for the intact pancreas of humans when giving somatostatin continuously [3, 9]. Whether this is a form of tachyphylaxis cannot be determined on the basis of our findings. Beyond this, we cannot explain why the inhibitory effect on amylase and lipase was limited to about 7 days.

An increase in secretion was observed beginning on the 5th postoperative day. This may be due to the beginning of oral intake. Although diverting of the pancreas juice from the anastomosis by means of a small catheter might have been favorable for both groups, we found differences in the clinical outcome between them. We observed two pancreas fistulas in the group without somatostatin and only one with somatostatin. Three postoperative bleedings occurred without and only one with somatostatin. The well-known pharmacologic properties of somatostatin may be the due to the lower incidence of bleeding complications in the somatostatin group [10].

There was one fatality due to bleeding in the group without somatostatin. The mortality rate was 4.16%.

The problems of measuring amylase in diseases of the pancreas are not discussed here.

The great range of exocrine pancreas secretion after duodeno-pancreatectomy is of interest. To measure this is difficult, but with the procedure presented here, it may be more feasible. For the first time we were able to demonstrate directly the inhibitory effects of somatostatin on the resected pancreas. This provides a rationale for the administration of somatostatin perioperatively in pancreas-resecting surgery.

References

1. Christ DW, Sitzmann JV, Cameron JL (1987) Improved hospital morbidity, mortality and survival after the Whipple procedure. Ann Surg 206:358
2. Creutzfeldt W, Lankisch PG, Fölsch UR (1975) Hemmung der sekretin- und cholecystokinin-, pankreozymininduzierten Saft- und Enzymsekretion und der Gallenblasenkontraktion beim Menschen durch Somatostatin. Dtsch Med Woschenschr 100:1135
3. Creutzfeldt W, Lembcke B, Fölsch UR (1987) Effect of somatostatin analogue on pancreatic secretion in humans. Am J Med 82:49
4. Cuthbertson DP (1982) Post-traumatic metobolism: a multidisciplinary challenge. Surg Clin North Am 58:1045
5. Faloona GR, Unger HR (1974) Glucagon. In: Jaffe BM, Behrmann MR (eds) Methods in hormone radioimmunoassay. Academic, New York, p 317
6. Grace PA, Pitt HA, Tompkins RK, Den Besten L, Longmire WP (1986) Decreased morbidity and mortality after pancreaticoduodenectomy. Am J Surg 151:141
7. Klempa I, Schwedes U, Usadel KH (1978) Verhütung von postoperativen pankreatischen Komplikationen nach Duodenopankreatektomie durch Somatostatin. Chirurg 50:427
8. Klempa I, Schwedes U, Encke A, Usadel KH (1989) Somatostatin therapy in pancreatic surgery. In: Raptis S, Rosenthal J, Gerich JE (eds) Proceedings of the 2nd international symposium on somatostatin. Attempto, Tübingen
9. Lembcke B, Creutzfeldt W, Schleser S, Ebert R, Shaw C, Koop I (1987) Effect of the somatostatin analoque Sandostatin (SMS 201-995) on gastrointestinal, pancreatic and biliary function and hormone release in normal men. Digestion 36:108
10. Reichlin S (1983) Somatostatin. N Engl J Med 309:1495–1556
11. Shaw JHF, Wolfe RR (1987) Whole body protein kinetics in severely ill septic patients: the response to glucose infusion and total nutritional support. Ann Surg 205:66
12. Shaw JHF, Wolfe RR (1988) Metabolic intervention in surgical patients. Ann Surg 207:274
13. Skyring AP, Singer A, Tornat P (1965) Treatment of acute pancreatitis with trasylol, report of controlled therapeutic trial. Br Med J II:627
14. Solomon ET (1987) Effect of somatostatin on exocrine pancreas. In: Reichlin S (ed) Somatostatin basic and clinical status. Plenum, New York
15. Van Heerden JA, McIlrath DC, Ilstrup DM, Weiland LH (1988) Total pancreatectomy for ductal adenocarcinoma of the pancreas: an update. World J Surg 12:658
16. Warshaw AL, Hawboldt MM (1988) Puzzling persistent hyperamylasemia, probably neither pancreatic nor pathologic. Am J Surg 155:453
17. Warshaw AL, Swanson RS (1988) Pancreatic cancer in 1988: possibilities and probabilities. Ann Surg 208:541
18. Willmore DW (1976) Hormonal response and their effect on metabolism. Surg. Clin North Am 56:999

Perioperative Inhibition of Pancreatic Secretion with Octreotide

M. Büchler[1], H. Friess, M. Hatzitheoklitos, W. Uhl, and H.G. Beger

Pancreatic diseases, especially cancer of the pancreas, show an increasing incidence [1–3]. Major pancreatic surgery, even nowadays, still carries a considerable risk of morbidity and even mortality. Although they have improved in recent years, mortality rates following pancreatic resection are between 3% and 10%, and complications including medical and surgical morbidity occur in one third to half of the patients [4–22].

Postoperative surgical complications such as peripancreatic fluid collections, abscess, fistula and consecutive sepsis are chiefly associated with exocrine pancreatic secretion [21]. They occur on the basis of pancreatic juice leaking from the pancreatic remnant and reaching the peripancreatic region or even the free abdominal cavity. The action of activated proteases such as trypsin or elastase leads to severe inflammation and may cause autodestruction of peripancreatic tissue including intestinal organs and major vessels. This pathomechanism explains the sometimes fatal outcome after leakage of a pancreatic anastomosis with sudden life-threatening hemorrhage [16].

Several concepts have been elaborated to avoid a pancreatic anastomosis and thereby prevent the risk of leakage by either taking out the whole pancreas in an operation for cancer [23, 24] or by occluding the major pancreatic duct [25–27]. None of these approaches were successful, and most pancreatic surgeons around the world still, or again, anastomose the remnant pancreas to the small intestine or stomach [4–13, 16–22].

The Role of Somatostatin

A fascinating concept to prevent complications following pancreatic resection is represented by the perioperative inhibition of exocrine pancreatic secretion by somatostatin or its analogs. The human hormone somatostatin has been demonstrated to strongly inhibit basal and stimulated exocrine pancreatic secretion in man and several animals [28–30]. This concept of blocking exocrine pancreatic secretion perioperatively was inaugurated by

[1] Department of Surgery, University of Ulm, Steinhoevelstrasse 9, W-7900 Ulm, FRG

Beger/Büchler/Malfertheiner (Eds.)
Standards in Pancreatic Surgery

Klempa et al. in 1979 [31]. In an open trial these authors used a continuous i.v. infusion of 300 µg/h of natural somatostatin perioperatively following Whipple resection. They reported a decreased complication rate, especially a lower occurrence of postoperative acute pancreatitis [31]. At that time it was not viable for this somatostatin treatment to become generally established because of the very short half-life of natural somatostatin (1 min) [28–30] and the need for continuous i.v. administration via an infusion pump. Another argument for many clinicians to renounce this concept was the high price of somatostatin in the late 1970s.

In the meantime, a synthetic somatostatin analog, namely octreotide (SMS 201-995), has become clinically available, which shows an increased potency with regard to the inhibition of pancreatic enzyme secretion [32, 33] and a much longer half-life (90 min) in comparison with the native hormone [34, 35].

Between 1989 and 1990, we therefore carried out a multicentric controlled randomized and double-blind trial with octreotide in patients undergoing major pancreatic resection. The results from this trial showed a significant reduction in clinically relevant postoperative complications [36].

The Role of Octreotide to Prevent Complications After Pancreatic Resection

In this multicentric trial [36] we recruited 322 patients from 18 surgical clinics in Germany [17] and Austria [1]. Patients suffering from pancreatic or periampullary tumors or from chronic pancreatitis suitable for elective pancreatic surgery (resection) were included (Table 1). They were randomly assigned the day before the operation to either a 7-day treatment of 3 × 100 µg/day octreotide subcutaneously (every 8 h) or three subcutaneous placebo injections per day for 7 days in a double-blinded study design. On the operation day, the treatment was started in each case at least 1 h before the operation. The dosage of 3 × 100 µg/day subcutaneously was

Table 1. Patients and indication for pancreatic operation

	Placebo patients (n = 121)	Octreotide patients (n = 125)
Age in years (median, range)	52 (20–80)	51 (19–75)
Sex (m/f)	82/39	92/33
Type of disease		
Chronic pancreatitis (%)	41	50
Pancreatic cancer (%)	28	30
Periampullary cancer (%)	21	11
Endocrine tumor (%)	3	4
Others (%)	7	5

chosen after a pilot trial [37] had shown that this dosage led to the maximal inhibition of pancreatic enzyme secretion in man.

According to general experience that the patients at risk following pancreatic surgery are those with a soft pancreas, we stratified our patients into two groups, namely patients with pancreatic or periampullary tumors (high-risk group) and those suffering from chronic pancreatitis (low-risk group).

Table 2. Definition of postoperative complications

Complication	Definition
Death	Within 90 days postoperatively
Leakage of anastomosis	Leakage of pancreatic, biliary or intestinal anastomosis as determined by X-ray or intraoperative (relaparotomy) findings
Pancreatic fistula	Concentration of amylase and lipase in the drainage fluid later than 3 days postoperatively of more than 3 times the serum concentration and a drainage volume of more than 10 ml/24 h at the same time
Abscess	Pus collection or an infected fluid collection revealed by ultrasound or CT-guided needle aspiration and microbiological culture or demonstrated by relaparotomy
Fluid collection	Collection of sterile fluid of at least 5×5 cm in diameter in ultrasound or CT which did not qualify as an abscess. Screening on day 4 and day 8 postoperatively
Shock	Systolic blood pressure of less than 80 mmHg for more than 20 min (later than 24 h postoperatively) which required continuous volume replacement and/or treatment with catecholamines
Sepsis	$\geqslant$ Four of the following criteria: a) bacterial-positive blood culture b) rectal temperature >38.5°C c) leukocytosis >12 000/mm^3 or leukopenia <3000/mm^3 d) thrombocytopenia <100 000/mm^3 e) metabolic acidosis (base excess >−4)
Pulmonary insufficiency	Arterial $PO_2 < 60$ mmHg, despite oxygen application (4 l/m) via the nose, or required prolonged postoperative mechanical ventilation (>24 h after the end of surgery) or reintubation
Renal insufficiency	Serum creatinine more than twice the preoperative value
Bleeding	Replacement of more than 3 units of blood later than 24 h after the end of surgery or the indication for relaparotomy due to intraabdominal or intraintestinal bleeding.
Acute pancreatitis	More than threefold increase in serum amylase or lipase later than 3 days after surgery, accompanied by morphological signs of acute pancreatitis in a contrast-enhanced CT scan. CT was mandatory in patients with a threefold increase in serum amylase or lipase on postoperative day 4 or after

According to our study protocol, we defined 11 typical complications (Table 2) after pancreatic resection, and each patient was followed for 90 days postoperatively. Of the 322 patients randomized the day before the operation, 76 patients were withdrawn from the study because pancreatic resection was found intraoperatively not to be possible, mostly on the basis of advanced tumor disease.

Finally 246 patients could be evaluated, 125 and 121 being assigned to the octreotide and placebo groups, respectively. Both groups were well-matched for age, sex, type of underlying disease, type of operation performed, and preoperative morbidity (Tables 1, 3). The majority of our 246 patients underwent either a pancreaticoduodenectomy (Whipple resection) [38], a duodenum preserving pancreatic head resection [39], or a pancreatic left resection (Table 3).

The overall mortality within 90 days following surgery was 4.5% (11/246 patients). Four (3.2%) and seven patients (5.8%) died in the octreotide and placebo group, respectively (Table 4). In the high-risk group (139 patients), mortality was 2.9% and 9.9% in the octreotide and placebo groups, respectively. According to the study protocol, 40 (32%) and 67 (55%) patients suffered from one or more postoperative complications in the octreotide and placebo groups, respectively (Table 4). This difference was significant at a level of $p < 0.005$.

Table 3. Type of operation in patients undergoing pancreatic surgery

Type of operation	Placebo patients (n = 121)	Octreotide patients (n = 125)
Whipple (%)	65	58
Duodenum preserving (%)		
Pancreatic head resection (%)	18	21
Left resection (%)	11	14
Pancreaticojejunostomy (%)	4	3
Enucleation (%)	1	1
Others (%)	1	3

Table 4. Mortality and complications

	Placebo patients (n = 121)	Octreotide patients (n = 125)
Mortality (n; %)	7 (5.8)	4 (3.2)
Complication rate (patients with one or more complication) (n; %)*	67 (55.4)	40 (32.0)

* Difference was significant; $p < 0.005$.

Table 5. Patients with one or more complications in the high-risk and low-risk groups

High-risk (tumors)[a] ($n = 139$)				Low-risk (chronic pancreatitis)[b] ($n = 107$)			
Octreotide ($n = 68$)		Placebo ($n = 71$)		Octreotide ($n = 57$)		Placebo ($n = 50$)	
n	%	*n*	%	*n*	%	*n*	%
26	38	46	65	14	25	21	42

[a] Difference was significant; $p < 0.01$.
[b] Difference was not significant.

According to our stratification in the high-risk group (tumors), the complication rate was 38% and 65% for octreotide and placebo, respectively ($p < 0.01$). Although the trend was similar in the low-risk group, there was no statistical difference in the complication rate between octreotide and placebo (Table 5). Patients with tumors (high-risk group) had the most benefit from octreotide injection with respect to the number and type of complications (Fig. 1). There was an obvious difference with respect to the criteria of death, fistula, abscess, shock, sepsis, pulmonary insufficiency, and postoperative pancreatitis (Fig. 1).

Interestingly, the postoperative increase in the serum pancreatic enzymes amylase and lipase was significantly lower postoperatively in the patients receiving octreotide than in the placebo group (Fig. 2).

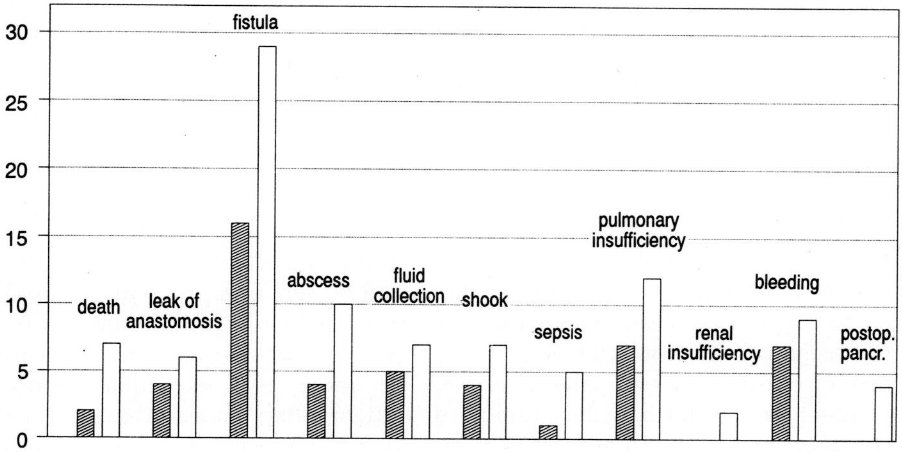

Fig. 1. Number and type of complications in patients in the high risk (tumors) group (*shaded blocks*, octreotide; *white blocks*, placebo)

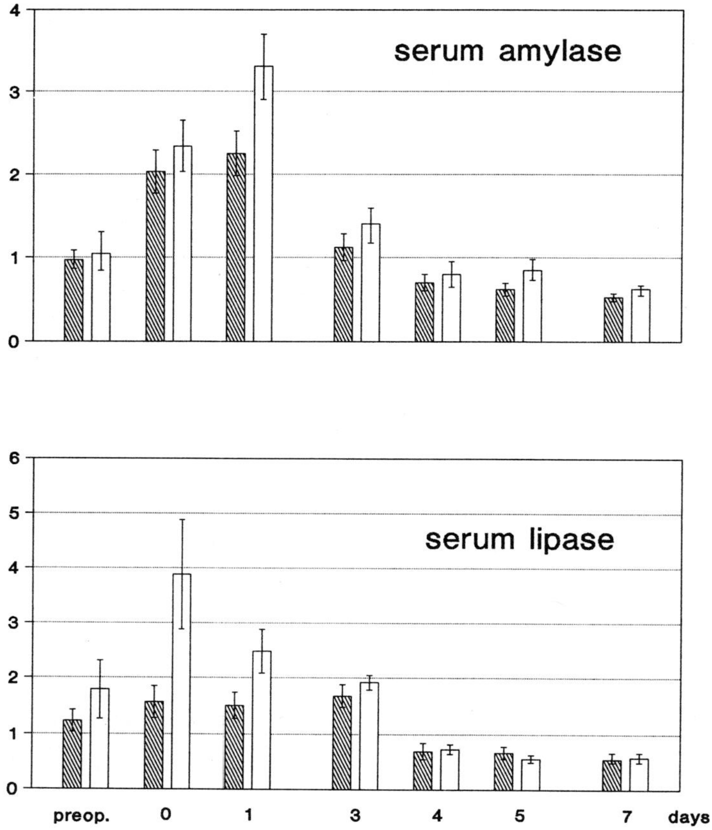

Fig. 2. Serum amylase (*upper graph*) and lipase (*lower graph*) concentrations before and following pancreatic resection (mean ± SEM) in 125 patients treated with octreotide (*shaded blocks*) and 121 patients treated with placebo (*white blocks*). The values on the y-axis are many times higher than the normal level of serum. D0 represents the enzym level in the evening after the operation

Comments

In major pancreatic surgery, the crucial risk factor is the pancreatic remnant and its anastomosis with the stomach or small bowel. This problem is caused by an ongoing exocrine pancreatic secretion of the pancreatic stump and by the technical difficulties of performing a proper and safe anastomosis with this often smooth and friable organ. We know, that particularly those patients with distal bile duct tumors or periampullary cancers have a high risk of postoperative breakdown of pancreatic anastomosis or leakage followed by fistula and/or sepsis [4–6, 8–10, 12, 17]. Therefore, these patients should constitute a suitable group for perioperative treatment with somatostatin or its analog octreotide. The correctness of defining risk groups in pancreatic surgery is underlined by our study results which show a significant reduction in postoperative complications in the high-risk group in contrast to the low-risk patients suffering from chronic pancreatitis, where no significant reduction of postoperative complications could be demonstrated using octreotide.

In 1979 the concept of inhibiting exocrine secretion perioperatively by intravenous continuous somatostatin infusion had already been put into practice [31]. In contrast to these authors, we used octreotide, an octapeptide analog of somatostatin, which was synthesized to be more specific, more potent, and longer acting in its inhibitory effects than native somatostatin [28–35, 37]. Particularly the longer half-life of octreotide in comparison with somatostatin-14 has made this compound useful for clinical application. Meanwhile, two other groups have used the somatostatin analog octreotide to prevent pancreatic fistula and acute pancreatitis following pancreatic transplantation [40, 41].

The most frequent complication after pancreatic resection is pancreatic fistula, which occurs in 10%–40% of patients retrospectively analyzed for postoperative complications [4–6, 8, 16, 17]. The prevalence of pancreatic fistulae in our multicentric trial was 27%, thus confirming these data from the literature. We were certainly expecting to reduce the occurrence of postoperative pancreatic fistulae by administering octreotide prophylactically, because somatostatin and its analogs have been shown to be effective even in the treatment of pancreatic fistulae [42–44]. Not only pancreatic fistulae as a direct consequence of uncontrolled postoperative exocrine secretion from the pancreatic remnant, but also other complications such as abscesses, acute pancreatitis, pulmonary insufficiency, shock, and sepsis, which represent local and systemic sequelae of a pancreatic leak, could be reduced by perioperative octreotide administration.

In conclusion, the perioperative administration of octreotide $3 \times 100\,\mu g$/day subcutaneously in patients undergoing elective pancreatic resection reduces the occurrence of typical postoperative complications, particularly in the group of patients suffering from pancreatic and periampullary tumors. It is therefore recommendable to include patients with a soft pancreas undergoing pancreatic resection in this treatment protocol. Finally, and interestingly, as we have learned from several animal trials inducing acute pancreatitis, somatostatin and its analogs were helpful if the drug was given before acute pancreatitis was induced in animals in the sense of providing prophylactic efficacy [45–48]. These data from acute pancreatitis in animals may also explain why octreotide is helpful in preventing postoperative complications following major pancreatic surgery because we can administer the drug prophylactically before trauma to the pancreas (through surgery) becomes effective.

References

1. Silverberg E, Lubera JA (1989) Cancer statistics 1989. Cancer J Clin 3:3–39
2. Gudjonsson B (1987) Cancer of the pancreas. 50 years of surgery. Cancer 60:2284–2303
3. Fontham E, Correa P, Cohn I Jr (1987) Epidemiology of cancer of the pancreas. In: Howard JM, Jordan GL Jr, Reber HA (eds) Surgical diseases of the pancreas. Lea and Febiger, Philadelphia, pp 613–626
4. Jordan GL Jr (1987) Pancreatic resection for pancreatic cancer. In: Howard JM, Jordan GL Jr, Reber HA (eds) Surgical diseases of the pancreas. Lea and Febiger, Philadelphia, pp 666–714
5. Moossa AR, Gadd M, Lavelle-Jones M (1986) Surgical treatment of exocrine pancreatic cancer. In: Go VLW, Gardner JD, Brooks FP, Lebenthal E, DiMagno EP, Scheele GA (eds) Exocrine pancreas. Biology, pathobiology and diseases. Raven, New York, pp 713–725
6. Howard JM (1987) Surgical treatment of chronic pancreatitis. In: Howard JM, Jordan GL Jr, Reber HA (eds) Surgical diseases of the pancreas. Lea and Febiger, Philadelphia, pp 496–521
7. Rossi RL, Rothschild J, Braasch JW, Munson JL, ReMine SG (1987) Pancreatoduodenectomy in the management of chronic pancreatitis. Arch Surg 122: 416–420
8. Crist DW, Sitzmann JV, Cameron JL (1987) Improved hospital morbidity, mortality, and survival after the Whipple procedure. Ann Surg 206:358–365
9. Peters JH, Carey LC (1991) Historical review of pancreaticoduodenectomy. Am J Surg 161:219–225
10. Prinz RA, Greenlee HB (1981) Pancreatic duct drainage in 100 patients with chronic pancreatitis. Ann Surg 194:313–320
11. Neoptolemos JP, Talbot IC, Carr-Locke DL et al. (1987) Treatment and outcome in 52 consecutive cases of ampullary carcinoma. Br J Surg 74:957–961
12. Robertson JFR, Imrie CW, Hole DJ, Carter DC, Blumgart LH (1987) Management of periampullary carcinoma. Br J Surg 74:816–819
13. Moossa AR (1987) Surgical treatment of chronic pancreatitis: an overview. Br J Surg 74:661–667
14. Van Heerden JA, McIllrath DC, Ilstrup DM, Weiland LH (1988) Total pancreatectomy for ductal adenocarcinoma of the pancreas: an update. World J Surg 12:658–662
15. Warshaw AL, Swanson RS (1988) What's new in general surgerys. Pancreatic cancer in 1988. Possibilities and probabilities. Ann Surg 208:541–553
16. Trede M, Schwall G (1988) The complications of pancreatectomy. Ann Surg 207:39–47
17. Pellegrini CA, Heck CF, Raper S, Way LW (1989) An analysis of the reduced morbidity and mortality rates after pancreatico duodenectomy. Arch Surg 124: 778–781
18. Bittner R, Roscher R, Safi F, Dopfer HP, Schölzel E, Beger HG (1989) Der Einfluß von Tumorgröße und Lymphknotenstatus auf die Prognose des Pankreascarcinoms. Chirurg 60:240–245
19. Grace PA, Pitt HA, Longmire WP (1990) Pylorus preserving pancreatoduodenectomy: an overview. Br J Surg 77:968–974
20. Singh SM, Longmire WP, Reber HA (1990) Surgical palliation for pancreatic cancer. Ann Surg 212:132–139
21. Grace PA, Pitt HA, Tompkins RK, DenBesten L, Longmire WP (1986) Decreased morbidity and mortality after pancreatoduodenectomy. Am J Surg 151:141
22. Spencer MP, Sarr MG, Nagorney DM (1990) Radical pancreatectomy for pancreatic cancer in the elderly. Ann Surg 212:140–143
23. Matsui Y et al. (1979) Ductal carcinoma of the pancreas: rationale for total pancreatectomy. Arch Surg 114:722

24. Brooks JR (1987) Total pancreatectomy for pancreatic cancer. In: Howard JM, Jordan GL Jr, Reber HA (eds) Surgical diseases of the pancreas. Lea and Febiger, Philadelphia, pp 715–724
25. Di Carlo V, Chiesa R, Pontiroli AE, Carlucci M, Staudacher C, Zerbi A, Cristallo M, Braga M, Pozza G (1989) Pancreatoduodenectomy with occlusion of the residual stump by neoprene injection. World J Surg 13:105–111
26. Waclawiczek HW, Lorenz D (1989) Der Schutz der pancreaticodigestiven Anastomose nach Pankreaskopfresektion durch Pankreasgangocclusion mit Fibrin(-kleber). Chirurg 60:403–409
27. Mackie JA Jr, Rhoads JE (1975) Pancreaticogastrostomy following radical pancreaticoduodenal resection. Bull Soc Int Chir 34:611
28. Konturek SJ, Tasler J, Obtulowic W et al. (1976) Effect of growth hormone release inhibiting hormone on hormones stimulating exocrine pancreatic secretion. J Clin Invest 58:1–6
29. Raptis S, Schlegel W, Lehmann E, Dollinger HC, Zoupas C (1978) Effects of somatostatin on the exocrine pancreas and the release of duodenal hormones. Metabolism 27:1321–1328
30. Creutzfeldt W, Lankisch PG, Fölsch UR (1975) Hemmung der Secretin und Cholecystokinin-Pancreozymin-induzierten Saft- und Enzymsekretion des Pankreas und der Gallenblasenkontraktion bei Menschen durch Somatostatin. Dtsch Med Wochenschr 100:1135–1138
31. Klempa J, Schwedes U, Usadel KH (1979) Verhütung von postoperativen pankreatitischen Komplikationen nach Duodenopankreatektomie durch Somatostatin. Chirurg 50:427–432
32. Lembcke B, Creutzfeldt W, Schleser S, Ebert R, Shaw C, Koop I (1987) Effect of the somatostatin analogue sandostatin (SMS 201-995) on gastrointestinal, pancreatic and biliary function and hormone release in normal men. Digestion 36:108–124
33. Bauer W, Briner U, Doepfner W et al. (1982) SMS 201-995: a very potent and selective octapeptide analogue of somatostatin with prolonged action. Life Sci 31:1133–1140
34. Pless J, Bauer W, Briner U et al. (1986) Chemistry and pharmacology of SMS 201-995, a long-acting octapeptide analogue of somatostatin. Scand J Gastroenterol 21 Suppl 119:55–64
35. Shiratori K, Watanabe SI, Takeuchi T (1991) Somatostatin analog, SMS 201-995, inhibits pancreatic exocrine secretion and release of secretin and cholecystokinin in rats. Pancreas 6:23–30
36. Büchler M, Frieß H, Klempa I, Hermanek P, Sulkowski U, Becker H, Schafmayer A, Baca I, Lorenz D, Meister R, Kremer B, Wagner P, Witte J, Zurmayer EL, Saeger HD, Rieck B, Dollinger P, Glaser K, Teichmann R, Konradt J, Gaus W, Dennerl HJ, Welzel D, Beger HG (1992) The role of somatostatin analogue octreotide in the prevention of postoperative complications following pancreatic resection. The results of a multicenter controlled trial. Am J Surg 163:125–131
37. Frieß H, Büchler M, Meschenmoser L et al. (1989) Effect of octreotide (SMS 201-995) on exocrine pancreatic function in man (Abstr). Pancreas 4:616
38. Whipple AO, Parsons WB, Mullins CR (1935) Treatment of carcinoma of the ampulla of Vater. Ann Surg 102:763–779
39. Beger HG, Büchler M, Bittner R, Oettinger W, Roscher R (1989) Duodenum-preserving resection of the head of the pancreas in severe chronic pancreatitis. Ann Surg 209:273–278
40. Starzl TE, Todo S, Tzakis A et al. (1989) Abdominal organ cluster transplantation for the treatment of upper abdominal malignancies. Ann Surg 210:374–386
41. Daloze P, Beauregard H, St Louis G et al. (1989) Clinical pancreas transplantation: a learning curve of its management. Transplant Proc 21:2858–2861
42. Pederzoli P, Bassi C, Falconi M, Albrigo R, Vantini I, Micciolo R (1986) Conservative treatment of external pancreatic fistulas with parenteral nutrition

alone or in combination with continuous intravenous infusion of somatostatin, glucagon or calcitonin. Surg Gynecol Obstet 163:428–432
43. Nubiola-Calonge P, Badia JM, Sancho J, Gil MJ, Segura M, Sitges-Serra A (1987) Blind evaluation of the effect of octreotide (SMS 201-995), a somatostatin analogue, on small-bowel fistula output. Lancet 2:672–674
44. Prinz RA, Pickleman J, Hoffman JP (1988) Treatment of pancreatic cutaneous fistula with a somatostatin analogue. Am J Surg 155:36–42
45. Lankisch PG, Koop H, Winckler K et al. (1977) Somatostatin therapy of acute experimental pancreatitis. Gut 18:713–716
46. Baxter JM, Jenkins SA, Day DW et al. (1985) Effects of somatostatin and a long-acting somatostatin analogue on the prevention and treatment of experimentally induced acute pancreatitis in the rat. Br J Surg 72:382–385
47. Mann NS, Mauch MJ (1981) Inhibitory effect of cycloheximide, somatostatin and 5-asa cytidine on acute experimental pancreatitis. Am J Proctol 32:24–32
48. Schwedes U, Althoff PH, Klempa I et al. (1979) Effect of somatostatin on bile-induced acute hemorrhagic pancreatitis in the dog. Horm Metab Res 11:655–661

The Management of Complications of Pancreatic Resection

J.M. Howard[1] and B.S. Kierstead

Introduction

Complications and death following pancreatic resection have been most frequent when the head of the pancreas is resected. It is the operation of pancreaticoduodenectomy, i.e., resection of the head of the pancreas, to which this report is directed.

The incidence of mortality and morbidity from resection of the head of the pancreas continues to diminish, at least in those large centers from which most current reports originate. This is due, in large part, to the establishment of specialized centers of expertise: expertise in the evaluation and management of patients with pancreatic disease. The assessment, operation, and follow-up care of the patient requiring pancreatic resection is best achieved by a multidisciplinary team. Paramount to the success of the team is a surgeon who maintains an ongoing interest in the field and who continues to maintain an active practice of pancreatic surgery.

Most resections of the head of the pancreas are for malignant disease. In general, the complication rates and the mortality rates for resection of benign pancreatic disease are lower than that for resection of malignant disease. In 1968 the senior author reported 41 consecutive Whipple resections without an operative mortality [1]. This report stimulated a renewed interest in pancreatic surgery and in the concentration of the experience in specialized centers. The success of a specialized service is clearly demonstrated by the report of Trede and associates, who in 1990 reported 118 consecutive resections of the head of the pancreas without an operative mortality [2].

Because survival of patients with pancreatic cancer has been disappointing, the magnitude of the operation has been increased. The authors, following the experience of Japanese colleagues, have broadened the resection to include skeletonization of the blood vessels and bile duct of the upper abdomen. This and the frequent use of intraoperative and postoperative irradiation, plus the inclusion of patients aged over 70 years has led to a slight increase in the overall hospital mortality rate. Today several

[1]Department of Surgery, Toledo Hospital, and Medical College of Ohio, Toledo, Ohio, USA

Beger/Büchler/Malfertheiner (Eds.)
Standards in Pancreatic Surgery

centers around the world are experiencing operative mortality rates of less than 5%, and this is a standard to which most surgeons should now be able to adhere. In a personal series of 189 patients there were five deaths in hospital (3%) and one death within 30 days of operation (0.5%).

The nature of the complications is clarifying, and to some extent changing, as experience evolves. Those complications to be considered in this report include operative hemorrhage, pancreatic and biliary fistulae, hepatic failure, infections, delayed gastric emptying, anastomotic ulcerations, postresection pancreatitis, delayed recurrent obstruction of the biliary tract, and delayed obstruction of the Roux-en-Y limb used for reconstruction.

Operative Hemorrhage

Intraoperative hemorrhage during resection of the head of the pancreas is usually preventable with care being taken to define the vascular anatomy before and during operation. Preoperative arteriography provides a useful road map and may sometimes prevent catastrophic accidents due to preexisting thrombosis of the major veins or to congenital anomalies, particularly of the arterial system. It is most useful in patients with tumors of the body of the gland, i.e., in those tumors in the vicinity of the celiac axis and the superior mesenteric vessels. Operative hemorrhage originates largely in the veins, specifically in the superior mesenteric and portal veins. The vena cava is seldom involved by pancreatic cancer, and bleeding from the vena cava is almost never a related problem. Serious operative hemorrhage may result because of tumor invasion of the portal or superior mesenteric vein. Such invasion makes adequate exposure of the vessels difficult, leading to hemorrhage and subsequent difficulty in careful repair of the torn vein. A key to the surgeon's technical skill in pancreatic surgery is how well he handles major venous bleeding: "If the surgeon cannot prevent or control venous bleeding, he should not be doing pancreatic surgery."

Bleeding occurs primarily under two circumstances. As the vessels of the hepatic triad are isolated small tears may occur in the portal vein before the vein is fully exposed and mobilized. This usually results from avulsion of small tributaries. Pressure over the bleeding area may well provide definitive treatment under this circumstance, although not infrequently the bleeding point must be exposed and the tear repaired. The second setting for major bleeding, more serious than the first, is bleeding from the superior mesenteric vein as it passes behind the pancreas or bleeding from the portal vein, along the superior border of the pancreas. As indicated, this may result from invasion by tumor with the invasion leading to hemorrhage as the pancreas is dissected off the vein. Usually the points of invasion can be identified prior to bleeding and the application of venous clamps will permit resection of the vein and its repair. The only two catastrophic hemorrhages which the senior author has experienced in pancreatic surgery resulted not from invasion of a patent vein, but from complete obstruction of the superior mesenteric vein. Division of important collaterals then led to development of acute portal hypertension with resultant bleeding from the large operative bed. Although this might be managed by mesenteric to vena caval shunting, it constitutes a very serious complication.

Control of hemorrhage from the mesenteric-portal system requires two competent surgeons, "plus additional hands." These individuals, plus the vascular instruments and vascular sutures, should be part of the original operative organization, not something that must be organized after the bleeding has started.

One patient had to be reoperated upon within 24 h for a life-threatening intra-abdominal hemorrhage after a Whipple resection. The bleeding point, almost missed at reexploration, was the superior epigastric artery at the site of penetration of the abdominal wall by a drain. When the abdominal incision was reopened, retractors compressed the bleeding site, thereby stopping the bleeding, and almost causing the surgeons to fail to localize the problem. Several similar observations have led the authors (a) to insert the drains at a distance from the epigastric artery and (b) carefully to inspect the insertion site from within the abdomen before closing.

Pancreatic Fistula

The postoperative development of a pancreatic fistula has constituted one of the more common and one of the more lethal complications of pancreatic resection. Several series have indicated that this is the underlying cause in a third of serious infections [3], 20% of delayed hemorrhage [4], and up to half of the postoperative fatalities [5]. Rates of fistula formation were earlier reported in 15%–20% of patients and an even higher incidence if the pancreatic duct was of small caliber. Numerous surgeons tried to reduce the incidence of fistula by performing anastomosis of the end of the transected pancreas to the end of the Roux-en-Y jejunal segment. Success was often reported.

In the centers of concentrated experience, the incidence of pancreatic fistula has now almost disappeared. Based on personal contact with K. Warren, the author now utilizes and teaches a single layer anastomosis between the mucosa of the transected pancreatic duct and the mucosa of a small opening in the side of the Roux-en-Y limb of jejunum. Anastomosis is made with 5.0 sutures such as derivatives of polyglycolic acid which are not digested for 6 weeks or more (F. Tian et al., to be published), or Prolene, which is permanent. The transected end of the distal pancreas is oversewn (Fig. 1) and is then sutured as an abutment to the side of the Roux-en-Y in order to prevent traction on the ductal anastomosis. The anastomosis of the duct itself is the crucial part of the technical maneuver and should be made with fine sutures on fine needles. Under no circumstances should the

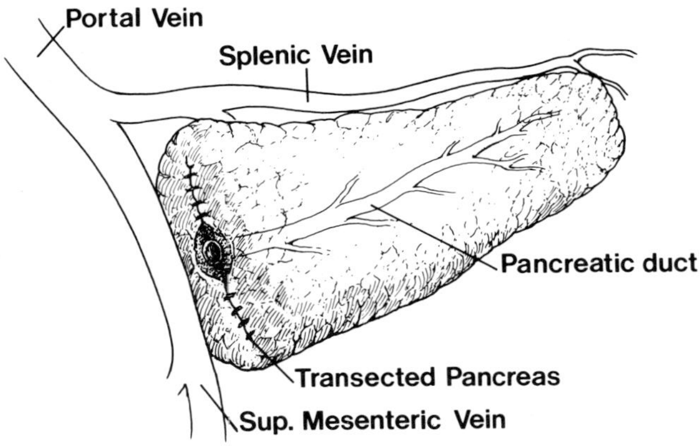

Fig. 1. The transected surface of the pancreas is oversewn with nonabsorbable or very slowly absorbable sutures. Care is taken not to occlude the duct of Wirsung. (From [10])

anastomosis be made with catgut. Plain catgut disintegrates in pancreatic juice within 48 h, and chronic catgut lasts only 1–2 days longer [6]. The anastomosis is usually intubated with a small polyethylene catheter which is brought out through the anterior wall of the Roux-en-Y to be sutured to the skin (Fig. 2). In utilizing the above mucosa to mucosa suture technique, the senior author has not experienced a pancreatic fistula within the past 30 resections. This is one setting in surgery in which technical skill is of great importance.

Near all pancreatic anastomoses, but not touching the anastomosis, a Jackson-Pratt drain is placed. If well drained, the subsequent development of a pancreatic fistula, initially signaled by bleeding along the drain site and hemodynamic instability, should not require operative reintervention. This is particularly true if there is a polyethylene catheter remaining in situ in the pancreatic duct, decompressing the pancreatic system. If the anastomosis has not been adequately drained, early operative drainage is mandatory. It is the author's observation, however, that if previously drained, reoperation may be an added insult to the patient without compensatory benefit.

Choledochojejunal Fistula

In several recent series choledochojejunal fistulae have been reported as occurring more frequently than pancreaticojejunal fistulae. The authors perform this anastomosis almost identically to that of the pancreaticojejunostomy (Fig. 2). A single layer of sutures approximate the end of the transected common duct to the side of the Roux-en-Y limb of the jejunum downstream from the pancreatic anastomosis. Again, the sutures of 4.0 or

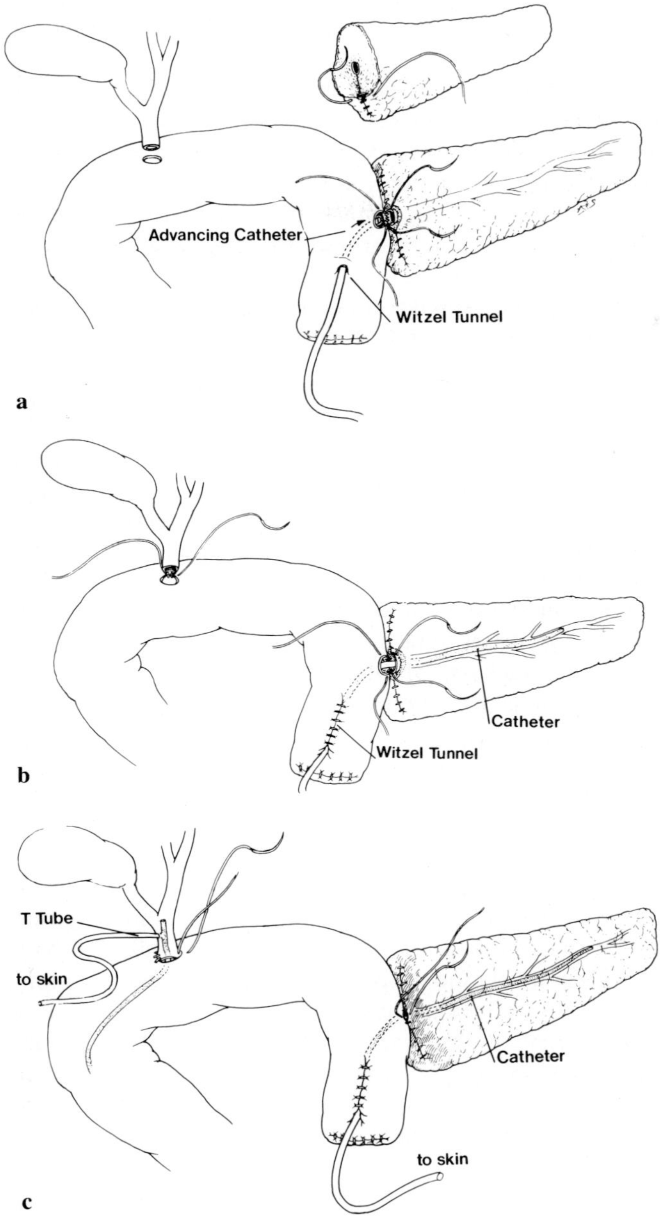

Fig. 2a–c. Pancreaticojejunostomy. **a** 5.0 polyglycholic acid or Prolene sutures are utilized to suture the posterior wall of the pancreatic duct to a small puncture wound of the jejunum. A small polyethylene catheter is positioned for cannulation of the anastomosis. **b** The catheter is then advanced through the incomplete anastomosis toward the tail of the pancreas. It is secured via a Witzel tunnel. **c** The anterior wall of the pancreaticojejunostomy is sutured. Additional sutures (not shown) are utilized to abut the transected surface of the pancreas to the jejunal wall. Downstream, the common bile duct is anastomosed to the jejunum, utilizing a similar technique. Catgut is not used in pancreatic anastomoses. (From [10])

5.0 caliber are of the slowly dissolving types such as Vicryl or Dexon or of the permanent synthetic type such as Prolene. Catgut is hazardous, with plain catgut dissolving in bile within 2–4 days, and with chromic catgut also dissolving rapidly, although more slowly than it does in the environment of pancreatic juice (F. Tian et al., to be published). Silk sutures, lasting indefinitely, have repeatedly been demonstrated to form foci or stones within the common bile duct and are therefore seldom utilized.

In order to prevent choledochojejunal fistulae it is important to maintain a good blood supply to the transected end of the common bile duct. The limited use of electrocautery and the preservation of the small vessels along the common duct are safeguards against ischemic necrosis of the suture lines. It has been observed that the hepatic duct has a better blood supply than does the common bile duct under these circumstances. Transection of the bile ducts above the cystic duct thus lends itself to a better blood supply to the transected duct, as well as permitting a more radical resection.

As with pancreatic anastomoses, drains should be placed near the anastomosis, but not touching it. If a small leak develops and persists, it may be that a fistulogram demonstrates the drain to be actually touching the anastomosis. Movement of the drain 1 cm away from the anastomosis may allow the leak to close. The leakage of bile into a well-drained bed is seldom life threatening, and under the above circumstances seldom requires reoperation.

Postoperative Hepatic Failure

In the authors' current experience, the most serious complication is hepatic failure following decompression of the obstructed biliary system. Characteristically, anastomosis of the common duct to the jejunum is followed by a drop in the serum bilirubin level and improvement in hepatic function. Sometimes, however, the serum bilirubin may fall for several days and then undergo a secondary rise. Further observations will probably demonstrate that this complication is seen more frequently in those patients with the highest preoperative serum bilirubin levels, and in those patients with "white bile" in the bile ducts at the time of operation. The authors transect the common bile duct and leave it open, unclamped, while the pancreatic resection is completed. Usually fresh bile drains into the peritoneal cavity under these circumstances, and it is of concern if this does not occur.

Among the patients with this complication at least two patterns are observed in the serum bilirubin concentrations. In the first there may be an initial drop in the serum bilirubin level followed by a progressive rise which may coincide with failure of other hepatic functions. The second pattern is a progressive or secondary rise in the bilirubin level which is followed by a plateau and then a fall in the bilirubin level. The initial complication has been the pattern of fatality in two of the authors' patients. The cause for the hepatic failure is uncertain. Perhaps it is sometimes due entirely to preoperative hepatic damage secondary to the prolonged obstruction of the common bile duct. In others, however, this does not seem to have been the case. Inquiry among colleagues has suggested that the liver has been replaced by lipid due to the excessive administration of glucose via hyperalimentation. In an effort to stimulate an increased flow of bile the authors have administered repeated doses of secretin or cholecystokinin, but the experience has not been adequate to permit conclusions. Repeatedly the question has arisen as to whether the increasing jaundice has reflected recurrent obstruction of the common bile duct. This has always been carefully assessed by cholangiography, and extrahepatic obstruction has not been found in any instance.

Currently the preoperative endoscopic placement of common duct stents, allowing the damaged liver to regain excretory function prior to operation, may minimize or prevent this problem [2]. Infection is also well known to cause damage to hepatic function and an abscess should be sought when hepatic failure threatens. In any case, in the authors' experience, a rising bilirubin level after resection seldom reflects a mechanical defect and reoperation will seldom be helpful in overcoming the complication.

Sepsis

In the immediate period after resection of the pancreas the most frequent cause of infection and fever is due to atelectasis. The next most common cause of infection is septicemia associated with an infected central venous catheter and these two sources need to be addressed before seriously considering intra-abdominal sepsis. Intra-abdominal or wound abscesses do not characteristically manifest themselves within the first few postoperative days. Should intraoperative sepsis be suspected it can usually be identified via computed tomography and can often be treated by a percutaneous drainage catheter inserted under computed tomographic guidance.

Failure of Gastric Emptying

Failure of gastric emptying after pancreatic resection is a well recognized complication. It apparently is more frequent after the pylorus-sparing operation, and it is even more frequent after palliative gastrojejunostomy for unresectable pancreatic cancer [7]. Prolonged gastric retention after pancreatic resection, in the authors' experience, is not a mechanical problem, but is due to a loss of gastric motility. Reoperation and repeated endoscopic investigations have not shown a mechanical etiology. Drugs such as ranitidine have been widely utilized without obvious benefit. As after gastric resection for ulcer, the best treatment is to support the patient and wait until gastric emptying spontaneously resumes. Meanwhile a feeding jejunostomy tube has often been inserted as part of the primary operation in the bad risk patient.

Anastomotic Ulceration

Marginal ulcer is seldom seen after resection of the head of the pancreas. Several decades ago vagotomy was recommended, but the authors do not utilize this and have not utilized it in many years. Marginal ulceration has not been noted in the patient with malignant disease and has seldom been noted in the patient who has had resection for benign disease. Nevertheless, continued observations as to its possible role after resection of benign pancreatic lesion or perhaps carcinoma of the duodenum or ampulla of Vater is needed.

Pancreatitis

An elevation of the serum amylase level 1 week after resection may well be an early sign of pancreatic fistula. Pancreatitis after the Whipple resection is rare and in most series is less than 2% [4, 8]. It is seldom a major problem. Obstruction of the pancreatic duct during the primary operation may be the most significant cause.

Delayed Recurrent Obstruction of the Biliary System

The gallbladder is frequently used for biliary decompression in a patient with *unresectable* cancer of the pancreas. This usually provides adequate decompression as the patient's life expectancy is short. When cholecystojejunostomy has been utilized in association with *resection* of cancer of the pancreas, recurrence of the cancer has occasionally been observed to block the cystic duct, thereby defeating the purpose of the original decompression. Obstruction of the biliary tract, developing months after the initial resection, is most likely due to recurrent cancer blocking the common bile duct, but it is a tragedy when a small recurrence, blocking the cystic duct, is overlooked.

In patients whose life expectancy is longer, for example, after resection of benign lesion of the head of the pancreas or carcinoma of the ampulla of Vater, the authors have seen a major complication in two patients. This resulted when the common duct was transected low, i.e., immediately above the duodenum, and the gallbladder was used for anastomosis to the jejunum. In this setting a segment of common duct, several centimeters in length, persisted between the transected end of the common duct and the proximal point of outflow of the cystic duct. This column filled with stagnant bile which was replaced by sediment and small stones, leading to cholangitis and obstructive jaundice. Reoperation for cholecystectomy and choledochojejunostomy was necessary.

As a generalization, the common bile duct provides a superior site for anastomosis.

Benign stricture of the choledochojejunostomy, associated with jaundice, has recently been observed in a patient who had had intraoperative and postoperative irradiation in addition to resection. Because of the Bilroth II component of the original postpancreatectomy reconstruction, endoscopic retrograde cholangiography may technically prove to be difficult or impossible, leaving transhepatic cholangiography as the least invasive approach to localization.

Delayed Obstruction of the Jejunal Segment Between the Pancreatic Jejunostomy and the Downstream Choledochojejunostomy

Two patients who had Whipple resections for benign disease were well for prolonged periods, after which they developed recurrent pancreatitis requiring repetitive hospitalizations. Ultimately reoperation was performed with the assumption that there was an obstruction at the pancreaticojejunostomy. To the contrary, operation demonstrated obstruction of the Roux-en-Y segment of jejunum, distal to the pancreaticojejunostomy but proximal to the choledochojejunostomy (Fig. 2). The obstruction resulted from adhesions to the under surface of the liver associated with acute flexion of the jejunal conduit at that point. Relief of the obstruction resulted in cure of the recurrent pancreatitis [9].

Miscellaneous Complications

Leakage of lymph into the peritoneal cavity is routine following pancreatic rescetion. Secondary to transection of the many periportal and pancreatic lymphatics, it cannot be avoided. With skeletonization of the mesenteric vessels, leakage of chyle via the Jackson-Pratt drains may result in a significant loss over a period of days or weeks. Continued parenteral replacement of lost protein and lipid may be needed. Continued support has resulted in spontaneous closure of the lymphatic fistulae.

Another complication resulting from extended pancreatectomy has been diarrhea. This has proved to be a significant problem, to be differentiated from the steatorrhea that may follow partial or total pancreatectomy. It is probable that the syndrome of 10–15 bowel movements per day may prove to be the result of resection of the celiac sympathetic ganglia along with the lymph nodes around the celiac axis. Although the diarrhea slowly lessens or disappears, it can prove disconcerting to the convalescing patient.

References

1. Howard, JM (1968) Pancreaticoduodenectomy: forty-one consecutive Whipple resections without an operative mortality. Ann Surg 168:629
2. Trede M, Schwall G, Saeger HD (1990) Survival after pancreatoduodenectomy: 118 consecutive resections without an operative mortality. Ann Surg 211: 447–458
3. Grace PA, Pitt HA, Tompkins RK, BenBesten L, Longmire WP (1986) Decreased morbidity and mortality after pancreatoduodenectomy. Am J Surg 151:141–149
4. Braasch JW, Gray BN (1977) Considerations that lower pancreatoduodenectomy mortality. Am J Surg 133:480–485
5. Gilsdorf RB, Spanos P (1973) Factors influencing morbidity and mortality in pancreatoduodenectomy. Ann Surg 177:332–337
6. Mizuma K, Lee PC, Howard JM (1977) The disintegration of surgical sutures on exposure to pancreatic juice. Ann Surg 186:718
7. Doberneck RC, Berndt GA (1987) Delayed gastric emptying after palliative gastrojejunostomy for carcinoma of the pancreas. Arch Surg 122:827–829
8. Warren KW, Choe DS, Plaza J, Relihan M (1975) Results of radical resection for periampullary cancer. Ann Surg 181:534–538
9. Howard JM Efferent limb obstruction after pancreaticojejunostomy: a late cause of pancreatitis following Whipple resection. Arch Surg 126:1157–1159, 1991
10. Howard JM (1990) Pancreaticoduodenectomy (Whipple resection) in the treatment of chronic pancreatitis. In: Beger HG, Büchler M, Ditschuneit H, Malfertheiner P (eds) Chronic pancreatitis. Springer, Berlin Heidelberg New York, pp 467–480

Hormonal Treatment of Pancreatic Fistulas

C. Bassi,[1] S. Vesentini, R. Girelli, M. Falconi L. Benetti, D. Lombardi, F. Nifosi, and P. Pederzoli

The past decade has witnessed a steady increase in surgical operations on the pancreas for a variety of diseases. This has transformed the external pancreatic fistula (EPF) from a rare complication into a relatively frequent event: fistulas are a complication to be expected in any surgical procedure on the gland [1, 2].

Their treatment has been revolutionized by the recent introduction of hormonal substances which inhibit pancreatic exocrine secretion, alongside the traditional conservative measures based on total parenteral nutrition (TPN) and/or enteral nutrition [3], allowing patients for whom surgery is indispensable to be operated on in a good nutritional state [1].

When defining strategies for the management of EPFs we should first of all bear in mind that the condition per se generally shows a tendency to heal spontaneously [2], and that any other therapeutic approach must be assessed not so much in terms of the closure rates obtained as in terms of closure time and costs [3].

In the absence of factors compromising any chance of achieving a conservative solution, it is essential to attempt some form of medical therapy based not only on adequate drainage of the fistula tract, but also on elimination of secretion-stmulating factors, inhibition of exocrine function, and prevention of septic and hemorrhagic complications.

Methods

The strong focus at our institute on developing knowledge and understanding of pancreatic disease (1669 operations performed up to 1990) have given us the opportunity over the years to observe 79 patients with high-output EPFs (range: 200–1200 cc/24 h), 25 of them referred by other centers.

Table 1 lists the causative factors and relative incidence of superinfection as assessed on the basis of pancreatic juice cultures. After fistulography, patients were conservatively treated according to various different regimens, as specified in Table 2. Surgery proved necessary in 14 cases.

[1] Surgical Department, University of Verona, Borgo Roma Hospital, 37134 Verona, Italy

Beger/Büchler/Malfertheiner (Eds.)
Standards in Pancreatic Surgery

Table 1. Causes of 79 cases of EPF and postoperative infections

Primary disease	No. (%)	Infection
Severe pancreatitis	37 (46.8)	36
Pancreatic abscess	16 (20.3)	14
Pancreatic cancer	11 (13.9)	6
Chronic pancreatitis	11 (13.9)	7
Others	4 (5.1)	4
Total	79 (100)	67 (84.8)

Table 2. Conservative treatment regimens in 79 cases of EPF: results and closure times

Patients	TPN + SST	TPN	TPN + GL	TPN + CT	TPN + SMS
Total	26[a]	20	12	7	14
Healed	20	19	12	6	7
Times (mean, days)	9.4	30.4	29.6	23.2	9.9
Surgery[b]	5	1	–	1	7

TPN, Total parenteral nutrition; GL, glucagon; SMS, somatostatin 201-995; SST, somatostatin; CT, calcitonin.
[a] One patient died in the course of treatment.
[b] All cases of complete rupture of duct of Wirsung.

Results

Of 79 cases, 65 (82.3%) were resolved with medical therapy. As early as in 1986 we demonstrated that the treatment of choice in this disease is a combination of TPN and naturally occurring somatostatin (SST) [3], which proved capable of healing seven of eight high-output external pancreatic fistulas within 12 days of treatment.

The time required for fistula tract closure was significantly shorter than that achieved with regimens consisting in TPN alone or in TPN plus glucagon or calcitonin. Later experience has confirmed the validity of our choice.

The advent of the new long-acting synthetic somatostatin octreotide (SMS 201-995), which has a long half-life and can be administered subcutaneously, has further facilitated conservative treatment. We evaluated the inhibitory effects of this compound on patients suffering from EPF and found them similar to those of the naturally occurring hormone [4].

Our results reveal that two factors are decisive for the success of conservative treatment [1–3, 5, 6]: (a) physiological outlet obstruction and/or complete rupture of Wirsung's duct, and (b) bacterial contamination. As regards the former, failures have occurred in almost all cases in which fistulography yielded evidence of complete rupture of Wirsung's duct as a result of severe pancreatitis. In these cases, surgery is almost always mandatory, while hormonal treatment is supportive.

The operation of choice is a Roux-en-Y bypass of the fistula tract in a defunctionalized jejunal loop at least 8 weeks after onset of the fistula, this being the time needed for consolidation of the fistula tract. In our experience radical pancreatic resection has never proved necessary.

As regards bacterial contamination, in our patient series infection of the fistula is very frequent (84.8%) and appears to be related to the cause of fistula formation. 67% of primarily infected cases (50 of 67) derived from diseases which were themselves septic, such as necrotizing pancreatitis and pancreatic abscess. In our series, however, there have been cases in which the pancreatic juice was originally sterile but later became contaminated, probably by ascending infection via drainages [7].

Microbiological investigations have revealed the presence of coagulase-positive *Staphylococcus aureus* in 29%, *Pseudomonas* in 24%, anaerobes in 23%, *Proteus* in 13%, *Escherichia coli* in 7%, *Klebsiella* in 6%, and enterococci and fungi in 4%. In most cases there was coloniziation of a polymicrobial type [7]. Eight cases (20%) of infected pancreatic fistulas in the course of conservative therapy with SMS or SST plus TPN presented us with a particular clinical picture characterized by disappearance of the output, fever, abdominal pain, and leukocytosis. We have defined this situation as "false closure," which can be resolved by either spontaneous or provoked re-opening of the fistula tract.

Specific antibiotic treatment (combined local and systemic) has enabled us to achieve healing, adding a subsequent course of inhibitory therapy with the fistula sterilized [1].

Discussion

The 1980s witnessed a radical change in the clinical and therapeutic approach to pancreatic fistulas. This is related to our greater understanding of the pathophysiology of pancreatic diseases, as well as to an effective increase in their incidence and in new surgical approaches.

The advent of alternative nutritional methods and of drugs inhibiting pancreatic secretion now enables us to tackle the problem of treatment of EPFs with a greater chance of achieving conservative healing. Somatostatin, both in the naturally occurring form and in the more recent synthetic form, appears to be a drug capable of meeting all therapeutic needs. Octreotide, in particular, has also been used for treating such patients in a home-care setting [8].

The chances of achieving conservative healing appear to be compromised by two factors: (a) obstruction of the physiological outlet for anatomical reasons or complete rupture of the duct of Wirsung, and (b) the presence of superinfection of the juice.

As reported elsewhere, infection appears to be so frequent that it can be regarded as almost inevitable [1, 2, 5, 6, 7] and capable of conditioning the success of any type of treatment. In 50 patients the fistula infection appeared to be related, from the outset, to a primary infection of pancreatic and peripancreatic tissue. In the remaining cases the course of the infection and the microbial species isolated were suggestive of an ascending infection via the drainages.

In contrast to the findings of other authors [6], the bacterial load of the juice appeared to be inversely proportional to the fistula output, suggesting that a reduced washout of the fistula tract should favor bacterial growth in the tract itself [1, 3, 4]. In fact, when patients with infected EPFs achieved a drastic reduction in fistula output by means of the use of SST or SMS, in eight cases we observed the clinical picture we define as "false closure". What actually happens is a rapid obliteration of the fistula tract due to the potent hormonal inhibitory action with formation of an abscess.

It thus clearly emerges that, when necessary, sterilization of the pancreatic juice must precede the hormonal therapy, since otherwise the latter may prove self-defeating.

In our opinion, the antibiotic can and must be used simultaneously via the drainages and systemically. The drug must be chosen on the basis of its proven antibiotic assay sensitivity, using agents which have shown good penetration into pancreatic juice [9].

In addition to microbiological tests, one should also do a morphological study of the pancreatic duct system by means of fistulography and/or ERCP. Such investigations have proved to be of decisive importance for the choice of medical and/or surgical therapy in these patients.

In conclusion, the correct treatment of EPFs involves the following procedures in chronological order: (a) thorough evaluation of 24-h fistula output; (b) analysis of pancreatic juice cultures; (c) anatomical study of the ductal system (fistulography and/or ERCP); (d) a targeted choice of antibiotic to be used both topically and systemically; (e) pancreatic rest and inhibition of secretion with TPN plus SST or SMS.

Alongside this therapeutic approach, certain authors have recently suggested the possibility of treatment with fibrin sealants, which are used progressively and with all due care, according to individual case requirements, to seal the fistula tract, ensuring physiological outflow [10]. This procedure warrants further study, as do other possible approaches to the inhibition of exocrine secretion, such as high-dose pancreatic enzymes [11] or the use of anti-CCK drugs, which are promising, among other reasons, because they can be administered orally.

References

1. Bassi C et al. (1989) Attualità in tema di fistole pancreatiche esterne: contributo clinico. In: Scritti in onore di Adamo Dagradi. Grafiche Fiorini, pp 137–142
2. Marrano D (1983) Le fistole pancreatiche. Atti della Società Italiana di Chirurgia; 85th congress. Masson, Milan, pp 279–329
3. Pederzoli P et al. (1986) Conservative treatment of external pancreatic fistulas with parenteral nutrition alone or in combination with continuous infusion of somatostatin, glucagon or calcitonin. Surg Gynecol Obstet 162:428–431
4. Falconi M et al. (1989) Risultati preliminari relativi all'effetto sulla secrezione pancreatica esocrina di una somatostatina long-acting (SMS 201-995). Atti XIII Congresso AISP 15A
5. Jordan JL (1987) Pancreatic fistula. In: Howard JH, Jordan JL, Reber HA (eds) Surgical diseases of the pancreas. Lea and Febiger, Philadelphia, pp 898–911
6. Zinner MJ et al. (1974) Pancreatic cutaneous fistulas. Surg Gynecol Obstet 138:710–714
7. Bassi C et al. (1989) Microbiological findings in severe pancreatitis. Surg Res Commun 5:1–4
8. Prinz RA et al. (1988) Treatment of pancreatic cutaneous fistulas with a somatostatin analogue. Am J Surg 155:36–42
9. Pederzoli M et al. (1990) Retroperitoneal and peritoneal drainage and lavage in the treatment of severe necrotizing pancreatitis. Surg Gynecol Obstet 170: 197–203
10. Costantino V et al. (1990) Treatment of pancreatic fistulas using fibrin sealant. Hepatopancreatic Biliary Surgery 2[Suppl]:174
11. Garcia-Pugés AM et al. (1988) Oral pancreatic enzymes accelerate closure of external pancreatic fistulae. Br J Surg 75:924–925

Subject Index